AF832566

CARDIAC ARRHYTHMIAS – NEW CONSIDERATIONS

Edited by **Francisco R. Breijo-Marquez**

Cardiac Arrhythmias – New Considerations
Edited by Francisco R. Breijo-Marquez

Published by InTech

Janeza Trdine 9, 51000 Rijeka, Croatia

Copyright © 2012 InTech

All chapters are distributed under the Creative Commons Attribution 3.0 license, which allows users to download, copy and build upon published articles even for commercial purposes, as long as the author and publisher are properly credited, which ensures maximum dissemination and a wider impact of our publications. After this work has been published by InTech, authors have the right to republish it, in whole or part, in any publication of which they are the author, and to make other personal use of the work. Any republication, referencing or personal use of the work must explicitly identify the original source.

As for readers, this license allows users to download, copy and build upon published chapters even for commercial purposes, as long as the author and publisher are properly credited, which ensures maximum dissemination and a wider impact of our publications.

Notice

Statements and opinions expressed in the chapters are these of the individual contributors and not necessarily those of the editors or publisher. No responsibility is accepted for the accuracy of information contained in the published chapters. The publisher assumes no responsibility for any damage or injury to persons or property arising out of the use of any materials, instructions, methods or ideas contained in the book.

Publishing Process Manager Bojan Rafaj

Technical Editor Teodora Smiljanic

Cover Designer InTech Design Team

Additional hard copies can be obtained from orders@intechopen.com

Cardiac Arrhythmias – New Considerations, Edited by Francisco R. Breijo-Marquez
p. cm.
ISBN 978-953-51-0126-0

We are IntechOpen, the world's leading publisher of Open Access books

Built by scientists, for scientists

4,100+
Open access books available

116,000+
International authors and editors

120M+
Downloads

151
Countries delivered to

Our authors are among the
Top 1%
most cited scientists

12.2%
Contributors from top 500 universities

WEB OF SCIENCE™

Selection of our books indexed in the Book Citation Index
in Web of Science™ Core Collection (BKCI)

Interested in publishing with us?
Contact book.department@intechopen.com

Numbers displayed above are based on latest data collected.
For more information visit www.intechopen.com

For EU product safety concerns:
IN TECH d.o.o., Prolaz Marije Krucifikse Kozulić 3, 51000 Rijeka, Croatia,
info@intechopen.com or visit our website at intechopen.com.

Meet the editor

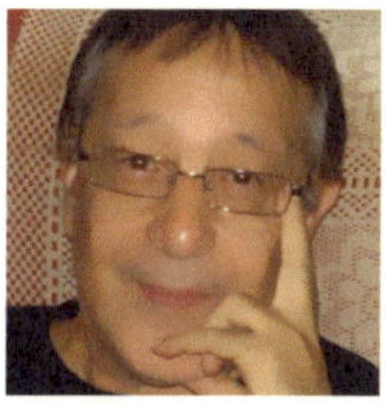

Professor Breijo-Marquez, Fr. obtained his Medical degree from Boston University, Massachusetts.U.S.A. He then pursued his postgraduate training in Cardiology at the University of Boston & Hartford (leave on personal grounds currently). On Nov 1995 he became a Fellow of the Commemorative Hospital. He obtained his American board in OBGYN on 1990. Currently he is a Professor and the chairman of the Department of Cardiology at Commemorative Hospital, Boston, MA. U.S.A (leave on personal grounds currently). He also is the Medical Director of CS. Abanilla, Spain from 2005 till present. He is a member ESC, AHA. His main interests are Clinical & Experimental Cardiology. He has a number of publications in different journals in Cardiology.

Contents

Preface XI

Part 1 Cardiac Arrhythmias and Genetics 1

Chapter 1 **Novel Genomic Approach to the Arrhytmogenic Sudden Cardiac Death 3**
Maria Brion, Beatriz Sobrino, Alejandro Blanco-Verea, Montserrat Santori, Rocio Gil and Angel Carracedo

Chapter 2 **Phenotypic Correlation of Genetic Mutations with Ventricular Arrhythmias 17**
Yamini Krishnan, Jerri Chen and Thomas V. McDonald

Part 2 The Cardiac Ion Channels 43

Chapter 3 **The Cardiac Ion Channels 45**
Thomas Jespersen

Chapter 4 **The Pathophysiological Implications of TRP Channels in Cardiac Arrhythmia 73**
Ryuji Inoue, Duan Yubin, Hu Yaopeng and Jun Ichikawa

Chapter 5 **Contributions of Ion Channels in Cardiac Arrhythmias 97**
Jing Hongjuan and Zhang Lu

Chapter 6 **L-Type Ca^{2+} Current in Cardiac Arrhythmias 121**
Gema Ruiz-Hurtado, Julio L. Alvarez and Jean-Pierre Benitah

Part 3 Pathophysiology of Cardiac Arrhythmia 149

Chapter 7 **Natural Protection Against Cardiac Arrhythmias During Hibernation: Significance of Adenosine 151**
Tulasi Ram Jinka

Chapter 8 **Neurohumoral Control of Heart Rate 167**
Jones Bernardes Graceli, Diego França Pedrosa and Ágata Lages Gava

Chapter 9 **Chronobiological Aspects of the Heart Rhythm Disorders at the Change of Pulmonary Ventilation in Rat Model 193**
Pavol Svorc, Alexander Marossy, Pavol Svorc, Jr., Sona Gresova, Marek Buzga and Benjamin L. Fulton

Chapter 10 **Late Ventricular Potentials in Cardiac and Extracardiac Diseases 227**
Ioana Mozoş, Corina Şerban and Rodica Mihăescu

Chapter 11 **Influence of Patern and Degree of Left Ventricular Hypertrophy on Cardiac Arrhythmias 257**
Juraj Kunisek

Chapter 12 **Sleep-Related Breathing Disorders and Cardiac Arrhythmia 267**
Ahmad Salah Hersi

Chapter 13 **Approach to Ventricular Arrhythmias in the Pediatric Intensive Care Unit 289**
Jong-Hau Hsu, Jiunn-Ren Wu, Zen-Kong Dai and I-Chen Chen

Chapter 14 **Psychological Approach to the Cardiac Arrhythmias: Focus on the Emotions 307**
Ana Myriam Sánchez Bonomo and Tereza Cristina Cavalcanti Ferreira de Araujo

Part 4 Uncommon Heart Rhythm Disorders 325

Chapter 15 **The Variations in Electrical Cardiac Systole and Its Impact on Sudden Cardiac Death 327**
F. R. Breijo-Marquez and M. Pardo Ríos

Chapter 16 **Bradycardia in Children During General Anaesthesia 343**
Judith A. Lens, Jeroen Hermanides, Peter L. Houweling, Jasper J. Quak and David R. Colnot

Chapter 17 **Spiral Waves, Obstacles and Cardiac Arrhythmias 357**
Daniel Olmos-Liceaga

Chapter 18 **Electrical Storm 377**
Federico Guerra, Matilda Shkoza, Marco Flori and Alessandro Capucci

Chapter 19 **Bradycardia Secondary to Cervical Spinal Cord Injury 395**
Farid Sadaka and Christopher Veremakis

Part 5 **Electrophysiology Study of the Heart: Mapping Procedure 403**

Chapter 20 **Electromagnetic Mapping During Complex RF Ablations 405**
Shimon Rosenheck, Jeffrey Banker, Alexey Weiss and Zehava Sharon

Chapter 21 **Novel Technologies for Mapping and Ablation of Complex Arrhythmias 443**
Louisa Malcolme-Lawes, Shahnaz Jamil-Copley and Prapa Kanagaratnam

Chapter 22 **The Future of Cardiac Mapping 461**
Pascal Fallavollita

Part 6 **Miscellaneous 479**

Chapter 23 **Mild Induced Therapeutic Hypothermia for Survivors of Cardiac Arrest 481**
Kevin Baker, John Prior, Karthik Sheka and Raymond A. Smego, Jr.

Chapter 24 **Arrhythmias in Pregnancy 497**
Marius Craina, Gheorghe Furău, Răzvan Niţu, Lavinia Stelea, Dan Ancuşa, Corina Şerban, Rodica Mihăescu and Ioana Mozoş

Chapter 25 **Development of Computer Aided Prediction Technology for Paroxysmal Atrial Fibrillation in Mobile Healthcare 515**
Desok Kim, Jae-Hyeong Park and Jun Hyung Kim

Preface

The book Cardiac Arrythmias contains a spectrum of different topics within the subject area presented in chapters written with a magnificent scientific rigour. Some of the topics include: the most prevalent causes of cardiac arrhythmias and their mechanisms of production; some emergent or almost unknown electrical cardiac disorders; ionic diseases; mapping and ablation techniques; and some original insights on psychological disorders related to cardiac arrythmias as well as some pathologies which can affect the heart in different ways, and vice versa. The book also includes the most current treatments of Cardiac Arrythmias.

It is my opinion as the editor that all the authors in this book have done an excellent job writing their chapters, which resulted in the publication becoming a proper textbook. I fervently hope that reading it will be as enjoyable and informative for all the readers as much as it has been for me. My sincere congratulations to all the authors for their work.

Prof. Dr. F. R. Breijo-Marquez,
Titular Professor of Clinical and Experimental Cardiology,
Boston, Massachusetts,
USA

Part 1

Cardiac Arrhythmias and Genetics

1

Novel Genomic Approach to the Arrhytmogenic Sudden Cardiac Death

Maria Brion, Beatriz Sobrino, Alejandro Blanco-Verea, Montserrat Santori, Rocio Gil and Angel Carracedo
Genomic Medicine Group, IDIS, CIBERER-University of Santiago, FPGMX
Spain

1. Introduction

Unfortunately, most of the common diseases in cardiology do not show traditional Mendelian genetics, they usually are complex genetic diseases resulting from the combination of multiple heritable and environmental factors. However, one of the cardiology dysfunction that can affect apparently healthy young adults or with any previous heart disease, such as sudden cardiac death (SCD), could be the first symptom of a Mendelian disease such as cardiomyopathies or channelopathies.
In many of the SCD cases, especially in case of young people, the cause of death cannot be explained neither after autopsy nor after laboratory tests. Inherited heart diseases such as hypertrophic cardiomyopathy (HCM), arrhythmogenic right ventricular cardiomyopathy (ARVC) and primary electrical diseases such as long QT syndrome (LQTS), Brugada syndrome (BrS) or catecholaminergic polymorphic ventricular tachycardia (CPVT), are the main cause of death in young adults with no previous clinical history. Most often these inherited cardiac disorders give rise to lethal ventricular arrhythmias and show an autosomal dominant mode of inheritance.
Genetic screening of the genes described as implicated in the different pathologies may help to determine the cause of death and to evaluate the potential risk of the relatives. Today we know which are the main causes of sudden cardiac death in young adults and we also know which are the genes responsible of these diseases in a high percentage of cases. The aim of this article is to present to the reader the estate of the art of the use of the new next generation sequencing technologies for the study of arrhythmogenic sudden cardiac deaths. We will discuss the different available technologies, and the different applications:
Candidate gene resequencing. We will describe the interesting genes to be studied and the different strategies available for their enrichment and sequencing
Whole exome resequencing. We will describe the application of this approach to those cases were we need to look for new genes.

2. Inherited arrhythmogenic diseases

There are various arrhythmogenic disorders, with different electrocardiographic patterns, which are not always present or are not evident in carriers of mutations implicated in the

pathology. In general these are diseases with low penetrance so the genetic study is of great importance in patients with personal or family history of sudden cardiac death.
The term inherited arrhythmogenic diseases typically includes cardiac diseases caused by mutations in ion channels and ion channel-controlling proteins such as the long-QT syndrome (LQTS), the short QT syndrome (SQTS), the Brugada syndrome (BrS) and catecholaminergic polymorphic ventricular tachycardia (CPVT). Ion channels are integral membrane proteins that regulate the flow of ions across the cell membrane. They consist of multimeric units generally encoded by different genes. The α subunit forms the pore and mediates ion current, while the β subunits are regulatory. Defects in these channels due to mutations in genes that encode proteins, or mutations in proteins associated with these channels may lead to an electrical disturbance in the heart linked to the development of channelopathies.

2.1 Long QT syndrome

The Long QT Syndrome (LQTS) is characterized by prolongation of the QT interval on the electrocardiogram, which indicates ventricular repolarisation unusually long, due either to a decrease in the K^+ flow of repolarisation or to a delayed entry of Na^+ into the myocyte.
The estimated incidence is between 1:2000 -1:5000 people (Hedley et al., 2009), and its penetrance is variable, ranging from sub clinical phenotypes with a QT interval at the limit, without arrhythmias or syncope (Napolitano et al., 2005; Priori et al., 1999; Vicent et al., 1992) to sudden cardiac death, being a major cause of sudden death in young people. To determine wheter the QT interval is prolonged the corrected QT interval (QTc) is used, which is calculated using the Bazzet formula $QTc = QT / \sqrt{RR}$ (Bazzet et al., 1920) Are considered abnormally prolonged QTc values when exceeding 440 ms in men and those over 460 ms in women (values corrected for heart rate). It is estimated that a patient with a QTc interval of 550 ms has a 63% higher risk of suffering a cardiac event that an individual with a value of QTc interval of 450 ms. (Zareba et al., 2008).
The LQTS shows a congenital form of the disease in about 85% of cases and a sporadic form which corresponds to 15% [85]. There is also an acquired form of QT prolongation caused mainly by drugs, both cardiac (e.g. antiarrhythmics) and other medications (e.g. antidepressants) or derived from an electrolyte imbalance. The congenital form shows two basic patterns of inheritance, one autosomal dominant called Romano-Ward syndrome and another autosomal recessive known as Jervell Lange-Nielsen syndrome, which presents with congenital deafness. To date 12 genes have been described in the pathology. The most common are genes that encode K + channels, KCNQ1, KCNH2, which represent about 40-55% and 35-45% of cases respectively, and the SCN5A gene coding for Na + channels which represents a 2 - 8% of cases (Hedley et al., 2009). The involvement of each of these genes leads to defined clinical phenotypes, so KCNQ1 gene leads to LQTS type 1 (LQT1), KCNH2 causes LQTS type 2 (LQT2) and SCN5A leads to LQTS3 (LQT3).

2.2 Short QT syndrome

The short QT syndrome (SQTS) has been recognized as a clinical entity characterized recently by a shortened QT interval that can lead to arrhythmias and sudden cardiac death (Gussak et al., 2000). Although there is no established consensus, it is accepted that a value between 320ms and 340 ms are considered short (although it could be considered normal 340ms) if there is a history of cardiac symptoms such as syncope or aborted sudden death. Nevertheless, as in LQTS, the transition zone of normal QT intervals to pathological intervals is difficult to establish (Schimpf et al., 2007).

In SQTS, mutations in genes encoding K^+ channels: KCNH2, KCNJ2, and KCNQ1, cause a gain of function of these channels and give rise to SQTS1, SQTS2and SQTS3 respectively. However, mutations in genes encoding α and β2 subunits of the Cav1.2 channel, the CACNB2 and CACNA1C genes, cause loss of function of these channels and give rise to SQTS4 and SQTS5 phenotype respectively (Hedley et al., 2009).

2.3 Brugada syndrome

Brugada Syndrome (BrS) is characterized by ST segment elevation in right precordial leads (V1-V3) of the electrocardiogram and can also be associated with an increase in PR interval and bundle branch block. Penetrance is also variable, and can trigger polymorphic ventricular tachycardia and / or ventricular fibrillation and sudden death. The distribution and incidence of this disease is difficult to determine because it is a syndrome recently described and because electrocardiographic manifestations are not always present. Campuzano et al. (2010) estimate a prevalence of approximately 35/100000 persons / year and they say that, although symptoms usually develop around the age of 40, sudden death can affect individuals of any age. They estimate sudden death affects 75% of the affected males, and between 20 and 50% of the affected people have a family history of sudden death.

The dominant pattern of inheritance is autosomal dominant with expression probably age dependent and incomplete penetrance. Today we have described more than 100 mutations in 7 different genes that give rise to the 7 types of BrS. These genes encode proteins of both Na + channels and other ion channels. The mutations affect the proper development of phases 1 and 2 of the cardiac action potential (Hedley et al., 2009b). It is estimated that 20-25% of BrS patients show mutations in the SCN5A gene (Schott et al., 1999), which also represents 5-10% of mutations found in cases of sudden cardiac death in adults and children (Hedley et al., 2009b) .

2.4 Catecholaminergic polymorphic ventricular tachycardia

Catecolaminergic polymorphic ventricular tachycardia (CPVT) occurs with a characteristic pattern of bidirectional or polymorphic tachycardia related to stress without structural cardiac abnormalities (Coumel et al., 1978). These clinical manifestations often occur during childhood and adolescence.

The CPVT has two modes of inheritance: autosomal dominant and recessive. The autosomal dominant form is caused by mutations in the gene encoding the ryanodine receptor RyR2, which is a large protein that forms the calcium release channel in sarcoplasmic reticulum. The recessive form of the disease is caused by mutations in the cardiac isoform calciquestrina gene (CASQ2), which binds to the ryanodine receptor and participates in the control of excitation-contraction (Ylänen et al., 2010). The steps of the molecular pathogenesis of CPVT are not entirely clear, but Mutations of the two interacting proteins, RyR2 and CASQ2, seem to result in inadequately controlled Ca2+ bursts into the sarcoplasm, with concomitant risk of delayed afterdepolarizations and triggered arrhythmia.

3. Genetic screening of arrhythmogenic diseases

The importance of knowing the molecular substrate in patients with inherited cardiac channelopathies is recognized and highlighted in the guidelines for the prevention of SCD developed by the American Heart Association, the American College of Cardiology, and the

European Society of Cardiology (Zipes et al., 2006). Screening for mutations in genes that encode cardiac ion channels associated with LQTS, SQTS, BrS, and CPVT is primarily sought in clinically affected patients to tailor risk stratification and management and to further identify family members (Priori et al., 2002a, b, 2003). However, genetic analysis is not yet available at most clinical centres and it is still mainly performed in finite research laboratories.

Our present understanding of human inherited arrhythmia diseases has become increasingly complex. Several clinical syndromes have been identified as human inherited arrhythmia diseases and at least 21 genes are known to cause these diseases. These genes and the associated syndromes are given in Table 1. Mutations associated with inherited arrhythmia syndromes occur in ion channel pore-forming proteins, associating subunit proteins and channel interacting proteins ,Ca2+ handling proteins, components of the ion cannel macromolecular complex, and regulatory pathways. Although most inherited arrhythmia syndromes are rare clinical findings, sometimes with just a single family described.

Several studies have been published trying to determine the effectiveness of genetic screening (Bai et al., 2009; Kapplinget et al., 2009) in terms of efficiency and cost. Bay et al. (2009) showed that the current cost of genetic testing for inherited cardiac channelopathies is reasonable for those who have a conclusive diagnosis and that these patients should have priority access to genetic screening (Fuster et al., 2008) However, until now these studies were limited by two main drawbacks, the reduced effectiveness of the techniques of genetic determination employed and the high cost of the same.

Gen	Symbol	Locus	CPVT	LQTS	SQTS	BrS
A kinase anchor protein (yotiao) 9	AKAP9	7q21-q22		x		
ankyrin 2	ANK2	4q25-q27		x		
calcium channel, voltage-dependent, L type, alpha 1C subunit	CACNA1C	12p13.3		x	x	x
calcium channel, voltage-dependent, beta 2 subunit	CACNB2	10p12			x	x
calsequestrin 2	CASQ2	1p13.3-p11	x			
caveolin 3	CAV3	3p25		x		
glycerol-3-phosphate dehydrogenase 1-like	GPD1L	3p22.3				x
hyperpolarization activated cyclic nucleotide-gated potassium channel 4	HCN4	15q24.1				x
potassium voltage-gated channel, Isk-related family, member 1	KCNE1	21q22.12		x		
potassium voltage-gated channel, Isk-related family, member 2	KCNE2	21q22.12		x		
potassium voltage-gated channel, Isk-related family, member 3	KCNE3	11q13.4				x
potassium voltage-gated channel, subfamily H, member 2	KCNH2	7q36.1		x	x	
potassium inwardly-rectifying channel, subfamily J, member 2	KCNJ2	17q24.3		x	x	
potassium inwardly-rectifying channel, subfamily J, member 5	KCNJ5	11q24		x		
potassium voltage-gated channel, KQT-like subfamily, member 1	KCNQ1	11p15.5		x	x	
ryanodine receptor 2	RYR2	1q43	x			
sodium channel, voltage-gated, type I, beta	SCN1B	19q13,1				x
sodium channel, voltage-gated, type III, beta	SCN3B	11q23,3				x
sodium channel, voltage-gated, type IV, beta	SCN4B	11q23.3		x		
sodium channel, voltage-gated, type V, alpha subunit	SCN5A	3p21		x		x
syntrophin, alpha 1	SNTA1	20q11.2		x		

Table 1. Genes related to arrhythmogenic sudden cardiac death

Today, with the development of the next generation sequencing strategies, these two problems are being overcome, so that on one hand, we managed to sequence as many genes as we want, detecting both, genetic variants already described and new variants not yet known; and on the other hand, we have significantly reduced the cost of each genetic screening and we hope that this reduction will still see increased in the future days.

The new next generation sequencing technologies are allowing us sequencing large number of DNA fragments or genes, using target resequencing strategies, in a fast, reliable and effective way. The selection of the genes will depend on the researcher's own interests, so that in our case, we could focus on those genes previously described as involved in arrhythmogenic heart diseases or we can make the sequencing of all genes and search exome mutations also in genes that have not previously been associated with the pathology. If we consider the aforementioned 21 genes as candidate genes to be sequenced, It would involve the sequencing of approximately 400 exons, accounting around 120.000 base pairs of coding DNA. This work, in terms of time and cost of each analysis represents a major handicap for the routine work of many small laboratories dedicated to genetic diagnosis of these pathologies. An indicative example of this type of analysis is the Familion test for Long QT syndrome (Kapplinger et al., 2009), a bidirectional DNA sequencing-based assay that comprises analysis of 73 polymerase chain reaction (PCR) amplicons to analyse the 3 major LQTS-susceptibility genes (KCNQ1 [LQT1], KCNH2 [LQT2], SCN5A [LQT3]) along with 2 minor genes (KCNE1 [LQT5] and KCNE2 [LQT6]). Kapplinger et al (2009) evaluated the Familion Test in 2500 unrelated LQTS cases and they found 903 positive genetic tests describing 562 putative mutations absent in 2600 reference alleles. They reported that despite the passage of 14 years since the first LQTS-causative mutations were discovered, still one-third of the mutations being discovered today are novel; therefore, this study is further evidence of the need for genetic screening strategies that allow us to detect both known mutations and new genetic variants, such as the sequencing. In addition, the study highlights the need for functional studies providing evidence on the possible pathogenicity for new genetic variants that are being described. Here we describe the implementation of a new research strategy using next generation sequencing, that allows the simultaneous study of the sequence of all the genes described in relation to arrhythmogenic disorders at risk of sudden cardiac death (candidate gene approach), or the study of the complete sequence of the human exome (whole exome approach), searching for genetic variants both in genes previously associated with sudden cardiac death and in new genes whose involvement in the fatal event is currently unknown

4. Next generation sequencing

Capillary electrophoresis based in Sanger sequencing is the technology widely used for analyzing genes involves in different pathologies. However, over the past five years, Next Generation Sequencing (NGS) technologies have became a reliable tool for massive parallel sequencing, overcoming the limitations in throughput and speed of capillary electrophoresis (Shendure & Ji, 2008; Metzer, 2010; Glenn , 2011) .

On this chapter we will focus on commercially available platforms: 454 (Roche), Illumina Genome Analyzer (Illumina Inc.), SOLiD and Ion Torrent (Life Technologies) (Table 2).

The 454 Genome Sequencer (Roche) was the first NGS platform available (Margulies et al., 2005). Small fragments of DNA are attached onto the surface of beads and amplified via emulsion PCR. Millions of beads are deposited onto a picotitre plate. Sequencing is performed in parallel by pyrosequencing, where the incorporation of a nucleotide by a DNA polymerase results in the release of a pyrophosphate, which initiates a series of downstream reactions that ultimately produce light by a luciferase. The light can be correlated with the nucleotide incorporated, because the nucleotides are added following a sequential order.

The Illumina Genome Analyzer (Illumina Inc.) relies on bridge PCR on a glass slide to amplify small fragments of DNA. In this approach, forward and reverse PCR primers are attached to a solid surface, and as a consequence, amplification products originating from any single template molecule remain immobilized and clustered to a physical position on the array. Sequencing chemistry is based on sequencing by synthesis with reversible terminators (Fedurco et al., 2006; Turcatti et al., 2008), where all fluorescently labeled four nucleotides are added simultaneously to the flow cell channels, along with the polymerase, for incorporation into the oligo-primed cluster fragments obtained after bridge PCR.

The SOLiD system (Life Technologies) is based on sequencing by ligation and the use of two-base encoded probes (Valouev et al., 2008). A universal sequencing primer is hybridized to templates and a pool of fluorescently labelled octamer probes containing all possible combination of A, C, G and T at positions 1-5, interrogates the sequence of the unknown template on each bead. Only the probe homologous to the first five bases of the template will be ligated to the universal sequencing primer. Up to ten cycles of ligation, detection and cleavage record the colour at every fifth position. Templates for sequencing are prepared via emulsion PCR.

In the case of the Ion PGM Sequencer (Life Technologies), sequence data are obtained by directly sensing the ions produced by template-directed DNA polymerase synthesis using all natural nucleotides on the ion chip. The ion chip contains ion-sensitive, field-effect transistor-based sensors in 1.2 million wells, which allow parallel and simultaneous detection of independent sequencing reactions (Rothberg et al., 2011). As 454 and SOLiD, template preparation is performed by emulsion PCR. Unlike the other technologies where the throughput is determined by the equipment, the Ion PGM throughput is determined by the chip used for sequencing (Table 2)

Very promising NGS approaches are the ones based on single molecule sequencing like Helicos Biosciences (Harris et al., 2008) and Pacific Biosciences (Eid et al., 2009), where sequencing is performing directly on the DNA, avoiding any amplification step. However, these platforms are not commercially available so they are only mentioned.

Instrument	Read length (bp)	Maximum Throughput	Run time
454-GS Junior	400	50 Mb	10 h
454-FLX+	700	900 Mb	23 h
Illumina-MiSeq	150+150	> 1 Gb	27 h
Illumina-GAII	150+150	95 Gb	14 days
Illumina-HiScanSQ	100+100	150 Gb	11 days
Illumina-HiSeq1000	100+100	300 Gb	11 days
Illumina-HiSeq2000	100+100	600 Gb	11 days
SOLiD-5500	75+35	90 Gb	7 days
SOLiD-5500xl	75+35	180 Gb	7 days
Ion PGM - 314 chip	200	>10 Mb	2 h
Ion PGM - 316 chip	200	>100 Mb	2 h

Table 2. Comparison of NGS platforms.

5. Target resequencing strategies

For some applications, it would be not necessary to sequence the whole genome, but sequence specific region or regions. This is the case of the study of: i) a disease phenotype previously mapped to a specific region of the genome, ii) candidate genes involve in a pathology or pathway, iii) whole exome. To reach these purposes it is necessary the combination of methods for targeted capture with massive parallel sequencing.

Methods for capturing the regions of interest are commercially available, but it is important to remind that, due to this field is in continuous and rapid evolution, before designing any experiment it will be necessary to check for latest approaches, in order to choose the more cost-effective strategy for each project (Turner et al., 2009; Mamanova et al., 2010).

Even considering the different capture strategies, the workflow for targeted resequencing for either candidate genes or exome sequencing is very similar. Genomic DNA is used to construct a library, which consists in small fragments of DNA flanqued by adaptors. Depending on the method used for capturing the regions of interest, the capture occurs before or after creating the library. Once the capture library is created, is clonally amplified followed by massive parallel sequencing.

During the process of capturing and library preparation it is possible to barcoding samples. This process enables the user to pool multiple samples per sequencing run, taking advantage of the high-throughput of the NGS platforms.

Capture strategies can be broadly grouped in two main groups, the first one is based on PCR, and the second one in the use of hybridization probes (Table 3).

1. PCR approaches:

   When a specific region has been previously mapped, long-PCRs using high-fidelity polymerases are used to analyze large kilobase-sized contiguous intervals (Yeager et al., 2008).

   Different strategies for amplified simultaneously hundreds of fragments of DNA have been developed over the last years. Access Array System (Fluidgm) uses a microfluidic chip with nanoliter scale chambers, where the simultaneous amplification of 48 different fragments in 48 samples is performed. By incorporating the adaptor sequences into the primer design the amplicon product is ready to go directly into clonal amplification (Voelkerding et al., 2010).

   Microdroplet-PCR technology developed by RainDance involves the use of emulsion PCR in a microfluidic device, creating droplets of primers in oil solution. The primer droplets that are targeted to different regions of the genome merge with separate droplets that contain fragmented genomic DNA and PCR reagents. These mixed droplets are thermal cycled in a single tube. The encapsulation of microdroplet PCR reactions prevents possible primer pair interactions allowing an efficient simultaneous amplification of up to 20,000 targeted sequences (Tewhey et al., 2009).

   Illumina and Life Technologies have followed similar strategies for capture regions for MiSeq and Ion PGM Sequencer, respectively. Illumina has launched the TrueSeq Custom Amplicon Kit for multiplex amplification of up to 384 amplicons per sample, and Life Technology has recently developed a multiplex PCR for amplified in a single tube up to 480 known as Ion AmpliSeq Cancer Panel. Currently, only the cancer panel is available, but it has been announced by the company that custom panels will be early available.

   Halo Genomics has developed two different strategies based on amplification methods, Selector and HaloPlex. The first one, Selector Target Enrichment system is based on multiple displacement amplification. This strategy produces circular DNA that is amplified in a whole genome amplification reaction. The resulting high molecular DNA product is compatible with all next generation sequencing library preparation protocols. For achieving this, DNA sample is first fragmented using restriction

enzymes, secondly the probe library is added and the probes hybridize with the targeted fragments. Each probe is an oligonucleotide designed to hybridize to both ends of a targeted DNA restriction fragment, thereby guiding the targeted fragments to form circular DNA molecules. The circular molecules are closed by ligation and then amplified. Next step is library preparation (Johansson et al., 2010).
In the case of HaloPlex technology, PCR products are ready for pooling and direct sequencing, it is not necessary to create the library after the capturing because the probes also contain a specific sequencing motif that is incorporated during the circularization. This motif allows the incorporation of specific adaptors and barcodes during the amplification. Currently, this product is optimized for Illumina.

2. Hybridization
Other strategy is capture by hybridization of specific probes complementary of the regions of interest. The first hybridization approaches were based on-array capture (Albert et al., 2007; Hodges et al., 2007; Ng et al., 2009). But to avoid the disadvantages of working with microarrays, currently methods are based in-solution capture. Fragment libraries are hybridized to biotinilated probes in solution and subsequently recovered with streptavidin-magnetic beads, amplified and sequence in the platform of choice (Gnirke et al., 2009; Bamshad., 2011).
All the vendors (Agilent, Nimblegen, Illumina and Life Technologies) offer kits either predesigned for specific application such as exome sequencing, cancer, etc or custom panels to be designed for the user (Table 3). There are different kits for different sizes of the region of interest that go from less than 100kb to up 60 Mb.

Approach	Method	Kits[a]	NGS - Compatibility[b]
PCR	Long-PCR	1	1, 2, 3, 4
	Access Array System (Fluidigm)	1	1, 2, 3, 4
	Microdroplet PCR (Raindance)	1, 2	1, 2, 3, 4
	AmpliSeq technology (Life Technologies)	2[c]	4
	TrueSeq Amplicon Kit (Illumina)	1	2
	HaloPlex (Halo Genomics)	1	2
	Selector (Halo Genomics)	1, 2	1, 2, 3, 4
In-solution hybridization	SureSelect (Agilent)	1, 3	2, 3
	SeqCap EZ (Nimblegen)	1, 3	1, 2, 3
	TrueSeq Enrichment Kit (Illumina)	1, 3	2
	TargetSeq (Life Technologies)	1, 3	3, 4

[a] Custom (1), specific gene panel (ej. cancer panel) (2), exome panel (3)
[b] 454 (1), Illumina (2), SOLiD (3), Ion PGM Sequencer (4).
[c] Custom early available

Table 3. Capture methods for targeted resequencing.

5.1 Candidate gene resequencing

In dealing with arrhythmogenic diseases at risk of sudden cardiac death, we can analyze those genes previously associated with the pathologies that explain a high percentage of cases, variable according to the pathology (Hedley et al., 2009ab; Kapplinget et al., 2009).

Therefore, as it was already used for SCD associated cardiomyoapties (Meder et al., 2011), the strategy with the arrhythmogenic diseases could be to capture the 21 genes mentioned above in Table 1. As it is shown in table 3, there are a great variety of strategies available. In addition, all commercially available kits have developed tools for designing specific primers or probes to capture the regions of interest.

For selecting both the capture method and the NGS platform many factors have to be evaluated: size of the region of interest, the coverage and accuracy needed, the number of samples and barcodes availability and DNA requirement. There is no an ideal method for all the situations.

5.2 Whole exome resequencing

The targeted resequencing of the subset of the genome that is protein coding is known as exome sequencing. This strategy is been a powerful approach for either identifying genes involve in Mendelian disorders or rare variants underlying the heritability of complex traits (Bamshad, 2011). Therefore, arrhythmogenic diseases such as the LQTS, the SQTS, the CPVT or the BrS, all genetic diseases with Mendelian inheritance, are appropriate candidates for this type of study.

All the vendors of in-solution hybridization methods have developed commercial kits for capturing whole exome. (Agilent, Illumina, LifeTechnologies, NimbleGen) (Table 3). Due to the throughput needed for obtaining enough coverage for variant calling, the platforms of choice for this application are Illumina GAII or superior and SOLiD 5500.

This approach has been successfully used since 2009 in at least 29 diseases, in which the genes involved in the disorders have been identified (Bamshad, 2011).

6. Genetic variant versus mutation

It should be kept in mind that this kind of genetic tests identifies the presence of a probable/possible arrythmogenic disease causing mutation for which the probability for pathogenesis and even the likelihood of sudden cardiac death is influenced by many factors, including rarity, conservation, topological location, co-segregation, functional studies, and so forth. According to Kapplinger et al. (2009), fewer than 25% of the previously published LQTS mutations have been characterized by heterologous expression studies to demonstrate the anticipated loss-of-function (LQT1 and LQT2) or gain-of-function (LQT3) conferred by the mutation. The rank of a new genetic variant detected in an afected individual as a pathogenic mutation must meet the following specifications:

a. The variant must disrupt either the open reading frame (i.e., missense, nonsense, insertion/deletion, or frame shift mutations) or the splice site (poly-pyrimidine tract, splice acceptor or splice donor recognition sequences). Considering the acceptor splice site as the 3 intronic nucleotides preceding an exón (designated as IVS-1, -2, or -3) and the donor splice site as the first 5 intronic nucleotides after an exon (designated as IVS+1, +2, +3, +4, or +5) (Rogan et al., 2003).
b. The variant must be absent in a representative cohort of healthy unrelated individuals with a minimum of 200 individuals and 400 alleles with a common population origin.
c. The variant must have been absent in all published databases listing the common polymorphisms in the studied genes and previously published reports or compendia of rare control variants.

Many of the possible new genetic variants described, although they meet the requirements listed above, may not have any pathogenic effect and the only real way to check would be through functional studies that prove this effect. Due to the difficulty in performing such studies in many of the functional proteins involved, during the last years several "in silico" tools have been created allowing us to infer the probability that a genetic variant is pathogenic or not. Unfortunately, different prediction algorithms use different information and each has its own strength and weakness. Since it has been suggested that investigators should use predictions from multiple algorithms instead of relying on a single one, Liu et al (2011) have developed dbNSFP (database for nonsynonymous SNPs functional predictions). It compiles prediction scores from four algorithms (SIFT, Polyphen2,LRT, and MutationTaster), along with a conservation score (PhyloP) and other related information, for every potential non synonymous variant in the human genome.

7. Conclusion

Despite the progress in knowledge of the mechanisms, risk factors, and management of SCD, it remains being a major public-health problem. One of the challenges is the accurate identification of the person at risk, especially in younger people where the sudden death is most of the times the first manifestation of the disease. Multimarker SCD risk scores including demographic, clinical and genetic variables should improve the identification of persons at risk (Adabag et al., 2010).

Although there are other processes affecting the electrical cardiac systole, pathologies considered in this chapter are the familiar diseases with a clear genetic inheritance in which genetic diagnosis has a great relevance.

Capturing strategies followed by NGS allowed us to accurately detect arrhythmogenic disease causing mutations in a fast and cost-efficient manner that will be suitable for daily clinical practice of genetic testing. Nevertheless, we cannot forget the need to use additional strategies proving their disease causality.

Additional benefits of great value in these genetically and phenotypically heterogeneous disease are: 1) the ability to detect both, known mutations and novel mutations, 2) the possibility of screening only selected gene exons or all exons in the human genome, and finally 3) the ability to detect individuals with multiple mutations.

8. Acknowledgments

Supported by grant PI10/00851 and grant EMER 07/018 from the Spanish Health Institute ISCIII to MB.

9. References

Adabag, A.S.; Luepker, R.V.; Roger, V.L.; Gersh, B.J (2010). Sudden cardiac death: epidemiology and risk factors. *Nat Rev Cardiol.*,7(4), pp. 216-225. ISSN: 1759-5002

Albert, TJ.; Molla, MN.; Muzny, DM.; Nazareth, L.; Wheeler, D.; Song, X.; Richmond, TA.; Middle, CM.; Rodesch, MJ.; Packard, CJ.; Weinstock, GM.& Gibbs, RA.(2007). Direct selection of human genomic loci by microarray hybridization. *Nat Methods*, Vol. 4, No. 11, pp. 903-905, ISSN 1548-7091

Bamshad, MJ.; Ng SB.; Bigham, AW.; Tabor, HK.; Emond, MJ.; Nickerson, DA. & Shendure J. (2011). Exome sequencing as a tool for Mendelian disease gene discovery. *Nat Rev Genet.* Vol. 12, No. 11, pp.745-755, ISSN 1471-0056

Bazzet, H. (1920). An analysis of the time relationship of electrocardiograms. *Heart,* Vol. 7, pp. 53-370.

Campuzano, O.; Beltrán-Alvarez, P.; Iglesias, A.; Scornik, F.; Pérez, G. & Brugada, R. (2010). Genetics and cardiac channelopathies. *Genet Med.* Vol. 12, No. 5, pp.260-267, ISSN 1098-3600

Coumel, P.; Fidelle, J.; Lucet, V.; Attuel, P. & Bouvrain, Y. (1978). Catecholamine-induced severe ventricular arrhythmias with Adams-Stokes syndrome in children: report of four cases. *Br Heart J,* Vol. 40(suppl), pp. 28-37, ISSN 0007-0769

Eid, J.; Fehr, A.; Gray, J.; Luong, K.; Lyle, J.; Otto, G.; Peluso, P.; Rank, D.; Baybayan, P.; Bettman, B.; Bibillo, A.; Bjornson, K.; Chaudhuri, B.; Christians, F.; Cicero, R.; Clark, S.; Dalal, R.; Dewinter, A.; Dixon, J.; Foquet, M.; Gaertner, A.; Hardenbol, P.; Heiner, C.; Hester, K.; Holden, D.; Kearns, G.; Kong, X.; Kuse, R.; Lacroix, Y.; Lin, S.; Lundquist, P.; Ma, C.; Marks, P.; Maxham, M.; Murphy, D.; Park, I.; Pham, T.; Phillips, M.; Roy, J.; Sebra, R.; Shen, G.; Sorenson, J.; Tomaney, A.; Travers, K.; Trulson, M.; Vieceli, J.; Wegener, J.; Wu, D.; Yang, A.; Zaccarin, D.; Zhao, P.; Zhong, F.; Korlach, J. & Turner, S. (2009). Real-time DNA sequencing from single polymerase molecules. *Science,* Vol. 323, No. 5910, pp. 133-138, ISSN 0036-8075

Fedurco, M.; Romieu, A.; Williams, S.; Lawrence, I. & Turcatti, G. (2006). BTA, a novel reagent for DNA attachment on glass and efficient generation of solid-phase amplified DNA colonies. *Nucleic Acids Res,* Vol. 34, No. 3, e22, ISNN 0305-1048

Fuster, O.R., Walsh, Poole-Wilson, KingIII, Roberts,Nash, Prystowsky. (2008). Hurst´s the heart. 12th edition. McGraw Hill.

Glenn, TC. (2011). Field guide to next-generation DNA sequencers. *Mol Ecol Resour,* Vol. 11, No. 5, pp. 759-769, ISSN 1755-098X

Gnirke, A.; Melnikov, A.; Maguire, J.; Rogov, P.; LeProust, EM.; Brockman, W.; Fennell, T.; Giannoukos, G.; Fisher, S.; Russ, C.; Gabriel, S.; Jaffe, DB.; Lander, ES.& Nusbaum, C. (2009). Solution hybrid selection with ultra-long oligonucleotides for massively parallel targeted sequencing. *Nat Biotechnol,* Vol. 27, No. 2, pp. 182-189, ISSN 1087-0156

Gussak, I.; Brugada, P.; Brugada, J.; Wright, R.S.; Kopecky, S.L.; Chaitman, B.R. & Bjerregaard, P. (2000). Idiopathic short QT interval: a new clinical syndrome? *Cardiology,* Vol. 94, No. 2, pp. 99-102, ISSN 0008-6312

Harris, TD.; Buzby, PR.; Babcock, H.; Beer, E.; Bowers, J.; Braslavsky, I.; Causey, M.; Colonell, J.; Dimeo, J.; Efcavitch, JW.; Giladi, E.; Gill, J.; Healy, J.; Jarosz, M.; Lapen, D.; Moulton, K.; Quake, SR.; Steinmann, K.; Thayer, E.; Tyurina, A.; Ward, R.; Weiss, H. & Xie, Z. (2008). Single-molecule DNA sequencing of a viral genome. *Science,* Vol. 320, No. 5872, pp. 106-109, ISSN 0036-8075

Hedley, P.L.; Jørgensen, P.; Schlamowitz, S.; Moolman-Smook, J.; Kanters, J.K.; Corfield, V.A. & Christiansen, M. (2009). The genetic basis of Brugada syndrome: a mutation update. *Hum Mutat,* Vol. 30, No. 9, pp. 1256-1266, ISSN 1059-7794

Hedley, P.L.; Jørgensen, P.; Schlamowitz, S.; Wangari, R.; Moolman-Smook, J.; Brink, P.A.; Kanters, J.K.; Corfield, V.A. & Christiansen, M. (2009). The genetic basis of long QT and short QT syndromes: a mutation update. *Hum Mutat*, Vol. 30, No. 11, pp. 1486-511, ISSN 1059-7794

Hodges, E.; Xuan, Z.; Balija, V.; Kramer, M.; Molla, MN.; Smith, SW.; Middle, CM.; Rodesch, MJ.; Albert, TJ.; Hannon, GJ. & McCombie, WR. (2007). Genome-wide in situ exon capture for selective resequencing. *Nat Genet*. Vol. 39, No. 12, pp. 1522-1527, ISSN 1061-4036

Johansson, H.; Isaksson, M.; Sörqvist, EF.; Roos, F.; Stenberg, J.; Sjöblom, T.; Botling, J.; Micke, P.; Edlund, K.; Fredriksson, S.; Kultima, HG.; Ericsson, O. & Nilsson, M. (2011). Targeted resequencing of candidate genes using selector probes. *Nucleic Acids Res*, Vol. 39, No. 2, e8, ISSN 0305-1048

Kapplinger, J.D.; Tester, D.J.; Salisbury, B.A.; Carr, J.L.; Harris-Kerr, C.; Pollevick, G.D.; Wilde, A.A. & Ackerman, M.J. (2009). Spectrum and prevalence of mutations from the first 2,500 consecutive unrelated patients referred for the FAMILION long QT syndrome genetic test. *Heart Rhythm*., Vol. 6, No. 9, pp. 1297-1303, ISSN 1547-5271

Liu, X. ; Jian, X. & Boerwinkle, E. (2011). dbNSFP: A Lightweight Database of Human Nonsynonymous SNPs and Their Functional Predictions. *Hum Mutat*,.Vol. 32, No. 8, pp. 894-899, ISSN 1059-7794

Mamanova, L.; Coffey, AJ.; Scott, CE.; Kozarewa, I.; Turner, EH.; Kumar, A.; Howard, E.; Shendure, J. & Turner, DJ. (2010). Target-enrichment strategies for next-generation sequencing. *Nat Methods*, Vol. 7, No. 2, pp. 111-118, ISSN 1548-7091

Margulies, M.; Egholm, M.; Altman, WE.; Attiya, S.; Bader, JS.; Bemben, LA.; Berka, J.; Braverman, MS.; Chen, YJ.; Chen, Z.; Dewell ,SB.; Du, L.; Fierro, JM.; Gomes, XV.; Godwin, BC.; He, W.; Helgesen, S.; Ho, CH.; Irzyk, GP.; Jando, SC.; Alenquer, ML.; Jarvie, TP.; Jirage, KB.; Kim, JB.; Knight, JR.; Lanza,,JR.; Leamon, JH.; Lefkowitz, SM.; Lei, M.; Li, J.; Lohman, KL.; Lu, H.; Makhijani, VB.; McDade, KE.; McKenna, MP.; Myers, EW.; Nickerson, E.; Nobile, JR.; Plant, R.; Puc, BP.; Ronan, MT.; Roth, GT.; Sarkis, GJ.; Simons, JF.; Simpson, JW.; Srinivasan, M.; Tartaro, KR.; Tomasz, A.; Vogt, KA.; Volkmer, GA.; Wang, SH.; Wang, Y.; Weiner, MP.; Yu, P.; Begley, RF. & Rothberg, JM. (2005). Genome sequencing in microfabricated high-density picolitre reactors. *Nature*, Vol. 437, No. 7057, pp. 376-380, ISSN 0028-0836

Meder, B.; Haas, J.; Keller, A.; Heid, C.; Just, S.; Borries, A.; Boisguerin, V.; Scharfenberger-Schmeer, M.; Stähler, P.; Beier, M.; Weichenhan, D.; Strom, T.M.; Pfeufer, A.; Korn, B.; Katus, H.A.; Rottbauer, W. (2011). Targeted next-generation sequencing for the molecular genetic diagnostics of cardiomyopathies. *Circ Cardiovasc Genet.*, 4(2), pp.110-122. ISSN: 1942-325X

Metzker, ML. (2010). Sequencing technologies - the next generation. *Nat Rev Genet*, Vol.11, No.1, pp. 31-46, ISSN 1471-0056

Napolitano, C.; Priori, S.G.; Schwartz, P.J.; Bloise, R.; Ronchetti, E.; Nastoli, J.; Bottelli, G.; Cerrone, M. & Leonardi, S. (2005). Genetic testing in the long QT syndrome: development and validation of an efficient approach to genotyping in clinical practice. *JAMA*, Vol. 294, No. 23, pp. 2975-2980, ISSN 0098-7484

Ng, SB.; Turner, EH.; Robertson, PD.; Flygare, SD.; Bigham, AW.; Lee, C.; Shaffer, T.; Wong, M.; Bhattacharjee, A.; Eichler, EE.; Bamshad, M.; Nickerson, DA.& Shendure, J. (2009). Targeted capture and massively parallel sequencing of 12 human exomes. *Nature*, Vol. 461, No. 7261, pp. 272-276, ISSN 0028-0836

Priori, S.G.; Napolitano C. & Schwartz P.J. (1999). Low penetrance in the long-QT syndrome: clinical impact. *Circulation*, Vol. 99, No. 4, pp. 529-533, ISSN 0009-7322

Priori, S.G.; Napolitano, C.; Gasparini, M.; Pappone, C.; Della Bella, P.; Giordano, U.; Bloise, R.; Giustetto, C.; De Nardis, R.; Grillo, M.; Ronchetti, E.; Faggiano, G.& Nastoli, J. (2002). Natural history of Brugada syndrome: insights for risk stratification and management. *Circulation*. Vol. 105, pp. 1342–1347, ISSN 0009-7322

Priori, S.G.; Napolitano, C.; Memmi, M.; Colombi, B.; Drago, F.; Gasparini, M.; DeSimone, L.; Coltorti, F.; Bloise, R.; Keegan, R.; Cruz Filho, F.E.; Vignati, G.; Benatar, A. & DeLogu, A. (2002). Clinical and molecular characterization of patients with catecholaminergic polymorphic ventricular tachycardia. *Circulation*. Vol. 106, pp. 69 –74, ISSN 0009-7322

Priori, S.G.; Schwartz, P.J.; Napolitano, C.; Bloise, R.; Ronchetti, E.; Grillo, M.; Vicentini, A.; Spazzolini, C.; Nastoli, J.; Bottelli, G.; Folli, R. & Cappelletti, D. (2003). Risk stratification in the long-QT syndrome. *N Engl J Med*. Vol. 348, pp. 1866–1874, ISSN 0028-4793

Rogan, P.K.; Svojanovsky, S. & Leeder, J.S. (2003). Information theory-based analysis of CYP2C19, CYP2D6 and CYP3A5 splicing mutations. *Pharmacogenetics,* Vol. 13, pp. 207–218, ISSN 0960-314X

Rothberg, JM.; Hinz, W.; Rearick, TM.; Schultz, J.; Mileski, W.; Davey, M.; Leamon, JH.; Johnson, K.; Milgrew, MJ.; Edwards, M.; Hoon, J.; Simons, JF.; Marran, D.; Myers, JW.; Davidson, JF.; Branting, A.; Nobile, JR.; Puc, BP.; Light, D.; Clark, TA.; Huber, M.; Branciforte, JT.; Stoner, IB.; Cawley, SE.; Lyons, M.; Fu, Y.; Homer, N.; Sedova, M.; Miao, X.; Reed, B.; Sabina, J.; Feierstein, E.; Schorn, M.; Alanjary, M.; Dimalanta, E.; Dressman, D.; Kasinskas, R.; Sokolsky, T.; Fidanza, JA.; Namsaraev, E.; McKernan, KJ.; Williams, A.; Roth, GT. & Bustillo, J. (2011). An integrated semiconductor device enabling non-optical genome sequencing. *Nature*. Vol. 475, No. 7356, pp.348-352, ISSN 0028-0836

Schimpf, R.; Borggrefe M. & Wolpert, C. (2008). Clinical and molecular genetics of the short QT syndrome. *Curr Opin Cardiol*, Vol. 23, No. 3, pp. 192-198, ISSN 0268-4705

Schott, J.J.; Alshinawi, C.; Kyndt, F.; Probst, V.; Hoorntje, T.M.; Hulsbeek, M.; Wilde, A.A.; Escande, D.; Mannens, M.M. & Le Marec, H. (1999). Cardiac conduction defects associate with mutations in SCN5A. *Nat Genet*, Vol. 23, No.1, pp. 20-21, ISSN 1061-4036

Shendure, J.& Ji H. (2008). Next-generation DNA sequencing.*Nat Biotechnol*, Vol. 26, No. 10, pp1135-1145, ISSN 1087-0156

Tewhey, R.; Warner, JB.; Nakano, M.; Libby, B.; Medkova, M.; David, PH.; Kotsopoulos, SK.; Samuels, ML.; Hutchison, JB.; Larson, JW.; Topol, EJ.; Weiner, MP.; Harismendy, O.; Olson, J.; Link, DR. & Frazer KA. (2010). Microdroplet-based PCR enrichment for large-scale targeted sequencing. *Nat Biotechnol*. Vol. 27, No. 11pp. 1025-1031, ISSN 1087-0156

Turcatti, G.; Romieu, A.; Fedurco, M. & Tairi, AP. (2008). A new class of cleavable fluorescent nucleotides: synthesis and optimization as reversible terminators for DNA sequencing by synthesis. *Nucleic Acids Res*, Vol. 36, No. 4, e25, ISSN 0305-1048

Turner, EH.; Ng, SB.; Nickerson, DA. & Shendure J. (2009). Methods for genomic partitioning. *Annu Rev Genomics Hum Genet*, Vol. 10, pp. 263-284, ISSN 1527-8204

Valouev, A.; Ichikawa, J.; Tonthat, T.; Stuart, J.; Ranade, S.; Peckham, H.; Zeng, K.; Malek, JA.; Costa, G.; McKernan, K.; Sidow, A.; Fire, A. & Johnson, SM. (2008). A high-resolution.; nucleosome position map of C. elegans reveals a lack of universal sequence-dictated positioning. *Genome Res*, Vol. 18, No. 7, pp. 1051-1063, ISSN 1088-9051

Vincent, G.M.; Timothy, K.W.; Leppert, M. & Keating, M. (1992). The spectrum of symptoms and QT intervals in carriers of the gene for the long-QT syndrome. *N Engl J Med*, Vol. 327, No. 12, pp. 846-852, ISSN 0028-4793

Voelkerding, KV.; Dames, S. & Durtschi, J.D. (2010). Next Generation Sequencing for Clinical Diagnostics-Principles and Application to Targeted Resequencing for Hypertrophic Cardiomyopathy. *Journal of Molecular Diagnostics* Vol. 12, No.5, pp. 539-551, ISSN 1525-1578

Yeager, M.; Xiao, N.; Hayes, RB.; Bouffard, P.; Desany, B.; Burdett, L.; Orr, N.; Matthews, C.; Qi, L.; Crenshaw, A.; Markovic ,Z.; Fredrikson, KM.; Jacobs, KB.; Amundadottir, L.; Jarvie, TP.; Hunter, DJ.; Hoover, R.; Thomas, G.; Harkins, TT.& Chanock SJ. (2008). Comprehensive resequence analysis of a 136 kb region of human chromosome 8q24 associated with prostate and colon cancers. *Hum Genet*, Vol. 124, No. 2, pp. 161-170, ISSN 0340-6717

Ylänen, K.; Poutanen, T.; Hiippala, A.; Swan, H.; Korppi, M. (2010). Catecholaminergic Polymorphic ventricular tachycardia. *Eur J Pediatr.*, 169(5), pp. 535-542. ISSN: 0340-6199

Zareba, W. & Cygankiewicz, I. (2008). Long QT syndrome and short QT syndrome. *Prog Cardiovasc Dis*, Vol. 51, No.3, pp. 264-278, ISSN 0033-0620

Zipes, D.P.; Camm, A.J.; Borggrefe, M.; Buxton, A.E.; Chaitman, B.; Fromer, M.; Gregoratos, G.; Klein, G.; Moss, A.J.; Myerburg, R.J.; Priori, S.G.; Quinones, M.A.; Roden, D.M.; Silka, M.J.; Tracy, C.; Smith, S.C. Jr, Jacobs, A.K.; Adams, C.D.; Antman, E.M.; Anderson, J.L.; Hunt, S.A.; Halperin, J.L.; Nishimura, R.; Ornato, J.P.; Page, R.L.; Riegel, B.; Priori, S.G.; Blanc, J.J.; Budaj, A.; Camm, A.J.; Dean, V.; Deckers, J.W.; Despres, C.; Dickstein, K.; Lekakis, J.; McGregor, K.; Metra, M.; Morais, J.; Osterspey, A.; Tamargo, J.L.; Zamorano, J.L.; American College of Cardiology ; American Heart Association Task Force ; & European Society of Cardiology Committee for Practice Guidelines. (2006). ACC/ AHA/ESC 2006 Guidelines for management of patients with ventricular arrhythmias and the prevention of sudden cardiac death: a report of the American College of Cardiology/American Heart Association Task Force and the European Society of Cardiology Committee for Practice Guidelines (Writing Committee to Develop Guidelines for Management of Patients With Ventricular Arrhythmias and the Prevention of Sudden Cardiac Death). *J Am Coll Cardiol*, Vol. 48, e247- e346, ISSN 0735-1097

2

Phenotypic Correlation of Genetic Mutations with Ventricular Arrhythmias

Yamini Krishnan, Jerri Chen and Thomas V. McDonald
Departments of Medicine and Molecular Pharmacology,
Wilf Family Cardiovascular Research Institute
Albert Einstein College of Medicine,
Einstein – Montefiore Cardiogenetics Program, Bronx, NY
USA

1. Introduction

Much progress has been made in identifying genetic loci linked to hereditary arrhythmia syndromes over the past decade and a half. Linkage analyses for Mendelian diseases have been powerful in the discovery phases. Considerable challenges remain however, for the clinician faced with individual patients and families when the clinical symptoms are atypical or intermediate and when novel mutations or polymorphisms are reported in the course of genetic testing. To unambiguously define the deleterious nature of any given mutation, additional functional analyses are required. Such studies should not only detect the functional consequence of mutations but also the degree of severity and mechanisms that bring about the deleterious behavior. These principles apply not only to cardiac arrhythmia syndromes but also to any hereditary genetic disease. In practice, this is not always feasible or possible with current technology. This is particularly problematic when standard genetically manipulable animals (mouse) differ considerably from human, as they do in cardiac electrophysiology. An additional obstacle occurs when the target organ is not amenable to biopsy without considerable risk (e.g. heart, brain, etc.). For evaluation of genetic mutations in cardiac arrhythmia syndromes, heterologous expression of affected genes has helped tremendously.

Hereditary arrhythmia syndromes include: the long QT syndrome, the Brugada syndrome, catecholaminergic polymorphic ventricular tachycardia, the short QT syndrome, and arrhythmogenic right ventricular dysplasia. We will restrict our discussion to the long QT syndrome; however, the basic principles of verifying functional consequences of mutations also applies to the other syndromes. In this chapter we will review the progress in characterizing arrhythmia-linked genetic mutations. Several areas of recent technical advancement have been achieved which we will discuss in detail. We will also highlight how biophysical, biochemical and cell-biological studies may be used to help inform clinicians in managing the more subtle and varied aspects of patients with specific mutations. Lastly, we will discuss how such studies may eventually point to therapeutic modalities that will lead to gene-specific, or personalized medicine.

2. Overview of the long QT syndrome

Congenital long QT syndrome (LQTS) was first described by Jervell and Lange-Nielsen in 1957, who presented a family in which four of six children were born deaf, had episodes of syncope, prolonged QT interval and early sudden death (Jervell & Lange-Nielsen, 1957). In 1963 and 1964, independent reports of a similar constellation of findings in patients, but without hearing loss, were made (Romano et al., 1963; Ward, 1964). Subsequently, these were classified as autosomal-recessive (Jervell-Lange-Nielsen syndrome, with hearing loss) and autosomal dominant (Romano-Ward syndrome) forms of LQTS. The incidence of hereditary LQTS has been estimated to be as high as 1 in 2500 (Crotti et al., 2008). Notably, disease severity varies widely—from patients who are mostly asymptomatic, to ones who suffer multiple episodes of syncope and/or sudden cardiac death at a young age.

The common pathophysiological feature of LQTS is delayed repolarization, manifest on electrocardiogram (ECG) as a prolonged QT interval corresponding to a prolonged action potential duration (APD). Delayed repolarization occurs either due to an excess of sodium (Na^+) or calcium (Ca^{2+}) influx, or to deficient potassium (K^+) efflux. This disruption in the normal ionic currents across the cell membrane undermines the highly regulated electrical activity in the heart required for normal, rhythmic beating, and leaves patients at risk for potentially lethal arrhythmias. Abnormal currents can result from congenital mutations in the ion channels, or from pharmacological agents and acquired disease that can alter cardiac ion channel function.

When a ventricular myocyte action potential is prolonged, abnormal depolarizations may develop, known as early afterdepolarizations (EAD) that occur during the plateau or repolarization phases of the action potential (i.e. a type of depolarization that occurs before an action potential has completed repolarization). An EAD can then trigger an action potential that is self-perpetuating, leading to a particularly deadly type of arrhythmia known as polymorphic ventricular tachycardia or "*torsade de pointes*" which may degenerate into ventricular fibrillation. Furthermore, intracardiac imbalances of ion currents may lead to disperson of refractoriness that may play a role in susceptibility to micro-reentry. Symptoms include syncope (fainting), palpitations and sudden cardiac death.

2.1 Linkage studies

The hereditary long QT syndrome (LQTS) is now recognized as a genetically heterogeneous disorder with at least 13 different proposed loci (Table 1). Most of the loci contain genes of cardiac ion channels, accessory subunits, or channel-associated scaffolding proteins. The approaches taken by researchers in the 1990s to initially characterize hereditary LQTS relied on classical genetics with pedigree analysis of large families using microsatellite markers and logarithm of odds (LOD) score calculation. LOD scores indicate the likelihood of linkage of two loci by comparing the calculated recombination frequency against chance. A positive LOD score signifies linkage, whereas a negative score signifies the absence of linkage. The major goal of the early studies was to connect symptomatic LQTS patients with a common genetic feature.

Originally, LQTS was thought to be a single-gene disorder linked to chromosome 11 (Keating et al., 1991a; Keating et al., 1991b). Subsequent refinement revealed that heterogeneity and multiple loci were involved (Worley et al., 1992; Benhorin et al., 1993). In 1994, analysis of multiple LQTS families using LOD scores showed that some had linkage to chromosome 7, others linked to chromosome 3, and both excluded chromosome 11 linkage (Jiang et al., 1994). Other of the families in the study did not show linkage to any of the three known loci, suggesting the existence of additional loci. Once the first three LQTS loci were identified, several groups worked to identify the genes responsible for the phenotypes. In

1995, Wang et al. used linkage analysis to show that locus LQT3 contained SCN5A, a Na^+ channel that was previously cloned and characterized in 1992 (Gellens et al., 1992; Wang et al., 1995a; Wang et al., 1995b).

Locus	Gene	Protein Function	Chromosome	Other Diseases
LQT1	KCNQ1	KvLQT1 K^+ channel α subunit	11p15.5	Short QT Syndrome (SQTS1) Familial Atrial Fibrillation (FAF)
LQT2	KCNH2	HERG K^+ channel α subunit	7q35-q36	SQT1
LQT3	SCN5A	Na^+ Channel α subunit	3p21	Brugada Syndrome (BrS1) Conduction & Sinus node disease
LQT4	ANK2	Ankyrin B adaptor protein	4q25-q27	LQTS
LQT5	KCNE1	minK β subunit	21q22.1-2	Atrial Fibrillation, Deafness
LQT6	KCNE2	MiRP1 β subunit	21q22.1-22.2	Hypothyroidism, Periodic paralysis
LQT7	KCNJ2	Kir2.1 K^+ Channel	17q23.1-q24.2	Andersen's Syndrome, myotonia
LQT8	CACNA1c	Ca^{2+} channel α subunit	12p13.3	Timothy Syndrome, BrS3
LQT9	CAV3	Caveolin 3 membrane scaffold	3p25	Cardiomyopathy
LQT10	SCN4B	Na^+ Channel β subunit	11q23	Conduction Disease
LQT11	AKAP9	Yotiao PKA scaffold	7q21-q22	LQTS
LQT12	SNTA1	Syntrophin α 1 scaffold protein	20q11.2	LQTS
LQT13	KCNJ5	Kir3.4 K^+ Channel	11q24	Neonatal hyper-insulinemia

Table 1. The Hereditary Long QT Syndrome Loci

In 1995 Curran et al. analyzed LQTS families using markers linked to locus LQT2 on chromosome 7q35-36 (Curran et al., 1995). Physical mapping using yeast artificial chromosomes (YACs) and fluorescent in situ hybridization (FISH) indicated that a candidate gene with homology to potassium ion channels (K^+ channels) resided in that position. This gene had been previously identified as the human *ether-à-go-go* related gene (HERG or KCNH2) (Warmke & Ganetzky, 1994). Patient sample analysis for mutations in HERG with single-strand conformation polymorphisms (SSCP) detected the presence of genetic variants and functional expression of the cDNA in *Xenopus* oocytes showed that HERG encoded a channel that carried the rapidly activating delayed rectifier K^+ current (I_{Kr}) and confirmed the deleterious nature of the mutations. Further positional cloning showed that LQT1 on chromosome 11 encoded KvLQT1/KCNQ1, another K^+ channel (Wang et al., 1996). Concurrently, Schott et al. used similar linkage techniques to map the LQT4 locus to chromosome 4q25-27 (Schott et al., 1995). The gene responsible for LQT4 was identified in 2003 by the Mohler group as ankyrin-B, a scaffolding protein which when mutated causes aberrant targeting of essential cardiac channel proteins (Mohler et al., 2004).

Identification of other LQTS loci was done through a variety of techniques ranging from classical genetics to modern genomic methods (Chevillard et al., 1993; Duggal et al., 1998; Abbott et al., 1999; Fodstad et al., 2004; Vatta et al., 2006; Ueda et al., 2008). The loci include other channel proteins such as the Kir2.1 channel encoded by KCNJ2 and the voltage-gated Cav1.2 calcium channel encoded by CACNA1c, K^+ channel accessory subunits (KCNE1 and KCNE2), as well as scaffolding proteins such as AKAP9 and syntrophin. While the genes are numerous and diverse, the overall themes of cardiac ion channel function/dysfunction and alterations in regulation unify the genetic causes of LQTS.

3. Heterologous expression of arrhythmia-linked genes

The ideal system for studying behavior of cardiac ion channels would be isolated cardiac myocytes that survive in culture for a long time period. Such primary cells however, entail significant risk to patients and are extremely difficult to maintain long term in culture. The next option is to express the channel proteins in a cell type that can be maintained and manipulated as necessary.

3.1 *Xenopus* oocytes

Xenopus laevis oocytes are an established system for studying ion channels using electrophysiological techniques. The procedure consists of creating cRNAs of the gene of interest followed by injection into oocytes, which contain all the necessary cellular machinery for protein expression (Gurdon et al., 1971; Barnard et al., 1982). Two-electrode voltage clamp is a relatively easy method to use with oocytes given their large size and provides a rapid way to functionally characterize many of the genes involved in LQTS, and many of the first studies utilized this method. *Xenopus* oocytes however, contain an endogenous K^+ channel similar to KCNQ1, thus confounding some of the early studies on KCNE1 and KCNQ1. Moreover, oocytes are maintained at 16-19ºC, a temperature that may permit mutant proteins to properly fold and traffic to the cell surface thereby masking a misfolding phenotype that would normally occur at human physiological temperatures. Such an occurrence was noted in the initial analysis of the cystic fibrosis transmembrane conductance regulator protein (CFTR)(Cheng et al., 1990; Denning et al., 1992).

3.2 Mammalian cultured cell systems

Another approach is to use immortalized mammalian cell lines such as human embryonic kidney (HEK 293), Chinese hamster ovary (CHO), or COS-7 cells. Unlike primary cell lines, immortalized cell lines can be propagated many times and maintain baseline characteristics. The cells are incubated at 37°C and contain all the necessary components for protein transcription, translation, trafficking and degradation. They are more amenable than oocytes for immunoblotting, immuno-precipitation, high-resolution immuno-fluorescence, trafficking assays, cell-surface expression assays, and patch clamp electrophysiology. The cells may also have endogenous K^+ current; however, the magnitude is small and does not usually interfere with measurements of over-expressed channels currents. Mammalian cell lines more closely mimic native systems than oocytes and are useful for analyzing biological consequences of LQTS mutations. A caveat to this system is that the LQT-linked channels may exist in macromolecular complexes in vivo. Such complexes may comprise accessory subunits and regulatory proteins, which may not be recapitulated by heterologous expression system.

3.3 Purified proteins for biochemistry and structural analysis

Functional expression in oocytes and cells allows the study of many aspects of mutations but the fundamental mechanism of mutational effects ultimately relies on structural analysis. The primary challenge is finding conditions under which a large quantity of protein can be expressed and purified. This process can be relatively straightforward for soluble, cytosolic proteins, but is more difficult for membrane proteins such as ion channels. Because of the large amount of protein needed for purification, transfection of mammalian cells, or even the use of stably transfected mammalian cells lines, may not be feasible. Alternative systems of expression have been developed for bacteria, yeast, and insect cells, but determining the best host for producing a particular protein is usually an empirical process.

One of the most commonly used expression systems is the bacteria *Escherichia coli*. There are several technical and economic advantages: the ease of introducing DNA via transformation with a plasmid expression vector, rapid growth, and simple growth media. Problems do exist, though, in expressing mammalian membrane proteins in bacteria. These include alternative translation, posttranslational modification and trafficking mechanisms. Certain limitations can be overcome by changing growth conditions, co-expressing necessary chaperones, or creating fusions with prokaryotic partners such as maltose-binding protein (MBP) or glutathione *S*-transferase (GST) to improve their solubility and stability. Even with these modifications, it can still be difficult to express the full length of a protein (for example, the full length of KCNQ1 is nearly 700 amino acids, and Nav1.5 is around 2000 amino acids). An alternative expression host is the yeast *Pichia pastoris*, which has a eukaryotic protein synthesis pathway and is capable of post-translational modifications, though it is not entirely equivalent to a mammalian system. The first (and thus far, only) mammalian K^+ channel to be crystallized was expressed in *P. pastoris*, whereas several previously crystallized bacterial channels were expressed in *E. coli* (Doyle et al., 1998; Jiang et al., 2002; Jiang et al., 2003; Long et al., 2005). A higher eukaryotic system that may be used is insect cells, with baculovirus as the vector for protein expression. Insect cells are even better equipped with the machinery needed for proper protein folding and for post-translational modifications. While they provide high expression levels and can be grown to high density, a disadvantage is that the growth media is more expensive than for bacteria or yeast.

If a system for high-yield expression and purification of a protein can be achieved, the protein can then be used in a multitude of biochemical and structural experiments. The highest resolution is crystal structure; however, this is a difficult and time consuming task. The difficulty of this task is evident in the small fraction of membrane proteins that have been crystallized, compared to soluble proteins. An alternative that has been used successfully is solution nuclear magnetic resonance (NMR) structure. Besides the obvious advantage of not needing crystals, NMR may yield structure that is closer to native form, since formation of crystals may impose non-native constraints on the protein.

4. Animal models of inherited human arrhythmias

Ideally, it is desirable to create an animal model of a disease—acquired or hereditary—in order to study pathophysiological mechanisms, and to design and test therapeutic options. To accomplish this it is important that the model recapitulate the human condition as closely as possible. For hereditary diseases it is necessary that the animal be genetically manipulable and that homologues of the genes of interest exist and be expressed in the same tissues as humans. Here we will discuss animal models that have been proposed and used for LQTS.

4.1 Rodent

Mice and rats are valuable systems for modeling a variety of human diseases, especially in terms of organ system pathophysiology and immune diseases. Since they can be easily genetically manipulated, they are good surrogates and provide clues to the hierarchy of genetic pathways and regulation that occur in the healthy and disease states.

Once the genetic loci were identified, investigators created knock-out (null) and knock-in mice to model the LQTS phenotype. The knock-out is done by creating an exogenous construct based on the sequence of the mouse gene, but where the relevant allele has been inactivated or nullified by inserting a stop codon or deletion/insertion to inhibit expression of the native protein. This construct is then injected into mouse embryos where homologous recombination occurs and the endogenous mouse gene is replaced by the null construct, which contains a marker so that recombinant mice may be distinguished. The recombinant mouse must then be bred to create heterozygous and homozygous null mice in subsequent generations. A knock-in mouse is created by a similar method, where the construct is a human gene (or mouse ortholog) that contains a known functional mutation. The engineered heterozygous mice will express one copy of endogenous mouse gene and one of the transgenic mutated gene.

There are at least 40 mouse models of LQTS genes. Two mouse models were created that disrupted exons 1 and 2 in KCNQ1 (Lee et al., 2000; Casimiro et al., 2001). Interestingly, the mouse with mutation in exon 1 did not show any ECG abnormalities. However, this mouse did have auditory-vestibular aspects of the Jervell and Lange-Nielsen syndrome. The mouse with KCNQ1 exon 2 disruption showed abnormal T-wave morphology on in vivo ECGs and inner ear abnormalities. In a third study, mice were created that expressed a dominant negative isoform of KCNQ1; these mice had QT prolongation on ECG as well as *torsade de pointes* arrhythmias (Demolombe et al., 2001). For KCNE1 null mice, the models exhibit deafness, but no baseline QT prolongation (Schulze-Bahr et al., 1997). One KCNE1 null mouse showed abnormal rate adaptation, which is similar to the phenotype seen in humans with KCNQ1/KCNE1 mutations upon exercise challenge (Charpentier et al., 1998; Warth & Barhanin, 2002). Mice express the HERG ortholog Merg1 in the heart. The Merg1 homozygous knock-out mouse is embryonic lethal as it dies early in development (London, 1998). A mouse model that expresses the dominant-negative HERG-G628S mutation showed a normal ECG phenotype (Babij et al., 1998).

While these studies yielded valuable information about pathogenesis of LQTS, they also highlighted how mice have limited value in studying inherited cardiac arrhythmias resulting from mutations in delayed rectifier K^+ current channels. Mice have a baseline heart rate of ~600 beats per minute. As such, they have a short action potential and repolarization phase that is largely dependent on the transient outward K^+ current (I_{to}) and have little to no I_{Ks} or I_{Kr} (Nerbonne, 2004; Milan & MacRae, 2005). So while they are genetically tractable, they may not be electrophysiologically similar enough to humans to provide a good model system. In contrast to the limitations of modeling human repolarization in the mouse, more success has been achieved for the depolarizing currents, which are more akin to those in the human. A LQTS mouse model generated by knock-in of an LQT3 mutation (KPQ deletion in SCN5A) (Nuyens et al., 2001). The transgenic mice had prolonged APD and polymorphic ventricular tachycardia.

Early studies of guinea pig ventricular myocytes revealed that two components making up the repolarization current I_{Kr} and I_{Ks} (Sanguinetti, 1990). This work was the original characterization of two repolarizing K^+ currents and forms the basis for many of the subsequent studies. Considering that isolated guinea pig ventricular myocytes was the in vitro system that launched a whole field of study, some groups have used an interesting approach by injecting adenoviral vectors containing wild-type or mutant KCNE1 or HERG into guinea pig myocardium (Hoppe et al., 2001). This group found that myocytes expressing the HERG G628S mutant, I_{Kr} was reduced, but action potential duration was not shortened however, beat-to-beat variability increased as did EADs. They also expressed the KCNE1-D76N mutant which suppressed I_{Ks}, significantly slowing repolarization, leading to frequent EADs and QT prolongation on ECG.

4.2 Rabbit

Given the limitations of rodent models, larger animals with cardiac electrophysiology more similar to humans might be considered. These included study of dogs, ferrets and rabbits. The Koren group has developed transgenic rabbits expressing human LQT mutations (Brunner et al., 2008). To create the transgenic rabbits the investigators injected embryos with a cDNA construct that contained either mutant HERG or KCNQ1 under a cardiac specific promoter, so that the transgene will only be active in the heart. These animals have enabled the investigators to gain significant insights by ECG analysis in awake freely moving animals, optical mapping of repolarization waves using voltage-sensitive dyes, and at the cellular level by recording from isolated rabbit myocytes. To date, this may be the most accurate model system that exists for hereditary LQTS.

4.3 Zebrafish

The newest model system to be explored is the zebrafish, *Danio rerio*. These are genetically tractable animals that expresses an endogenous ortholog of HERG (zERG) (Langheinrich et al., 2003). zERG is expressed specifically in both heart chambers of zebrafish embryos, is similarly composed of six transmembrane domains, and displays a particularly high degree of amino acid conservation in the S6 helix and pore domain. One specific mutant that was characterized named *breakdance* displayed prolonged ventricular APD, spontaneous EADs, and 2:1 atrio-ventricular block in the embryonic stages of development. The group of Scholz et al. expressed cloned zERG in *Xenopus* oocytes and showed current characteristics similar to the human channel however the details of its kinetics and gating were distinctly different (Scholz et al., 2009). Arnaout et al. recently performed a forward genetic screen and identified two zebrafish HERG mutants s213 and s290. They showed that homozygous animals had virtually no ventricular contraction and impaired calcium handling in the ventricles. Heterozygous animals showed increased APD and prolonged QT-interval on ECG (Arnaout et al., 2007). These studies show that given the conserved channel function, zebrafish does represent a valuable genetic model system to investigate HERG channel mutations.

4.4 Primary isolated myocytes

To find a more native system to study ion channels, researchers have sought methods to isolate and maintain primary cardiac myocytes. Primary isolated myocytes are best suited for short-term culture (approximately four days) and electrophysiological or immunofluorescence experiments that require only a low yield of viable cells (10s compared to 10,000s needed for biochemistry experiments) (Nuss & Marban, 1994). Some of the technical challenges involved include obtaining fresh healthy heart samples, appropriate and not over-digestion of the tissue by enzymes, purification of myocytes from fibroblasts and matrix, calcium tolerance of the freshly isolated myocytes, and finding the correct conditions for culture. Most adult myocytes have been isolated from mouse, rat, guinea pig, and rabbit since the animals are readily available and economical. Fresh human heart samples for cardiomyocyte isolation are difficult to obtain routinely for ethical reasons. Rat neonatal cardiomyocytes have provided a fairly easy-to-obtain and widely applicable system in recent years (Chlopcikova et al., 2001). Since the rat neonatal cardiomyocytes may only transiently express the relevant channel, another approach is to use adenoviral or lentiviral vectors containing the cDNA of interest to infect the cells and allow adequate expression for study in a more native system. Comparing the behavior of wild type HERG and KCNQ1 channels with previously characterized deleterious mutants in rat neonatal myocytes has confirmed initial phenotypic characterization (Li et al., 2001; Lin et al., 2010). These groups found that the wild-type and mutant channel behaved generally the same as in cultured cells with some slight differences. Additionally some groups used the neonatal cardiomyocyte system to understand localization and interaction of the HERG, KCNQ1 and β accessory subunits (Rasmussen et al., 2004; Wu et al., 2006).

5. Human phenotypic studies

5.1 Locus-specific triggers

While QT interval prolongation puts patients at risk for abnormal heart rhythms, most patients are asymptomatic on a daily basis, with arrhythmias triggered by certain conditions or stimuli. In a 2001 study of 670 patients with known symptomatic LQT1, LQT2, or LQT3, a correlation between genotype and one of three specific triggers: exercise, emotion, or sleep was found. LQT1 patients had most events (syncope, cardiac arrest, or sudden death) triggered by exercise (62% of cases), while LQT2 patients had most events triggered by emotion (43% of cases), and LQT3 patients had most events during sleep (39% of cases) (Schwartz et al., 2001). In another study exercise induced significant further prolongation of QTc in LQT1 patients compared to LQT2 (Takenaka et al., 2003). In mice with an LQT3 knock-in mutation, bradycardia induced by cholinergic stimulation provoked *torsade de pointes*, while physical stress, mental stress, isoproterenol, and atropine did not (Fabritz et al., 2010). In female LQT2 patients, the post-partum period is a time of increased risk for arrhythmia (Khositseth et al., 2004). These efforts to categorize locus-specific triggers help clinicians in initial diagnostic phases and to better advise patients diagnosed with a specific LQTS genotype. There are some overlaps in triggers; for example, a certain percentage of LQT2 patients have cardiac events triggered by exercise. One study found a correlation of mutation location within HERG and the type of trigger causing symptoms: pore-loop mutations correlated with arousal-triggered events, non-pore mutations more often associated with exercise-triggered events (Kim et al., 2010).

5.2 Therapeutic approaches

Currently, there are five main avenues for treatment for adult patients with LQTS: (1) β-blockers, (2) gene-specific therapy, (3) pacemakers, (4) left cervico-thoracic sympathetic ganglionectomy, and (5) implanted cardio-verter defibrillators (ICDs). The primary goal of these therapies is to prevent life-threatening ventricular tachyarrhythmias and sudden cardiac death.

Given the correlation of LQTS locus and specific arrhythmia triggers, an important part of LQTS management is avoidance of triggers. LQT1 patients are advised to avoid competitive and endurance athletics, especially swimming. LQT2 patients are advised to reduce exposure to startle-stimuli, such as loud alarm clocks. LQT3 patients may have a pacemaker implanted to prevent bradycardia during sleep. For all patients with a LQTS diagnosis, the first line treatments demand avoidance of all potentially QT-prolonging drugs and the correction of electrolyte imbalances or other precipitating metabolic conditions.

Pharmacological treatment may used in combination with trigger avoidance. β-blocker therapy is widely used for treatment of LQT1 and LQT2, having been associated with significant risk-reduction in adult and pediatric cases and is considered a treatment with very low risk of adverse effects (Goldenberg et al., 2010). Mortality of patients on β-blockers is around 0.5% (Schwartz, Priori et al., 2001; Priori et al., 2004). Channel blockers or openers may also be used, though they can be pro-arrhythmic if not properly monitored. A study examining the effects of the K^+ channel opener nicorandil on canine models of LQT1, 2 and 3 showed that the drug may be effective in shortening the QT interval and preventing *torsade de pointes* in LQT1 and LQT2, but not LQT3 (Shimizu & Antzelevitch, 2000). For LQT3 patients where cardiac events are more likely to happen at low heart rates, β-blocker therapy is generally less helpful. LQT3 who have mutations in SCN5A where the defect is a persistent late current, channel blockers such as mexilitene, or flecainide are potentially helpful (Rosero et al., 1997).

Novel approaches include potassium supplementation for LQT2 patients. In vitro experiments have showed that proper intracellular K^+ concentration is a requirement for normal HERG channel trafficking to the membrane, and that extracellular potassium modulates HERG current (Guo et al., 2009; Wang et al., 2009). These findings correlate with earlier studies that focused on HERG current density, showing that I_{Kr} current paradoxically increased when extracellular K^+ concentration was increased (Sanguinetti & Jurkiewicz, 1992). One group administered spironolactone to eight LQT2 patients for four weeks, and observed a decrease in QT interval, (Etheridge et al., 2003) while another treated seven subjects with potassium supplementation and had similar findings (Compton et al., 1996). Such approaches may be considered in LQT2 patients.

Invasive therapies include left cardiac sympathetic denervation (LCSD), stellate ganglionectomy, and implantable cardioverter defibrillators (ICDs). LCSD involves the removal or ablation of the first four thoracic ganglia (which includes the stellate ganglion). In a 2004 study that included 174 high-risk, symptomatic LQTS patients who underwent LCSD, post-surgical QT intervals were shortened, and there was a 91% reduction in cardiac events over eight years of follow-up (Schwartz et al., 2004). These types of surgical interventions decrease sympathetic stimulation to the heart and may be recommended for patients who have not experienced cardiac arrest, but still experience syncope while on β-blocker therapy. ICD placement in such patients may be problematic because they may receive an intolerably high number of shocks. ICDs are most appropriate for patients who have already had an episode of cardiac arrest and are at higher risk for recurrence.

5.3 Male / female differences

To date, all LQTS loci are autosomal and not sex-linked. There are however, interesting differences between male and female LQTS patients. The QTc for women during the reproductive years (age 16-45) is longer than that for men of the same age (Bazett, 1920).

Women also have a higher resting heart rate than men (Ashman, 1942; Jose & Collison, 1970). The QTc intervals for males and females under age 16 are comparable as are those of post-menopausal women and men of the same age (Locati et al., 1998). There is also an increased risk for women of reproductive age with LQT1 and LQT2 mutations to have arrhythmic events (Zareba et al., 1995); (Lehmann et al., 1997). These findings implicate differential affects of the sex hormone pathways on cardiac electrophysiology.
Interestingly, there is an increased risk of having a cardiac event for female LQT1 and LQT2 patients in the immediate post-partum period (Seth et al., 2007). Another recent report described a patient with KCNE1 mutation who experienced aborted sudden cardiac death in the post-partum period (Nakajima et al., 2010). The current recommendation is to continue β-blocker therapy throughout the pregnancy and post-partum period to avoid cardiac events. While LQT1 and LQT2 mutations seem to adversely affect women more, the LQT3 (and Brugada syndrome mutations) event rate is greater in men (Priori et al., 2003). Among LQT3 genotyped individuals, men have a longer QTc than women. Another important condition where there are significant male/female differences is in acquired LQTS that may occur with drugs that block K^+ channels, mainly HERG. Multiple studies found that women are more likely to have adverse events when taking a QT-prolonging medication (Woosley & Sale, 1993; Drici et al., 1996; Reinoehl et al., 1996). This should be a key consideration when prescribing medications to patients with LQTS and in the general population.

6. New model systems: Induced patient-specific stem cells (iPSCs)

A novel model that has been under recent investigation to better understand the pathophysiology of LQTS is induced patient-specific stem cells. This process consists of obtaining skin cells (dermal fibroblasts) from patients with known LQTS mutations as well as unaffected control subjects, culturing them, de-differentiating them into pluripotent stem cells, and re-differentiating them into cardiomyocytes in vitro. The dermal fibroblasts are infected with retroviruses or lentiviruses containing specific transcription factors that convert and reprogram the dermal cell to a pluripotent stem cell without affecting the other genomic DNA containing the LQTS mutation. The pluripotent stem cells are then given specific growth factors in a precise order and grown on feeder cells until they form embryoid bodies: aggregates of cells that can differentiate into cardiomyocytes of three distinct types: "nodal", "atrial" and "ventricular" (Zhang et al., 2009). The cells were also shown to have cardiomyocyte architecture including sarcomeric organization of actin, myosin and other components, albeit immature.
In 2010, Moretti et al. characterized cells derived from a LQT1 patient who had the mutation R190Q in KCNQ1. They showed that these cells exhibited a prolonged APD due to reduced I_{Ks} current density (Moretti et al., 2010). Itzhaki et al. derived cardiomyocytes from a patient with an LQT2 mutation in HERG (A614V); these cells also showed a prolonged APD and reduction in I_{Kr} (Itzhaki et al., 2011). They used microelectrode arrays to record from groups of mutant cells and showed an increased incidence of EADs. To study mutations in the calcium channel, the group of Yazawa and colleagues were able to derive iPSCs from patients with LQT8 (Timothy syndrome) (Yazawa et al., 2011). They found that the mutation-carrying cells contracted slowly and irregularly, had exaggerated calcium influx with prolonged APD in ventricular type cells. These studies were able to confirm previous findings of channel dysfunction in a more native setting.

Two notable caveats with the iPSC approach are that the differentiated cells are immature and may not express the full complement of ion channels and accessory or regulatory proteins and cellular architecture as does an adult cardiomyocyte and that the differentiated cells may be heterogeneous. A challenge is to develop a selection method or purification scheme to isolate the induced cardiomyocytes in larger and more uniform quantities.

The iPSC system holds particular promise in determining the effect of potentially deleterious mutations in proteins other than ion channels such as regulatory or scaffolding proteins. This system may also be of particular utility in analysis of mutations non-coding areas (introns promoters, splice-sites and untranslated mRNA sequences). For therapeutics, iPSCs may provide a platform to test new potential pharmacologic approaches in a more native and genotype-specific setting prior to testing in animals and humans.

7. Mechanisms of deleterious mutations

LQTS mutations cause alterations in cardiac ionic currents that result in delayed action potential repolarization. The delay can be caused by sustained inward sodium or calcium currents, or impaired outward K^+ current. Mutations to ion channels or their regulatory proteins alter channel function such that an increase or decrease in current occurs; the mechanism by which the mutation causes these functional changes can be categorized into several classes: (1) changes in biophysical properties, (2) changes in channel synthesis and processing, and (3) changes channel regulation.

7.1 Biophysical

Biophysical defects are caused by mutation to channel subunits that result in channel gain or loss of function. Several biophysical parameters affect how much current a channel carries: the structure of the channel pore, channel gating, and the stability of the channel in the open versus closed states.

To discuss the effects on channel structure, we will focus on voltage-gated K^+ channels as an example (see Figure 1). The pore of a K^+ channel subunit is composed of two transmembrane helices (S5 and S6) and an intervening loop; when tetramerized, the loops form the K^+ selectivity filter that extends into the ion conduction pathway, while the helices line the remainder of the pore (Doyle, Morais Cabral et al., 1998; Jiang, Lee et al., 2002; Jiang, Lee et al., 2003; Long, Campbell et al., 2005). The structure of the selectivity filter is rigid as ion selectivity is based on size; it holds the same conformation regardless of whether the channel is open or closed. The pore-lining transmembrane helices though, move in response to changes in membrane voltage; when the channel is closed, the intracellular end of the helices prevent ions from accessing the selectivity filter, and when the channel is open, the helices are positioned such that ions can enter the pore. Deleterious mutations have been identified in the pore region. They presumably alter the structure of this sensitive region such that ions cannot access the selectivity filter, or cannot pass through the selectivity filter.

A second region that may be affected is the voltage sensor. The S4 transmembrane domain of a K^+ channel is lined with positively charged amino acids. A change in the membrane potential causes movement in the voltage-sensor, and subsequently the pore region to which it is linked. Mutation to the voltage-sensing domain can result in delayed or impaired channel opening. Analysis of several LQT1 mutations in the S4 domain revealed a depolarizing shift in voltage-dependent activation of the channel, which indicates that a larger driving force was required to open the mutant channels (Henrion et al., 2009). Though

S4 contains the voltage-sensing residues, transmembrane domains S1 to S4 are structurally clustered together as the voltage-sensing domain; thus, mutations to residues in S1, S2, and S3 have also been associated with LQTS.

Unlike in K^+ channels, where loss-of-function mutations are the pathophysiologial defect, in Na^+ channels, gain-of-function mutations lead to an increased Na^+ current that maintain the cell in a depolarized state. Na^+ channels are responsible for the rapid influx of Na^+ ions in phase 0 of the action potential; this phase is extremely short-lived (milliseconds) as Na^+ channels normally rapidly inactivate. Mutations that alter Na^+ channel inactivation (rather than activation or deactivation) account for the majority of LQT3 . A defect in inactivation leads to a persistent Na^+ current throughout the action potential duration, which delays repolarization. Several cytoplasmic regions of the Na^+ channel are responsible for inactivation, and mutations in these regions lead to persistent current (Jones & Ruben, 2008).

Biophysical mutations can act in a dominant-negative manner in patients with one wild-type allele and one mutant allele. Because K^+ channels are composed of four separate, identical channel subunits, wild-type and mutant subunits randomly combine together. Mutations that act in a dominant-negative manner may affect the function of channels that contain even one mutant subunit; less severe mutations may result in heteromeric channels with normal function or a partial defect. Sodium and calcium channels, however, are encoded such that the entire pore-forming channel is translated into a single polypeptide. Therefore, a patient who inherits a single mutant allele will have roughly 50% normal and 50% mutant channels. The mechanisms for dominant phenotype in these cases resides in the fact that LQTS mutations in sodium and calcium channels are "gain-of-function" which cannot be overcome by expression of the normal allele.

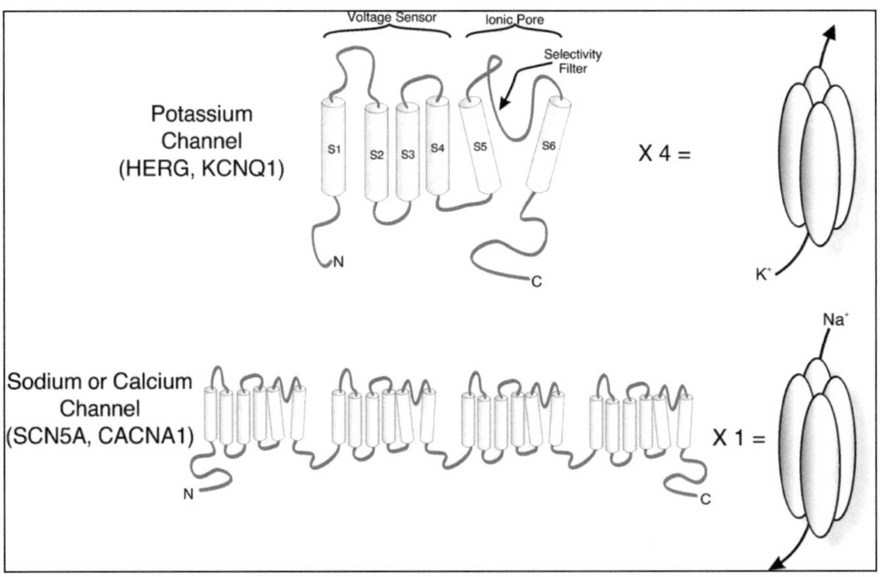

Fig. 1. Schematic representation of K^+ (top) and sodium or calcium (bottom) channel proteins. Note that four identical subunits combine to form a single unit for K^+ channels. Sodium and calcium channels are encoded as a singe polypeptide that is compised of four domains that are homologous the single subunit of a K^+ channel. S1 through S6 signify the transmembrane helices

7.2 Cell biological processes

7.2.1 Errors in synthesis

The first steps in channel synthesis include transcription of RNA in the nucleus and post-transcriptional modifications (capping, addition of a poly-A tail, splicing, and editing). The mature mRNA is then targeted to ribosomes on the endoplasmic reticulum to begin protein translation. Several classes of mutations can change mRNA stability and negatively affect abundance of functional protein. These include frame-shift and premature termination codons. These types of mutations may cause mRNA instability and subsequent degradation, a process called nonsense-mediated decay (NMD). NMD has been shown to be an underlying mechanism in other diseases. This phenomenon has been implicated as a cause recurrent intrauterine fetal death or LQTS in mutations of HERG (Bhuiyan et al., 2008) (Zarraga et al., 2011). Similarly NMD has been implicated to play a role in LQT3 mutation of the Na^+ channel SCN5A (Teng et al., 2009). It is certainly conceivable that mutations, yet to be described, may also introduce new binding motifs for micro-RNAs that would alter stability and the mRNA and hence, protein synthesis.

7.2.2 Errors in trafficking

In general, defective protein trafficking is emerging as an important disease mechanism that concerns a variety of cell types. A newly synthesized channel goes through numerous processing steps before it ultimately reaches the membrane and is functional. At the earliest stage, some signaling systems may affect channel synthesis itself (Chen et al., 2009; Chen et al., 2010; Sroubek & McDonald, 2011). After the channel is synthesized at the endoplasmic reticulum (ER) it must fold to attain its tertiary structure and then assemble with other subunits to form the functional macromolecular complex. Folding is a complex process involving helper proteins called chaperones, which work in iterations to achieve the final proper conformation. Once the protein is properly folded it may be glycosylated and it leaves the ER through vesicle transport to arrive at the Golgi. At the Golgi the glycoslyations may be further modified and finally the channel leaves the Golgi in vesicles bound for the plasma membrane.

Mutations may cause channel proteins to fold improperly; these mis-folded proteins may be recognized by the quality-control system and marked for degradation by the proteasome. This causes a trafficking error, and mis-folded protein may accumulate in the ER or Golgi membrane. Though severe mis-folding results in a non-functional channel (for example, mutations that prevent tetramerization of channel subunits), milder mutations may allow for a functional channel to fold, yet still be retained intracellularly. This is in theory possible, but under most circumstances it is difficult to test because functional experiments such as electrophysiology require proper trafficking. Mutations in HERG and KCNQ1 that affect trafficking can be loss-of-function and many of them can act in a dominant-negative fashion interfering with associated normal allele subunits. While tetramerization has been studied for these channels, the mechanisms are incompletely understood. Given a situation where wild-type and mutant subunits are co-expressed, the heterogeneous pool of tetrameric channels may express a range of current density from zero to the full wild-type amount. This could explain why some trafficking mutations have a more severe phenotype than others.

It is worth considering LQTS mutation-associated trafficking errors in HERG. A trafficking defect is the most common cellular phenotype for LQT2 mutants (Anderson et al., 2006). Particular attention has been paid to the HERG cytoplasmic C-terminal portion where analysis of various LQT2 mutations has revealed that this segment is critical for tetrameric assembly and proper trafficking. While many of these studies have focused on the C-terminus of HERG, it is important to note that trafficking defective mutants have also been found throughout the N-terminus as well as the transmembrane domains (Balijepalli et al., 2010). Complex mechanisms for the forward trafficking (from ER to Golgi) of HERG have been suggested. Recently, Delisle et al. showed that HEK cell expressed HERG undergoes COPII-dependent ER export and also endosomal trafficking which determine its plasma membrane expression (Delisle et al., 2009). They also showed that this atypical trafficking route is mediated by small GTPases such as Sar1 and Rab11b. More recent trafficking studies show that LQT2 mutants may be subjected to quality-control in the ER-Golgi intermediate compartment (ERGIC) (Smith et al., 2011). It has also been shown that trafficking defective LQT2 mutants are subsequently degraded by the ER-associated degradation pathway (ERAD) and the ubiquitin proteasome pathway (Kagan et al., 2000; Gong et al., 2005). While this picture is incomplete (studies rely on heterologous expression), it does give us insight into the points during synthesis where HERG is particularly susceptible and how mutations affect its maturation.

Recent studies have examined the role of extracellular potassium in the endocytosis and degradation of HERG. Recently, the work of Guo and colleagues has provided a biochemical basis and mechanistic approach to study the behavior of HERG in low-potassium conditions. The 155 kDa form of HERG undergoes endocytic internalization from the plasma membrane and proteasomal degradation through a mechanism involving caveolin (Massaeli et al., 2010). Further work was done by Massaeli and colleagues who studied the behavior of pore-lining mutations in HERG under zero-potassium conditions. They found that alanine mutants at certain positions in the pore helix and selectivity filters abolished the low-potassium induced degradation. This is an interesting mechanism since arrhythmias are often precipitated by electrolyte disturbances such as hypokalemia (Berthet et al., 1999).

7.3 Regulation

In addition to intrinsic channel defects, there are many regulatory proteins that interact with channels to modulate their activity. Since LQT1 and LQT2 patients often have arrhythmias precipitated by physical or emotional stress, it is important to consider the human stress response affect these channels. The α- and β-adrenergic systems are activated during stress. The β-adrenergic system involves the β-adrenergic receptor, a hetero-trimeric G-protein, and cyclic adenosine monophosphate (cAMP), a second messenger that ultimately activates protein kinase A (PKA). HERG current is acutely reduced by PKA signaling due to direct phosphorylation of the channel. Furthermore, cAMP can interact with the HERG channel directly in a manner that partially abrogates the suppressive effects of phosphorylation. An added complexity to this signaling pathway is the interaction between 14-3-3, a scaffolding protein, and HERG (Kagan et al., 2002; Kagan & McDonald, 2005)). 14-3-3 dynamically binds proteins (including HERG) upon phosphorylation, primarily by PKA. When this occurs with HERG, channel activation is accelerated and current augmented. An LQT2 mutation has been described in which the deleterious effect is disruption of 14-3-3 binding (Choe et al., 2006). An A-kinase anchoring protein (AKAP) is likely involved in targeting PKA to HERG in a macromolecular complex, which may intensify current modulation (Li et al., 2008). The Kass group showed S27 in the KCNQ1 N-terminus is phosphorylated by PKA and this causes an increase in current. They also showed that a AKAP Yotiao targets PKA to the channel complex (Marx et al., 2002). These studies demonstrate an important, specific, and tightly controlled form of regulation by the components of the β-adrenergic pathway in relation to the two K^+ channels.

In contrast to the β-adrenergic system, the α-adrenergic system involves phospholipase C, which hydrolyzes the membrane lipid phosphatidyl inositol-4,5-bisphosphate (PIP_2) into the signaling molecules inositol 1,4,5-trisphosphate (IP_3) and the second messenger diacylglycerol (DAG). DAG and calcium go on to activate protein kinase C (PKC) isoforms. An acute decrease in the PIP_2 concentration, which occurs upon α-adrenergic stimulation, reduces HERG currents (Bian et al., 2001). This effect is dependent on consumption of PIP_2 at the membrane and direct binding of PIP_2 to HERG but occurs independently of calcium signaling or PKC activity (Bian et al., 2004; Bian & McDonald, 2007)). PKC regulation of HERG remains an active area of investigation where conclusive results await (Thomas, 2003) (Cockerill et al., 2007). For KCNQ1/KCNE1 and I_{Ks}, Varnum et al. showed that PKC stimulation decreased in I_{Ks} due to KCNE1 phosphorylation at serine-102 (Varnum et al., 1993). The mechanism of this I_{Ks} downregulation remained unclear until the Abbott group showed that PKC downregulates I_{Ks} current through inducing endocytosis (Kanda et al., 2011). Another group studied the regulation of I_{Ks} by PIP_2 and showed that application of PIP_2 delayed rundown of I_{Ks} in excised patch recordings (Loussouarn et al., 2003).

7.4 Correlation of mutational mechanisms with clinical phenotype and the approach to genetic testing results

Different channel mutations cause a range of clinical phenotypes, from very mild (asymptomatic) to severe (sudden cardiac death at a young age). Though some generalizations can be made correlating the mechanism by which a mutation acts and severity of clinical phenotype, the task is made difficult by the extensive list of implicated residues and their broad distribution across each gene. As one may expect, mutations to channel pore loops are generally severe, since they directly impact on channel conductance. A study of 858 LQT2 patients in 2009 revealed that patients with mutation to the pore region of HERG (S5 - pore loop - S6) had significantly higher rates of cardiac events than patients with mutations in the S1 - S4 transmembrane domains or the N- or C-termini, with the difference increasing with increasing age. The study also explored possible differences between types of mutations and found that in the C-terminus, patients with non-missense mutations were at significantly higher risk than those with missense mutations (Shimizu et al., 2009).

It is still difficult, though, to predict what type of cellular defect a certain mutation may case. Mutations that affect trafficking are not clustered in any particular region, and mutations that cause biophysical defects can also affect trafficking. K^+ channel mutations are complicated by the ability to form wild-type/mutant heteromultimeric channels that exhibit different levels of defect depending on the number of mutant subunits. Functional analysis by in vitro expression of mutant channels is the only way to fully assess the cellular phenotype of a mutation. Additional genetic and environmental influences exist such that two patients with the same mutation may differ in clinical presentation. We do not yet know all the different factors that may affect the relative expression of mutant versus wild-type channels in a heterozygous patient, such that the distribution is not a 50/50 mix. One patient may express significantly differing amounts of normal or mutant allele subunits, and therefore have a variable clinical phenotype. For K^+ channels, there is an overlap between the I_{Kr} and I_{Ks} currents in their role during repolarization (known as "repolarization reserve"), so the clinical presentation of a patient may be mild unless the unaffected current is also compromised by environmental factors.

A computational prediction tool called KvSNP for voltage-gated K^+ channel genes to predict the severity of possible disease-causing mutations has been published (Stead et al., 2011). Two recent case studies illustrate the complexity of patient presentation and how prediction databases, although initially valuable, have limitations. Each case involved patients with QT prolongation noted on ECG, yet mild clinical history until presentation with sudden cardiac death in early adulthood. One patient had the LQT1 mutation KCNQ1-S277L, located in the S5 pore helix just proximal to the pore loop, predicted by KvSNP to be a severe mutation. The location suggests a biophysical defect, but thorough analysis revealed a combination of trafficking defect with a partially dominant-negative biophysical effect on heteromultimeric channels that managed to traffic properly to the membrane. The second patient had the LQT2 mutation HERG-G816V, located in the C-terminal region adjacent to a cyclic-nucleotide binding domain important for HERG regulation. This mutation was not predicted to be severe, yet functional analysis showed abnormal trafficking and significantly reduced current. Given the severe cellular defects, one would not predict a generally mild clinical phenotype. Both patients presented with sudden death when they experienced a second exogenous insult such as drug-induced blockade or electrolyte disturbance that reduced their remaining repolarizing current (Chen et al., 2011; Krishnan et al., 2011).

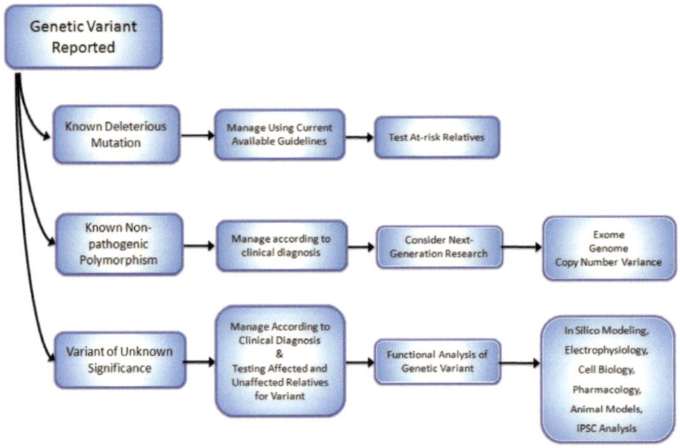

Fig. 2. A general approach to managing families with suspected hereditary arrhythmia syndromes after receiving genetic testing results.

These reports highlight the challenge that clinicians face upon receiving genetic testing results for patients suspected of having a hereditary cause of cardiac arrhythmia. The results from clinical laboratories may be given as clear-cut pathogenic deleterious mutations that have been reported in the literature. Such cases are relatively straightforward and further testing of at-risk family members is indicated with treatment and management dictated by the clinical presentation and recommendations for the documented mutation. Alternatively, the testing result may be read as a known non-pathogenic polymorphism that has been documented in normal populations. In this instance the clinician must guide therapy to the clinical diagnosis and consider whether the patient warrants further investigation such as analysis of copy number variance or various "omics" studies (whole exome or genome sequencing), which presently comprise investigative research studies. The third possibility is that genetic testing results are given as possible deleterious mutation or variants of unknown significance. This is a difficult puzzle for the clinician to solve. An initial step might be to search mutational or polymorphism genetic databases for reports of the given variant, but the commercial laboratories usually perform this task. Another is to submit the reported variant to in silico analysis as described above (KvSNP), but remaining aware of the potential inaccuracies. More desirable is to perform one or more of the several functional analyses outlined above. Although this will entail collaboration with an academic laboratory, it will provide more solid evidence for, or against the variant being deleterious. Figure 2 illustrates a suggested algorithm for the approach of genetic testing results.

7.5 Exploring novel therapeutic modalities

One of the greatest challenges in LQTS is developing new therapeutic modalities aimed at the root cause of the defect instead of managing or preventing arrhythmias. One example is designing methods that correct the trafficking defective phenotype in many LQT2 cases. Work by January and colleagues have sought to use pharmacological methods to rescue trafficking deficient HERG mutants (Gong, 2006). In some LQT2 mutations trafficking can be partially rescued in heterologous systems by lower temperature, glycerol or DMSO, which act as non-specific chaperones. HERG channel blocking drugs E-4031, astemizole and cisapride have also been shown to rescue some mutant-related trafficking defects, but functionality was abolished since the channel pore was blocked. As is the case for many in-vitro studies, the results are hard to translate into clinical therapies at present. Similar therapeutic models are in development for cystic fibrosis and rescue of CFTR trafficking mutants, but the same difficulties prevail (Becq et al., 2011). The ideal goal is to achieve a trafficking rescue without pore blockage. Encouraging results have been reported by Rajamani et al. who showed that the antihistamine fexofenadine was able to rescue some trafficking-deficient HERG mutants without channel block (Rajamani et al., 2002).

Other efforts have utilized functional screens to discover small molecules that would suppress the long-QT phenotype irrespective of mechanism. An interesting approach has been reported using the *breakdance* (see section 4.3) mutant to screen for molecules that would rescue the phenotype (Peal et al., 2010). The investigators isolated 2 compounds that shortened the APD. The mechanisms by which these drugs work remain unclear as does the application of these drugs to mammals or later to humans. Nevertheless, this provides a good starting point and shows the utility of zebrafish as a genetic model in a high-throughput screen.

8. Conclusion

Modern medical genetics has advanced the diagnosis and treatment of hereditary arrhythmia syndromes greatly in the past 15 years. Future advances will include recognition of modifying genetic and environmental factors that influence penetrance and severity. There is also hope for novel gene- and mutation-specific therapies. An achievable goal in the sort-term will be clear delineation of genetic mutations and variants that presently reported to clinicians that patients and families with possible hereditary arrhythmias.

9. Acknowledgment

Authors YK and JC contributed equally. The authors are supported by grants from the NIH (1F30HL096279 to YK; 1F30HL096296 to JC; and HL093440 and 1RC1HL100756 to TVM).

10. References

Abbott, G. W., Sesti, F., Splawski, I., Buck, M. E., Lehmann, M. H., Timothy, K. W., Keating, M. T. & Goldstein, S. A. (1999). MiRP1 forms IKr potassium channels with HERG and is associated with cardiac arrhythmia. *Cell* 97(2): 175-187.

Anderson, C. L., Delisle, B. P., Anson, B. D., Kilby, J. A., Will, M. L., Tester, D. J., Gong, Q., Zhou, Z., Ackerman, M. J. & January, C. T. (2006). Most LQT2 mutations reduce Kv11.1 (hERG) current by a class 2 (trafficking-deficient) mechanism. *Circulation* 113(3): 365-373.

Arnaout, R., Ferrer, T., Huisken, J., Spitzer, K., Stainier, D. Y., Tristani-Firouzi, M. & Chi, N. C. (2007). Zebrafish model for human long QT syndrome. *Proc Natl Acad Sci U S A* 104(27): 11316-11321.

Ashman, R. (1942). The normal duration of the QT intercal. *Am Heart J* 23: 522.

Babij, P., Askew, G. R., Nieuwenhuijsen, B., Su, C. M., Bridal, T. R., Jow, B., Argentieri, T. M., Kulik, J., DeGennaro, L. J., Spinelli, W. & Colatsky, T. J. (1998). Inhibition of cardiac delayed rectifier K+ current by overexpression of the long-QT syndrome HERG G628S mutation in transgenic mice. *Circ Res* 83(6): 668-678.

Balijepalli, S. Y., Anderson, C. L., Lin, E. C. & January, C. T. (2010). Rescue of mutated cardiac ion channels in inherited arrhythmia syndromes. *J Cardiovasc Pharmacol* 56(2): 113-122.

Barnard, E. A., Miledi, R. & Sumikawa, K. (1982). Translation of exogenous messenger RNA coding for nicotinic acetylcholine receptors produces functional receptors in Xenopus oocytes. *Proc R Soc Lond B Biol Sci* 215(1199): 241-246.

Bazett, H. C. (1920). The time relations of the blood-pressure changes after excision of the adrenal glands, with some observations on blood volume changes. *J Physiol* 53(5): 320-339.

Becq, F., Mall, M. A., Sheppard, D. N., Conese, M. & Zegarra-Moran, O. (2011). Pharmacological therapy for cystic fibrosis: from bench to bedside. *J Cyst Fibros* 10 Suppl 2: S129-145.

Benhorin, J., Kalman, Y. M., Medina, A., Towbin, J., Rave-Harel, N., Dyer, T. D., Blangero, J., MacCluer, J. W. & Kerem, B. S. (1993). Evidence of genetic heterogeneity in the long QT syndrome. *Science* 260(5116): 1960-1962.

Berthet, M., Denjoy, I., Donger, C., Demay, L., Hammoude, H., Klug, D., Schulze-Bahr, E., Richard, P., Funke, H., Schwartz, K., Coumel, P., Hainque, B. & Guicheney, P. (1999). C-terminal HERG mutations: the role of hypokalemia and a KCNQ1-associated mutation in cardiac event occurrence. *Circulation* 99(11): 1464-1470.

Bhuiyan, Z. A., Momenah, T. S., Gong, Q., Amin, A. S., Ghamdi, S. A., Carvalho, J. S., Homfray, T., Mannens, M. M., Zhou, Z. & Wilde, A. A. (2008). Recurrent intrauterine fetal loss due to near absence of HERG: clinical and functional characterization of a homozygous nonsense HERG Q1070X mutation. *Heart Rhythm* 5(4): 553-561.

Bian, J., Cui, J. & McDonald, T. V. (2001). HERG K(+) channel activity is regulated by changes in phosphatidyl inositol 4,5-bisphosphate. *Circ Res* 89(12): 1168-1176.

Bian, J. S., Kagan, A. & McDonald, T. V. (2004). Molecular analysis of PIP2 regulation of HERG and IKr. *Am J Physiol Heart Circ Physiol* 287(5): H2154-2163.

Bian, J. S. & McDonald, T. V. (2007). Phosphatidylinositol 4,5-bisphosphate interactions with the HERG K(+) channel. *Pflugers Arch* 455(1): 105-113.

Brunner, M., Peng, X., Liu, G. X., Ren, X. Q., Ziv, O., Choi, B. R., Mathur, R., Hajjiri, M., Odening, K. E., Steinberg, E., Folco, E. J., Pringa, E., Centracchio, J., Macharzina, R. R., Donahay, T., Schofield, L., Rana, N., Kirk, M., Mitchell, G. F., Poppas, A., Zehender, M. & Koren, G. (2008). Mechanisms of cardiac arrhythmias and sudden death in transgenic rabbits with long QT syndrome. *J Clin Invest* 118(6): 2246-2259.

Casimiro, M. C., Knollmann, B. C., Ebert, S. N., Vary, J. C., Jr., Greene, A. E., Franz, M. R., Grinberg, A., Huang, S. P. & Pfeifer, K. (2001). Targeted disruption of the Kcnq1 gene produces a mouse model of Jervell and Lange-Nielsen Syndrome. *Proc Natl Acad Sci U S A* 98(5): 2526-2531.

Charpentier, F., Merot, J., Riochet, D., Le Marec, H. & Escande, D. (1998). Adult KCNE1-knockout mice exhibit a mild cardiac cellular phenotype. *Biochem Biophys Res Commun* 251(3): 806-810.

Chen, J., Sroubek, J., Krishnan, Y., Li, Y., Bian, J. & McDonald, T. V. (2009). PKA phosphorylation of HERG protein regulates the rate of channel synthesis. *Am J Physiol Heart Circ Physiol* 296(5): H1244-1254.

Chen, J., Chen, K., Sroubek, J., Wu, Z. Y., Thomas, D., Bian, J. S. & McDonald, T. V. (2010). Post-transcriptional control of human ether-a-go-go-related gene potassium channel protein by alpha-adrenergic receptor stimulation. *Mol Pharmacol* 78(2): 186-197.

Chen, J., Weber, M., Um, S. Y., Walsh, C. A., Tang, Y. & McDonald, T. V. (2011). A Dual Mechanism for IKs Current Reduction bu the Pathogenic Mutation KCNQ1-S277L. *Pacing Clin Electrophysiol* In Press.

Cheng, S. H., Gregory, R. J., Marshall, J., Paul, S., Souza, D. W., White, G. A., O'Riordan, C. R. & Smith, A. E. (1990). Defective intracellular transport and processing of CFTR is the molecular basis of most Cystic Fibrosis. *Cell* 63: 827-834.

Chevillard, C., Attali, B., Lesage, F., Fontes, M., Barhanin, J., Lazdunski, M. & Mattei, M. G. (1993). Localization of a Potassium Channel Gene (KCNE1) to 21q22.1-q22.2 by in Situ Hybridization and Somatic Cell Hybridization. *Genomics* 15: 243-245.

Chlopcikova, S., Psotova, J. & Miketova, P. (2001). Neonatal rat cardiomyocytes--a model for the study of morphological, biochemical and electrophysiological characteristics of the heart. *Biomed Pap Med Fac Univ Palacky Olomouc Czech Repub* 145(2): 49-55.

Choe, C. U., Schulze-Bahr, E., Neu, A., Xu, J., Zhu, Z. I., Sauter, K., Bahring, R., Priori, S., Guicheney, P., Monnig, G., Neapolitano, C., Heidemann, J., Clancy, C. E., Pongs, O. & Isbrandt, D. (2006). C-terminal HERG (LQT2) mutations disrupt IKr channel regulation through 14-3-3epsilon. *Hum Mol Genet* 15(19): 2888-2902.

Cockerill, S. L., Tobin, A. B., Torrecilla, I., Willars, G. B., Standen, N. B. & Mitcheson, J. S. (2007). Modulation of hERG potassium currents in HEK-293 cells by protein kinase C. Evidence for direct phosphorylation of pore forming subunits. *J Physiol* 581(Pt 2): 479-493.

Compton, S. J., Lux, R. L., Ramsey, M. R., Strelich, K. R., Sanguinetti, M. C., Green, L. S., Keating, M. T. & Mason, J. W. (1996). Genetically defined therapy of inherited long-QT syndrome. Correction of abnormal repolarization by potassium. *Circulation* 94(5): 1018-1022.

Crotti, L., Celano, G., Dagradi, F. & Schwartz, P. J. (2008). Congenital long QT syndrome. *Orphanet journal of rare diseases* 3: 18.

Cui, J., Melman, Y., Palma, E., Fishman, G. I. & McDonald, T. V. (2000). Cyclic AMP regulates the HERG K(+) channel by dual pathways. *Curr Biol* 10(11): 671-674.

Curran, M., Splawski, I., Timothy, K., Vincent, G. M., Green, E. D. & Keating, M. T. (1995). A Molecular Basis for Cardiac Arrhythmia: HERG Mutations Cause Long QT Syndrome. *Cell* 80: 795-803.

Delisle, B. P., Underkofler, H. A., Moungey, B. M., Slind, J. K., Kilby, J. A., Best, J. M., Foell, J. D., Balijepalli, R. C., Kamp, T. J. & January, C. T. (2009). Small GTPase determinants for the Golgi processing and plasmalemmal expression of human ether-a-go-go related (hERG) K+ channels. *J Biol Chem* 284(5): 2844-2853.

Demolombe, S., Lande, G., Charpentier, F., van Roon, M. A., van den Hoff, M. J., Toumaniantz, G., Baro, I., Guihard, G., Le Berre, N., Corbier, A., de Bakker, J., Opthof, T., Wilde, A., Moorman, A. F. & Escande, D. (2001). Transgenic mice overexpressing human KvLQT1 dominant-negative isoform. Part I: Phenotypic characterisation. *Cardiovasc Res* 50(2): 314-327.

Denning, G. M., Anderson, M. P., Amara, J. F., Marshall, J., Smith, A. E. & Welsh, M. J. (1992). Processing of mutant cystic fibrosis transmembrane conductance regulator is temerature sensitive. *Nature* 358: 761-764.

Doyle, D. A., Morais Cabral, J., Pfuetzner, R. A., Kuo, A., Gulbis, J. M., Cohen, S. L., Chait, B. T. & MacKinnon, R. (1998). The structure of the potassium channel: molecular basis of K+ conduction and selectivity. *Science* 280(5360): 69-77.

Drici, M. D., Burklow, T. R., Haridasse, V., Glazer, R. I. & Woosley, R. L. (1996). Sex hormones prolong the QT interval and downregulate potassium channel expression in the rabbit heart. *Circulation* 94(6): 1471-1474.

Duggal, P., Vesely, M. R., Wattanasirichaigoon, D., Villafane, J., Kaushik, V. & Beggs, A. H. (1998). Mutation of the Gene for IsK Associated with Both Jervell and Lange-Nielsen and Romano-Ward Forms of Long-QT Syndrome. *Circulation* 97: 142-146.

Etheridge, S. P., Compton, S. J., Tristani-Firouzi, M. & Mason, J. W. (2003). A new oral therapy for long QT syndrome: long-term oral potassium improves repolarization in patients with HERG mutations. *J Am Coll Cardiol* 42(10): 1777-1782.

Fabritz, L., Damke, D., Emmerich, M., Kaufmann, S. G., Theis, K., Blana, A., Fortmuller, L., Laakmann, S., Hermann, S., Aleynichenko, E., Steinfurt, J., Volkery, D., Riemann, B., Kirchhefer, U., Franz, M. R., Breithardt, G., Carmeliet, E., Schafers, M., Maier, S. K., Carmeliet, P. & Kirchhof, P. (2010). Autonomic modulation and antiarrhythmic therapy in a model of long QT syndrome type 3. *Cardiovasc Res* 87(1): 60-72.

Fodstad, H., Swan, H., Auberson, M., Gautschi, I., Loffing, J., Schild, L. & Kontula, K. (2004). Loss-of-function mutations of the K(+) channel gene KCNJ2 constitute a rare cause of long QT syndrome. *J Mol Cell Cardiol* 37(2): 593-602.

Gellens, M. E., George, A. L., Jr., Chen, L. Q., Chahine, M., Horn, R., Barchi, R. L. & Kallen, R. G. (1992). Primary structure and functional expression of the human cardiac tetrodotoxin-insensitive voltage-dependent sodium channel. *Proc Natl Acad Sci U S A* 89(2): 554-558.

Goldenberg, I., Bradley, J., Moss, A., McNitt, S., Polonsky, S., Robinson, J. L., Andrews, M. & Zareba, W. (2010). Beta-blocker efficacy in high-risk patients with the congenital long-QT syndrome types 1 and 2: implications for patient management. *J Cardiovasc Electrophysiol* 21(8): 893-901.

Gong, Q., Keeney, D. R., Molinari, M. & Zhou, Z. (2005). Degradation of trafficking-defective long QT syndrome type II mutant channels by the ubiquitin-proteasome pathway. *J Biol Chem* 280(19): 19419-19425.

Gong, Q., Jones, M.A., Zhou, Z. (2006). Mechanisms of pharmacological rescue of trafficking defective hERG mutant channels in human long QT syndrome. *J Biol Chem* 281(7): 4069-4074.

Guo, J., Massaeli, H., Xu, J., Jia, Z., Wigle, J. T., Mesaeli, N. & Zhang, S. (2009). Extracellular K+ concentration controls cell surface density of IKr in rabbit hearts and of the HERG channel in human cell lines. *J Clin Invest* 119(9): 2745-2757.

Gurdon, J. B., Lane, C. D., Woodland, H. R. & Marbaix, G. (1971). Use of frog eggs and oocytes for the study of messenger RNA and its translation in living cells. *Nature* 233(5316): 177-182.

Henrion, U., Strutz-Seebohm, N., Duszenko, M., Lang, F. & Seebohm, G. (2009). Long QT syndrome-associated mutations in the voltage sensor of I(Ks) channels. *Cell Physiol Biochem* 24(1-2): 11-16.

Hoppe, U. C., Marban, E. & Johns, D. C. (2001). Distinct gene-specific mechanisms of arrhythmia revealed by cardiac gene transfer of two long QT disease genes, HERG and KCNE1. *Proc Natl Acad Sci U S A* 98(9): 5335-5340.

Itzhaki, I., Maizels, L., Huber, I., Zwi-Dantsis, L., Caspi, O., Winterstern, A., Feldman, O., Gepstein, A., Arbel, G., Hammerman, H., Boulos, M. & Gepstein, L. (2011). Modelling the long QT syndrome with induced pluripotent stem cells. *Nature* 471(7337): 225-229.

Jervell, A. & Lange-Nielsen, F. (1957). Congenital deaf-mutism, functional heart disease with prolongation of the Q-T interval and sudden death. *American heart journal* 54(1): 59-68.

Jiang, C., Atkinson, D., Towbin, J. A., Splawski, I., Lehmann, M. H., Li, H., Timothy, K., Taggart, R. T., Schwartz, P. J., Vincent, G. M., Moss, A. J. & Keating, M. T. (1994). Two long QT syndrom loci map to chromosomes 3 and 7 with evidence for further heterogeneity. *Nature Genetics* 8: 141-147.

Jiang, Y., Lee, A., Chen, J., Cadene, M., Chait, B. T. & MacKinnon, R. (2002). The open pore conformation of potassium channels. *Nature* 417(6888): 523-526.

Jiang, Y., Lee, A., Chen, J., Ruta, V., Cadene, M., Chait, B. T. & MacKinnon, R. (2003). X-ray structure of a voltage-dependent K+ channel. *Nature* 423(6935): 33-41.

Jones, D. K. & Ruben, P. C. (2008). Biophysical defects in voltage.gated sodium channels associated with long QT and Brugada syndromes. *Channels (Austin)* 2(2): 70-80.

Jose, A. D. & Collison, D. (1970). The normal range and determinants of the intrinsic heart rate in man. *Cardiovasc Res* 4(2): 160-167.

Kagan, A., Yu, Z., Fishman, G. I. & McDonald, T. V. (2000). The dominant negative LQT2 mutation A561V reduces wild-type HERG expression. *J Biol Chem* 275(15): 11241-11248.

Kagan, A., Melman, Y. F., Krumerman, A. & McDonald, T. V. (2002). 14-3-3 amplifies and prolongs adrenergic stimulation of HERG K+ channel activity. *EMBO J* 21(8): 1889-1898.

Kagan, A. & McDonald, T. V. (2005). Dynamic control of hERG/I(Kr) by PKA-mediated interactions with 14-3-3. *Novartis Found Symp* 266: 75-89; discussion 89-99.

Kanda, V. A., Purtell, K. & Abbott, G. W. (2011). Protein kinase C downregulates I(Ks) by stimulating KCNQ1-KCNE1 potassium channel endocytosis. *Heart Rhythm*.

Keating, M., Atkinson, D., Dunn, C., Timothy, K., Vincent, G. M. & Leppert, M. (1991a). Linkage of a cardiac arrhythmia, the long QT syndrome, and the Harvey ras-1 gene. *Science* 252(5006): 704-706.

Keating, M., Dunn, C., Atkinson, D., Timothy, K., Vincent, G. M. & Leppert, M. (1991b). Consistent linkage of the long-QT syndrome to the Harvey ras-1 locus on chromosome 11. *Am J Hum Genet* 49(6): 1335-1339.

Khositseth, A., Tester, D. J., Will, M. L., Bell, C. M. & Ackerman, M. J. (2004). Identification of a common genetic substrate underlying postpartum cardiac events in congenital long QT syndrome. *Heart Rhythm* 1(1): 60-64.

Kiehn, J. (2000). Regulation of the cardiac repolarizing HERG potassium channel by protein kinase A. *Trends Cardiovasc Med* 10(5): 205-209.

Kim, J. A., Lopes, C. M., Moss, A. J., McNitt, S., Barsheshet, A., Robinson, J. L., Zareba, W., Ackerman, M. J., Kaufman, E. S., Towbin, J. A., Vincent, M. & Goldenberg, I. (2010). Trigger-specific risk factors and response to therapy in long QT syndrome type 2. *Heart Rhythm* 7(12): 1797-1805.

Krishnan, Y., Zheng, R., Walsh, C., Tang, Y. & McDonald, T. V. (2011). Partially dominant mutant channel defect corresponding with intermediate Long-QT2 phenotype. *Pacing Clin Electrophysiol* In Press.

Langheinrich, U., Vacun, G. & Wagner, T. (2003). Zebrafish embryos express an orthologue of HERG and are sensitive toward a range of QT-prolonging drugs inducing severe arrhythmia. *Toxicol Appl Pharmacol* 193(3): 370-382.

Lee, M. P., Ravenel, J. D., Hu, R. J., Lustig, L. R., Tomaselli, G., Berger, R. D., Brandenburg, S. A., Litzi, T. J., Bunton, T. E., Limb, C., Francis, H., Gorelikow, M., Gu, H., Washington, K., Argani, P., Goldenring, J. R., Coffey, R. J. & Feinberg, A. P. (2000). Targeted disruption of the Kvlqt1 gene causes deafness and gastric hyperplasia in mice. *J Clin Invest* 106(12): 1447-1455.

Lehmann, M. H., Timothy, K. W., Frankovich, D., Fromm, B. S., Keating, M., Locati, E. H., Taggart, R. T., Towbin, J. A., Moss, A. J., Schwartz, P. J. & Vincent, G. M. (1997). Age-Gender Influence on the Rate-Corrected QT Interval and the QT-Heart Rate Relation in Families With Gentotypically Characterized Long QT Syndrome. *J Am Coll Cardiol* 29(1): 93-99.

Li, R. A., Miake, J., Hoppe, U. C., Johns, D. C., Marban, E. & Nuss, H. B. (2001). Functional consequences of the arrhythmogenic G306R KvLQT1 K+ channel mutant probed by viral gene transfer in cardiomyocytes. *J Physiol* 533(Pt 1): 127-133.

Li, Y., Sroubek, J., Krishnan, Y. & McDonald, T. V. (2008). A-kinase anchoring protein targeting of protein kinase A and regulation of HERG channels. *J Membr Biol* 223(2): 107-116.

Lin, E. C., Holzem, K. M., Anson, B. D., Moungey, B. M., Balijepalli, S. Y., Tester, D. J., Ackerman, M. J., Delisle, B. P., Balijepalli, R. C. & January, C. T. (2010). Properties of WT and mutant hERG K(+) channels expressed in neonatal mouse cardiomyocytes. *Am J Physiol Heart Circ Physiol* 298(6): H1842-1849.

Locati, E. H., Zareba, W., Moss, A. J., Schwartz, P. J., Vincent, G. M., Lehmann, M. H., Towbin, J. A., Priori, S. G., Napolitano, C., Robinson, J. L., Andrews, M., Timothy, K. & Hall, W. J. (1998). Age- and Sex-Related Differences in Clinical Manifestations in Patients With Congenital Long-QT Syndrome: Findings From the International LQTS Registry. *Circulation* 87: 2237-2244.

London, B. (1998). QT interval prolongation and arrhythmias in heterozygous Merg1-targeted mice. *Circulation (New York, N.Y.)* 98: 279.

Long, S. B., Campbell, E. B. & Mackinnon, R. (2005). Crystal structure of a mammalian voltage-dependent Shaker family K+ channel. *Science* 309(5736): 897-903.

Loussouarn, G., Park, K. H., Bellocq, C., Baro, I., Charpentier, F. & Escande, D. (2003). Phosphatidylinositol-4,5-bisphosphate, PIP2, controls KCNQ1/KCNE1 voltage-gated potassium channels: a functional homology between voltage-gated and inward rectifier K+ channels. *EMBO J* 22(20): 5412-5421.

Marx, S. O., Kurokawa, J., Reiken, S., Motoike, H., D'Armiento, J., Marks, A. & Kass, R. S. (2002). Requirement of a Macromolecular Signaling Complex for beta Adrenergic Receptor Modulation of the KCNQ1-KCNE1 Potassium Channel. *Science* 295: 496-499.

Massaeli, H., Sun, T., Li, X., Shallow, H., Wu, J., Xu, J., Li, W., Hanson, C., Guo, J. & Zhang, S. (2010). Involvement of caveolin in low K+-induced endocytic degradation of cell-surface human ether-a-go-go-related gene (hERG) channels. *J Biol Chem* 285(35): 27259-27264.

Milan, D. J. & MacRae, C. A. (2005). Animal models for arrhythmias. *Cardiovasc Res* 67(3): 426-437.

Mohler, P. J., Splawski, I., Napolitano, C., Bottelli, G., Sharpe, L., Timothy, K., Priori, S. G., Keating, M. T. & Bennett, V. (2004). A cardiac arrhythmia syndrome caused by loss of ankyrin-B function. *Proc Natl Acad Sci U S A* 101(24): 9137-9142.

Moretti, A., Bellin, M., Welling, A., Jung, C. B., Lam, J. T., Bott-Flugel, L., Dorn, T., Goedel, A., Hohnke, C., Hofmann, F., Seyfarth, M., Sinnecker, D., Schomig, A. & Laugwitz, K. L. (2010). Patient-specific induced pluripotent stem-cell models for long-QT syndrome. *N Engl J Med* 363(15): 1397-1409.

Nakajima, T., Kaneko, Y., Manita, M., Iso, T. & Kurabayashi, M. (2010). Aborted Cardiac Arrest in a Patient Carrying KCNE1 D85N Variant during the Postpartum Period. *Internal Medicine* 49(17): 1875-1878.

Nerbonne, J. M. (2004). Studying cardiac arrhythmias in the mouse--a reasonable model for probing mechanisms? *Trends Cardiovasc Med* 14(3): 83-93.

Nuss, H. B. & Marban, E. (1994). Electrophysiological properties of neonatal mouse cardiac myocytes in primary culture. *J Physiol* 479 (Pt 2): 265-279.

Nuyens, D., Stengl, M., Dugarmaa, S., Rossenbacker, T., Compernolle, V., Rudy, Y., Smits, J. F., Flameng, W., Clancy, C. E., Moons, L., Vos, M. A., Dewerchin, M., Benndorf, K., Collen, D., Carmeliet, E. & Carmeliet, P. (2001). Abrupt rate accelerations or premature beats cause life-threatening arrhythmias in mice with long-QT3 syndrome. *Nat Med* 7(9): 1021-1027.

Peal, D. S., Peterson, R. T. & Milan, D. (2010). Small molecule screening in zebrafish. *J Cardiovasc Transl Res* 3(5): 454-460.

Priori, S. G., Schwartz, P. J., Napolitano, C., Bloise, R., Ronchetti, E., Grillo, M., Vicentini, A., Spazzolini, C., Nastoli, J., Bottelli, G., Folli, R. & Cappelletti, D. (2003). Risk stratification in the long-QT syndrome. *N Engl J Med* 348(19): 1866-1874.

Priori, S. G., Napolitano, C., Schwartz, P. J., Grillo, M., Bloise, R., Ronchetti, E., Moncalvo, C., Tulipani, C., Veia, A., Bottelli, G. & Nastoli, J. (2004). Association of long QT syndrome loci and cardiac events among patients treated with beta-blockers. *JAMA* 292(11): 1341-1344.

Rajamani, S., Anderson, C. L., Anson, B. D. & January, C. T. (2002). Pharmacological rescue of human K(+) channel long-QT2 mutations: human ether-a-go-go-related gene rescue without block. *Circulation* 105(24): 2830-2835.

Rasmussen, H. B., Moller, M., Knaus, H. G., Jensen, B. S., Olesen, S. P. & Jorgensen, N. K. (2004). Subcellular localization of the delayed rectifier K(+) channels KCNQ1 and ERG1 in the rat heart. *Am J Physiol Heart Circ Physiol* 286(4): H1300-1309.

Reinoehl, J., Frankovich, D., Machado, C., Kawasaki, R., Baga, J. J., Pires, L. A., Steinman, R. T., Fromm, B. S. & Lehmann, M. H. (1996). Probucol-associated tachyarrhythmic events and QT prolongation: importance of gender. *Am Heart J* 131(6): 1184-1191.

Romano, C., Gemme, G. & Pongiglione, R. (1963). [Rare Cardiac Arrythmias of the Pediatric Age. Ii. Syncopal Attacks Due to Paroxysmal Ventricular Fibrillation. (Presentation of 1st Case in Italian Pediatric Literature)]. *La Clinica pediatrica* 45: 656-683.

Rosero, S. Z., Zareba, W., Robinson, J. L. & Moss, A. J. (1997). Gene-Specific Therapy for Long-QT Syndrome. *Annals of Noninvasive Electrocardiology* 2(3): 274-278.

Sanguinetti, M. C. & Jurkiewicz, N. K. (1992). Role of external Ca2+ and K+ in gating of cardiac delayed rectifier K+ currents. *Pflugers Arch* 420(2): 180-186.

Sanguinetti, M. C. a. J., N.K. (1990). Two Components of Cardiac Delayed Rectifier K+ current *J Gen Physiol*.

Scholz, E. P., Niemer, N., Hassel, D., Zitron, E., Bürgers, H. F., Bloehs, R., Seyler, C., Scherer, D., Thomas, D., Kathöfer, S., Katus, H. A., Rottbauer, W. A. & Karle, C. A. (2009). Biophysical properties of zebrafish ether-à-go-go related gene potassium channels. *Biochemical and Biophysical Research Communications* 381(2): 159-164.

Schott, J., Charpentier, F., Peltier, S., Foley, P., Droulin, E., Bouhour, J., Donnelly, P., Vergnaud, G., Bachner, L., Moisan, J., Le Marec, H. & Pascal, O. (1995). Mapping of a Gene for Long QT Syndrome to Chromosome 4q25-27. *Am J Hum Genet* 57: 1114-1122.

Schulze-Bahr, E., Wang, Q., Wedekind, H., Haverkamp, W., Chen, Q., Sun, Y., Rubie, C., Hordt, M., Towbin, J. A., Borggrefe, M., Assmann, G., Qu, X., Somberg, J. C., Breithardt, G., Oberti, C. & Funke, H. (1997). KCNE1 mutations cause jervell and Lange-Nielsen syndrome. *Nat Genet* 17(3): 267-268.

Schwartz, P. J., Priori, S. G., Spazzolini, C., Moss, A. J., Vincent, G. M., Napolitano, C., Denjoy, I., Guicheney, P., Breithardt, G., Keating, M. T., Towbin, J. A., Beggs, A. H., Brink, P., Wilde, A. A., Toivonen, L., Zareba, W., Robinson, J. L., Timothy, K. W., Corfield, V., Wattanasirichaigoon, D., Corbett, C., Haverkamp, W., Schulze-Bahr, E., Lehmann, M. H., Schwartz, K., Coumel, P. & Bloise, R. (2001). Genotype-phenotype correlation in the long-QT syndrome: gene-specific triggers for life-threatening arrhythmias. *Circulation* 103(1): 89-95.

Schwartz, P. J., Priori, S. G., Cerrone, M., Spazzolini, C., Odero, A., Napolitano, C., Bloise, R., De Ferrari, G. M., Klersy, C., Moss, A. J., Zareba, W., Robinson, J. L., Hall, W. J., Brink, P. A., Toivonen, L., Epstein, A. E., Li, C. & Hu, D. (2004). Left cardiac sympathetic denervation in the management of high-risk patients affected by the long-QT syndrome. *Circulation* 109(15): 1826-1833.

Seth, R., Moss, A. J., McNitt, S., Zareba, W., Andrews, M. L., Qi, M., Robinson, J. L., Goldenberg, I., Ackerman, M. J., Benhorin, J., Kaufman, E. S., Locati, E. H., Napolitano, C., Priori, S. G., Schwartz, P. J., Towbin, J. A., Vincent, G. M. & Zhang, L. (2007). Long QT syndrome and pregnancy. *J Am Coll Cardiol* 49(10): 1092-1098.

Shimizu, W. & Antzelevitch, C. (2000). Effects of a K(+) channel opener to reduce transmural dispersion of repolarization and prevent torsade de pointes in LQT1, LQT2, and LQT3 models of the long-QT syndrome. *Circulation* 102(6): 706-712.

Shimizu, W., Moss, A. J., Wilde, A. A., Towbin, J. A., Ackerman, M. J., January, C. T., Tester, D. J., Zareba, W., Robinson, J. L., Qi, M., Vincent, G. M., Kaufman, E. S., Hofman, N., Noda, T., Kamakura, S., Miyamoto, Y., Shah, S., Amin, V., Goldenberg, I., Andrews, M. L. & McNitt, S. (2009). Genotype-phenotype aspects of type 2 long QT syndrome. *J Am Coll Cardiol* 54(22): 2052-2062.

Smith, J. L., McBride, C. M., Nataraj, P. S., Bartos, D. C., January, C. T. & Delisle, B. P. (2011). Trafficking-deficient hERG K channels linked to long QT syndrome are regulated by a microtubule-dependent quality control compartment in the ER. *Am J Physiol Cell Physiol* 301(1): C75-85.

Sroubek, J. & McDonald, T. V. (2011). Protein kinase A activity at the endoplasmic reticulum surface is responsible for augmentation of human ether-a-go-go-related gene product (HERG). *J Biol Chem* 286(24): 21927-21936.

Stead, L. F., Wood, I. C. & Westhead, D. R. (2011). KvSNP: accurately predicting the effect of genetic variants in voltage-gated potassium channels. *Bioinformatics* 27(16): 2181-2186.

Takenaka, K., Ai, T., Shimizu, W., Kobori, A., Ninomiya, T., Otani, H., Kubota, T., Takaki, H., Kamakura, S. & Horie, M. (2003). Exercise stress test amplifies genotype-phenotype correlation in the LQT1 and LQT2 forms of the long-QT syndrome. *Circulation* 107(6): 838-844.

Teng, S., Gao, L., Paajanen, V., Pu, J. & Fan, Z. (2009). Readthrough of nonsense mutation W822X in the SCN5A gene can effectively restore expression of cardiac Na+ channels. *Cardiovasc Res* 83(3): 473-480.

Thomas, D. (2003). Regulation of HERG potassium channel activation by protein kinase C independent of direct phosphorylation of the channel protein. *Cardiovascular Research* 59(1): 14-26.

Ueda, K., Valdivia, C., Medeiros-Domingo, A., Tester, D. J., Vatta, M., Farrugia, G., Ackerman, M. J. & Makielski, J. C. (2008). Syntrophin mutation associated with long QT syndrome through activation of the nNOS-SCN5A macromolecular complex. *Proc Natl Acad Sci U S A* 105(27): 9355-9360.

Varnum, M. D., Busch, A. E., Bond, C. T., Maylie, J. & Adelman, J. P. (1993). The min K channel underlies the cardiac potassium current IKs and mediates species-specific responses to protein kinase C. *Proc Natl Acad Sci U S A* 90(24): 11528-11532.

Vatta, M., Ackerman, M. J., Ye, B., Makielski, J. C., Ughanze, E. E., Taylor, E. W., Tester, D. J., Balijepalli, R. C., Foell, J. D., Li, Z., Kamp, T. J. & Towbin, J. A. (2006). Mutant caveolin-3 induces persistent late sodium current and is associated with long-QT syndrome. *Circulation* 114(20): 2104-2112.

Wang, L., Dennis, A. T., Trieu, P., Charron, F., Ethier, N., Hebert, T. E., Wan, X. & Ficker, E. (2009). Intracellular potassium stabilizes human ether-a-go-go-related gene channels for export from endoplasmic reticulum. *Mol Pharmacol* 75(4): 927-937.

Wang, Q., Shen, J., Li, Z., Timothy, K., Vincent, G. M., Priori, S. G., Schwartz, P. J. & Keating, M. T. (1995a). Cardiac sodium channel mutations in patients with long QT syndrome, an inherited cardiac arrhythmia. *Hum Mol Genet* 4(9): 1603-1607.

Wang, Q., Shen, J., Splawski, I., Atkinson, D., Li, Z., Robinson, J. L., Moss, A. J., Towbin, J. A. & Keating, M. T. (1995b). SCN5A Mutations Associated with an Inherited Cardiac Arrhythmia, Long QT Syndrome. *Cell* 80: 805-811.

Wang, Q., Curran, M. E., Splawski, I., Burn, T. C., Millholland, J. M., VanRaay, T. J., Shen, J., Timothy, K. W., Vincent, G. M. & de Jager, T. (1996). Positional cloning of a novel potassium channel gene: KvLQT1 mutations cause cardiac arrhythmias. *Nature Genetics* 12: 17-23.

Ward, O. C. (1964). A New Familial Cardiac Syndrome in Children. *Journal of the Irish Medical Association* 54: 103-106.

Warmke, J. W. & Ganetzky, B. (1994). A family of potassium channel genes related to eag in Drosophila and mammals. *Proc Natl Acad Sci U S A* 91(8): 3438-3442.

Warth, R. & Barhanin, J. (2002). The multifaceted phenotype of the knockout mouse for the KCNE1 potassium channel gene. *Am J Physiol Regul Integr Comp Physiol* 282(3): R639-648.

Woosley, R. L. & Sale, M. (1993). QT interval: a measure of drug action. *Am J Cardiol* 72(6): 36B-43B.

Worley, K. C., Towbin, J. A., Zhu, X. M., Barker, D. F., Ballabio, A., Chamberlain, J., Biesecker, L. G., Blethen, S. L., Brosnan, P., Fox, J. E. & et al. (1992). Identification of new markers in Xp21 between DXS28 (C7) and DMD. *Genomics* 13(4): 957-961.

Wu, D. M., Jiang, M., Zhang, M., Liu, X. S., Korolkova, Y. V. & Tseng, G. N. (2006). KCNE2 is colocalized with KCNQ1 and KCNE1 in cardiac myocytes and may function as a negative modulator of I(Ks) current amplitude in the heart. *Heart Rhythm* 3(12): 1469-1480.

Yazawa, M., Hsueh, B., Jia, X., Pasca, A. M., Bernstein, J. A., Hallmayer, J. & Dolmetsch, R. E. (2011). Using induced pluripotent stem cells to investigate cardiac phenotypes in Timothy syndrome. *Nature* 471(7337): 230-234.

Zareba, W., Moss, A. J., le Cessie, S., Locati, E. H., Robinson, J. L., Hall, W. J. & Andrews, M. L. (1995). Risk of cardiac events in family members of patients with long QT syndrome. *J Am Coll Cardiol* 26(7): 1685-1691.

Zarraga, I. G., Zhang, L., Stump, M. R., Gong, Q., Vincent, G. M. & Zhou, Z. (2011). Nonsense-mediated mRNA decay caused by a frameshift mutation in a large kindred of type 2 long QT syndrome. *Heart Rhythm* 8(8): 1200-1206.

Zhang, J., Wilson, G. F., Soerens, A. G., Koonce, C. H., Yu, J., Palecek, S. P., Thomson, J. A. & Kamp, T. J. (2009). Functional cardiomyocytes derived from human induced pluripotent stem cells. *Circ Res* 104(4): e30-41.

Part 2

The Cardiac Ion Channels

3

The Cardiac Ion Channels

Thomas Jespersen
Danish Arrhythmia Research Centre
Department of Biomedical Sciences
University of Copenhagen
Denmark

1. Introduction

Action potentials are mediated by transient changes in ion conductance across the cell surface membrane. These changes in conductance are primarily mediated by ion channels. Ion channels are membrane-embedded proteins that selectively pass specific ions upon opening. Some ion channels are constitutively open; however, most channels open following stimulation, such as through voltage changes, intracellular messengers, neurotransmitters, or shear stress. In the heart, voltage gated ion channels, conducting sodium, calcium and potassium ions, are primarily important in generating and shaping the action potential as well as exchangers and pumps that contribute to ion fluxes.

The most prominent features of the cardiac action potential is the synchronised depolarisation of all the cardiomyocytes and the very long lasting depolarisation period, which in humans lasts 200-450 ms, depending on the beating frequency. The electrical impulse is generated in the pacemaker cells in the sinoatrial node located at the junction of the superior vena cava and right atrium. The electrical signal spreads to the right and left atria, thereby initiating muscular contraction and resulting in additional filling of the ventricles. When the depolarisation reaches the atrioventricular node, conduction is slowed before the depolarisation progresses to the ventricular cardiomyocytes. The electrical impulse is spread to the ventricles through a specialised conduction system formed by the His bundle branches and the Purkinje fibres, resulting in the depolarisation of the ventricular cardiomyocytes within a relatively short time span. The very long cardiac action potential mediates a long lasting increase in cytosolic calcium and, thereby, a long lasting contraction. Furthermore, the long action potential duration makes the myocardium refractory, whereby under normal physiological conditions no new action potentials will disturb the ongoing contraction. After the depolarisation phase and the plateau phase, the myocardium repolarises such that the contraction cesses and the ventricular chambers can be refilled. Disturbances in this highly fine-tuned electrical-contraction pattern - termed arrhythmia - can be detrimental since unorganised electrical impulse propagation in the musculature will lead to uncoordinated muscle contraction and therefore a loss of pumping function (Jespersen, 2011).

The cardiac action potential is the summarised output of several different types of ion channels. The functional significance of the different ion channels depends on both the subcardial location and the biophysical configuration of the channels, as well as the physiological demands to be fulfilled. This is illustrated by the fact that the action potential morphology differs whether it is recorded in nodal tissue, in atria or else in either the subendocardial or subepicardial myocytes in the ventricle.

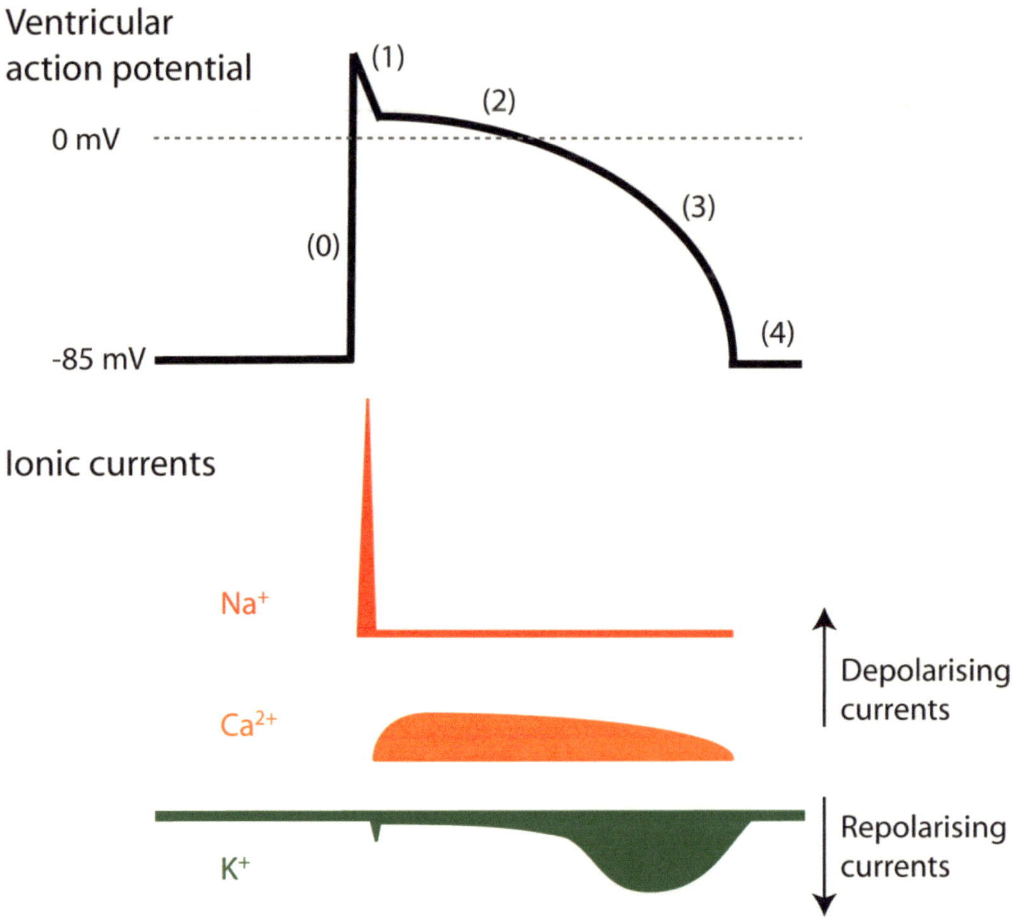

Fig. 1. Ionic currents shape the cardiac action potential. Illustration of a ventricular action potential and the underlying currents.

Ion channels consist of a central protein, named the α-subunit, where ions pass through a pore. Cardiac sodium and calcium channel α-subunits are composed of a single protein constituting a functional channel, while the potassium channels are tetrameric complexes of either homomeric or heteromeric composition. The pore contains a selectivity filter which ensures, for most channels, a high selectivity of one ion over the others (Hille, 2001). The opening, closing and inactivation of the channels are managed in a number of different ways. The voltage-gated channels contain a voltage sensor - primarily located in transmembrane segment 4 - which detects voltage changes, thereby initiating a conformational change in the protein leading to the opening and closing of the channel (Gouaux & Mackinnon, 2005). The inactivation of channel conductance - which is important for the physiological functions of a number of the cardiac channels - can be induced either by fast intramolecular changes or by slower extramolecular regulation, such as through the binding of calcium ions to calmodulin, which interacts with the channel. A number of different classes of proteins interact with the cardiac ion channels. Closely associated proteins which are believed to be specific to the ion channels are termed β-subunits. β-subunits can regulate both surface expression and opening and inactivation kinetics (Isom *et al.*, 1992). Many of these β-subunits have been suggested as being promiscuous since they can interact with several different α-subunits (Panaghie & Abbott, 2006). In addition to the β-subunits, a growing number of regulatory and scaffolding proteins have been found to interact with the different cardiac ion channel complexes.

This chapter will provide an overview of the major cardiac currents, the protein complexes constituting the ion channels and the regulatory mechanisms of these channels which are of crucial importance for controlling the progression, synchronisation and rhythmicity of the cardiac action potentials.

1.1 Impulse generation

The sinoatrial node, the atrioventricular node and the purkinje fibres all show spontaneous beating activity, but because the sinoatrial node normally has the highest frequency this is considered the primary pacemaker of the heart. The automaticity of the sinoatrial node is thus the basis for the rhythm and rate of the heart. The nodal action potential is initiated by a slow increase in depolarisation - driven by a sodium influx - followed by a faster depolarisation due to a calcium influx and terminated by a potassium ion efflux (reviewed by Mangoni & Nargeot, 2008a).

One of the important ion currents participating in generating the spontaneous impulse is the hyperpolarisation activated current I_f (f for 'funny'), which is conducted through the hyperpolarisation-activated cyclic nucleotide-gated channels (HCN) of which four members are known (HCN1-4). HCN4 is the primary expressed pacemaker channel, but HCN1 and HCN2 are also present in the sinoatrial node (Marionneau *et al.*, 2005; Moosmang *et al.*, 1999; Moroni *et al.*, 2001; Shi *et al.*, 1999; Sizarov *et al.*, 2011). HCN channels are permeable to both sodium and potassium (Xue *et al.*, 2002). However, as the channels deactivate at depolarising potentials, the predominant conductance is an inward sodium current. These channels are activated by cyclic nucleotides and hyperpolarisation potentials negative to ~-55 mV (Gauss *et al.*, 1998; Ludwig *et al.*, 1998; Santoro *et al.*, 1998). The one transmembrane spanning β-subunit, KCNE2 (MiRP1), has been reported to increase the surface expression and accelerate the kinetics of the HCN channels and has, therefore, been proposed as playing a role in generating the pacemaker signal (Macri *et al.*, 2002; Qu *et al.*, 2004; Yu *et al.*, 2001).

In the sinoatrial and atrioventricular nodes, the activation of the HCN channels leads to a gradual depolarisation. This depolarisation is counteracted by an acetylcholine-activated potassium current ($I_{K,Ach}$) conducted through the G-protein coupled inward rectifier (GIRK) (Noma & Trautwein, 1978). The cardiac $I_{K,Ach}$ channels are heteromeric complexes consisting of Kir3.1 (GIRK1) and Kir3.4 (GIRK4) subunits (Wickman *et al.*, 1999). The Kir3 channels are activated by various heptahelical receptors coupled to G proteins of the pertussis toxin class (G_i/G_o). Upon receptor activation, the heterotrimeric G protein complex is dissociated in its α and ßγ subunits, where the latter interacts with Kir3 subunits inducing an increased open probability of the channel complex (Logothetis *et al.*, 1987). The activation of cardiac GIRK

channels by acetylcholine, adenosine and ATP mediates a negative chronotropic effect (Friel & Bean, 1990; Kurachi *et al.*, 1986a; Kurachi *et al.*, 1986b; Medina *et al.*, 2000; Ravens & Dobrev, 2003). Vagal stimulation activates cardiac muscarinic M2 receptors whereby $I_{K,Ach}$ increases. This results in a slowing of the depolarising phase of the sinoatrial action potential and thereby provides a reduced action potential frequency. In contrast, the sympathetic stimulation of β-adrenergic receptors in the sinoatrial node mediates a positive chronotropic effect by increasing the cAMP levels, which reduces the GIRK-mediated current and - at the same time - increases the activity of the HCN and Ca^{2+} channels (see below), whereby the diastolic depolarisation phase is shortened and the spike frequency is increased (Baruscotti *et al.*, 2005; Bucchi *et al.*, 2003; DiFrancesco & Tromba, 1988; DiFrancesco, 1993; Noma *et al.*, 1980; Zaza *et al.*, 1996). Although HCN and GIRK channel regulation is considered central to setting the firing frequency of the sinoatrial node, other ion channels, including the ryanodine receptors (calcium-activated calcium channels located in the sarcoplasmic reticulum), I_{ST} channels with unknown molecular correlates and voltage-gated sodium channels (probably of the neuronal type) have also been found to play a role (Lakatta & DiFrancesco, 2009; Mangoni & Nargeot, 2008b).
The increasing depolarisation triggers the activation of T-type and L-type calcium channels (Fermini & Nathan, 1991; Hagiwara *et al.*, 1988; Vuill & Hancox, 2002), whereby an action potential is generated. The repolarisation of the nodal cells is controlled by voltage-gated potassium channels. Both the rapid and slow inward rectifying current (I_{Kr} and I_{Ks}) as well as the transient outward current (I_{To}) are present, but further investigation is necessary to establish the relative and spatial importance of these currents (Mangoni & Nargeot, 2008b). As both the calcium and potassium currents play prominent roles in shaping the atrial and ventricular action potentials, they will be described below.

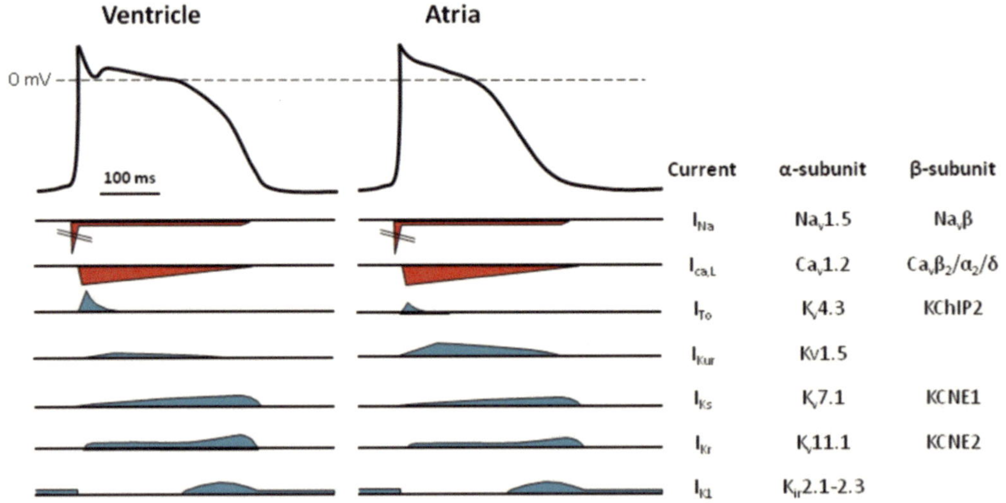

Fig. 2. The major ion channels responsible for the ventricular and atrial action potentials. An illustration of the different depolarising (red) and repolarising (blue) currents underlying the action potential in the ventricle and the atria. The current names, together with the major proteins constituting the channels conducting these currents, are listed to the right.

1.2 The atrial and ventricular action potentials

The majority of the ion channels responsible for determining the action potential in atrial and ventricular myocytes are the same (Nerbonne & Kass, 2005). However, the relative expression level and means of being regulated differ for several of them (Gaborit *et al.*, 2007). The action potential can be divided into 5 phases (Fig. 1). Propagation and the rapid depolarisation (phase 0) of the cardiac action potential is mediated by a voltage-gated sodium current. $Na_v1.5$ is the predominant α-subunit responsible for conducting the sodium current, but recently several reports have suggested other channels within the same voltage-gated sodium channel family to be important. The fast activation of the sodium channels drives the membrane potential towards the equilibrium potential of sodium - which is quite positive - depolarising the membrane. Partial repolarisation (phase 1), after a few milliseconds, happens due to inactivation of the sodium channels together with the somewhat slower activation of L-type calcium channels (Striessnig, 1999). The depolarising sodium and calcium currents are countered by a repolarising potassium flux. In the ventricular subepicardium, the transient outward potassium current (I_{To}) - conducted through a multimeric complex with Kv4.x α-subunits - induces a notch in the beginning of the plateau phase (phase 2). In the atria, the ultra-rapid potassium current (I_{Kur}) - conducted through the Kv1.5 channels, potentially together with I_{To} - induces a partial repolarisation early in the action potential. The L-type calcium channels undergo a slow calcium and voltage-dependent inactivation and, at the same time, an increase in the rapid and slow delayed rectifier potassium currents, I_{Kr} and I_{Ks}, respectively, is observed. This moves the action potential into phase 3. The inward rectifier current I_{K1} participates in the latter part of phase 3, together with I_{Kr} and I_{Ks}, in driving the membrane potential towards the equilibrium potential of potassium and thereby terminating the action potential. I_{Kr} is conducted through human the ether-a-go-go-related gene channel 1 (hERG1, also called Kv11.1), while I_{Ks} is conducted through the Kv7.1/KCNE1 channels and I_{K1} through the Kir2.x channels. Together with the sodium potassium exchanger 1 (NCX1), I_{K1} is the current that is primarily responsible for setting the resting membrane potential (phase 4). Several other ion channels, including the K_{ATP} channels, the T-type calcium channels, the GIRK channels and the small conductance potassium channels, have been reported to be present in atrial and ventricular myocytes, but a thorough review these channels is beyond the scope of this chapter .

2. Sodium channels

The primary determinant in depolarising the surface membrane in the atrial and ventricular myocytes is the sodium current. the activation of the sodium channels leads to a very fast depolarisation of the myocytes, changing the membrane potential from approximately -85 mV to approximately +25 mV within 10th of milliseconds (Petitprez *et al.*, 2008) (phase 0, Fig. 1). The sodium channels inactivate equally fast and only a small fraction of the channels are open during what remains of the action potential (Fig. 3).

2.1 $Na_v1.5$ voltage-gated sodium channels

The voltage-gated sodium channel $Na_V1.5$ is the primary component in generating the cardiac sodium current. This is proved by the fact that several cardiac syndromes, including long QT syndrome and Brugada Syndrome, have been linked to mutations in SCN5A, which is the gene encoding $Na_v1.5$ (Jespersen, 2011; Tfelt-Hansen *et al.*, 2009). The $Na_v1.5$ protein is a relatively large glycosylated membrane protein consisting of 2015 or 2016 residues (depending on the splice variant) with a molecular weight of ~220 kilo Dalton (Makielski *et al.*, 2003). The $Na_v1.5$ protein comprises 4 homologue domains (I to IV), each consisting of 6 transmembrane segments (TM1 to TM6) forming a functional channel (Fig. 3). The channel can be found in three confirmations: closed, open and inactivated. Around the resting membrane potential, the majority of channels are in the closed state. When a depolarising pulse reaches the $Na_v1.5$ channels - which are embedded in the cardiomyocyte plasma membrane - the channels undergo a very fast transition, rendering the channels open.

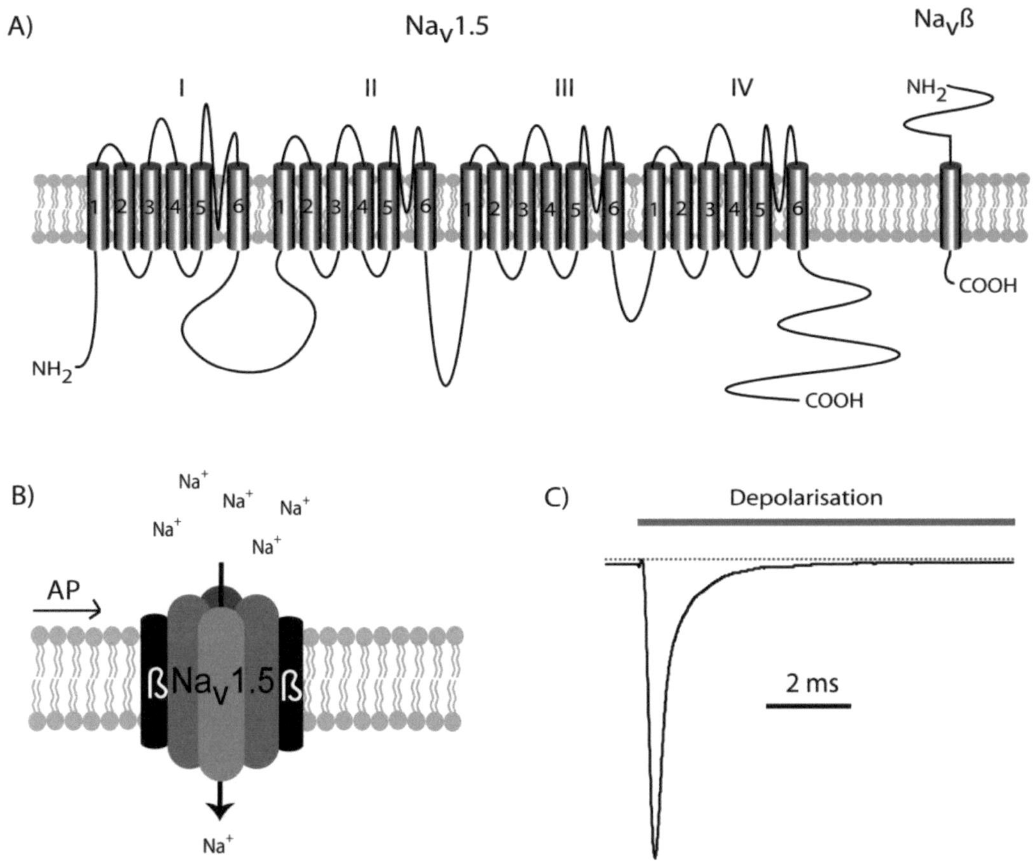

Fig. 3. The cardiac $Na_v1.5$ sodium channel. A) The SCN5A gene is transcribed into the large $Na_v1.5$ protein containing 24 transmembrane domains. B) This protein can fold up into a functional channel, but it is believed to be modulated by the Navβ one-transmembrane spanning β-subunits *in vivo*. When an action potential (AP) induces a depolarisation of the membrane, $Na_v1.5$ is activated and a transient influx of sodium begins. C) Illustration of the current conducted through $Na_v1.5$ channels following a depolarising pulse. The channels will activate very quickly, but as soon as the action potential has commenced a fast inactivation is also initiated. After approximately 10 milliseconds, only a small fraction of the channels will be open.

This opening is, however, only transient as the inactivation of the channels is also a fast process, beginning immediately after depolarisation and making almost all of the channel complexes non-conducting after a few milliseconds. Although the vast majority of sodium conductance is within the first few milliseconds of the action potential sustained - or late - the inward sodium current is also observed. This sustained current, which is in the range of 5 ‰ of the peak current, participates in determining the action potential duration, which is illustrated in long QT syndrome 3 patients who have mutations in *SCN5A* resulting in an increased sustained sodium current (~1-3 % of peak current) (Bennett *et al.*, 1995). In cardiomyocytes with an increased sustained sodium current, the depolarising power of this current will lead to a longer depolarisation time and as the QT interval reflects the ventricular action potential duration, a prolonged QT interval is observed. This sodium ion selectivity is due to peptide sequences located in the pore between TM5 and TM6, while TM4 is involved in the activation of the channel. Furthermore, an intracellular sequence between domain 3 and 4 is important for the inactivation (West *et al.*, 1992).

2.2 $Na_v\beta1$-$\beta4$ subunits interact with $Na_v1.5$

Four sodium channel β-subunits, $Na_v\beta1$-$\beta4$, are encoded by *SCN1-4B* and have been identified (Meadows & Isom, 2005). *SCN1-4B* all comprise large extracellular immunoglobulin-like domains, a single transmembrane spanning segment and intracellular C-terminal domains. The β-subunits have been found implicated in sodium channel expression at the cell surface, the modulation of channel gating and the voltage dependency of the sodium current. All *SCNB* transcripts are present in the heart, but thorough investigations of protein expression have not been performed (Gaborit *et al.*, 2007; Olesen *et al.*, 2011). *In vivo* investigations of the cardiac role of $Na_v\beta$s are restricted to knock-out mice, and the reported *in vitro* effects inflicted by these β-subunits often depend on the cellular expression system applied; further studies in native settings are needed. However, the fact that mutations in the genes underlying the β-subunits have been linked to a number of arrhythmic disorders (reviewed in detail by Abriel, 2010) underlines the importance of these proteins in the heart.

SCN1B is spliced into two variants, β1 (Isom *et al.*, 1992) and β1A in rats (Kazen-Gillespie *et al.*, 2000), and β1B in humans (Qin *et al.*, 2003). While the rat and human β1 proteins have a high degree of similarity, the alternatively spliced part of rβ1A and hβ1B only shows a 33% sequence homology. In heterologous expression systems, the two most consistent findings with Navβ1 co-expressed with $Na_v1.5$ are a positive voltage shift in the steady-state inactivation and an increase in peak current (Dhar *et al.*, 2001; Herfst *et al.*, 2003; Qu *et al.*, 1995). *SCN1B* mutations have been associated with atrial fibrillation and Brugada syndrome, both of which can be caused by a reduced sodium conductance, indicating that the *in vitro* observations can - at least to some extent - be translated into a functional myocyte context (Watanabe *et al.*, 2008; Watanabe *et al.*, 2009).

In most studies, the expression of $Na_v\beta2$ in various cell systems does not promote changes in the electrophysiological properties of $Na_v1.5$, but it has been suggested that $Na_v\beta2$ is involved in linking sialic acids to $Na_v1.5$, which alters the activation properties (Johnson & Bennett, 2006). *SCN2B* mutations have been found in patients with atrial fibrillation (Watanabe *et al.*, 2009). The $Na_v\beta3$ subunit is reported to modify a number of biophysical properties - depending on expression system - including both activation and inactivation voltage dependence, as well as reducing the sustained current of $Na_v1.5$ (Fahmi *et al.*, 2001; Ko *et al.*, 2005). *SCN3B* knock-down mice show a reduced sodium current and a negative voltage shift in steady-state inactivation, indicating that this subunit augments sodium conductance in the heart. The observations are supported by the fact that mutations in *SCN3B* have been associated with both Brugada Syndrome and atrial fibrillation (Hu *et al.*, 2009; Olesen *et al.*, 2011).

The studies performed with heterologous expression systems and transgenic mice have so far been inconclusive in determining the role of $Na_v\beta4$ in the heart. However, *SCN4B* mutations have been linked to both long QT syndrome and sudden infant death syndrome, as *in vitro* electrophysiological investigations revealed an increased sustained current of $Na_v1.5$ when these $Na_v\beta4$ mutant proteins were co-expressed (Medeiros-Domingo *et al.*, 2007; Tan *et al.*, 2010).

2.3 Phosphorylation of $Na_v1.5$

Phosphorylation is a well-known regulatory mechanism of ion channels, often resulting in altered biophysical properties. Protein kinase C (PKC) activation provokes a drastic reduction in $Na_v1.5$ current amplitude as well as a negative shift in steady-state inactivation (Qu *et al.*, 1994). This effect is believed to be primarily mediated through the phosphorylation of serine residue 1503 (Murray *et al.*, 1997; Qu *et al.*, 1996). The function of glycerol 3-phosphate dehydrogenase 1-like (GPD1L) has recently been linked to the PKC phosphorylation of $Na_v1.5$ (Valdivia *et al.*, 2009). GPD1L catalyses the conversion of glycerol-3-phosphate to dihydroxyacetone phosphate. Glycerol-3-phosphate stimulates - through several intermediate proteins - PKC and thereby feeds the PKC-mediated phosphorylation of $Na_v1.5$. Mutations in GPD1L have been associated to Brugada (London *et al.*, 2007; Weiss *et al.*, 2002) and sudden infant death syndromes (Van Norstrand *et al.*, 2007), and Valdivia and colleagues have shown this to be related to the decreased activity of GPD1L, inducing higher PKC activity and a reduced sodium current (Valdivia *et al.*, 2009).

The tyrosine phosphorylation of $Na_v1.5$ has also been found to promote changes in the channel kinetics. The cardiac-expressed protein kinase Fyn induces a depolarising shift in steady-state inactivation (Ahern *et al.*, 2005). By mutating tyrosine residue 1495, located in the linker between domains 3 and 4 and in close proximity to residues involved in inactivation (Patton *et al.*, 1992), the authors found the effect of Fyn to be abolished. In contrast, the expression of the protein tyrosine phosphatase PTPH1 - which is also expressed in the heart - induced a hyperpolarisation shift in steady-state inactivation (Jespersen *et al.*, 2006). PTPH1 interacts with the 14-3-3β regulatory protein suggest that 14-3-3β functions as a regulator or adapter protein of the phosphatase (Zhang *et al.*, 1997). Another member of the 14-3-3 family, namely 14-3-3η, has been found to interact with the Nav1.5 cytoplasmic I inter-domain, modifying the biophysical properties of the channel (Allouis *et al.*, 2006). Whether or not this interaction modulates the level of $Na_v1.5$ phosphorylation is unknown.

2.4 Plasma membrane stability of $Na_v1.5$

$Na_v1.5$ holds a C-terminal PDZ domain-binding motif. This domain binds syntrophin, which again interacts with dystrophin (Gavillet *et al.*, 2006). The most prominent role of dystrophin is to provide a structural link between the cytoskeleton and the extracellular matrix in order to maintain muscle integrity. However, experiments performed by Abriel and co-workers on dystrophin-deficient mdx mice indicated the cardiac sodium channel to be regulated through a syntrophin/dystrophin complex (Gavillet *et al.*, 2006). A significant reduction in $Na_v1.5$ protein and current levels - together with ECG alterations - was found when the hearts from these mdx mice were analysed. The functional importance of this interaction has been confirmed in humans, where mutations in α1-syntrophin have been associated with long QT syndrome and sudden infant death syndrome (Cheng *et al.*, 2009; Ueda *et al.*, 2008; Wu *et al.*, 2008).

For an increasing number of ion channels, Nedd4/Nedd4-like ubiquitin-protein ligase mediated internalisation has been found to be important (review by Abriel & Staub, 2005). This class of protein ligases - counting 9 members - interacts with membrane proteins holding a PY-motif (Staub *et al.*, 1996). Ubiquitin is a 76 amino acid protein which can be covalently linked to lysine residues on target proteins, marking them for internalisation, followed by either degradation or intracellular storage (Hershko & Ciechanover, 1998; Hicke, 1999). $Na_v1.5$ is regulated by Nedd4/Nedd4-like mediated ubiquitylation (Rougier *et al.*, 2005; van Bemmelen *et al.*, 2004). *In vitro* electrophysiological experiments revealed that a down-regulation in current density - without altering the biophysical properties - to be was induced by Nedd4-2 through a PY-motif located in the C-terminal tail of $Na_v1.5$. Nedd4-2 induces an increase in the ubiquitylation of $Na_v1.5$, which leads to a drastic redistribution, where Nav1.5 proteins are almost absent from the surface membrane but are instead found in intracellular compartments.

2.5 Other sodium channels in the heart

Although $Na_v1.5$ is the most important sodium channel in the heart, other voltage-gated sodium channels may also play a role in generating the cardiac I_{Na}. Neuronal sodium channels do, in contrast to $Na_v1.5$, have a very high sensitivity to tetrodotoxin. This has been used to investigate the potential function of neuronal voltage-gated sodium channels in the heart. Although present at a relatively low mRNA level (Gaborit *et al.*, 2007) neuronal sodium channels have been suggested to play a role in electrical-chemical coupling, as low tetrodotoxin concentrations lead to a reduction in sercoplasmic reticulum calcium release (Torres *et al.*, 2010) and thereby reduce left ventricular functioning (Maier *et al.*, 2002). Brette & Orchad found that TTX-sensitive I_{Na} makes up approximately 15% of the total I_{Na} in isolated rat ventricular cells, which decreased the rate of the depolarisation of the action potential by 10% (Brette & Orchard, 2006). Further, the sodium current in Purkinje fibres has been shown to be sensitive to low concentrations of tetrodotoxin (Carmeliet, 1987), indicating that the neuronal sodium channels participate in the propagation of the cardiac action potential.

Recently, genome-wide association studies have revealed that *SCN10A* - encoding the $Na_v1.8$ sodium channel - seems to participate in determining the conduction velocity in both atria (PR interval) and the ventricles (QRS duration) (Chambers *et al.*, 2010; Holm *et al.*, 2010; Pfeufer *et al.*, 2010). $Na_v1.8$ has a low sensitivity to tetrodotoxin, as with $Na_v1.5$, and it can therefore be speculated that this channel has been overlooked up until now.

3. L-type calcium channels

The fast depolarisation (phase 0) driven by the influx of sodium through the voltage-gated sodium channels triggers the activation of voltage-gated calcium channels. Both voltage-gated T-type and L-type calcium channels have been reported to be expressed in the heart. The T-type channels are low voltage-activated transient Ca^{2+} channels which are functionally expressed during development, while they are drastically down-regulated in adult myocytes (Ono & Iijima, 2010). However, these T-type calcium channels may still play a role in impulse generation in the sinoatrial node (Hagiwara *et al.*, 1988). The long lasting,

high voltage-activated L-type Ca^{2+} channels are both abundant and ubiquitously expressed in the heart (Bodi *et al.*, 2005). These voltage-dependent calcium channels (VDCC) bind dihydropyridine and have, therefore, also been named dihydropyridine receptors (Taira *et al.*, 1987; Tanabe *et al.*, 1987). The L-type Ca^{2+} channels are the primary source of extracellular calcium influx. The opening of L-type Ca^{2+} channels is delayed when compared with Na^+ channels and in contrast to the voltage-gated sodium channels, the L-type Ca^{2+} channels inactivate slowly (<100 ms) in a voltage- and calcium-dependent manner (Bean, 1985). This slowly inactivated calcium current is - together with the fine-tuned regulation of sodium and potassium conductance - the basis for the action potential plateau observed in ventricular myocytes (phase 2). The ryanodine receptor calcium channels (RYR2) - which are located in the sarcoplasmic reticulum in close proximity to the L-type Ca^{2+} channels - is activated by the calcium influx (Bers, 2004). This RYR2-mediated sarcoplasmic calcium release is the major contributor in the activation of the contractile machinery (Bers, 2002).
The cardiac L-type calcium channel consists of a pore-forming α-subunit, the $Ca_v1.2$ protein, which is encoded by Cacna1c. $Ca_v1.2$ has a similar topology to $Na_v1.5$ (Fig. 3). A functional cardiac channel complex is composed of four polyproteins which, apart from Cav1.2, form the β and α_2/δ auxiliary subunits (Bodi *et al.*, 2005). The α_2 and δ subunits are encoded by the same gene and are separated by proteolytic cleavage (De Jongh *et al.*, 1990). Several different isoforms of this protein are known. The α_2/δ subunits are linked together by a disulphide bridge and are closely associated with the $Ca_v1.2$ α-subunit by surface interaction. The α_2 subunit is entirely extracellular, and the δ subunit has a single transmembrane region with a very short intracellular part. The α_2/δ subunits have been suggested to increase the membrane density of the channel complex, and mice lacking this gene have a tendency to have bradycardia (Ivanov *et al.*, 2004). All four calcium channel β-subunits (CACNB1-4) are known to modify the currents; however, it has been suggested that β_2 is the primary subunit in the heart (Colecraft *et al.*, 2002). The β-subunits play a prominent role in the trafficking of the channel complexes to the cell surface membrane (Bichet *et al.*, 2000; Chen *et al.*, 2004; Van *et al.*, 2004). Furthermore, the absence of β-subunits renders the channel insensitive to β-adrenergic stimulation (Mikala *et al.*, 1998).
One of the important regulatory mechanisms of L-type calcium channels is cAMP-dependent phosphorylation, which increases the amplitude of the calcium current (McDonald *et al.*, 1994). An increase in cAMP is induced by the β-adrenergic control of cardiac functions. β-adrenergic stimulation thereby leads to an increased calcium influx through the L-type channels, which facilitates an increased calcium release from the ryanodine receptors. Other important regulators of L-type calcium channels are calmodulin-dependent protein kinase II (CaMKII) (Maier & Bers, 2007) and calcium-induced inactivation through binding to calmodulin (Bodi *et al.*, 2005).

4. Potassium channels

In the heart, potassium conductance is conducted through a number of different potassium channels. All of the potassium channels described below consist of six transmembrane domains - except for Kir2.x which has two - and assembles into tetrameric complexes, which can either be homo- or heteromeric (Nerbonne & Kass, 2005) (Fig. 4). In the early phase of the action potential, the transient outward potassium current (I_{To}) is important in the atria and in subepicardial ventricular myocytes. The ultra-rapid potassium current (I_{Kur}) - which is also a fast activating current present early on in the action potential - is predominantly expressed in the atria. The rapid and slow delayed rectifier potassium currents, I_{Kr} and I_{Ks}, respectively, are, together with the inward rectifier current I_{K1}, the primary currents responsible for repolarising the myocyte membranes in the final part of the action potential and thereby terminating it (phase 3). All three of these currents are important in both atria and the ventricles.

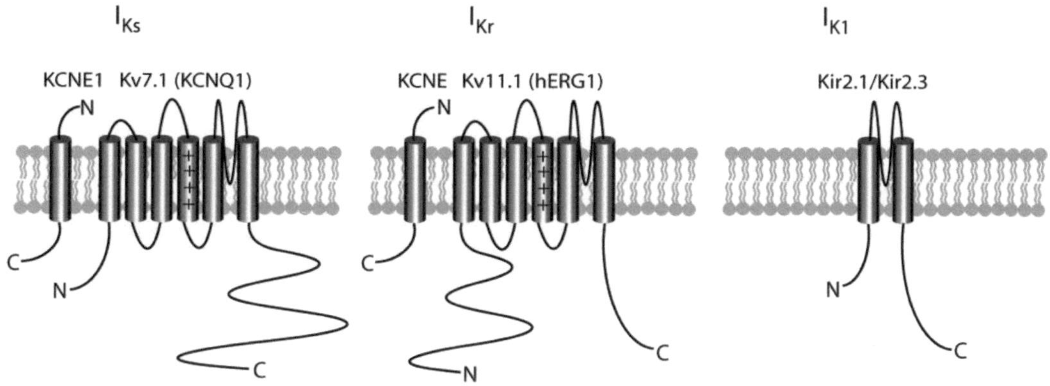

Fig. 4. Topology of the major repolarising potassium channels and their β-subunits.

4.1 The transient outward (Kv4.x/I_{To}) potassium channels

The transient outward current I_{To} is composed of two different components, namely a calcium-dependent chloride current and a calcium-independent potassium current. While the molecular components underlying the chloride current are unknown, several recently published reports have revealed a detailed picture of the proteins involved in forming the potassium transient outward current (reviewed by Patel & Campbell, 2005). This current can be divided into a rapidly activating and inactivating current - named $I_{To,f}$ - and a current with slow recovery kinetics - named $I_{To,s}$. $I_{To,s}$, conducted through Kv1.4 channels - which are regulated by Kvβ cytosolic proteins (Morales *et al.*, 1995). Kv1.4 channels are expressed throughout the ventricular wall as well as in the atria, where it is suggested that they participate to a minor extent with I_{To} (Calloe *et al.*, 2010; Calloe *et al.*, 2011). The $I_{To,f}$ channels activate rapidly (in the order of milliseconds) in a voltage-dependent manner and are inactivated through a somewhat slower process (in the order of tens of milliseconds). The pore-forming subunit in $I_{To,f}$ which is predominantly present in larger mammals is Kv4.3, which when co-expressed with the Kv channel interacting protein 2 (KChiP2) recapitulates most of the features of the native current (An *et al.*, 2000; Deschenes *et al.*, 2002). Kv4.3 is homogenously expressed in the ventricle. The KChiP2 auxiliary protein potentiates the current conducted through the Kv4.3 channels by promoting cell surface expression. In fact, in human and canine ventricles, a transmural expression gradient of KChiP2 has been found to correlate with a much higher $I_{To,f}$ in the subepicardial layer than in the subendocardial layer (Calloe *et al.*, 2010; Deschenes *et al.*, 2002; Gaborit *et al.*, 2007; Soltysinska *et al.*, 2009; Zicha *et al.*, 2004). This large expression of $I_{To,f}$ is responsible for the characteristic notch (phase 1 repolarisation) observed in subepicardial cardiomyocytes (Calloe *et al.*, 2009; Di Diego *et al.*, 2002). $I_{To,f}$ is also prominently expressed in the atria, where it likewise participates in early repolarisation (Calloe *et al.*, 2010; Calloe *et al.*, 2011; Gaborit *et al.*, 2007). While KChIP2 has the most prominent effect on Kv4.3 channels, with altered current levels as well as inactivation and recovery parameters (Patel & Campbell, 2005), other auxiliary subunits have also been shown to be important for $I_{To,f}$. Dipeptidyl aminopeptidase-related proteins (DPPs) affect the biophysical properties of the Kv4.3 channels in a manner very similar to KCHiP2 proteins, with the important difference that they also accelerate activation, thereby providing current properties resembling native $I_{To,f}$ (Cotella *et al.*, 2010; Nadal *et al.*, 2003; Radicke *et al.*, 2005). Kvβ cytosolic proteins, which increase the expression of Kv4.3, have been suggested to regulate this transient outward potassium current (Yang *et al.*, 2001). KCNE β-subunits, of which 5 different subtypes exit, have also been suggested to interact with Kv4.3/KCHiP2 channels as they modify the channel kinetics in *in vitro* studies (Radicke *et al.*, 2006; Radicke *et al.*, 2008). Recently, mutations in KCNE3 and KCNE5 have been linked to Brugada syndrome, which is a syndrome associated with an increased risk of ventricular fibrillation (Brugada & Brugada, 1992; Delpon *et al.*, 2008; Ohno *et al.*, 2011). Both KCNE3 and KCNE5 decrease the I_{To} current level when co-expressed, and as the mutations found in Brugada Syndrome patients provide an increase in current level compared to controls, it is suggested that this inhibitory effect of I_{To} is important in maintaining the current balance between the sodium and potassium currents in the early part of the ventricular action potential.

4.2 The ultra-rapid (Kv1.5/I_{Kur}) potassium channels

The ultra rapid potassium current I_{Kur} is well-expressed in the atria, where it contributes to repolarisation (Amos *et al.*, 1996). This current activates early during an action potential and inactivates slowly. Hence, I_{Kur} is an important repolarising current throughout most of the atrial action potential. The molecular constituent of I_{Kur} is the Kv1.5 potassium channel (Wang *et al.*, 1993). Although, I_{Kur} has predominantly been reported in atria, this current has also been suggested to play a role in canine and human ventricles (Calloe *et al.*, 2010; Nielsen *et al.*, 2007; Sridhar *et al.*, 2007).

4.3 The fast delayed rectifier (hERG1/I_{Kr}) potassium channels

The rapid delayed rectifier current I_{Kr} is present in nodal tissue, atria, purkinje fibres and ventricles. The molecular correlate of I_{Kr} is the ether-a-go-go-related gene 1 product ERG1, also termed Kv11.1 (Sanguinetti *et al.*, 1995; Trudeau *et al.*, 1995). It is the unique biophysical features - with fast inactivation followed by slow deactivation - of the ERG1 potassium channel which makes it pivotal in cardiac repolarisation (Grunnet, 2010; Spector *et al.*, 1996). Upon depolarisation, the ERG1 channels open but inactivate very quickly and at the same time display marked inward rectification (Grunnet *et al.*, 2008b). This means that the ERG1 channel complexes conduct a minor potassium current during the initial depolarisation and the plateau phase of the cardiac action potential. However, when the membrane potential moves slightly towards the repolarisation potential - partly due to L-type calcium channel inactivation and partly due to I_{Ks} activation - then ERG1 channels are released from inactivation. As ERG1 channels only slowly progress into a closed state (deactivation) – and, therefore, are kept in an open state (Piper *et al.*, 2005) - a relatively large potassium current is conducted and the membrane potential is accelerated towards the resting membrane potential. The inactivation of ERG1 channels is called C-type inactivation, which involves a change at the extracellular mouth of the pore modulated by the extracellular potassium concentration (Baukrowitz & Yellen, 1995). A low concentration of potassium will lead to a pore collapse. Hence, the external potassium concentration is an important regulator of potassium conductance, where low concentrations will reduce activity and high concentrations will increase activity. Loss-of-function mutations in hERG1 are associated with long QT syndrome type 2 (Sanguinetti *et al.*, 1996a), while gain-of-function mutations have been found in short QT syndrome type 1 (Brugada *et al.*, 2004; Cordeiro *et al.*, 2005; Grunnet *et al.*, 2008a).

Two splice variants of ERG1 have been reported. The originally identified ERG1 protein is termed ERG1a while an alternatively spliced variant, termed ERG1b, has a much shorter intracellular N-terminal with a unique 36 residue sequence (Lees-Miller *et al.*, 1997; London *et al.*, 1997). ERG1b displays different deactivation kinetics to ERG1a (Lees-Miller *et al.*, 1997; London *et al.*, 1997). The co-expression of mRNA levels corresponding to the levels found in the human ventricles of the two variants alter several of the kinetic parameters (Larsen *et al.*, 2008), and this may explain a reported dispersion of I_{Kr} deactivation kinetics observed between myocytes isolated from the subepicardium and the mid-myocardium (Szabo *et al.*, 2005).

The membrane-spanning KCNE2 β-subunits have been found to modify the kinetics of the hERG1 channel (Abbott *et al.*, 1999; McDonald *et al.*, 1997). KCNE2/hERG1 expression in heterologous expression systems has been found to provide currents partly resembling native I_{Kr}, and as KCNE2 mutations found in long QT syndrome patients alter the channel properties it has been suggested that KCNE2 interacts with ERG1 in the heart (Abbott *et al.*, 1999). However, another report has not found KCNE2 to act as an essential constituent of the ERG1 channel complex carrying native I_{Kr} (Weerapura *et al.*, 2002).

4.4 The slow delayed rectifier (Kv7.1/I_{Ks}) potassium channels

The KCNQ1 gene, encoding Kv7.1 proteins, was cloned by Wang and co-workers using linkage analyses on genomic material from Long QT syndrome patients (Wang *et al.*, 1996), and was, therefore, originally named KvLQT1. The voltage-gated Kv7.1 channel is progressively opened by increasing membrane depolarisations. The channel gives rise to slowly activating and deactivating potassium currents. Upon longer depolarising steps, a fraction of the KCNQ1 channels inactivate (Pusch, 1998). KCNQ1 potassium channels are expressed in several tissues throughout the body and regulate key physiological functions. The two most important roles of KCNQ1 channels are: i) the repolarisation of the cardiac tissue following an action potential, and ii) water and salt transport across epithelial tissues (reviewed by Jespersen *et al.*, 2005).

The five relatively small one-transmembrane spanning KCNE proteins - KCNE1-5 - have been found to be highly promiscuous with respect to modulating the biophysical properties of Kv potassium channels as well as HCN pacemaker channels (McCrossan & Abbott, 2004). All five members of the KCNE family modify the properties of Kv7.1 channels (Jespersen *et al.*, 2005). The co-expression of Kv7.1 with KCNE1 - formerly known as minK - recapitulates native I_{Ks} (Barhanin *et al.*, 1996; Sanguinetti *et al.*, 1996b), which not only plays a pivotal role in repolarising the myocardium but which is also important in transporting potassium across the strial marginal cells in the inner ear (Sunose *et al.*, 1997). The co-assembly of Kv7.1 and KCNE1 results in an increase in single channel conductance, a positive shift in the voltage activation threshold, the slowing of activation and deactivation, and an almost complete absence of inactivation (Splawski *et al.*, 1997). In long QT syndromes 1 and 5, which are caused by mutations in Kv7.1 and KCNE1, a reduced I_{Ks} current is observed (Wang *et al.*, 1996; Wang *et al.*, 1999).

I_{Ks} is the only potassium current which is upregulated with increased beating frequency. The upregulation of I_{Ks} is orchestrated by sympathetic mediated β-adrenergic receptor activation. The β-adrenergic receptor activation results in an increased level of cAMP and PKA stimulation, which interacts with the I_{Ks} channel complex through an A-kinase anchoring protein (AKAP) called 'yotiao' (Marx *et al.*, 2002; Potet *et al.*, 2001). PKA and protein phosphatase 1 interact with the C-terminal tail of KCNQ1 through yotiao, which leads to a phosphorylation of serine 27 in the N-terminus. cAMP-induced regulation of Kv7.1 is dependent on KCNE1 and Long QT mutations in both KCNQ1 and KCNE1 have been shown to disrupt this regulation (Kurokawa *et al.*, 2004; Marx *et al.*, 2002). The β-adrenergic activation increases the activation and slows the deactivation kinetics of I_{Ks}, and these features - together with the increased beating frequencies - have been suggested to underlie the profoundly augmented cardiac I_{Ks} current (Marx *et al.*, 2002; Terrenoire *et al.*, 2005). I_{Ks} is therefore essential for action potential shortening at increased beating frequencies. The importance of β-adrenergic stimulation is underlined by the fact that in humans I_{Ks} is almost absent without sympathetic stimulation (Jost *et al.*, 2005).

KCNE2-5 β-subunits also interact with Kv7.1 channels, modifying the biophysical parameters (Angelo *et al.*, 2002; Bendahhou *et al.*, 2005; Grunnet *et al.*, 2002; Jespersen *et al.*, 2004; Mazhari *et al.*, 2002; Tinel *et al.*, 2000). Although KCNE2 is primarily believed to be of importance in the stomach, it has also been suggested as modifying I_{Ks} properties in the heart (Jiang *et al.*, 2009; Wu *et al.*, 2006). A polymorphism in KCNE4 has been associated with atrial fibrillation through a proposed gain-of-function mechanism (Ma *et al.*, 2007), but solid evidence is still missing concerning a potential physiological function of the Kv7.1/KCNE4 interaction in the heart. KCNE5 expression drastically reduces the I_{Ks} current amplitude (Angelo *et al.*, 2002). A KCNE5 mutation found in a patient with atrial fibrillation has been shown to increase I_{Ks} and it has therefore been suggested that KCNE5 β-subunits regulate the current conducted through Kv7.1/KCNE1 channels (Ravn *et al.*, 2005; Ravn *et al.*, 2008).

Under pathophysiological conditions, such as during ischemia, cell volume and pH may undergo considerable alterations. KCNQ1 channels have been found to be activated by a drastic increase in extracellular hyperosmolarity in cardiomyocytes (Sasaki *et al.*, 1994; Vandenberg *et al.*, 1996). In heterologous expression systems, it has been shown that hyperosmolar-induced swelling increases the Kv7.1 current while hyperosmolar shrinkage decreases the current (Grunnet *et al.*, 2003). The ability of Kv7.1 to sense volume changes depends on an intact cytoskeleton which interacts with the N-terminal part of Kv7.1. As with volume changes, internal and external acidification also modifies the Kv7.1 current density. Homomeric KCNQ1 channels are inhibited by both intracellular and extracellular acidic pH (Freeman *et al.*, 2000; Peretz *et al.*, 2002; Unsold *et al.*, 2000). KCNE β-subunits enforce differential effects on the Kv7.1 channel complex following acidification. While KCNE3 renders Kv7.1 insensitive to external acidification, KCNE2 induces an increase in the current level following such acidification, which seems to be determined by the extracellular and transmembrane domains of KCNE2 (Heitzmann *et al.*, 2007). The pH-dependent regulation induced by KCNE1 has been disputed, as both a small decrease (Peretz *et al.*, 2002) and an increase (Heitzmann *et al.*, 2007) in current amplitude has been found; however, both external and internal acidification seem to modify the Kv7.1/KCNE1 current kinetics by changing the slow activation kinetics to an instantaneous onset (Heitzmann *et al.*, 2007; Unsold *et al.*, 2000).

4.5 The inward rectifier (Kir2.X/I_{K1}) potassium channels

The resting membrane potential of cardiomyocytes - being between -80 and -90 mV - is close to the equilibrium potential of potassium, partly due to relatively large resting K^+ conductance through inward rectifier potassium channels (I_{Kir}) (phase 4) (Dhamoon & Jalife,

2005). I_{Kir} channels are composed of four pore-forming subunits, being either homomeric or heteromeric and characterised by a preferentially conducting current at potentials below -50 mV (Lu, 2004). I_{Kir} is not, in contrast to the above described currents, voltage gated. The inward rectification profile, where much less current is passing when the membrane is depolarised than when it is repolarised, is not an inherent property of the channel protein itself, but reflects strong voltage dependence of channel block by intracellular cations, such as Mg^{2+} and polyamines (Ficker *et al.*, 1994; Lopatin *et al.*, 1994; Matsuda *et al.*, 1987; Vandenberg, 1987). The primary inward rectifying current responsible for terminating the action potential - as well as for setting the resting membrane potential - is I_{K1}, constituted by Kir2.1 and, to a lesser extent, the Kir2.2 and Kir2.3 proteins (Preisig-Muller *et al.*, 2002; Zaritsky *et al.*, 2001). Regional differences in the expression of I_{K1} have been described (Dhamoon *et al.*, 2004; Samie *et al.*, 2001) (Samie *et al.*, 2001; Dhamoon *et al.*, 2004) and the modulation of this current affects cardiac excitability and arrhythmogenesis (Nakamura *et al.*, 1998; Plaster *et al.*, 2001; Poelzing & Veeraraghavan, 2007; Warren *et al.*, 2003).
I_{K1} channels, such as ERG1 (I_{Kr}) channels, are regulated by extracellular potassium (Dhamoon *et al.*, 2004; Hume & Uehara, 1985; Knot *et al.*, 1996). Increased extracellular potassium augments potassium conductance - even though the potassium driving force is decreased - while a decreased concentration reduces the current. This biophysical property of I_{K1} and I_{Kr} channels is important in a clinical setting, as a patient with hypokalaemia will have a reduction in two of the three major repolarising cardiac currents which will lead to action potential prolongation as potentially being the trigger of arrhythmia. Another important regulator of the I_{K1} function is phosphatidylinositol 4,5-bisphosphate (PIP2) (Soom *et al.*, 2001; Takano & Kuratomi, 2003). PIP_2 is a quantitatively minor membrane component, although its local concentration may be relatively high. PIP is a key signalling phospholipid, whereby its hydrolysis by phospholipase C as well as its phosphorylation by PI3 kinases generates important second messengers. PIP2 binds directly to Kir channels, where it stabilises the open state. PIP2 has a high affinity with Kir2.X channels, which probably underlies the almost constitutive active I_{K1} (Lopes *et al.*, 2002).

5. Summary

The length and morphology of cardiac action potential are shaped by the expression and fine-tuning of a number of ion channels. Sodium channels are responsible for the rapid depolarisation of the myocardium. The influx of sodium is followed by an influx of calcium through L-type calcium channels, contributing to keeping the depolarisation for several hundred milliseconds. The cardiac action potential is terminated by an increased efflux of potassium driving the membrane potential towards repolarisation. The dynamic properties of the action potential are obtained through a number of regulatory mechanisms maintaining the delicate balance between the different depolarising and repolarising ionic currents. Many of the primary regulatory mechanisms - such as β-subunits and phosphorylation sites - have been established. However, below the direct channel interacting proteins there is a whole network of modulatory mechanisms, and we are only just on the brink of discovering their role in regulating the cardiac action potential.

6. References

Abbott GW, Sesti F, Splawski I, Buck ME, Lehmann MH, Timothy KW, Keating MT, & Goldstein SA (1999). MiRP1 forms IKr potassium channels with HERG and is associated with cardiac arrhythmia. *Cell* 97, 175-187.

Abriel H (2010). Cardiac sodium channel Na(v)1.5 and interacting proteins: Physiology and pathophysiology. *J Mol Cell Cardiol* 48, 2-11.

Abriel H & Staub O (2005). Ubiquitylation of ion channels. *Physiology (Bethesda)* 20, 398-407.

Ahern CA, Zhang JF, Wookalis MJ, & Horn R (2005). Modulation of the cardiac sodium channel NaV1.5 by Fyn, a Src family tyrosine kinase. *Circ Res* 96, 991-998.

Allouis M, Le BF, Wilders R, Peroz D, Schott JJ, Noireaud J, Le MH, Merot J, Escande D, & Baro I (2006). 14-3-3 is a regulator of the cardiac voltage-gated sodium channel Nav1.5. *Circ Res* 98, 1538-1546.

Amos GJ, Wettwer E, Metzger F, Li Q, Himmel HM, & Ravens U (1996). Differences between outward currents of human atrial and subepicardial ventricular myocytes. *J Physiol* 491 (Pt 1), 31-50.

An WF, Bowlby MR, Betty M, Cao J, Ling HP, Mendoza G, Hinson JW, Mattsson KI, Strassle BW, Trimmer JS, & Rhodes KJ (2000). Modulation of A-type potassium channels by a family of calcium sensors. *Nature* 403, 553-556.

Angelo K, Jespersen T, Grunnet M, Nielsen MS, Klaerke DA, & Olesen SP (2002). KCNE5 induces time- and voltage-dependent modulation of the KCNQ1 current. *Biophys J* 83, 1997-2006.

Barhanin J, Lesage F, Guillemare E, Fink M, Lazdunski M, & Romey G (1996). K(V)LQT1 and lsK (minK) proteins associate to form the I(Ks) cardiac potassium current. *Nature* 384, 78-80.

Baruscotti M, Bucchi A, & DiFrancesco D (2005). Physiology and pharmacology of the cardiac pacemaker ("funny") current. *Pharmacol Ther* 107, 59-79.

Baukrowitz T & Yellen G (1995). Modulation of K+ current by frequency and external [K+]: a tale of two inactivation mechanisms. *Neuron* 15, 951-960.

Bean BP (1985). Two kinds of calcium channels in canine atrial cells. Differences in kinetics, selectivity, and pharmacology. *J Gen Physiol* 86, 1-30.

Bendahhou S, Marionneau C, Haurogne K, Larroque MM, Derand R, Szuts V, Escande D, Demolombe S, & Barhanin J (2005). In vitro molecular interactions and distribution of KCNE family with KCNQ1 in the human heart. *Cardiovasc Res* 67, 529-538.

Bennett PB, Yazawa K, Makita N, & George AL, Jr. (1995). Molecular mechanism for an inherited cardiac arrhythmia. *Nature* 376, 683-685.

Bers DM (2002). Cardiac excitation-contraction coupling. *Nature* 415, 198-205.

Bers DM (2004). Macromolecular complexes regulating cardiac ryanodine receptor function. *J Mol Cell Cardiol* 37, 417-429.

Bichet D, Cornet V, Geib S, Carlier E, Volsen S, Hoshi T, Mori Y, & De WM (2000). The I-II loop of the Ca2+ channel alpha1 subunit contains an endoplasmic reticulum retention signal antagonized by the beta subunit. *Neuron* 25, 177-190.

Bodi I, Mikala G, Koch SE, Akhter SA, & Schwartz A (2005). The L-type calcium channel in the heart: the beat goes on. *J Clin Invest* 115, 3306-3317.

Brette F & Orchard CH (2006). No apparent requirement for neuronal sodium channels in excitation-contraction coupling in rat ventricular myocytes. *Circ Res* 98, 667-674.

Brugada P & Brugada J (1992). Right bundle branch block, persistent ST segment elevation and sudden cardiac death: a distinct clinical and electrocardiographic syndrome. A multicenter report. *J Am Coll Cardiol* 20, 1391-1396.

Brugada R, Hong K, Dumaine R, Cordeiro J, Gaita F, Borggrefe M, Menendez TM, Brugada J, Pollevick GD, Wolpert C, Burashnikov E, Matsuo K, Wu YS, Guerchicoff A,

Bianchi F, Giustetto C, Schimpf R, Brugada P, & Antzelevitch C (2004). Sudden death associated with short-QT syndrome linked to mutations in HERG. *Circulation* 109, 30-35.

Bucchi A, Baruscotti M, Robinson RB, & DiFrancesco D (2003). I(f)-dependent modulation of pacemaker rate mediated by cAMP in the presence of ryanodine in rabbit sino-atrial node cells. *J Mol Cell Cardiol* 35, 905-913.

Calloe K, Cordeiro JM, Di Diego JM, Hansen RS, Grunnet M, Olesen SP, & Antzelevitch C (2009). A transient outward potassium current activator recapitulates the electrocardiographic manifestations of Brugada syndrome. *Cardiovasc Res* 81, 686-694.

Calloe K, Nof E, Jespersen T, Diego JM, Chlus N, Olesen SP, Antzelevitch C, & Cordeiro JM (2011). Comparison of the Effects of a Transient Outward Potassium Channel Activator on Currents Recorded from Atrial and Ventricular Cardiomyocytes. *J Cardiovasc Electrophysiol* 22:1057-66.

Calloe K, Soltysinska E, Jespersen T, Lundby A, Antzelevitch C, Olesen SP, & Cordeiro JM (2010). Differential effects of the transient outward K(+) current activator NS5806 in the canine left ventricle. *J Mol Cell Cardiol* 48, 191-200.

Carmeliet E (1987). Voltage-dependent block by tetrodotoxin of the sodium channel in rabbit cardiac Purkinje fibers. *Biophys J* 51, 109-114.

Chambers JC, Zhao J, Terracciano CM, Bezzina CR, Zhang W, Kaba R, Navaratnarajah M, Lotlikar A, Sehmi JS, Kooner MK, Deng G, Siedlecka U, Parasramka S, El-Hamamsy I, Wass MN, Dekker LR, de Jong JS, Sternberg MJ, McKenna W, Severs NJ, de SR, Wilde AA, Anand P, Yacoub M, Scott J, Elliott P, Wood JN, & Kooner JS (2010). Genetic variation in SCN10A influences cardiac conduction. *Nat Genet* 42, 149-152.

Chen YH, Li MH, Zhang Y, He LL, Yamada Y, Fitzmaurice A, Shen Y, Zhang H, Tong L, & Yang J (2004). Structural basis of the alpha1-beta subunit interaction of voltage-gated Ca2+ channels. *Nature* 429, 675-680.

Cheng J, Van Norstrand DW, Medeiros-Domingo A, Valdivia C, Tan BH, Ye B, Kroboth S, Vatta M, Tester DJ, January CT, Makielski JC, & Ackerman MJ (2009). Alpha1-syntrophin mutations identified in sudden infant death syndrome cause an increase in late cardiac sodium current. *Circ Arrhythm Electrophysiol* 2, 667-676.

Colecraft HM, Alseikhan B, Takahashi SX, Chaudhuri D, Mittman S, Yegnasubramanian V, Alvania RS, Johns DC, Marban E, & Yue DT (2002). Novel functional properties of Ca(2+) channel beta subunits revealed by their expression in adult rat heart cells. *J Physiol* 541, 435-452.

Cordeiro JM, Brugada R, Wu YS, Hong K, & Dumaine R (2005). Modulation of I(Kr) inactivation by mutation N588K in KCNH2: a link to arrhythmogenesis in short QT syndrome. *Cardiovasc Res* 67, 498-509.

Cotella D, Radicke S, Bortoluzzi A, Ravens U, Wettwer E, Santoro C, & Sblattero D (2010). Impaired glycosylation blocks DPP10 cell surface expression and alters the electrophysiology of Ito channel complex. *Pflugers Arch* 460, 87-97.

De Jongh KS, Warner C, & Catterall WA (1990). Subunits of purified calcium channels. Alpha 2 and delta are encoded by the same gene. *J Biol Chem* 265, 14738-14741.

Delpon E, Cordeiro JM, Nunez L, Thomsen PE, Guerchicoff A, Pollevick GD, Wu Y, Kanters JK, Larsen CT, Hofman-Bang J, Burashnikov E, Christiansen M, & Antzelevitch C

(2008). Functional effects of KCNE3 mutation and its role in the development of Brugada syndrome. *Circ Arrhythm Electrophysiol* 1, 209-218.

Deschenes I, DiSilvestre D, Juang GJ, Wu RC, An WF, & Tomaselli GF (2002). Regulation of Kv4.3 current by KChIP2 splice variants: a component of native cardiac I(to)? *Circulation* 106, 423-429.

Dhamoon AS & Jalife J (2005). The inward rectifier current (IK1) controls cardiac excitability and is involved in arrhythmogenesis. *Heart Rhythm* 2, 316-324.

Dhamoon AS, Pandit SV, Sarmast F, Parisian KR, Guha P, Li Y, Bagwe S, Taffet SM, & Anumonwo JM (2004). Unique Kir2.x properties determine regional and species differences in the cardiac inward rectifier K+ current. *Circ Res* 94, 1332-1339.

Dhar MJ, Chen C, Rivolta I, Abriel H, Malhotra R, Mattei LN, Brosius FC, Kass RS, & Isom LL (2001). Characterization of sodium channel alpha- and beta-subunits in rat and mouse cardiac myocytes. *Circulation* 103, 1303-1310.

Di Diego JM, Cordeiro JM, Goodrow RJ, Fish JM, Zygmunt AC, Perez GJ, Scornik FS, & Antzelevitch C (2002). Ionic and cellular basis for the predominance of the Brugada syndrome phenotype in males. *Circulation* 106, 2004-2011.

DiFrancesco D (1993). Pacemaker mechanisms in cardiac tissue. *Annu Rev Physiol* 55, 455-472.

DiFrancesco D & Tromba C (1988). Muscarinic control of the hyperpolarization-activated current (if) in rabbit sino-atrial node myocytes. *J Physiol* 405, 493-510.

Fahmi AI, Patel M, Stevens EB, Fowden AL, John JE, III, Lee K, Pinnock R, Morgan K, Jackson AP, & Vandenberg JI (2001). The sodium channel beta-subunit SCN3b modulates the kinetics of SCN5a and is expressed heterogeneously in sheep heart. *J Physiol* 537, 693-700.

Fermini B & Nathan RD (1991). Removal of sialic acid alters both T- and L-type calcium currents in cardiac myocytes. *Am J Physiol* 260, H735-H743.

Ficker E, Taglialatela M, Wible BA, Henley CM, & Brown AM (1994). Spermine and spermidine as gating molecules for inward rectifier K+ channels. *Science* 266, 1068-1072.

Freeman LC, Lippold JJ, & Mitchell KE (2000). Glycosylation influences gating and pH sensitivity of I(sK). *J Membr Biol* 177, 65-79.

Friel DD & Bean BP (1990). Dual control by ATP and acetylcholine of inwardly rectifying K+ channels in bovine atrial cells. *Pflugers Arch* 415, 651-657.

Gaborit N, Le BS, Szuts V, Varro A, Escande D, Nattel S, & Demolombe S (2007). Regional and tissue specific transcript signatures of ion channel genes in the non-diseased human heart. *J Physiol* 582, 675-693.

Gauss R, Seifert R, & Kaupp UB (1998). Molecular identification of a hyperpolarization-activated channel in sea urchin sperm. *Nature* 393, 583-587.

Gavillet B, Rougier JS, Domenighetti AA, Behar R, Boixel C, Ruchat P, Lehr HA, Pedrazzini T, & Abriel H (2006). Cardiac sodium channel Nav1.5 is regulated by a multiprotein complex composed of syntrophins and dystrophin. *Circ Res* 99, 407-414.

Gouaux E & Mackinnon R (2005). Principles of selective ion transport in channels and pumps. *Science* 310, 1461-1465.

Grunnet M (2010). Repolarization of the cardiac action potential. Does an increase in repolarization capacity constitute a new anti-arrhythmic principle? *Acta Physiol (Oxf)* 198 Suppl 676, 1-48.

Grunnet M, Diness TG, Hansen RS, & Olesen SP (2008a). Biophysical characterization of the short QT mutation hERG-N588K reveals a mixed gain-and loss-of-function. *Cell Physiol Biochem* 22, 611-624.

Grunnet M, Hansen RS, & Olesen SP (2008b). hERG1 channel activators: a new anti-arrhythmic principle. *Prog Biophys Mol Biol* 98, 347-362.

Grunnet M, Jespersen T, MacAulay N, Jorgensen NK, Schmitt N, Pongs O, Olesen SP, & Klaerke DA (2003). KCNQ1 channels sense small changes in cell volume. *J Physiol* 549, 419-427.

Grunnet M, Jespersen T, Rasmussen HB, Ljungstrom T, Jorgensen NK, Olesen SP, & Klaerke DA (2002). KCNE4 is an inhibitory subunit to the KCNQ1 channel. *J Physiol* 542, 119-130.

Hagiwara N, Irisawa H, & Kameyama M (1988). Contribution of two types of calcium currents to the pacemaker potentials of rabbit sino-atrial node cells. *J Physiol* 395, 233-253.

Heitzmann D, Koren V, Wagner M, Sterner C, Reichold M, Tegtmeier I, Volk T, & Warth R (2007). KCNE beta subunits determine pH sensitivity of KCNQ1 potassium channels. *Cell Physiol Biochem* 19, 21-32.

Herfst LJ, Potet F, Bezzina CR, Groenewegen WA, Le MH, Hoorntje TM, Demolombe S, Baro I, Escande D, Jongsma HJ, Wilde AA, & Rook MB (2003). Na+ channel mutation leading to loss of function and non-progressive cardiac conduction defects. *J Mol Cell Cardiol* 35, 549-557.

Hershko A & Ciechanover A (1998). The ubiquitin system. *Annu Rev Biochem* 67, 425-479.

Hicke L (1999). Gettin' down with ubiquitin: turning off cell-surface receptors, transporters and channels. *Trends Cell Biol* 9, 107-112.

Hille B (2001). *Ion Channels of Excitable Membranes,* third ed. Sunderland, Mass: Sinauer Associates.

Holm H, Gudbjartsson DF, Arnar DO, Thorleifsson G, Thorgeirsson G, Stefansdottir H, Gudjonsson SA, Jonasdottir A, Mathiesen EB, Njolstad I, Nyrnes A, Wilsgaard T, Hald EM, Hveem K, Stoltenberg C, Lochen ML, Kong A, Thorsteinsdottir U, & Stefansson K (2010). Several common variants modulate heart rate, PR interval and QRS duration. *Nat Genet* 42, 117-122.

Hu D, Barajas-Martinez H, Burashnikov E, Springer M, Wu Y, Varro A, Pfeiffer R, Koopmann TT, Cordeiro JM, Guerchicoff A, Pollevick GD, & Antzelevitch C (2009). A mutation in the beta 3 subunit of the cardiac sodium channel associated with Brugada ECG phenotype. *Circ Cardiovasc Genet* 2, 270-278.

Hume JR & Uehara A (1985). Ionic basis of the different action potential configurations of single guinea-pig atrial and ventricular myocytes. *J Physiol* 368, 525-544.

Isom LL, De Jongh KS, Patton DE, Reber BF, Offord J, Charbonneau H, Walsh K, Goldin AL, & Catterall WA (1992). Primary structure and functional expression of the beta 1 subunit of the rat brain sodium channel. *Science* 256, 839-842.

Ivanov SV, Ward JM, Tessarollo L, McAreavey D, Sachdev V, Fananapazir L, Banks MK, Morris N, Djurickovic D, vor-Henneman DE, Wei MH, Alvord GW, Gao B, Richardson JA, Minna JD, Rogawski MA, & Lerman MI (2004). Cerebellar ataxia, seizures, premature death, and cardiac abnormalities in mice with targeted disruption of the Cacna2d2 gene. *Am J Pathol* 165, 1007-1018.

Jespersen T (2011). Regulation and physiological function of Na(v)1.5 and KCNQ1 channels. *Acta Physiol (Oxf)* 202 Suppl 683, 1-26.

Jespersen T, Gavillet B, van Bemmelen MX, Cordonier S, Thomas MA, Staub O, & Abriel H (2006). Cardiac sodium channel Na(v)1.5 interacts with and is regulated by the protein tyrosine phosphatase PTPH1. *Biochem Biophys Res Commun* 348, 1455-1462.

Jespersen T, Grunnet M, & Olesen SP (2005). The KCNQ1 potassium channel: from gene to physiological function. *Physiology (Bethesda)* 20, 408-416.

Jespersen T, Rasmussen HB, Grunnet M, Jensen HS, Angelo K, Dupuis DS, Vogel LK, Jorgensen NK, Klaerke DA, & Olesen SP (2004). Basolateral localisation of KCNQ1 potassium channels in MDCK cells: molecular identification of an N-terminal targeting motif. *J Cell Sci* 117, 4517-4526.

Jiang M, Xu X, Wang Y, Toyoda F, Liu XS, Zhang M, Robinson RB, & Tseng GN (2009). Dynamic partnership between KCNQ1 and KCNE1 and influence on cardiac IKs current amplitude by KCNE2. *J Biol Chem* 284, 16452-16462.

Johnson D & Bennett ES (2006). Isoform-specific effects of the beta2 subunit on voltage-gated sodium channel gating. *J Biol Chem* 281, 25875-25881.

Jost N, Virag L, Bitay M, Takacs J, Lengyel C, Biliczki P, Nagy Z, Bogats G, Lathrop DA, Papp JG, & Varro A (2005). Restricting excessive cardiac action potential and QT prolongation: a vital role for IKs in human ventricular muscle. *Circulation* 112, 1392-1399.

Kazen-Gillespie KA, Ragsdale DS, D'Andrea MR, Mattei LN, Rogers KE, & Isom LL (2000). Cloning, localization, and functional expression of sodium channel beta1A subunits. *J Biol Chem* 275, 1079-1088.

Knot HJ, Zimmermann PA, & Nelson MT (1996). Extracellular K(+)-induced hyperpolarizations and dilatations of rat coronary and cerebral arteries involve inward rectifier K(+) channels. *J Physiol* 492 (Pt 2), 419-430.

Ko SH, Lenkowski PW, Lee HC, Mounsey JP, & Patel MK (2005). Modulation of Na(v)1.5 by beta1-- and beta3-subunit co-expression in mammalian cells. *Pflugers Arch* 449, 403-412.

Kurachi Y, Nakajima T, & Sugimoto T (1986a). Acetylcholine activation of K+ channels in cell-free membrane of atrial cells. *Am J Physiol* 251, H681-H684.

Kurachi Y, Nakajima T, & Sugimoto T (1986b). On the mechanism of activation of muscarinic K+ channels by adenosine in isolated atrial cells: involvement of GTP-binding proteins. *Pflugers Arch* 407, 264-274.

Kurokawa J, Motoike HK, Rao J, & Kass RS (2004). Regulatory actions of the A-kinase anchoring protein Yotiao on a heart potassium channel downstream of PKA phosphorylation. *Proc Natl Acad Sci U S A* 101, 16374-16378.

Lakatta EG & DiFrancesco D (2009). What keeps us ticking: a funny current, a calcium clock, or both? *J Mol Cell Cardiol* 47, 157-170.

Larsen AP, Olesen SP, Grunnet M, & Jespersen T (2008). Characterization of hERG1a and hERG1b potassium channels-a possible role for hERG1b in the I (Kr) current. *Pflugers Arch* 456, 1137-1148.

Lees-Miller JP, Kondo C, Wang L, & Duff HJ (1997). Electrophysiological characterization of an alternatively processed ERG K+ channel in mouse and human hearts. *Circ Res* 81, 719-726.

Logothetis DE, Kurachi Y, Galper J, Neer EJ, & Clapham DE (1987). The beta gamma subunits of GTP-binding proteins activate the muscarinic K+ channel in heart. *Nature* 325, 321-326.

London B, Michalec M, Mehdi H, Zhu X, Kerchner L, Sanyal S, Viswanathan PC, Pfahnl AE, Shang LL, Madhusudanan M, Baty CJ, Lagana S, Aleong R, Gutmann R, Ackerman MJ, McNamara DM, Weiss R, & Dudley SC, Jr. (2007). Mutation in glycerol-3-phosphate dehydrogenase 1 like gene (GPD1-L) decreases cardiac Na+ current and causes inherited arrhythmias. *Circulation* 116, 2260-2268.

London B, Trudeau MC, Newton KP, Beyer AK, Copeland NG, Gilbert DJ, Jenkins NA, Satler CA, & Robertson GA (1997). Two isoforms of the mouse ether-a-go-go-related gene coassemble to form channels with properties similar to the rapidly activating component of the cardiac delayed rectifier K+ current. *Circ Res* 81, 870-878.

Lopatin AN, Makhina EN, & Nichols CG (1994). Potassium channel block by cytoplasmic polyamines as the mechanism of intrinsic rectification. *Nature* 372, 366-369.

Lopes CM, Zhang H, Rohacs T, Jin T, Yang J, & Logothetis DE (2002). Alterations in conserved Kir channel-PIP2 interactions underlie channelopathies. *Neuron* 34, 933-944.

Lu Z (2004). Mechanism of rectification in inward-rectifier K+ channels. *Annu Rev Physiol* 66, 103-129.

Ludwig A, Zong X, Jeglitsch M, Hofmann F, & Biel M (1998). A family of hyperpolarization-activated mammalian cation channels. *Nature* 393, 587-591.

Ma KJ, Li N, Teng SY, Zhang YH, Sun Q, Gu DF, & Pu JL (2007). Modulation of KCNQ1 current by atrial fibrillation-associated KCNE4 (145E/D) gene polymorphism. *Chin Med J (Engl)* 120, 150-154.

Macri V, Proenza C, Agranovich E, Angoli D, & Accili EA (2002). Separable gating mechanisms in a Mammalian pacemaker channel. *J Biol Chem* 277, 35939-35946.

Maier LS & Bers DM (2007). Role of Ca2+/calmodulin-dependent protein kinase (CaMK) in excitation-contraction coupling in the heart. *Cardiovasc Res* 73, 631-640.

Maier SK, Westenbroek RE, Schenkman KA, Feigl EO, Scheuer T, & Catterall WA (2002). An unexpected role for brain-type sodium channels in coupling of cell surface depolarization to contraction in the heart. *Proc Natl Acad Sci USA* 99, 4073-4078.

Makielski JC, Ye B, Valdivia CR, Pagel MD, Pu J, Tester DJ, & Ackerman MJ (2003). A ubiquitous splice variant and a common polymorphism affect heterologous expression of recombinant human SCN5A heart sodium channels. *Circ Res* 93, 821-828.

Mangoni ME & Nargeot J (2008). Genesis and regulation of the heart automaticity. *Physiol Rev* 88, 919-982.

Marionneau C, Couette B, Liu J, Li H, Mangoni ME, Nargeot J, Lei M, Escande D, & Demolombe S (2005). Specific pattern of ionic channel gene expression associated with pacemaker activity in the mouse heart. *J Physiol* 562, 223-234.

Marx SO, Kurokawa J, Reiken S, Motoike H, D'Armiento J, Marks AR, & Kass RS (2002). Requirement of a macromolecular signaling complex for beta adrenergic receptor modulation of the KCNQ1-KCNE1 potassium channel. *Science* 295, 496-499.

Matsuda H, Saigusa A, & Irisawa H (1987). Ohmic conductance through the inwardly rectifying K channel and blocking by internal Mg2+. *Nature* 325, 156-159.

Mazhari R, Nuss HB, Armoundas AA, Winslow RL, & Marban E (2002). Ectopic expression of KCNE3 accelerates cardiac repolarization and abbreviates the QT interval. *J Clin Invest* 109, 1083-1090.

McCrossan ZA & Abbott GW (2004). The MinK-related peptides. *Neuropharmacology* 47, 787-821.

McDonald TF, Pelzer S, Trautwein W, & Pelzer DJ (1994). Regulation and modulation of calcium channels in cardiac, skeletal, and smooth muscle cells. *Physiol Rev* 74, 365-507.

McDonald TV, Yu Z, Ming Z, Palma E, Meyers MB, Wang KW, Goldstein SA, & Fishman GI (1997). A minK-HERG complex regulates the cardiac potassium current I(Kr). *Nature* 388, 289-292.

Meadows LS & Isom LL (2005). Sodium channels as macromolecular complexes: implications for inherited arrhythmia syndromes. *Cardiovasc Res* 67, 448-458.

Medeiros-Domingo A, Kaku T, Tester DJ, Iturralde-Torres P, Itty A, Ye B, Valdivia C, Ueda K, Canizales-Quinteros S, Tusie-Luna MT, Makielski JC, & Ackerman MJ (2007). SCN4B-encoded sodium channel beta4 subunit in congenital long-QT syndrome. *Circulation* 116, 134-142.

Medina I, Krapivinsky G, Arnold S, Kovoor P, Krapivinsky L, & Clapham DE (2000). A switch mechanism for G beta gamma activation of I(KACh). *J Biol Chem* 275, 29709-29716.

Mikala G, Klockner U, Varadi M, Eisfeld J, Schwartz A, & Varadi G (1998). cAMP-dependent phosphorylation sites and macroscopic activity of recombinant cardiac L-type calcium channels. *Mol Cell Biochem* 185, 95-109.

Moosmang S, Biel M, Hofmann F, & Ludwig A (1999). Differential distribution of four hyperpolarization-activated cation channels in mouse brain. *Biol Chem* 380, 975-980.

Morales MJ, Castellino RC, Crews AL, Rasmusson RL, & Strauss HC (1995). A novel beta subunit increases rate of inactivation of specific voltage-gated potassium channel alpha subunits. *J Biol Chem* 270, 6272-6277.

Moroni A, Gorza L, Beltrame M, Gravante B, Vaccari T, Bianchi ME, Altomare C, Longhi R, Heurteaux C, Vitadello M, Malgaroli A, & DiFrancesco D (2001). Hyperpolarization-activated cyclic nucleotide-gated channel 1 is a molecular determinant of the cardiac pacemaker current I(f). *J Biol Chem* 276, 29233-29241.

Murray KT, Hu NN, Daw JR, Shin HG, Watson MT, Mashburn AB, & George AL, Jr. (1997). Functional effects of protein kinase C activation on the human cardiac Na+ channel. *Circ Res* 80, 370-376.

Nadal MS, Ozaita A, Amarillo Y, Vega-Saenz de ME, Ma Y, Mo W, Goldberg EM, Misumi Y, Ikehara Y, Neubert TA, & Rudy B (2003). The CD26-related dipeptidyl aminopeptidase-like protein DPPX is a critical component of neuronal A-type K+ channels. *Neuron* 37, 449-461.

Nakamura TY, Artman M, Rudy B, & Coetzee WA (1998). Inhibition of rat ventricular IK1 with antisense oligonucleotides targeted to Kir2.1 mRNA. *Am J Physiol* 274, H892-H900.

Nerbonne JM & Kass RS (2005). Molecular physiology of cardiac repolarization. *Physiol Rev* 85, 1205-1253.

Nielsen NH, Winkel BG, Kanters JK, Schmitt N, Hofman-Bang J, Jensen HS, Bentzen BH, Sigurd B, Larsen LA, Andersen PS, Haunso S, Kjeldsen K, Grunnet M, Christiansen

M, & Olesen SP (2007). Mutations in the Kv1.5 channel gene KCNA5 in cardiac arrest patients. *Biochem Biophys Res Commun* 354, 776-782.

Noma A, Kotake H, & Irisawa H (1980). Slow inward current and its role mediating the chronotropic effect of epinephrine in the rabbit sinoatrial node. *Pflugers Arch* 388, 1-9.

Noma A & Trautwein W (1978). Relaxation of the ACh-induced potassium current in the rabbit sinoatrial node cell. *Pflugers Arch* 377, 193-200.

Ohno S, Zankov DP, Ding WG, Itoh H, Makiyama T, Doi T, Shizuta S, Hattori T, Miyamoto A, Naiki N, Hancox JC, Matsuura H, & Horie M (2011). KCNE5 (KCNE1L) variants are novel modulators of Brugada syndrome and idiopathic ventricular fibrillation. *Circ Arrhythm Electrophysiol* 4, 352-361.

Olesen MS, Jespersen T, Nielsen JB, Liang B, Moller DV, Hedley P, Christiansen M, Varro A, Olesen SP, Haunso S, Schmitt N, & Svendsen JH (2011). Mutations in sodium channel beta-subunit SCN3B are associated with early-onset lone atrial fibrillation. *Cardiovasc Res* 89, 786-793.

Ono K & Iijima T (2010). Cardiac T-type Ca(2+) channels in the heart. *J Mol Cell Cardiol* 48, 65-70.

Panaghie G & Abbott GW (2006). The impact of ancillary subunits on small-molecule interactions with voltage-gated potassium channels. *Curr Pharm Des* 12, 2285-2302.

Patel SP & Campbell DL (2005). Transient outward potassium current, 'Ito', phenotypes in the mammalian left ventricle: underlying molecular, cellular and biophysical mechanisms. *J Physiol* 569, 7-39.

Patton DE, West JW, Catterall WA, & Goldin AL (1992). Amino acid residues required for fast Na(+)-channel inactivation: charge neutralizations and deletions in the III-IV linker. *Proc Natl Acad Sci USA* 89, 10905-10909.

Peretz A, Schottelndreier H, haron-Shamgar LB, & Attali B (2002). Modulation of homomeric and heteromeric KCNQ1 channels by external acidification. *J Physiol* 545, 751-766.

Petitprez S, Jespersen T, Pruvot E, Keller DI, Corbaz C, Schlapfer J, Abriel H, & Kucera JP (2008). Analyses of a novel SCN5A mutation (C1850S): conduction vs. repolarization disorder hypotheses in the Brugada syndrome. *Cardiovasc Res* 78, 494-504.

Pfeufer A, van NC, Marciante KD, Arking DE, Larson MG, Smith AV, Tarasov KV, Muller M, Sotoodehnia N, Sinner MF, Verwoert GC, Li M, Kao WH, Kottgen A, Coresh J, Bis JC, Psaty BM, Rice K, Rotter JI, Rivadeneira F, Hofman A, Kors JA, Stricker BH, Uitterlinden AG, van Duijn CM, Beckmann BM, Sauter W, Gieger C, Lubitz SA, Newton-Cheh C, Wang TJ, Magnani JW, Schnabel RB, Chung MK, Barnard J, Smith JD, Van Wagoner DR, Vasan RS, Aspelund T, Eiriksdottir G, Harris TB, Launer LJ, Najjar SS, Lakatta E, Schlessinger D, Uda M, Abecasis GR, Muller-Myhsok B, Ehret GB, Boerwinkle E, Chakravarti A, Soliman EZ, Lunetta KL, Perz S, Wichmann HE, Meitinger T, Levy D, Gudnason V, Ellinor PT, Sanna S, Kaab S, Witteman JC, Alonso A, Benjamin EJ, & Heckbert SR (2010). Genome-wide association study of PR interval. *Nat Genet* 42, 153-159.

Piper DR, Hinz WA, Tallurri CK, Sanguinetti MC, & Tristani-Firouzi M (2005). Regional specificity of human ether-a'-go-go-related gene channel activation and inactivation gating. *J Biol Chem* 280, 7206-7217.

Plaster NM, Tawil R, Tristani-Firouzi M, Canun S, Bendahhou S, Tsunoda A, Donaldson MR, Iannaccone ST, Brunt E, Barohn R, Clark J, Deymeer F, George AL, Jr., Fish FA, Hahn A, Nitu A, Ozdemir C, Serdaroglu P, Subramony SH, Wolfe G, Fu YH, & Ptacek LJ (2001). Mutations in Kir2.1 cause the developmental and episodic electrical phenotypes of Andersen's syndrome. *Cell* 105, 511-519.

Poelzing S & Veeraraghavan R (2007). Heterogeneous ventricular chamber response to hypokalemia and inward rectifier potassium channel blockade underlies bifurcated T wave in guinea pig. *Am J Physiol Heart Circ Physiol* 292, H3043-H3051.

Potet F, Scott JD, Mohammad-Panah R, Escande D, & Baro I (2001). AKAP proteins anchor cAMP-dependent protein kinase to KvLQT1/IsK channel complex. *Am J Physiol Heart Circ Physiol* 280, H2038-H2045.

Preisig-Muller R, Schlichthorl G, Goerge T, Heinen S, Bruggemann A, Rajan S, Derst C, Veh RW, & Daut J (2002). Heteromerization of Kir2.x potassium channels contributes to the phenotype of Andersen's syndrome. *Proc Natl Acad Sci USA* 99, 7774-7779.

Pusch M (1998). Increase of the single-channel conductance of KvLQT1 potassium channels induced by the association with minK. *Pflugers Arch* 437, 172-174.

Qin N, D'Andrea MR, Lubin ML, Shafaee N, Codd EE, & Correa AM (2003). Molecular cloning and functional expression of the human sodium channel beta1B subunit, a novel splicing variant of the beta1 subunit. *Eur J Biochem* 270, 4762-4770.

Qu J, Kryukova Y, Potapova IA, Doronin SV, Larsen M, Krishnamurthy G, Cohen IS, & Robinson RB (2004). MiRP1 modulates HCN2 channel expression and gating in cardiac myocytes. *J Biol Chem* 279, 43497-43502.

Qu Y, Isom LL, Westenbroek RE, Rogers JC, Tanada TN, McCormick KA, Scheuer T, & Catterall WA (1995). Modulation of cardiac Na+ channel expression in Xenopus oocytes by beta 1 subunits. *J Biol Chem* 270, 25696-25701.

Qu Y, Rogers J, Tanada T, Scheuer T, & Catterall WA (1994). Modulation of cardiac Na+ channels expressed in a mammalian cell line and in ventricular myocytes by protein kinase C. *Proc Natl Acad Sci USA* 91, 3289-3293.

Qu Y, Rogers JC, Tanada TN, Catterall WA, & Scheuer T (1996). Phosphorylation of S1505 in the cardiac Na+ channel inactivation gate is required for modulation by protein kinase C. *J Gen Physiol* 108, 375-379.

Radicke S, Cotella D, Graf EM, Banse U, Jost N, Varro A, Tseng GN, Ravens U, & Wettwer E (2006). Functional modulation of the transient outward current Ito by KCNE beta-subunits and regional distribution in human non-failing and failing hearts. *Cardiovasc Res* 71, 695-703.

Radicke S, Cotella D, Graf EM, Ravens U, & Wettwer E (2005). Expression and function of dipeptidyl-aminopeptidase-like protein 6 as a putative beta-subunit of human cardiac transient outward current encoded by Kv4.3. *J Physiol* 565, 751-756.

Radicke S, Vaquero M, Caballero R, Gomez R, Nunez L, Tamargo J, Ravens U, Wettwer E, & Delpon E (2008). Effects of MiRP1 and DPP6 beta-subunits on the blockade induced by flecainide of Kv4.3/KChIP2 channels. *Br J Pharmacol* 154, 774-786.

Ravens U & Dobrev D (2003). Cardiac sympathetic innervation and control of potassium channel function. *J Mol Cell Cardiol* 35, 137-139.

Ravn LS, Aizawa Y, Pollevick GD, Hofman-Bang J, Cordeiro JM, Dixen U, Jensen G, Wu Y, Burashnikov E, Haunso S, Guerchicoff A, Hu D, Svendsen JH, Christiansen M, &

Antzelevitch C (2008). Gain of function in IKs secondary to a mutation in KCNE5 associated with atrial fibrillation. *Heart Rhythm* 5, 427-435.

Ravn LS, Hofman-Bang J, Dixen U, Larsen SO, Jensen G, Haunso S, Svendsen JH, & Christiansen M (2005). Relation of 97T polymorphism in KCNE5 to risk of atrial fibrillation. *Am J Cardiol* 96, 405-407.

Rougier JS, van Bemmelen MX, Bruce MC, Jespersen T, Gavillet B, Apotheloz F, Cordonier S, Staub O, Rotin D, & Abriel H (2005). Molecular determinants of voltage-gated sodium channel regulation by the Nedd4/Nedd4-like proteins. *Am J Physiol Cell Physiol* 288, C692-C701.

Samie FH, Berenfeld O, Anumonwo J, Mironov SF, Udassi S, Beaumont J, Taffet S, Pertsov AM, & Jalife J (2001). Rectification of the background potassium current: a determinant of rotor dynamics in ventricular fibrillation. *Circ Res* 89, 1216-1223.

Sanguinetti MC, Curran ME, Spector PS, & Keating MT (1996a). Spectrum of HERG K+-channel dysfunction in an inherited cardiac arrhythmia. *Proc Natl Acad Sci USA* 93, 2208-2212.

Sanguinetti MC, Curran ME, Zou A, Shen J, Spector PS, Atkinson DL, & Keating MT (1996b). Coassembly of K(V)LQT1 and minK (IsK) proteins to form cardiac I(Ks) potassium channel. *Nature* 384, 80-83.

Sanguinetti MC, Jiang C, Curran ME, & Keating MT (1995). A mechanistic link between an inherited and an acquired cardiac arrhythmia: HERG encodes the IKr potassium channel. *Cell* 81, 299-307.

Santoro B, Liu DT, Yao H, Bartsch D, Kandel ER, Siegelbaum SA, & Tibbs GR (1998). Identification of a gene encoding a hyperpolarization-activated pacemaker channel of brain. *Cell* 93, 717-729.

Sasaki N, Mitsuiye T, Wang Z, & Noma A (1994). Increase of the delayed rectifier K+ and Na(+)-K+ pump currents by hypotonic solutions in guinea pig cardiac myocytes. *Circ Res* 75, 887-895.

Shi W, Wymore R, Yu H, Wu J, Wymore RT, Pan Z, Robinson RB, Dixon JE, McKinnon D, & Cohen IS (1999). Distribution and prevalence of hyperpolarization-activated cation channel (HCN) mRNA expression in cardiac tissues. *Circ Res* 85, e1-e6.

Sizarov A, Devalla HD, Anderson RH, Passier R, Christoffels VM, & Moorman AF (2011). Molecular analysis of patterning of conduction tissues in the developing human heart. *Circ Arrhythm Electrophysiol* 4, 532-542.

Soltysinska E, Olesen SP, Christ T, Wettwer E, Varro A, Grunnet M, & Jespersen T (2009). Transmural expression of ion channels and transporters in human nondiseased and end-stage failing hearts. *Pflugers Arch* 459, 11-23.

Soom M, Schonherr R, Kubo Y, Kirsch C, Klinger R, & Heinemann SH (2001). Multiple PIP2 binding sites in Kir2.1 inwardly rectifying potassium channels. *FEBS Lett* 490, 49-53.

Spector PS, Curran ME, Zou A, Keating MT, & Sanguinetti MC (1996). Fast inactivation causes rectification of the IKr channel. *J Gen Physiol* 107, 611-619.

Splawski I, Tristani-Firouzi M, Lehmann MH, Sanguinetti MC, & Keating MT (1997). Mutations in the hminK gene cause long QT syndrome and suppress IKs function. *Nat Genet* 17, 338-340.

Sridhar A, da Cunha DN, Lacombe VA, Zhou Q, Fox JJ, Hamlin RL, & Carnes CA (2007). The plateau outward current in canine ventricle, sensitive to 4-aminopyridine, is a constitutive contributor to ventricular repolarization. *Br J Pharmacol* 152, 870-879.

Staub O, Dho S, Henry P, Correa J, Ishikawa T, McGlade J, & Rotin D (1996). WW domains of Nedd4 bind to the proline-rich PY motifs in the epithelial Na+ channel deleted in Liddle's syndrome. *EMBO J* 15, 2371-2380.

Striessnig J (1999). Pharmacology, structure and function of cardiac L-type Ca(2+) channels. *Cell Physiol Biochem* 9, 242-269.

Sunose H, Liu J, & Marcus DC (1997). cAMP increases K+ secretion via activation of apical IsK/KvLQT1 channels in strial marginal cells. *Hear Res* 114, 107-116.

Szabo G, Szentandrassy N, Biro T, Toth BI, Czifra G, Magyar J, Banyasz T, Varro A, Kovacs L, & Nanasi PP (2005). Asymmetrical distribution of ion channels in canine and human left-ventricular wall: epicardium versus midmyocardium. *Pflugers Arch* 450, 307-316.

Taira N, Takahashi K, & Hosono M (1987). Effect of DHP-218, a novel dihydropyridine phosphonate, on atrioventricular nodal conductivity compared with its vascular effect in dogs. *J Cardiovasc Pharmacol* 10, 274-279.

Takano M & Kuratomi S (2003). Regulation of cardiac inwardly rectifying potassium channels by membrane lipid metabolism. *Prog Biophys Mol Biol* 81, 67-79.

Tan BH, Pundi KN, Van Norstrand DW, Valdivia CR, Tester DJ, Medeiros-Domingo A, Makielski JC, & Ackerman MJ (2010). Sudden infant death syndrome-associated mutations in the sodium channel beta subunits. *Heart Rhythm* 7, 771-778.

Tanabe T, Takeshima H, Mikami A, Flockerzi V, Takahashi H, Kangawa K, Kojima M, Matsuo H, Hirose T, & Numa S (1987). Primary structure of the receptor for calcium channel blockers from skeletal muscle. *Nature* 328, 313-318.

Terrenoire C, Clancy CE, Cormier JW, Sampson KJ, & Kass RS (2005). Autonomic control of cardiac action potentials: role of potassium channel kinetics in response to sympathetic stimulation. *Circ Res* 96, e25-e34.

Tfelt-Hansen J, Winkel BG, Grunnet M, & Jespersen T (2009). Inherited Cardiac Diseases Caused by Mutations in the Nav1.5 Sodium Channel. *J Cardiovasc Electrophysiol* 21:107-15.

Tinel N, Diochot S, Borsotto M, Lazdunski M, & Barhanin J (2000). KCNE2 confers background current characteristics to the cardiac KCNQ1 potassium channel. *EMBO J* 19, 6326-6330.

Torres NS, Larbig R, Rock A, Goldhaber JI, & Bridge JH (2010). Na+ currents are required for efficient excitation-contraction coupling in rabbit ventricular myocytes: a possible contribution of neuronal Na+ channels. *J Physiol* 588, 4249-4260.

Trudeau MC, Warmke JW, Ganetzky B, & Robertson GA (1995). HERG, a human inward rectifier in the voltage-gated potassium channel family. *Science* 269, 92-95.

Ueda K, Valdivia C, Medeiros-Domingo A, Tester DJ, Vatta M, Farrugia G, Ackerman MJ, & Makielski JC (2008). Syntrophin mutation associated with long QT syndrome through activation of the nNOS-SCN5A macromolecular complex. *Proc Natl Acad Sci USA* 105, 9355-9360.

Unsold B, Kerst G, Brousos H, Hubner M, Schreiber R, Nitschke R, Greger R, & Bleich M (2000). KCNE1 reverses the response of the human K+ channel KCNQ1 to cytosolic pH changes and alters its pharmacology and sensitivity to temperature. *Pflugers Arch* 441, 368-378.

Valdivia CR, Ueda K, Ackerman MJ, & Makielski JC (2009). GPD1L links redox state to cardiac excitability by PKC-dependent phosphorylation of the sodium channel SCN5A. *Am J Physiol Heart Circ Physiol* 297, H1446-H1452.

van Bemmelen MX, Rougier JS, Gavillet B, Apotheloz F, Daidie D, Tateyama M, Rivolta I, Thomas MA, Kass RS, Staub O, & Abriel H (2004). Cardiac voltage-gated sodium channel Nav1.5 is regulated by Nedd4-2 mediated ubiquitination. *Circ Res* 95, 284-291.

Van Norstrand DW, Valdivia CR, Tester DJ, Ueda K, London B, Makielski JC, & Ackerman MJ (2007). Molecular and functional characterization of novel glycerol-3-phosphate dehydrogenase 1 like gene (GPD1-L) mutations in sudden infant death syndrome. *Circulation* 116, 2253-2259.

Van PF, Clark KA, Chatelain FC, & Minor DL, Jr. (2004). Structure of a complex between a voltage-gated calcium channel beta-subunit and an alpha-subunit domain. *Nature* 429, 671-675.

Vandenberg CA (1987). Inward rectification of a potassium channel in cardiac ventricular cells depends on internal magnesium ions. *Proc Natl Acad Sci USA* 84, 2560-2564.

Vandenberg JI, Rees SA, Wright AR, & Powell T (1996). Cell swelling and ion transport pathways in cardiac myocytes. *Cardiovasc Res* 32, 85-97.

Wang Q, Curran ME, Splawski I, Burn TC, Millholland JM, VanRaay TJ, Shen J, Timothy KW, Vincent GM, de JT, Schwartz PJ, Toubin JA, Moss AJ, Atkinson DL, Landes GM, Connors TD, & Keating MT (1996). Positional cloning of a novel potassium channel gene: KVLQT1 mutations cause cardiac arrhythmias. *Nat Genet* 12, 17-23.

Wang Z, Fermini B, & Nattel S (1993). Sustained depolarization-induced outward current in human atrial myocytes. Evidence for a novel delayed rectifier K+ current similar to Kv1.5 cloned channel currents. *Circ Res* 73, 1061-1076.

Wang Z, Tristani-Firouzi M, Xu Q, Lin M, Keating MT, & Sanguinetti MC (1999). Functional effects of mutations in KvLQT1 that cause long QT syndrome. *J Cardiovasc Electrophysiol* 10, 817-826.

Warren M, Guha PK, Berenfeld O, Zaitsev A, Anumonwo JM, Dhamoon AS, Bagwe S, Taffet SM, & Jalife J (2003). Blockade of the inward rectifying potassium current terminates ventricular fibrillation in the guinea pig heart. *J Cardiovasc Electrophysiol* 14, 621-631.

Watanabe H, Darbar D, Kaiser DW, Jiramongkolchai K, Chopra S, Donahue BS, Kannankeril PJ, & Roden DM (2009). Mutations in sodium channel beta1- and beta2-subunits associated with atrial fibrillation. *Circ Arrhythm Electrophysiol* 2, 268-275.

Watanabe H, Koopmann TT, Le SS, Yang T, Ingram CR, Schott JJ, Demolombe S, Probst V, Anselme F, Escande D, Wiesfeld AC, Pfeufer A, Kaab S, Wichmann HE, Hasdemir C, Aizawa Y, Wilde AA, Roden DM, & Bezzina CR (2008). Sodium channel beta1 subunit mutations associated with Brugada syndrome and cardiac conduction disease in humans. *J Clin Invest* 118, 2260-2268.

Weerapura M, Nattel S, Chartier D, Caballero R, & Hebert TE (2002). A comparison of currents carried by HERG, with and without coexpression of MiRP1, and the native rapid delayed rectifier current. Is MiRP1 the missing link? *J Physiol* 540, 15-27.

Weiss R, Barmada MM, Nguyen T, Seibel JS, Cavlovich D, Kornblit CA, Angelilli A, Villanueva F, McNamara DM, & London B (2002). Clinical and molecular heterogeneity in the Brugada syndrome: a novel gene locus on chromosome 3. *Circulation* 105, 707-713.

West JW, Patton DE, Scheuer T, Wang Y, Goldin AL, & Catterall WA (1992). A cluster of hydrophobic amino acid residues required for fast Na(+)-channel inactivation. *Proc Natl Acad Sci USA* 89, 10910-10914.

Wickman K, Krapivinsky G, Corey S, Kennedy M, Nemec J, Medina I, & Clapham DE (1999). Structure, G protein activation, and functional relevance of the cardiac G protein-gated K+ channel, IKACh. *Ann N Y Acad Sci* 868, 386-398.

Wu DM, Jiang M, Zhang M, Liu XS, Korolkova YV, & Tseng GN (2006). KCNE2 is colocalized with KCNQ1 and KCNE1 in cardiac myocytes and may function as a negative modulator of I(Ks) current amplitude in the heart. *Heart Rhythm* 3, 1469-1480.

Wu G, Ai T, Kim JJ, Mohapatra B, Xi Y, Li Z, Abbasi S, Purevjav E, Samani K, Ackerman MJ, Qi M, Moss AJ, Shimizu W, Towbin JA, Cheng J, & Vatta M (2008). alpha-1-syntrophin mutation and the long-QT syndrome: a disease of sodium channel disruption. *Circ Arrhythm Electrophysiol* 1, 193-201.

Xue T, Marban E, & Li RA (2002). Dominant-negative suppression of. *Circ Res* 90, 1267-1273.

Yang EK, Alvira MR, Levitan ES, & Takimoto K (2001). Kvbeta subunits increase expression of Kv4.3 channels by interacting with their C termini. *J Biol Chem* 276, 4839-4844.

Yu H, Wu J, Potapova I, Wymore RT, Holmes B, Zuckerman J, Pan Z, Wang H, Shi W, Robinson RB, El-Maghrabi MR, Benjamin W, Dixon J, McKinnon D, Cohen IS, & Wymore R (2001). MinK-related peptide 1: A beta subunit for the HCN ion channel subunit family enhances expression and speeds activation. *Circ Res* 88, E84-E87.

Yuill KH & Hancox JC (2002). Characteristics of single cells isolated from the atrioventricular node of the adult guinea-pig heart. *Pflugers Arch* 445, 311-320.

Zaritsky JJ, Redell JB, Tempel BL, & Schwarz TL (2001). The consequences of disrupting cardiac inwardly rectifying K(+) current (I(K1)) as revealed by the targeted deletion of the murine Kir2.1 and Kir2.2 genes. *J Physiol* 533, 697-710.

Zaza A, Robinson RB, & DiFrancesco D (1996). Basal responses of the L-type Ca2+ and hyperpolarization-activated currents to autonomic agonists in the rabbit sino-atrial node. *J Physiol* 491 (Pt 2), 347-355.

Zhang SH, Kobayashi R, Graves PR, Piwnica-Worms H, & Tonks NK (1997). Serine phosphorylation-dependent association of the band 4.1-related protein-tyrosine phosphatase PTPH1 with 14-3-3beta protein. *J Biol Chem* 272, 27281-27287.

Zicha S, Xiao L, Stafford S, Cha TJ, Han W, Varro A, & Nattel S (2004). Transmural expression of transient outward potassium current subunits in normal and failing canine and human hearts. *J Physiol* 561, 735-748.

4

The Pathophysiological Implications of TRP Channels in Cardiac Arrhythmia

Ryuji Inoue, Duan Yubin, Hu Yaopeng and Jun Ichikawa
Department of Physiology, Fukuoka University School of Medicine
Japan

1. Introduction

The cardiac arrhythmia is a common cause of morbidity and mortality in the present world, especially in developed countries. The etiology of cardiac arrhythmia is quite broad involving both hereditary and secondary backgrounds. An increasing number of rare but lethal arrhythmogenic mutations have been identified by genome-wide association assays in genes associated with cardiac excitation, conduction and morphogenesis. Such well-characterized examples include causative mutations in voltage-dependent Na^+, Ca^{2+} or K^+ channel (Na_v, Ca_v, K_v) genes for the prolongation of QT interval which sometimes result in premature sudden death and may act as predisposing factors to drug-induced arrhythmia (Chen et al., 1998; Roden, 2004; Saenen & Vrints, 2008; Towbin & Vatta, 2001; Zareba et al., 2004). Furthermore, some of heart malformations (e.g. atrial septal defect) and idiopathic cardiomyopathy (e.g. dilated cardiomyopathy) with symptoms of arrhythmias have also proved to have some genetic linkage to impaired impulse conduction (Benson et al., 1999; Bonne, et al.,2001; Schott et al., 1998). However, much more prevalent are rhythm disturbances and conduction failures occurring in 'remodeling' hearts which progressively undergo structural and electrical changes in prolonged metabolically and mechanically stressed states, e.g. chronic heart failure and myocardial infarction (Nattel, 2007; Olson, 2005). The well-known consequences of cardiac remodeling are; altered expression and gating properties of ion channels shaping the action potential and generating pace-making activities; reduced electrical coupling which leads to aberrant conduction of excitation. These changes are thought to work as the 'substrates' increasing the risk of lethal cardiac arrhythmia (Janse, 2004; Nattel, 2007). It has also been known that abnormal handling of intracellular Ca^{2+} occurring in the remodeled heart may cause spontaneous membrane depolarizations triggering ectopic excitations (Dobrev, 2010; Janse, 2004; Nattel, 2007). However, the available knowledge is still limited largely to ion channels/transporters/pumps whose roles in the cardiac excitation-contraction cycle have relatively been well established.

The transient receptor potential (TRP) channels constitute a newly-emerging non-selective cation channel (NSCC) superfamily activated by a plethora of physico-chemical stimuli other than voltage change. Because of this unique activation profile as well as the ability to permeate Ca^{2+} (except for TRPM4/TRPM5), TRP channels have attracted great attention as promising candidate molecules elucidating a variety of biological functions and disorders associated with slow sustained Ca^{2+} influx initiated by neurohormonal factors, pheromones, mechanical (membrane stretch/bending, osmotic change, shear force etc.) and thermal (from cold through cool and warm to heat) stresses, noxious stimuli (acid, respiratory irritants and toxicants) and many gustatory and pungent/cooling agents (camphor, citral, capsaicin, eucalyptol, icilin, menthol, allicin, mustard oil, sweet, umami and bitter tastants etc.) (Holzer, 2011; Vay et al., 2011; Wu et al., 2010). In the cardiovascular system, recent investigations have revealed pathophysiological implications of TRP channels in vasospasm, hypertension, occlusive vascular diseases, cardiac hypertrophy, cardiomyopathy and cardiac arrhythmia (Dietrich et al., 2010; Inoue et al, 2009b; Watanabe et al., 2008). Especially, as will be described below, involvement of some TRP channels in abnormal intracellular Ca^{2+} handling and increased responses to mechanical and noxious stresses may make them particularly relevant to the pathogenesis of acquired cardiac arrhythmias tightly associated with cardiac hypertrophy and failure, myocardial infarction and atrial fibrillation (Nattel, 2007; Ter Keurs & Boyden, 2007).

This chapter will deal with the arrhythmogenic potential of several TRP isoforms identified in the cardiovascular system, with brief introduction to the general concepts of cardiac arrhythmia and its connection to cardiac diseases and with several examples in which the roles of TRP channels have been established or suggested.

2. Factors contributing to cardiac arrhythmia

Cardiac arrhythmia is the abnormality of cardiac rhythm, the highly coordinated and integrated electrophysiological behavior of multiple ion channels/transporters/exchangers residing in tens of billions of myocytes and non-myoctes consisting of the heart. Clinically, cardiac arrhythmia can be defined as any anomalous excitations out of normal sinus control, and is conventionally classified into bradyarrhythmia (<50 beats per minute) and tachyarrhythmia (>100). Faulty or abnormal excitation of sinus node and various extents of conduction blocks mainly explain the former. In contrast, ectopic excitations occurring outside the sinus node (triggered activity, ectopic automaticity) and perpetuation of spiral/scroll waves rotating around a central core/filament (reentry) are thought to contribute to the latter. Although the mechanism remains still incompletely understood, shortened refractoriness, slowed and anisotropic conduction facilitate the occurrence of reentry (Jalife, 2000). Thus, altered expression or activities of ion channels contributing to the upstroke (Na_v) and repolarization of action potential (K_v) as well as those determining the conduction velocity and cell-to-cell coupling [Na_v and connexins (Cx), respectively] are involved in the reentrant mechanism.

Ectopic excitations result from premature depolarizations before the next normal excitation arrives. Early afterdepolarization (EAD) occurs before the repolarization of action potential completely terminates, thereby prolonging it and evoking premature action potentials due to re-opening of Na_v and/or Ca_v channels. This is a mechanistic background for the initiation of a specific form of polymorphic ventricular arrhythmias (Torsades de pointes) observed in both congenital and drug-induced Long QT syndromes; the function of 'repolarization reserve', i.e. K_v channels, is compromised, or residual activity of Na_v channel sustains because of its incomplete inactivation (Roberts & Gollob, 2010).

Delayed afterdepolarization (DAD) is thought to reflect the generation of transient inward currents (I_{ti}) activated by diastolic Ca^{2+} release from the sarcoplasmic reticulum (SR) of myocytes (Venetucci et al., 2008). If the magnitude of DAD exceeds the threshold of Na_v channel activation, an extrasystolic discharge of action potentials occurs. Sustained discharges from one or more foci may propagate around to cause tachyarrhythmias (focal excitation). In ventricular myocytes from rabbit failing heart which shows spontaneous ventricular tachyarrhythima, I_{ti} has been ascribed exclusively to enhanced forward-mode Na^+/Ca^{2+} exchanger type 1 (NCX1) current (Pogwizd et al., 2001; Pogwizd & Bers, 2004). However, there is evidence that implicates Ca^{2+}-dependent Cl^- and nonselective cationic conductances in the genesis of DAD (Han & Ferrier, 1992; Hill et al., 1988; Kass et a., 1978; Laflamme & Becker, 1996; Wu & Anderson, 2000). The mechanism underlying the diastolic Ca^{2+} release is likely to reflect Ca^{2+} overload into the sarcoplasmic reticulum (SR) caused by a net increase in Ca^{2+} uptake into the SR (increased Ca^{2+} influx and SRECA2a Ca^{2+}-ATPase activity), or the dysfunction of ryanodine type 2 receptor (RyR2) which may, especially when intensively phosphorylated by protein kinase A (Wehrens et al., 2003) or Ca^{2+}/calmodulin-dependent kinase II (Ai et al, 2005), causes a diastolic Ca^{2+} leak from the SR (Bers, 2006). Thus, under excessive sympathetic activities (hard exercise, mental stress, chronic heart diseases) or upon the application of drugs increasing the cAMP level (caffeine, catecholamines, phosphodiesterase inhibitors) or $[Na^+]_i$ (digitalis) in cardiomyocytes which increase Ca^{2+} loading into the SR, the occurrence of DAD and resultant tachyarrhythmias may be greatly enhanced (Pogwizd, 2003; Sipido, 2007; Venetucci, 2008). In addition, in some pathological settings such as unphysiologically decreased extracellular K^+ level and excessive sympathetic activity, ectopic automaticity, particularly in the Purkinje fiber, can also be abnormally increased to cause tachyarrhythmias (Osadchii, 2010).

Clinical significance of mechanical loading in inducing arrhythmia has been well recognized (Dean & Lab, 1989). It is widely accepted that both acute and chronic stretch of myocardial tissue significantly affects its electrophysiological properties to increase the propensity for arrhythmia (Janse, 2003; Ravens, 2003). Experimentally, a transient diastolic stretch of isolated left ventricle was shown to induce ventricular arrhythmia which was inhibited by micromolar Gd^{3+} (Hansen *et al.* 1991; Stancy *et al*, 1992). Atrial fibrillation elicited by an acute increase in intra-atrial pressure in isolated rabbit hearts was also found effectively blocked by MSCC blockers, Gd^{3+} and a *Tarantula* toxin GsMTx-4 (Franz and Bode, 2003; Suchyna, 2000). At the single cell level, Kamkin *et al.* (2000a) demonstrated that direct stretch of a ventricular myocyte could cause membrane depolarization and prolongation of action potential resembling EAD, which, at extensive stretch, led to an extrasystolic depolarization. This stretch-induced depolarization was attributed to the activation of Gd^{3+}-sensitive mechanosensitive NSCCs (MSCCs) (Hamill & Martinac, 2001; Inoue et al., 2009b). The stretch sensitivity of MSCCs was significantly enhanced in hypertrophied cardiomyocytes with increased susceptibility to stretch-induced arrhythmia (Kamkin et al., 2000a). Considering that the heart is continuously subjected to hemodynamic stresses and deformation due to contraction, mechanical stresses may play a significant role in the causality and severity of arrhythmia, particularly under pressure- and volume-overloaded conditions.

3. Connection of cardiac diseases to cardiac remodeling and arrhythmia

The cardiac remodeling can be defined as the restructuring and reactivation of differentiated cardiac tissues comprised of myocytic and non-myocytic populations, and is initiated and progressed by a complex interplay of genetic, environmental and aging factors (Cohn, et al., 2000; Fedak, et al., 2005; Swynghedauw, 1999). Chronic heart failure, myocardial infarction and atrial fibrillation (AF) are three common pathological states accompanying the remodeling process with arrhythmic changes; in which excessively activated sympathetic nervous and renin-angiotensin-aldosterone systems, increased generation of inflammatory cytokines and reactive oxygen/nitrogen species, and sustained mechanical stresses likely play active roles. The remodeling process is initially 'adaptive' to compensate the impaired pumping function, but gradually becomes 'maladaptive' with disturbances in rhythm formation and conduction as common clinical complications.

The key consequences of cardiac remodeling associated with the appearance of arrhythmia include both structural and electrical alterations. Enhanced collagen synthesis promotes the fibrotic replacement of damaged myocardial tissues thereby increasing the electrical heterogeneity. Altered expression and activities of ion channels, transporters and exchangers also bring about significant changes in the shape of action potential and its conduction properties as well as induce the susceptibility to premature excitations (Nattel, et al., 2007; Janse, 2004).

In chronic heart failure, the major electrophysiological changes are pronounced prolongation of action potential which often accompanies EAD-like membrane oscillations. These changes likely occur through decreased expression or activity of transient outward current (I_{to}; K_v4,3) and voltage-dependent K^+ channels forming the repolarization phase of action potential (I_{Kr}, I_{Ks}) (Bers, 2006; Janse, 2004; Nattel, et al.,2007; Ravens, 2010). The reduced inward rectifying K^+ current (I_{K1}) may also destabilize the membrane (i.e. increases the diastolic membrane resistance) and thereby enhance extrasystolic depolarizing responses (DAD) (Nattel, et al., 2007; Pogwitz et al, 2001). Furthermore, upregulation of hyperpolarization-activated current (I_f) and its mRNA (HCN2/4) (Cerbai, 1994; Fernandez-Velasco et al., 2003) and reduced expression of gap junction channel (Cx43; Dupont et al, 2001) have been reported to contribute to abnormally enhanced automaticity and impaired conduction, respectively. However, more notable changes observed in failing heart are abnormalities in intracellular Ca^{2+} handling (Bers, 2006; Janse, 2004). Despite a reduction in the SR Ca^{2+} content due to decreased expression of SERCA2a, the propensity for triggered activity based on DAD is enhanced. This likely reflects the other two major changes in Ca^{2+} handling, i.e. (1) the increased Ca^{2+} sensitivity of RyR2 under intensive phosphorylation by protein kinase A (however controversial now; Wehrens et al, 2003) or Ca^{2+}/calmodulin kinase II (Ai et al, 2005) which causes diastolic Ca^{2+} leak from the SR, and (2) upregulation of Na^+/Ca^{2+} exchanger (NCX1) protein which can carry depolarizing inward currents in the diastole. It has been suggested that increased β-adrenergic drive, which is prominent in chronic heart failure, may greatly facilitate the occurrence of DAD by increasing the Ca^{2+} content in the SR above the threshold of spontaneous Ca^{2+} release (Bers, 2006; Pogwizd, 2003).

Myocardial infarction is initiated by a sudden cessation of blood supply to heart tissues (i.e. myocardial ischemia), most frequently by thrombotic obstruction of coronary arteries. The time course of ischemic changes in the heart is variable and complex, and can mechanistically be distinguished between early and late acute phases, and subsequent postinfarction period vulnerable to structural and electrical remodeling (Clements-Jewery et al., 2005; Janse & Wit, 1989; Nattel et al., 2007). In acute phases, rapid depletion of intracellular ATP and accumulation of intracellular ADP, extracellular K^+ and lactate occur because of anaerobic glycolysis, and loss of intracellular K^+ and intracellular acidosis follows. The extracellular accumulation of K^+ leads to the depolarization of myocyte membrane that attenuates the amplitude and upstroke velocity of action potential (facilitated Na_v inactivation) and the shortening of action potential duration (due to enhanced K_v activities) or refractoriness. Simultaneously, intercellular accumulation and release of many biochemical substances occurs including catecholamines, ATP, lysophosphatidylcholine, cytokines (e.g., TNFα), reactive oxygen species (ROS), and platelet-activating factors (Clements-Jewery et al., 2005; de Jong & Dekker, 2010). All these possess arrhythmogenic potential to induce ventricular premature excitations (DAD, EAD) and reentry. In postinfarction period, down-regulation of K^+ channels (I_{to}, I_{Ks}, I_{Kr}, I_{K1}) occurs in border-zones adjacent to infarct areas which impairs the repolarization of action potential leading to EAD, and altered intracellular Ca^{2+} handling facilitates spontaneous subcellular Ca^{2+} release events that can trigger arrhythmic episodes (Nattel, et al., 2007).

Atrial fibrillation (AF) is a common supraventicular tachyarrhythmia with rapid and highly irregular firing, being closely associated with aging and cardiovascular diseases such as heart failure, myocardial infarction, valvular diseases and hypertension (Nattel et al, 2007; Ravens, 2010). AF per se is thought to serve as an arrhythmogenic remodeling process, because the occurrence of AF itself progressively aggravates electrophysiological features and facilitates fibrotic changes of atrial tissues in favor of more frequent and sustained occurrences. This clinical feature is described "AF begets AF" and experimentally confirmed by the finding that rapid atrial pacing causes significant shortening of atrial refractoriness and persistent AF (Wijffels, et al. 1995). The major arrhythmogenic changes found for AF are marked shortening of action potential duration which reduces the refractoriness and increases the susceptibility to reentry (Nattel et al, 2007; Ravens, 2010). In AF, this change is combined with abnormal Ca^{2+} handling with increased Ca^{2+} release from the SR and augmented NCX1 expression which facilitates ectopic premature depolarizations (i.e. DAD) that serve as a trigger to initiate the reentry (Dobrev, 2010). Both reduced/increased or unchanged expression of gap-junction channels have been reported, but their increased regional heterogeneity may contribute to various extents of conduction failure and reentry (Nattel, et al., 2007).

4. TRP channels and cardiac arrhythmia

The above considerations strongly suggest that, although alterations in the genesis and conduction properties of action potential are undoubtedly of central importance, other factors, e.g. Ca^{2+} overload, increased stretch sensitivity and noxious stimuli generated in ischemia/reperfusion, may also play a vital role in arrhythmogenicity. It is also possible that structural remodeling (necrotic/apoptotic and fibrotic changes) may contribute to the electrical heterogeneity of the myocardium which may act as the pro-arrhythmic substrates for altered conduction and reentry. As described above, Ca^{2+}- and stretch-sensitivities, nociception as well as association to remodeling are the hallmark features of TRP channel members (Inoue et al., 2009b; Nishida & Kurose, 2008; Watanabe et al., 2008; Wu et al, 2010; Vay et al., 2011). Therefore, in the following, we would like to discuss about the pathophysiological relevance of several TRP isoforms particularly in these aspects of acquired arrhythmogenicity (see Table 1).

	Intrinsic activator/modulator	possible arrhythmogenic mechanisms	chemical agonists	inhibitors
		Cardiomyocyte		
TRPC1	store depletion, stretch?, GPCR stimulation (TRPC1/TRPC4 or C5), Ca^{2+}/CaM	strecth-induced EAD/DAD in hypertrophy?		Gd^{3+}, SKF, GsMTX-4?
TRPC3	const-act., store depletion, GPCR stimulation, BDNF, DAG, oxidative stress (TRPC3/C4), Ca^{2+}/CaM, PKC, PKG, Src	oxidative stress? and other mediators (ATP, UTP) during ischemia/reperfusion		Gd^{3+}, La^{3+}, SKF, 2-APB, flufenamate, Pyr-3
TRPC5	const-act, store depletion, GPCR stimulation, LPC、S1P、EGF, neurosteroids, oxdized phospholipids, Ca^{2+}/CaM, PGE_2、S-nitrosylation, thioredoxin, oxidative stress (H_2O_2)	possible relation to ischemia/oxidative stress in failing heart	Gd^{3+}, SKF, GsMTX-4?	Gd^{3+}, La^{3+} (high), SKF, 2-APB, BTP-2, ML-7, ML-9, propfol, halothane, chloroform
TRPC6	store depletion, stretch?, GPCR stimulation, GF, DAG, 20-HETE, PIP_3/PIP_2, Ca^{2+}/CaM, CaMKII, PKC, PKG、Fyn	stretch-inudced EAD/DAD in hypertrophy?	flufenamate	Gd^{3+}, La^{3+}, SKF, 2-APB, ML-9, ML-7, GsMTX-4?
TRPM2	oxidative stress (e.g. H_2O_2), ADPR, cADPR, NAADP, AMP, $[Ca^{2+}]$i, pH	oxidative stress in ischemia/reperfusion?		flufenamate, ACA, 2-APB
TRPM4	$[Ca^{2+}]_i$, GPCR stimulation, PIP_2, MgATP, ATP, ADP, AMP, voltage, PKC、CaM, spermine,	familial conduction block (PFHBI, ICCD), stretch-inudced EAD/DAD?, QT-elongation in hypertrophy, DAD in AF?	decavanadate, BTP-2	Gd^{3+}, flufenamate, clotrimazol, 9-PA
		cardiac fibroblast		
TRPC6	see above	anti-fibrogenesis	see above	see above
TRPM7	const-act, GPCR stimulation, $[Mg^{2+}]_i$, MgATP, ATP, CTP, GTP, UTP, pH, PIP_2, cAMP, PKA, spermine,	fibrogenesis in AF	2-APB (high)	Gd^{3+}, SKF, 2-APB (low), LOE908,
		respiratory sensory neuron		
TRPA1	cold (<17°C), $[Ca^{2+}]_i$, alkalosis, stretch, GPCR, PIP_2, PKA.	autonomic imbalance	**environmental irritants** (**acrolein**), allicin, allyl isothocyanate, citral, NSAIDs, eugenol, cinnamaldehyd, 2-APB, GsMTX-4	HC-030031
TRPV1	heat (>43°C)、acidity (pH<5.9)、12-HETE, 12-LOX metabolites, anandamide, chemokines、GPCR (e.g. bradykinin, ATP, PAR2)、NGF, GDNF, PKA, PKC, PI3K, Ca^{2+}/CaM, CaMK II, src, calcineurin, Ras/MAPK, SCF	autonomic imbalance	**enviromental irritants,** capsaicin, 2-APB、camphor, allicin, citral, resiniferatoxin, gingerol, eugenol, EtOH	capasazeine, ABT-102, AMG-517, GRC-6211, MK-2295, SB-366791, SB-705498,

Table 1. Arrhythmogenic TRP channels

Abbreviations; CaM, calmodulin: GPCR, G-protein-coupled receptor (Gq-coupled): const-act, constitutively active: BDNF, brain-derived neurotrophic factor: DAG, diacylglycerol: PKC, protein kinase C: PKG, protein kinase G: LPC, lysophosphatidylcholine: S1P, sphingosin 1-phosphate: EGF, epidermal growth factor: PGE2, prostaglandin E2: 20-HETE, 20-hydroxytetraenoic acid: PIP3, phosphatidylinositol 3,4,5-trisphospate: PIP2, phosphatidylinositol 4,5-trisphospate: CaMKII, calmodulin-dependent kinase II: ADPR, ADP ribose: cADPR, cyclic ADP ribose: NAADP, nicotinic acid adenine dinucleotide phosphate: PKA, protein kinase A: 12-HETE, 12-hydroxy-5,8,10,14-eicosatetraenoic acid: LOX, lipooxygenase: PAR2, Proteinase-activated receptor 2: NGF, nerve growth factor: GDNF, glial cell-line derived neurotrophic factor: MAPK, mitogen-activated protein kinase: SCF, stem cell factor: SKF, SK&F96365: BTP-2, 4-methyl-4 -[3,5-bis(trifluoromethyl)-1H-pyrazol-1-yl]-1,2,3-thiadiazole-5-carboxanilide: Pyr-2, Ethyl-1-(4-(2,3,3-trichloroacrylamide)phenyl)-5-(trifluoroluoromethyl)-1H-pyrazole-4-carboxylate: 2-APB, 2-aminoethoxydiphenyly boroate, 9-PA, 9-phenanthrol.

4.1 Stretch-induced arrhythmia in pathological settings

As described above, acute stretch of cardiac muscle can induce arrhythmic responses in both atrium and ventricle, which are inhibited by widely used MSCC blockers Gd^{3+} and GsMTx-4. This has led to the speculation that activation of nonselective cationic MSCCs causes premature depolarizations. There are at least three candidates for these MSCCs in TRPs expressed in the heart, i.e. TRPC1, TRPC6 and TRPM4.

In both heterologous and native overexpression systems, TRPC1 and TRPC6 have been found to activate in response to mechanical stimuli (Maroto *et al.*,2005; Spassova *et al.*, 2006). Albeit controversial (e.g. Inoue *et al.*, 2009a), the so-called MSCC-selective peptide blocker GsMTx-4 has been found to inhibit the mechanical activation of both TRPC1- and TRPC6-mediated MSCC activities (Maroto *et al.*,2005; Spassova *et al.*, 2006). TRPC1 and TRPC6 are ubiquitously expressed in whole myocardial tissues (Huang et al, 2009; Ward et al., 2008), and GsMTx-4 suppresses stretch-induced force development and concomitant $[Ca^{2+}]_i$ increase in mouse left ventricular trabecular muscle (Ward et al., 2008) and pressure-induced atrial fibrillation (Franz and Bode, 2003). Moreover, the expression of TRPC1 and TRPC6 is greatly increased in hypertrophied heart under prolonged pressure overload (Kuwahara, et al; 2006; Ohba, et al., 2007), where the susceptibility to mechanically-induced arrhythmia is also enhanced (Kamkin et al., 2000a). All these observations favor the view that TRPC1 and TRPC6 contribute to stretch-induced arrhythmias as MSCCs in some pathological settings. However, there is controversy over the mechanosensitivity of these two TRPC channels. In knock-out mice deficient in TRPC1 or TRPC6 expression, pressure-induced vasoconstriction (myogenic response), which is believed to reflect the depolarizing effects of MSCC activation, was found intact (Dietrich et al., 2005; Gottlieb et al., 2007). Although this fact could not totally negate the roles of these TRP channels in the heart, it is essential to test whether mechanical activation of myocardial MSCCs and mechanical arrhythmogenicity are indeed impaired in these knock-out mice or vice versa in TRPC1- or TRPC6-overexpressing mice. Alternatively, it may also deserve to test the possible involvement of a recently identified GsMTx-4-sensitive MSCC, Piezo1/Piezo2, in stretch-induced arrhythmia in the heart (Bae et al., 2011).

In cerebral arterial myocytes, TRPM4 has been proposed as a MSCC responsible for myogenic response (Earley et al., 2004). However, again, the results from TRPM4-deficient mice do not support this role (for more detail, see below) (Mathar et al., 2010). Nevertheless,

it is noteworthy that TRPM4 can be secondarily activated by mechanical stretch through stretch-induced Ca^{2+} release from ryanodine-sensitive stores in arterial myocytes (Morita et al., 2007), since similar axial stretch-induced Ca^{2+} release from the SR has been demonstrated in cardiomyocytes (Iribe, et al., 2009). Considering that heart wall is periodically distended by diastolic filling pressure, this mechanosensitive mechanism may have considerable pathophysiological significance for the genesis of DAD in remodeled heart in which the expression of TRPM4 and Ca^{2+} loading into SR are prominently enhanced (see below).
It has been shown that repeated cyclic stretch induces hypertrophic responses of cardiac myocytes, which are significantly attenuated by antagonists for a PLC-linked G-protein coupled receptor (GPCR), angiotensin type 1 (AT_1) receptor (Komuro and Yazaki, 1993). This is explained by direct mechanical activation of unoccupied AT_1 receptor as demonstrated by the substituted cysteine accessibility mapping technique (Yasuda et al., 2008). Similar mechanical activation also appears to occur for many other PLC-linked GPCRs including endothelin ET_A, vasopressin V_{1A} and muscarinic M_5 receptors (Mederos y Schnitzler *et al.*, 2008). TRPC6 and its homologue TRPC3 are activated by stimulation of PLC-coupled GPCRs via generation of diacylglycerol (DAG) (Hofmann, et al., 1999) and Ca^{2+} influx through activated TRPC3 and TRPC6 channels has been shown to be essential for hypertrophic responses of caridomyocyte via calcineurin/NFAT pathway (Kuwahra et al., 2006; Bush et al., 2006; Onohara et al., 2006). In failing hearts where pressure overload is sustained, the release of catecholamines from sympathetic nerves and adrenal gland is increased (see above), and the production of angiotensin II (AngII) and expression of AT_1 receptor and angiotensin converting enzyme are greatly enhanced (Goette, A et al., 2000; Ihara M et al, 2000; Kaprielian RR et al., 1997). Moreover, the mechanosensitivity of TRPC6 channel is remarkably enhanced by the simultaneous stimulation of PLC-linked GPCRs via concerted actions of two lipid messengers DAG and 20-HETE (Inoue et al., 2009a). Thus, taken together, it is highly conceivable that sustained mechanical loads promote the hypertrophic remodeling of cardiomyocytes through synergistic interplay between excessive activation of GPCR-PLC pathways and enhanced receptor/mechanical activation of TRPC6 (and TRPC3) channels. This would in turn exacerbate Ca^{2+} overload into the myocyte SR to increase the propensity for pro-arrhythmic depolarizations. Consistent with this scenario, cardiac-specific TRPC6 transgenic mice have been found to exhibit much increased susceptibility to mechanical stress with increased incidence of sudden death accompanied by severe macroscopic and histological signs of cardiomyopathy (Kuwahara et al., 2006). The same study also found that expression of TRPC6 was several-fold upregulated in human failing heart. Obviously, detailed electrophysiological analyses are required to corroborate whether the above changes could indeed induce the arrhythmogenicity.

4.2 Ca^{2+}-dependent arrhythmia

Abnormal Ca^{2+} handling or cycling in cardiac tissues is the main cause for arrhythmia (Ter Keurs & Boyden, 2007). As briefly introduced above, diastolic Ca^{2+} release (or leak) from the SR is a key event to initiate arrhythmogenic premature depolarizations DAD. Presently, the mechanism whereby DAD is generated by the Ca^{2+} release can be accounted for by the activation of three ionic conductances which can generate I_{ti} near the resting membrane potential; an electrogenic forward-mode NCX1 current which allows the influx of three Na^+ ions in exchange of one Ca^{2+} efflux after the repolarization has completed; and Ca^{2+}-activated Cl^- and nonselective cation channel (CAN) currents. Although the most accepted hypothesis suggests that I_{ti} is carried exclusively by enhanced forward-mode NCX1 inward current in failing ventricle (Pogwizd, et al. 2001; Pogwizd, 2003; Wu and Anderson, 1999), there is also experimental evidence suggesting the involvement of Ca^{2+}-activated Cl^- current (Han et al., 1996; Laflamme et al., 1996) and CAN (Hill et al., 1988; Kass et a., 1978; Wu & Anderson, 2000) in the genesis of I_{ti}.

CAN constitutes a large heterogenous family of cation channels with varying unitary conductances, Ca^{2+}-sensitivities, voltage dependence and regulations, and distributes broadly in neurons, smooth muscle, heart, exocrine and endocrine glands, and other epithelial tissues (Siemen, 1993). The most frequently recorded CAN from cardiac tissues, first identified in a cultured rat neonatal ventricular myocyte (Colquhoun, 1981), is a 20-40pS channel with almost equal selectivity over monovalent cations and poor permeability to divalent cations (Guinamard et al, 2006). Albeit rather great variations, these cardiac CANs are activated by the micro- to mili-molar range of Ca^{2+} and voltage-dependent. The molecular identification that best fits this type of CAN is now thought to be TRPM4 protein (Launay et al., 2002). Expressed TRPM4 channel shows a ~25pS conductance (in near-physiological ionic milieu), is monovalent cation-selective, and, in cell-free conditions, undergoes Ca^{2+}-dependent activation and depolarization-dependent enhancement of open probability only in their unphysiologically high ranges. However, it has been found that the Ca^{2+}- and voltage-sensitivities of TRPM4 rapidly shift to their much higher ranges immediately after the excision of patch membrane ('desensitization' or 'rundown'), and this is substantially prevented by pretreatment with MgATP, protein kinase C activators, maneuvers replenishing phosphatidylinositol 4,5-bisphosphate and increased temperature (Nilius, 2006). These findings suggest that, in vivo, TRPM4 may be more effectively regulated by physiological ranges of $[Ca^{2+}]_i$ and membrane potential. Expressed TRPM4 channel also undergoes negative regulation of free adenosine nucleotide phosphates (efficacy; ADP > ATP = AMP), and is subject to spermine block, so that severe ischemic conditions might affect this channel activity (Nilius et al., 2004).

In human, cardiac expression of TRPM4 is ubiquitous in the order of abundance; Purkinje fibers, septum, atrium, left and right ventricles (Kruse *et al.*, 2009). Guinamard *et al* (2002) found that expression of TRPM4-like CAN, which was virtually absent at the time of cell isolation, was progressively enhanced in rat dedifferentiating ventricular myocytes with the time of culture. Studies from the same group also found that purinergic receptor activation by ATPγS, PKC activators and DAG, all of which act as interventions to facilitate cardiac remodeling, enhanced the occurrence of TRPM4-like channel in cultured ventricular myocytes. This led to the postulation that remodeling of ventricular myocytes in response to excessive hypertrophic signals may enhance the activity of TRPM4 thereby increasing arrhythmogenic propensity mostly likely by increasing DAD. Consistent with this, in the hypertrophic heart of spontaneously hypertensive rat, the elongation of Q-T interval in electrocardiogram has been reported together with increased expression of TRPM4 protein and density of CAN (Guinamard *et al.*, 2006). Recent reports indicate that TRPM4 is more abundantly expressed in atrium and sinoatrial node (Demion et al, 2007; Guinamard, 2004; Kruse et al., 2009), where DAD-based tachyarrhythmias have been well established (Dobrev, 2010; Guinamard 2006; Nattel 2007; Raves, 2010). However, TRPM4-deficient mice showed no obvious abnormalities in heart rate, cardiac output, ejection fraction and cardiac contractility at basal conditions questioning a vital role of TRPM4 in physiological regulation of cardiac functions (Mathar *et al.*, 2009). Rather unexpectedly, the genetic deletion of TRPM4 caused postnatal development of high blood pressure due to increased sympathetic catecholamine secretion. These seemingly paradoxical observations might point to the pathological contribution of TRPM4 to arrhythmogenicity in diseased remodeling heart rather than to normal rhythm formation, in which the expression and activity of TRPM4 are enhanced.

A recent genetic analysis of human families with lethal conduction failure has found a gain-of-function mutation (c.19G→A in exon 1 or p.E7K) in the N-terminal domain of TRPM4 channel (PFHBI; progressive familial heart block type I) (Kruse et al., 2009). More recently, other TRPM4 mutations with very similar biological impacts (p.R164W, p.A432T, p.G844D) have also been assigned to autosomal dominant isolated cardiac conduction block (ICCD) of Lebanese and French families (Liu et al., 2010). Biochemical and immunocytochemical data suggested that these mutations increase the cell surface expression of TRPM4 protein due to desregulated SUMOylation/deSUMOylation process which results in impaired endocytotic protein degradation. The accompanying electrophysiological changes for these mutations are consistent with the biochemical/immunicytochemical data; the density of whole-cell CAN current was increased with little noticeable changes in macroscopic Ca^{2+} sensitivity and voltage dependence or in unitary conductance and open probability at single channel level. These results suggest that the number of functional channels were increased without altered biophysical properties. The precise pathogenic mechanism for these mutations to cause conduction block remains unclear. However, RT-PCR analysis indicated the highest expression of TRPM4 in Purkinje fiber, and detailed immunohistochemical examination showed strongly TRPM4-positive subendocardial bundles of Purkinje fibers branching and penetrating toward subepithelial layer (Kruse et al., 2009; Liu et al., 2010). These morphological findings, combined with a broadened QRS complex in ECG in both PFHBI and ICCD patients, led the authors to speculate that elevated TRPM4 expression may increase the membrane leak conductance thereby disabling action potential propagation along the Purkinje fibers. There are several previous studies showing that Ca^{2+} overload causes membrane oscillations in Purkinje fibers due to increased spontaneous Ca^{2+} release when Na^+ extrusion via Na^+/K^+-ATPase was pharmacologically inhibited (Kass et al., 1978; Kass & Tsien, 1982; Lederer & Tsien, 1976). Considering that TRPM4 may also act as a Na^+ entry pathway in response to GPCR stimulation (Launay, et al., 2002), the resultant increase in $[Na^+]_i$ might then elevate $[Ca^{2+}]_i$ via the reversed mode operation of NCX1 in Purkinje fiber cells (Bers, 2006; Pogwizd, 2003). This would not only facilitate Ca^{2+} overload and DAD generation due to increased TRPM4 channel activation, but could also induce cell death leading to cardiac injury/remodeling if the elevation of $[Ca^{2+}]$ would persist. Fibrotic replacement observed in the His-Purkinje fiber system of a PFHBI patient (Kruse et al., 2009) may support the latter possibility. Thus, the depolarizing and Na^+-permeating properties of TRPM4 channel could bring about both acute (induction of DAD) and chronic (conduction block due to remodeling) pro-arrhythmic effects.

4.3 Arrhythmia associated with ischemia and oxidative stress

In the acute phases of myocardial infarction, many arrhythmogenic substances are released (see above). ATP and UTP are amongst these, being released from cardiomycytes during ischemia and may promote the occurrence of ventricular tachyarrhythmias (Dutta et al., 2004; Kuzmin et al., 1998). In vitro, ATP can induce DAD-based arrhythmic depolarizations in single cadiomyocytes when combined with Ca^{2+} increasing agents such as catecholamines (Song & Belardinelli, 1994). In voltage-clamped adult ventricular myocytes, ATP/UTP can activate a sustained inward current via P2Y2 receptor and enhance the opening of 14 and 23pS single channel activities in a PLC-dependent manner. TRPC3 and TRPC7 proteins from rat ventricular myocytes immunocoprecipitated, and the macroscopic current induced by

ATP was suppressed by intracellular application of anti-TRPC3 antibody from the patch pipette (Alvarez et al., 2008). These findings are collectively interpreted as indicating that ATP/UTP may cause arrhythmia by activating TRPC3/TRPC7 heterotetrameric Ca^{2+} and Na^{+} entry channels whereby to facilitate intracellular Ca^{2+} overloading and trigger electrical activities. Consistent with this scenario, the same researchers' group has recently shown that flash photolysis of caged ATP can evoke one or even a train of extrasystolic contractions. Further, intraperitoneal injection of creatine, which is capable of buffering a sudden ATP/UTP release and clinically exhibits anti-arrhythmic effects, markedly reduced ventricular tachyarrhythmias and early death events in a rat coronary-ligature myocardial infarction model. These ameliorating effects of creatine were defective in an inactive creatine analogue β-guanidinopropionate (Vassort et al., 2010). Cell surface expression of TRPC3 was found tightly controlled by vesicular trafficking, cytoskeletal actin dynamics and interaction with caveolar or subsarcolemmal proteins and molecules (Groschner K, et al., 2005). And PLC stimulation by AngII in cardiomycytes was reported to facilitate the recruitment of TRPC3 complexed with NCX1 to cell membrane, resulting in the reverse mode Ca^{2+} entry through NCX1 (Eder et al., 2007). Thus, although the precise connection between TRPC3 (and possibly TRPC7) channel activation by ATP and arrhythmogenicty is unclear, the above mechanism may have particular pathophysiological significance in Ca^{2+}-dependent arrhythmogenesis during postinfaction remodeling period or sudden ischemic insult of hypertrophied heart, where enhanced expression of TRPC3 and sympathetic nerve activity play pivotal roles. Seemingly in line with these results, a recent independent study has reported that cardiomyocytes from TRPC3-overexressing mice show an increased susceptibility to apoptotic death due to Ca^{2+} overload when subjected to hypoxia/reoxgenation (Shan et al., 2007).

Oxidative stress causes tissue damage in a variety of pathological states including aging, cancer, neurogenerative disorders, autoimmune diseases, atherosclerosis and ischemia/reperfusion injury of myocardium (Chandra et al., 2000; Langley et al., 2004; Misra et al., 2009). Many reactive oxygen spices (ROS; $O_2^{-}\cdot$,$\cdot OH$, H_2O_2, NO, $\cdot ONOO^{-}$) are generated as the result of ischemia and reoxygenation and may confer the susceptibility to arrhythmia in direct and indirect ways (via modifying autonomic nerve activity (Danson et al., 2006; Misra et al., 2009). Several TRP members including TRPM2, TRPM7, TRPC5 and a TRPC3/TRPC4 heterooligomer are known to be activated by oxidative stresses (Miller & Zhang, 2011; Naylor et al., 2011; Poteser et al., 2006). TRPM2 is the first reported ROS-sensitive Ca^{2+}-permeable nonselective cation channel activated by H_2O_2, ADP-ribose, TNFα, and β-amyloid peptide, and is implicated in both physiological functions and pathophysiology including oxidant (H_2O_2)-induced cell damage/death in pancreatic β-cells and neurons. TRPM2 is positively regulated by intracellular Ca^{2+}, and its cell damaging action appears to be mediated at least in part by sustained $[Ca^{2+}]_i$ elevation (Takahashi et al., 2011). In myocardial infarction, reperfusion injury and congestive heart failure, elevated plasma levels of TNFα have been reported (Sack et al., 2000). TNFα can activate both cytotoxic and cytoprotective signaling pathways in many cell types including mitochondrial ROS production through the recruitment of caspase-8 into the death-inducing signaling complex (Kroemer et al., 2007; Zhu et al., 2006). Further, altered redox state changes the activity of cardiac ion channels and transporters regulating Ca^{2+} dynamics in the cardiomyocyte, i.e. L-type Ca_v, RyR2, NCX1 and SERCA2a (Zima & Blatter, 2006). In keeping with these observations, activation of TRPM2 by oxidative stress (H_2O_2) has been found to cause apoptotic/necrotic changes in single cardiomyocytes with ultrastructural changes characteristic of cardiac ischemia/reperfusion injury (Yang et al, 2006). Although whether these changes are pro-arrhythmic remains to be explored, it is possible that sustained $[Ca^{2+}]_i$ elevation through activated TRPM2 channel would disturb basal Ca^{2+} homeostasis underlying rhythmic excitations in cardiomyocytes thereby inducing Ca^{2+}-dependent arrhythmogenicity. The arrhythmogenic effect of TRPM2 may not necessarily be restricted to direct cell-damaging actions via sustained $[Ca^{2+}]_i$ elevation. It could occur indirectly through the production of inflammatory cytokines from ambient immune cells, as was demonstrated in an animal model of inflammatory bowel syndrome (Yamamoto et al., 2008).

In addition, expression of TRPC4 and TRPC5 was found to increase 2-3-fold in cultured rat cardiomyocytes subjected to downregulation of SERCA by siRNA technology which mimics the remodeling process of diseased heart (Seth et al., 2004). TRPC5 is known to be activated by many noxious stimuli such as H_2O_2 and LPC (Flemming et al., 2006; Naylor et al., 2011), and thus could act as a pro-arrhythmic mediator in ischemic remodeling heart. This possibility will be an intriguing subject of future investigation, together with other TRP isoforms implicated in the pathogenesis of cardiomyopathy (TRPV2, TRPC7; Iwata et al., 2003; Satoh et al., 2007).

4.4 Arrhythmia related to fibrosis

Cardiac fibroblasts occupy about 70% of whole cardiac cell populations, and, once placed in pathological states such as myocardial injury, oxidative stress and excessive mechanical stretch, start to proliferate and differentiate into the active phenotype 'myofibroblast'. Activated myofibroblasts secrete extracellular matrix proteins (e.g. collagen), matrix metaloproteinases, cytokines and growth factors thereby promoting the pathological restructuring of diseased heart with fibrotic replacement of damaged myocardial tissue (Souders, et al., 2009). Cardiac fibroblasts have a shallow resting membrane potential (-30 - -10mV) and are non-excitable themselves, but show mechanically-induced depolarizations well synchronized with spontaneous contractions of myocardium (Kamkin et al, 2000b; Kamkin et al, 2003). These electrophysiological properties allow them, by coupling electrically to myocytes as a leaky capacitor, to modify the electrical properties of myocyte action potential and its propagation (Yue et al., 2011). In contrast, fibrotic tissues generated by myofibroblasts act as a physical barrier insulating the spread of electrical currents between the bundles of cardiomyocytes. Thus, disturbances in the myocyte-fibroblast coupling and alterations in myocardial architecture due to spatially inhomogenous fibrosis can lead to cardiac arrhythmias associated with reentry or conduction block.

It has been known that fibrotic remodeling is a fundamental process underlying the perpetuation of AF. Atrial fibrosis is dependent on Ca^{2+}, but what source of Ca^{2+} is involved therein had been elusive. A recent study of Du *et al.* (2010) demonstrated that upregulation of TRPM7, a constitutively active Ca^{2+}/Mg^{2+} entry channel (Wu et al, 2010), and resultant Ca^{2+} influx was crucial for the progression of atrial fibrosis in AF patients. This was supported by the following evidence; (1) human atrial fibroblasts express TRPM7 protein abundantly, and show basal Ca^{2+} influx and spontaneously active Ca^{2+}-permeable inward currents with the fingerprint features of heterologously expressed TRPM7 channels [potentiation by low pH and inhibition/potentiation by low/high concentrations of 2-aminoethoxydiphenyly boroate (2-APB) respectively: Li et al., 2006, 2007]; (2) TRPM7-like current and accompanying Ca^{2+} influx were strikingly increased in parallel with the upregulation of TRPM7 expression in differentiated fibroblasts from AF patients; (3) all these changes were largely eliminated by knockdown of TRPM7 expression with small hairpin RNA; and (4) in vitro promotion of myofibroblastic differentiation by TGF-β1, a major stimulator of atrial fibrosis, was correlated with the upregulation of TRPM7. Although in this study a direct linkage between Ca^{2+} influx through TRPM7 channel, the fibrogenesis and arrhythmogenesis in AF have not been explored, the above results may provide a new therapeutic target against the progression of AF, by disclosing an essential role of TRPM7-asscociated Ca^{2+} influx in fibroblast proliferation and differentiation.

In rat neonatal cardiac fibroblasts, endothelin-1 (ET-1) or AngII can induce myofibroblastic differentiation and collagen synthesis via the $G\alpha_{12/13}$ signaling. ET-1 (via ET_A receptor) and AngII can also selectively enhance the expression of TRPC6, thereby increasing basal Ca^{2+} influx in the fibroblasts. Importantly, increased TRPC6 expression is causally correlated with anti-fibrotic effects via calcineurin/NFAT pathway (Nishida et al., 2007). The upregulation of TRPC6 likely occurs through the $G_{12/13}$- (Rac/NOX)-ROS-JNK signaling, which is reminiscent of TRPC6-mediated abnormal proliferation of pulmonary artery smooth muscle cells induced by platelet-derived growth factor, a pathogenic model of pulmonary artery hypertension (Yu et al., 2003). The concentrations of ET-1 or AngII required to upregulate TRPC6 are significantly higher than those for the differentiation of fibroblasts (Nishida et al., 2007). Thus, in an intriguing contrast to the pro-fibrotic role of TRPM7, the anti-fibrotic effects of enhanced TRPC6 channel activity may serve as a negative feedback mechanism to limit excessive fibrogenesis via ET-1/AngII signaling during cardiac remodeling. It remains to be determined whether this mechanism works beneficially in human AF patients or other fibrosis-associated arrhythmias.

4.5 Arrhythmia related to autonomic imbalance

The cardiac rhythm is under tight control of the autonomic nervous system. For instance, baroreceptors monitor blood pressure fluctuations and transmit the information to the brainstem vasomotor center via parasympathetic afferents, which then modulates the cardiac pumping force and rate via sympathetic efferents. The renin-angiotensin-aldosterone system is another well-established system centrally controlled via sympathetic nerves (via β_1-adrenoceptor). It fulfills a long-term control of body fluid and electrolyte balance, thereby effectively regulating the cardiac output (Guyenet, 2006). Any disturbances in these centrally-mediated autonomic regulations could therefore become the substrates for cardiac arrhythmias (Danson, et al., 2006; Janse 2004; Nattel, et al., 2007). Accumulating evidence however suggests that nociceptive reflexes via respiratory sensory neurons (e.g. C-fibers in nose and lung) have also some pathophysiological impact on cardiac functions through centrally-mediated autonomic mechanisms, as exemplified by air pollutant-induced changes in 'repolarization' parameters of ECG (Henneberger et al., 2005). The sensory nerve endings in respiratory airways contain two TRP members sensing noxious stimuli, i.e. TRPV1 and TRPA1 which likely participate in airway chemosensation and inflammation (Bessac & Jordt, 2008). It has thus been postulated that these TRP isoforms may be involved in nociceptive signaling in the respiratory system (Vay et al., 2011).

Two recent studies have revealed intriguing associations between respiratory sensory TRP channels and arrhythmogenicity. In one experimental model, activation of respiratory sensory neurons by inhalation of concentrated ambient particles significantly affected the cardiac rhythm with decreased heart rate, and shortened QT interval and P wave duration. Abrogation of these cardiac effects by a selective TRPV1 antagonist capsazepine suggested that TRPV1-mediated autonomic reflexes play a central role therein (Ghelfi et al., 2008). In another study employing a gaseous pollutant (Hazari et al., 2011), one-day exposure of rats to diesel exhaust gas resulted in increased heart rate with pro-arrhythmic ECG changes of prolonged action potential and shorted repolarization. Notably, these rats showed much heightened sensitivity to aconitine challenge that can induce moderate to lethal ventricular tachyarrhythmias dose-dependently. This pro-arrhythmic change was prevented by pretreatment with a TRPA1 antagonist HC-030031 or by sympathetic blockade with guanethidine, suggesting the involvement of increased sympathetic drive. In addition, partial involvement of TRPV1 in moderate aconitine-induced tachyarrhythmias was also suggested by pharmacological inhibition with a selective TRPV1 antagonist SB-366791. Although detailed mechanisms underlying remain unclear, these results clearly point to the pro-arrhythmic risk of environmentally-induced autonomic imbalance in which sensory chemosensing channels TRPA1 and TRPV1 may play a pivotal role.

5. Conclusions and therapeutic implications

The evidence presented above has disclosed that the unique activation profile (e.g. stretch- and Ca^{2+}-sensitivities, neurohormonal activation, sensitivity to noxious stimuli) and permeability to Ca^{2+} and Na^{+} (TRPM4/TRPM5 are however virtually Ca^{2+}-impermeable) render several TRP channels contribute to the acquired arrhythmogenesis during cardiac remodeling and other pathological processes. The examples so far available implicates, at least, TRPC1 and TRPC6 (and possibly their homologues) in stretch-induced arrhythmias in both acute and chronic manners, TRPM4 in Ca^{2+}-dependent arrhythmia and familial conduction block, TRPC3 and TRPM2 in ischemia-induced arrhythmia, TRPA1 and TRPV1 in autonomic imbalance-induced arrhythmia, and TRPM7 and TRPC6 in fibrosis-related arrhythmogenicity, especially in AF, as pro-fibrotic and anti-fibrotic factors respectively. Although the mechanism of the actions of each TRP isoform appears variable in different pathophysiological settings, these new lines of evidence have certainly put forward our essential understanding about the pathogenesis of commonly observed arrhythmias associated with cardiac diseases accompanying structural and electrical remodeling. Simultaneously it may open an avenue toward exploiting an entirely new generation of anti-arrhythmic drugs for increased mechanosensitivity, abnormal Ca^{2+} handling, oxidative stress, or nociception.

When considering the actual strategy for developing such drugs, however, there are at least two not easily tractable problems. The serious lack of structure-based chemical knowledge about the selectivity and efficacy for most TRP members is the first obvious one, although substantial progress is going on for analgesic therapy based on TRPV1 pharmacology (Szallasi et al., 2007). Virtually all drugs so far shown to be effective for cardiovascular TRP isoforms appear to be non-specific or have only narrow ranges of concentrations for their relatively selective actions, as exemplified by a pyrazole compound Pyr-3 for TRPC3 which reportedly inhibits experimentally-induced cardiac hypertrophy (Kiyonaka et al., 2009). The second type of difficulty for exploiting TRP-selective drugs is that connecting one TRP isoform to one end-function is almost always irrelevant oversimplification. This is because signaling pathways linked to TRPs appear to form a complex interwoven network with high degrees of divergence and convergence and with numerous feed-back and -forward regulations. In addition to this, activation of TRP channels depends intimately on local lipid dynamics in the cell membrane, which dramatically changes by lipid composition, voltage, temperature, membrane stretch, and enzyme-assisted catalysis (Hardie, 2007; Inoue et al.,

2009b). In the current absence of good knowledge about lipid physiology/pathophysiology for membrane proteins, these disadvantages would make it difficult to pharmacologically manipulate the gating of TRP channels. In this context, recent observations that activation of the cGMP-PKG signaling by nitric oxide, atrial natriuretic peptides and their structural and functional mimetics attenuate hypertrophic cardiac remodeling partly via inhibition of TRP channels (Inoue et al., 2010; Tsai & Kass, 2009) may provide a promising alternative maneuver to ameliorate the acquired arrhythmogenicity. Activation of this pathway is also known to improve myocardial damage after myocardial infarction (Burley et al., 2007; Garcia-Dorado et al., 2009). Obviously, there is much to be learned about the pathogenic roles and therapeutic potential of cardiovascular TRP channels for cardiac arrhythmias.

6. Acknowledgment

Part of this work is supported by Grants-in-aid for Scientific Research on Innovative Areas (No.22136008) and Scientific Research (C) (No. 21590246), and a grant from Seizon Kagaku Institute to R.I.

7. References

Ai, X., Curran, J. W., Shannon, T. R., Bers, D. M., & Pogwizd, S. M. (2005). Ca^{2+}/calmodulin-dependent protein kinase modulates cardiac ryanodine receptor phosphorylation and sarcoplasmic reticulum Ca^{2+} leak in heart failure. *Circ Res, 97*(12), pp. 1314-1322.

Alvarez, J., Coulombe, A., Cazorla, O., Ugur, M., Rauzier, J. M., Magyar, J., et al. (2008). ATP/UTP activate cation-permeable channels with TRPC3/7 properties in rat cardiomyocytes. *Am J Physiol Heart Circ Physiol, 295*(1), pp. H21-28.

Bae, C., Sachs, F.,& Gottlieb, P.A.(2011). The Mechanosensitive ion channel Piezo1 is inhibited by the peptide GsMTx4. *Biochemistry,50,* pp. 6295–6300.

Benson, D. W., Silberbach, G. M., Kavanaugh-McHugh, A., Cottrill, C., Zhang, Y., Riggs, S., et al. (1999). Mutations in the cardiac transcription factor NKX2.5 affect diverse cardiac developmental pathways. *J Clin Invest, 104*(11), pp. 1567-1573.

Bers, D. M. (2006). Altered cardiac myocyte Ca regulation in heart failure. *Physiology (Bethesda), 21,* pp. 380-387.

Bessac, B. F., & Jordt, S. E. (2008). Breathtaking TRP channels: TRPA1 and TRPV1 in airway chemosensation and reflex control. *Physiology (Bethesda), 23,* pp. 360-370.

Bonne, G., Di Barletta, M. R., Varnous, S., Becane, H. M., Hammouda, E. H., Merlini, L., et al. (1999). Mutations in the gene encoding lamin A/C cause autosomal dominant Emery-Dreifuss muscular dystrophy. *Nat Genet, 21*(3), pp. 285-288.

Burley, D. S., Ferdinandy, P., & Baxter, G. F. (2007). Cyclic GMP and protein kinase-G in myocardial ischaemia-reperfusion: opportunities and obstacles for survival signaling. *Br J Pharmacol, 152*(6), pp. 855-869.

Bush, E.W., Ho, D.B., Papst, P.J. *et al.* (2006). Canonical transient receptor potential channels promote cardiomyocyte hypertrophy through activation of calcineurin signaling. *J Biol Chem,* 281, pp.33487-96.

Cerbai, E., Barbieri, M., & Mugelli, A. (1994). Characterization of the hyperpolarization-activated current, I(f), in ventricular myocytes isolated from hypertensive rats. *J Physiol, 481 (Pt 3)*, pp. 585-591.

Chandra, J., Samali, A., & Orrenius, S. (2000). Triggering and modulation of apoptosis by oxidative stress. *Free Radic Biol Med, 29*(3-4), pp. 323-333.

Chen, Q., Kirsch, G. E., Zhang, D., Brugada, R., Brugada, J., Brugada, P., et al. (1998). Genetic basis and molecular mechanism for idiopathic ventricular fibrillation. *Nature, 392*(6673), pp. 293-296.

Clements-Jewery, H., Hearse, D. J., & Curtis, M. J. (2005). Phase 2 ventricular arrhythmias in acute myocardial infarction: a neglected target for therapeutic antiarrhythmic drug development and for safety pharmacology evaluation. *Br J Pharmacol, 145*(5), pp. 551-564.

Cohn, J. N., Ferrari, R., & Sharpe, N. (2000). Cardiac remodeling--concepts and clinical implications: a consensus paper from an international forum on cardiac remodeling. Behalf of an International Forum on Cardiac Remodeling. *J Am Coll Cardiol, 35*(3), pp. 569-582.

Colquhoun, D., Neher, E., Reuter, H., & Stevens, C. F. (1981). Inward current channels activated by intracellular Ca in cultured cardiac cells. *Nature, 294*(5843), pp. 752-754.

Danson, E. J., & Paterson, D. J. (2006). Reactive oxygen species and autonomic regulation of cardiac excitability. *J Cardiovasc Electrophysiol, 17 Suppl 1*, pp. S104-S112.

de Jong, J. S., & Dekker, L. R. (2010). Platelets and cardiac arrhythmia. *Front Physiol, 1*, article 166, pp. 1-8.

Dean, J. W., & Lab, M. J. (1989). Arrhythmia in heart failure: role of mechanically induced changes in electrophysiology. *Lancet, 1*(8650), pp. 1309-1312.

Demion, M., Bois, P., Launay, P., & Guinamard, R. (2007). TRPM4, a Ca^{2+}-activated nonselective cation channel in mouse sino-atrial node cells. *Cardiovasc Res, 73*(3), pp. 531-538.

Dietrich, A., Kalwa, H., & Gudermann, T. (2010). TRPC channels in vascular cell function. *Thromb Haemost, 103*(2), pp. 262-270.

Dietrich, A., Kalwa, H., Storch, U., Mederos y Schnitzler, M., Salanova, B., Pinkenburg, O., et al. (2007). Pressure-induced and store-operated cation influx in vascular smooth muscle cells is independent of TRPC1. *Pflugers Arch, 455*(3), pp. 465-477.

Dobrev, D. Atrial Ca^{2+} signaling in atrial fibrillation as an antiarrhythmic drug target. *Naunyn Schmiedebergs Arch Pharmacol, 381*(3), pp. 195-206.

Du, J., Xie, J., Zhang, Z., Tsujikawa, H., Fusco, D., Silverman, D., et al. (2010). TRPM7-mediated Ca2+ signals confer fibrogenesis in human atrial fibrillation. *Circ Res, 106*(5), pp. 992-1003.

Dupont, E., Matsushita, T., Kaba, R. A., Vozzi, C., Coppen, S. R., Khan, N., et al. (2001). Altered connexin expression in human congestive heart failure. *J Mol Cell Cardiol, 33*(2), pp. 359-371.

Dutta, A. K., Sabirov, R. Z., Uramoto, H., & Okada, Y. (2004). Role of ATP-conductive anion channel in ATP release from neonatal rat cardiomyocytes in ischaemic or hypoxic conditions. *J Physiol, 559*(Pt 3), pp. 799-812.

Earley, S., Waldron, B. J., & Brayden, J. E. (2004). Critical role for transient receptor potential channel TRPM4 in myogenic constriction of cerebral arteries. *Circ Res, 95*(9), pp. 922-929.

Eder, P., Probst, D., Rosker, C., Poteser, M., Wolinski, H., Kohlwein, S. D., et al. (2007). Phospholipase C-dependent control of cardiac calcium homeostasis involves a TRPC3-NCX1 signaling complex. *Cardiovasc Res, 73*(1), pp. 111-119.

Fedak, P. W., Verma, S., Weisel, R. D., & Li, R. K. (2005). Cardiac remodeling and failure: from molecules to man (Part I). *Cardiovasc Pathol, 14*(1), pp. 1-11.

Fernandez-Velasco, M., Goren, N., Benito, G., Blanco-Rivero, J., Bosca, L., & Delgado, C. (2003). Regional distribution of hyperpolarization-activated current (If) and hyperpolarization-activated cyclic nucleotide-gated channel mRNA expression in ventricular cells from control and hypertrophied rat hearts. *J Physiol, 553*(Pt 2), pp. 395-405.

Flemming, P. K., Dedman, A. M., Xu, S. Z., Li, J., Zeng, F., Naylor, J., et al. (2006). Sensing of lysophospholipids by TRPC5 calcium channel. *J Biol Chem, 281*(8), pp. 4977-4982.

Franz, M. R., & Bode, F. (2003). Mechano-electrical feedback underlying arrhythmias: the atrial fibrillation case. *Prog Biophys Mol Biol, 82*(1-3), pp. 163-174.

Garcia-Dorado, D., Agullo, L., Sartorio, C. L., & Ruiz-Meana, M. (2009). Myocardial protection against reperfusion injury: the cGMP pathway. *Thromb Haemost, 101*(4), pp. 635-642.

Ghelfi, E., Rhoden, C. R., Wellenius, G. A., Lawrence, J., & Gonzalez-Flecha, B. (2008). Cardiac oxidative stress and electrophysiological changes in rats exposed to concentrated ambient particles are mediated by TRP-dependent pulmonary reflexes. *Toxicol Sci, 102*(2), pp. 328-336.

Goette, A., Staack, T., Rocken, C., Arndt, M., Geller, J. C., Huth, C., et al. (2000). Increased expression of extracellular signal-regulated kinase and angiotensin-converting enzyme in human atria during atrial fibrillation. *J Am Coll Cardiol, 35*(6), pp. 1669-1677.

Gottlieb, P., Folgering, J., Maroto, R., Raso, A., Wood, T. G., Kurosky, A., et al. (2008). Revisiting TRPC1 and TRPC6 mechanosensitivity. *Pflugers Arch, 455*(6), pp. 1097-1103.

Groschner, K., & Rosker, C. (2005). TRPC3: a versatile transducer molecule that serves integration and diversification of cellular signals. *Naunyn Schmiedebergs Arch Pharmacol, 371*(4), pp. 251-256.

Guinamard, R., Chatelier, A., Demion, M., Potreau, D., Patri, S., Rahmati, M., et al. (2004). Functional characterization of a Ca^{2+}-activated non-selective cation channel in human atrial cardiomyocytes. *J Physiol, 558*(Pt 1), pp. 75-83.

Guinamard, R., Chatelier, A., Lenfant, J., & Bois, P. (2004). Activation of the Ca^{2+}-activated nonselective cation channel by diacylglycerol analogues in rat cardiomyocytes. *J Cardiovasc Electrophysiol, 15*(3), pp. 342-348.

Guinamard, R., Demion, M., Chatelier, A., & Bois, P. (2006). Calcium-activated nonselective cation channels in mammalian cardiomyocytes. *Trends Cardiovasc Med, 16*(7), pp. 245-250.

Guinamard, R., Demion, M., Magaud, C., Potreau, D., & Bois, P. (2006). Functional expression of the TRPM4 cationic current in ventricular cardiomyocytes from spontaneously hypertensive rats. *Hypertension, 48*(4), pp. 587-594.

Guinamard, R., Rahmati, M., Lenfant, J., & Bois, P. (2002). Characterization of a Ca^{2+}-activated nonselective cation channel during dedifferentiation of cultured rat ventricular cardiomyocytes. *J Membr Biol, 188*(2), pp. 127-135.

Guyenet, P. G. (2006). The sympathetic control of blood pressure. *Nat Rev Neurosci, 7*(5), pp. 335-346.

Hamill, O. P., & Martinac, B. (2001). Molecular basis of mechanotransduction in living cells. *Physiol Rev, 81*(2), pp. 685-740.

Han, X., & Ferrier, G. R. (1992). Ionic mechanisms of transient inward current in the absence of Na^{+}-Ca^{2+} exchange in rabbit cardiac Purkinje fibres. *J Physiol, 456*, pp. 19-38.

Hansen, D. E., Borganelli, M., Stacy, G. P., Jr., & Taylor, L. K. (1991). Dose-dependent inhibition of stretch-induced arrhythmias by gadolinium in isolated canine ventricles. Evidence for a unique mode of antiarrhythmic action. *Circ Res, 69*(3), pp. 820-831.

Hardie, R. C. (2007). TRP channels and lipids: from Drosophila to mammalian physiology. *J Physiol, 578*(Pt 1), pp. 9-24.

Hazari, M. S., Haykal-Coates, N., Winsett, D. W., Krantz, Q. T., King, C., Costa, D. L., et al. (2011). TRPA1 and sympathetic activation contribute to increased risk of triggered cardiac arrhythmias in hypertensive rats exposed to diesel exhaust. *Environ Health Perspect, 119*(7), pp. 951-957.

Henneberger, A., Zareba, W., Ibald-Mulli, A., Ruckerl, R., Cyrys, J., Couderc, J. P., et al. (2005). Repolarization changes induced by air pollution in ischemic heart disease patients. *Environ Health Perspect, 113*(4), pp. 440-446.

Hill, J. A., Jr., Coronado, R., & Strauss, H. C. (1988). Reconstitution and characterization of a calcium-activated channel from heart. *Circ Res, 62*(2), pp. 411-415.

Hofmann, T., Obukhov, A. G., Schaefer, M., Harteneck, C., Gudermann, T., & Schultz, G. (1999). Direct activation of human TRPC6 and TRPC3 channels by diacylglycerol. *Nature, 397*(6716), pp. 259-263.

Holzer, P. TRP channels in the digestive system. (2011). *Curr Pharm Biotechnol, 12*(1), pp. 24-34.

Huang, H., Wang, W., Liu, P., Jiang, Y., Zhao, Y., Wei, H., et al. (2009). TRPC1 expression and distribution in rat hearts. *Eur J Histochem, 53*(4), pp. 217-223.

Ihara, M., Urata, H., Shirai, K., Ideishi, M., Hoshino, F., Suzumiya, J., et al. (2000). High cardiac angiotensin-II-forming activity in infarcted and non-infarcted human myocardium. *Cardiology, 94*(4), pp. 247-253.

Inoue, R., Jensen, L. J., Jian, Z., Shi, J., Hai, L., Lurie, A. I., et al. (2009a). Synergistic activation of vascular TRPC6 channel by receptor and mechanical stimulation via phospholipase C/diacylglycerol and phospholipase A_2/ω-hydroxylase/20-HETE pathways. *Circ Res, 104*(12), pp. 1399-1409.

Inoue, R., Jian, Z., & Kawarabayashi, Y. (2009b). Mechanosensitive TRP channels in cardiovascular pathophysiology. *Pharmacol Ther, 123*(3), pp. 371-385.

Inoue, R., Shi, J., Jian, Z., Imai, Y. (2010) Regulation of cardiovascular TRP channel functions along the NO-cGMP-PKG axis. *Expert Review of Clinical Pharmacology, 3(3), pp.347-360.*

Iribe, G., Ward, C. W., Camelliti, P., Bollensdorff, C., Mason, F., Burton, R. A., et al. (2009). Axial stretch of rat single ventricular cardiomyocytes causes an acute and transient increase in Ca2+ spark rate. *Circ Res, 104*(6), pp. 787-795.

Iwata, Y., Katanosaka, Y., Arai, Y., Komamura, K., Miyatake, K., & Shigekawa, M. (2003). A novel mechanism of myocyte degeneration involving the Ca2+-permeable growth factor-regulated channel. *J Cell Biol, 161*(5), pp. 957-967.

Jalife, J. (2000). Ventricular fibrillation: mechanisms of initiation and maintenance. *Annu Rev Physiol, 62*, pp. 25-50.

Janse, M. J. (2004). Electrophysiological changes in heart failure and their relationship to arrhythmogenesis. *Cardiovasc Res, 61*(2), pp. 208-217.

Janse, M. J., Coronel, R., Wilms-Schopman, F. J., & de Groot, J. R. (2003). Mechanical effects on arrhythmogenesis: from pipette to patient. *Prog Biophys Mol Biol, 82*(1-3), pp. 187-195.

Janse, M. J., & Wit, A. L. (1989). Electrophysiological mechanisms of ventricular arrhythmias resulting from myocardial ischemia and infarction. *Physiol Rev, 69*(4), pp. 1049-1169.

Kamkin, A., Kiseleva, I., & Isenberg, G. (2000a). Stretch-activated currents in ventricular myocytes: amplitude and arrhythmogenic effects increase with hypertrophy. *Cardiovasc Res, 48*(3), pp. 409-420.

Kamkin, A., Kiseleva, I., Isenberg, G., Wagner, K. D., Gunther, J., Theres, H., et al. (2003). Cardiac fibroblasts and the mechano-electric feedback mechanism in healthy and diseased hearts. *Prog Biophys Mol Biol, 82*(1-3), pp. 111-120.

Kamkin, A., Kiseleva, I., Wagner, K. D., Leiterer, K. P., Theres, H., Scholz, H., et al. (2000b). Mechano-electric feedback in right atrium after left ventricular infarction in rats. *J Mol Cell Cardiol, 32*(3), pp. 465-477.

Kaprielian, R. R., Dupont, E., Hafizi, S., Poole-Wilson, P. A., Khaghani, A., Yacoub, M. H., et al. (1997). Angiotensin II receptor type 1 mRNA is upregulated in atria of patients with end-stage heart failure. *J Mol Cell Cardiol, 29*(8), pp. 2299-2304.

Kass, R. S., & Tsien, R. W. (1982). Fluctuations in membrane current driven by intracellular calcium in cardiac Purkinje fibers. *Biophys J, 38*(3), pp. 259-269.

Kass, R. S., Tsien, R. W., & Weingart, R. (1978). Ionic basis of transient inward current induced by strophanthidin in cardiac Purkinje fibres. *J Physiol, 281*, pp. 209-226.

Kiyonaka, S., Kato, K., Nishida, M., Mio, K., Numaga, T., Sawaguchi, Y., et al. (2009). Selective and direct inhibition of TRPC3 channels underlies biological activities of a pyrazole compound. *Proc Natl Acad Sci U S A, 106*(13), pp. 5400-5405.

Komuro, I., & Yazaki, Y. (1993). Control of cardiac gene expression by mechanical stress. *Annu Rev Physiol, 55*, pp. 55-75.

Kroemer, G., Galluzzi, L., & Brenner, C. (2007). Mitochondrial membrane permeabilization in cell death. *Physiol Rev, 87*(1), pp. 99-163.

Kruse, M., Schulze-Bahr, E., Corfield, V., Beckmann, A., Stallmeyer, B., Kurtbay, G., et al. (2009). Impaired endocytosis of the ion channel TRPM4 is associated with human progressive familial heart block type I. *J Clin Invest, 119*(9), pp. 2737-2744.

Kuwahara, K., Wang, Y., McAnally, J., Richardson, J. A., Bassel-Duby, R., Hill, J. A., et al. (2006). TRPC6 fulfills a calcineurin signaling circuit during pathologic cardiac remodeling. *J Clin Invest, 116*(12), pp. 3114-3126.

Kuzmin, A. I., Lakomkin, V. L., Kapelko, V. I., & Vassort, G. (1998). Interstitial ATP level and degradation in control and postmyocardial infarcted rats. *Am J Physiol, 275*(3 Pt 1), pp. C766-771.

Laflamme, M. A., & Becker, P. L. (1996). Ca^{2+}-induced current oscillations in rabbit ventricular myocytes. *Circ Res, 78*(4), pp. 707-716.

Langley, B., & Ratan, R. R. (2004). Oxidative stress-induced death in the nervous system: cell cycle dependent or independent? *J Neurosci Res, 77*(5), pp. 621-629.

Launay, P., Fleig, A., Perraud, A. L., Scharenberg, A. M., Penner, R., & Kinet, J. P. (2002). TRPM4 is a Ca2+-activated nonselective cation channel mediating cell membrane depolarization. *Cell, 109*(3), pp. 397-407.

Lederer, W. J., & Tsien, R. W. (1976). Transient inward current underlying arrhythmogenic effects of cardiotonic steroids in Purkinje fibres. *J Physiol, 263*(2), pp. 73-100.

Li, M., Du, J., Jiang, J., Ratzan, W., Su, L. T., Runnels, L. W., et al. (2007). Molecular determinants of Mg2+ and Ca2+ permeability and pH sensitivity in TRPM6 and TRPM7. *J Biol Chem, 282*(35), pp. 25817-25830.

Li, M., Jiang, J., & Yue, L. (2006). Functional characterization of homo- and heteromeric channel kinases TRPM6 and TRPM7. *J Gen Physiol, 127*(5), pp. 525-537.

Liu, H., El Zein, L., Kruse, M., Guinamard, R., Beckmann, A., Bozio, A., et al. (2010). Gain-of-function mutations in TRPM4 cause autosomal dominant isolated cardiac conduction disease. *Circ Cardiovasc Genet, 3*(4), pp. 374-385.

Maroto, R., Raso, A., Wood, T. G., Kurosky, A., Martinac, B., & Hamill, O. P. (2005). TRPC1 forms the stretch-activated cation channel in vertebrate cells. *Nat Cell Biol, 7*(2), pp. 179-185.

Mathar, I., Vennekens, R., Meissner, M., Kees, F., Van der Mieren, G., Camacho Londono, J. E., et al. (2010). Increased catecholamine secretion contributes to hypertension in TRPM4-deficient mice. *J Clin Invest, 120*(9), pp. 3267-3279.

Mederos y Schnitzler, M., Storch, U., Meibers, S., Nurwakagari, P., Breit, A., Essin, K., et al. (2008). Gq-coupled receptors as mechanosensors mediating myogenic vasoconstriction. *Embo J, 27*(23), pp. 3092-3103.

Miller, B. A., & Zhang, W. (2010). TRP channels as mediators of oxidative stress. *Adv Exp Med Biol, 704*, pp. 531-544.

Misra, M. K., Sarwat, M., Bhakuni, P., Tuteja, R., & Tuteja, N. (2009). Oxidative stress and ischemic myocardial syndromes. *Med Sci Monit, 15*(10), pp. RA209-219.

Morita, H., Honda, A., Inoue, R., Ito, Y., Abe, K., Nelson, M. T., et al. (2007). Membrane stretch-induced activation of a TRPM4-like nonselective cation channel in cerebral artery myocytes. *J Pharmacol Sci, 103*(4), pp. 417-426.

Nattel, S., Maguy, A., Le Bouter, S., & Yeh, Y. H. (2007). Arrhythmogenic ion-channel remodeling in the heart: heart failure, myocardial infarction, and atrial fibrillation. *Physiol Rev, 87*(2), pp. 425-456.

Naylor, J., Al-Shawaf, E., McKeown, L., Manna, P. T., Porter, K. E., O'Regan, D., et al. (2011). TRPC5 channel sensitivities to antioxidants and hydroxylated stilbenes. *J Biol Chem, 286*(7), pp. 5078-5086.

Nilius, B., Prenen, J., Voets, T., & Droogmans, G. (2004). Intracellular nucleotides and polyamines inhibit the Ca2+-activated cation channel TRPM4b. *Pflugers Arch, 448*(1), pp. 70-75.

Nilius, B., & Vennekens, R. (2006). From cardiac cation channels to the molecular dissection of the transient receptor potential channel TRPM4. *Pflugers Arch, 453*(3), pp. 313-321.

Nishida, M., & Kurose, H. (2008). Roles of TRP channels in the development of cardiac hypertrophy. *Naunyn Schmiedebergs Arch Pharmacol, 378*(4), pp. 395-406.

Nishida, M., Onohara, N., Sato, Y., Suda, R., Ogushi, M., Tanabe, S., et al. (2007). Galpha12/13-mediated up-regulation of TRPC6 negatively regulates endothelin-1-induced cardiac myofibroblast formation and collagen synthesis through nuclear factor of activated T cells activation. *J Biol Chem, 282*(32), pp. 23117-23128.

Ohba, T., Watanabe, H., Murakami, M., Takahashi, Y., Iino, K., Kuromitsu, S., et al. (2007). Upregulation of TRPC1 in the development of cardiac hypertrophy. *J Mol Cell Cardiol, 42*(3), pp. 498-507.

Olson, T. M., Michels, V. V., Ballew, J. D., Reyna, S. P., Karst, M. L., Herron, K. J., et al. (2005). Sodium channel mutations and susceptibility to heart failure and atrial fibrillation. *Jama, 293*(4), pp. 447-454.

Onohara, N., Nishida, M., Inoue, R., Kobayashi, H., Sumimoto, H., Sato, Y., et al. (2006). TRPC3 and TRPC6 are essential for angiotensin II-induced cardiac hypertrophy. *Embo J, 25*(22), pp. 5305-5316.

Osadchii, O. E. (2010). Mechanisms of hypokalemia-induced ventricular arrhythmogenicity. *Fundam Clin Pharmacol, 24*(5), pp. 547-559.

Poteser M, Graziani A, Rosker C, Eder P, Derler I, Kahr H, Zhu MX, Romanin C, Groschner K (2006). TRPC3 and TRPC4 associate to form a redox-sensitive cation channel. Evidence for expression of native TRPC3-TRPC4 heteromeric channels in endothelial cells. *J Biol Chem*, 12;281(19), pp.13588-95.

Pogwizd, S. M. (2003). Clinical potential of sodium-calcium exchanger inhibitors as antiarrhythmic agents. *Drugs, 63*(5), pp. 439-452.

Pogwizd, S. M., & Bers, D. M. (2004). Cellular basis of triggered arrhythmias in heart failure. *Trends Cardiovasc Med, 14*(2), pp. 61-66.

Pogwizd, S. M., Schlotthauer, K., Li, L., Yuan, W., & Bers, D. M. (2001). Arrhythmogenesis and contractile dysfunction in heart failure: Roles of sodium-calcium exchange, inward rectifier potassium current, and residual beta-adrenergic responsiveness. *Circ Res, 88*(11), pp. 1159-1167.

Ravens, U. Antiarrhythmic therapy in atrial fibrillation. (2010). *Pharmacol Ther, 128*(1), pp. 129-145.

Ravens, U. Novel pharmacological approaches for antiarrhythmic therapy. (2010). *Naunyn Schmiedebergs Arch Pharmacol, 381*(3), pp. 187-193.

Ravens, U. (2003). Mechano-electric feedback and arrhythmias. *Prog Biophys Mol Biol, 82*(1-3), pp. 255-266.

Roberts, J. D., & Gollob, M. H. (2010). The genetic and clinical features of cardiac channelopathies. *Future Cardiol, 6*(4), pp. 491-506.

Roden, D. M. (2004). Drug-induced prolongation of the QT interval. *N Engl J Med, 350*(10), pp. 1013-1022.

Sack, M. N., Smith, R. M., & Opie, L. H. (2000). Tumor necrosis factor in myocardial hypertrophy and ischaemia--an anti-apoptotic perspective. *Cardiovasc Res, 45*(3), pp. 688-695.

Saenen, J. B., & Vrints, C. J. (2008). Molecular aspects of the congenital and acquired Long QT Syndrome: clinical implications. *J Mol Cell Cardiol, 44*(4), pp. 633-646.

Satoh, S., Tanaka, H., Ueda, Y., Oyama, J., Sugano, M., Sumimoto, H., et al. (2007). Transient receptor potential (TRP) protein 7 acts as a G protein-activated Ca^{2+} channel mediating angiotensin II-induced myocardial apoptosis. *Mol Cell Biochem, 294*(1-2), pp. 205-215.

Schott, J. J., Alshinawi, C., Kyndt, F., Probst, V., Hoorntje, T. M., Hulsbeek, M., et al. (1999). Cardiac conduction defects associate with mutations in SCN5A. *Nat Genet, 23*(1), pp. 20-21.

Seth, M., Sumbilla, C., Mullen, S. P., Lewis, D., Klein, M. G., Hussain, A., et al. (2004). Sarco(endo)plasmic reticulum Ca2+ ATPase (SERCA) gene silencing and remodeling of the Ca2+ signaling mechanism in cardiac myocytes. *Proc Natl Acad Sci U S A, 101*(47), pp. 16683-16688.

Shan, D., Marchase, R. B., & Chatham, J. C. (2008). Overexpression of TRPC3 increases apoptosis but not necrosis in response to ischemia-reperfusion in adult mouse cardiomyocytes. *Am J Physiol Cell Physiol, 294*(3), pp. C833-841.

Siemen, D. (1993). Nonselective cation channels. *Exs, 66*, pp. 3-25.

Sipido, K. R., Bito, V., Antoons, G., Volders, P. G., & Vos, M. A. (2007). Na/Ca exchange and cardiac ventricular arrhythmias. *Ann N Y Acad Sci, 1099*, pp. 339-348.

Song, Y., & Belardinelli, L. (1994). ATP promotes development of afterdepolarizations and triggered activity in cardiac myocytes. *Am J Physiol, 267*(5 Pt 2), pp. H2005-2011.

Souders, C. A., Bowers, S. L., & Baudino, T. A. (2009). Cardiac fibroblast: the renaissance cell. *Circ Res, 105*(12), pp. 1164-1176.

Spassova, M. A., Hewavitharana, T., Xu, W., Soboloff, J., & Gill, D. L. (2006). A common mechanism underlies stretch activation and receptor activation of TRPC6 channels. *Proc Natl Acad Sci U S A, 103*(44), pp. 16586-16591.

Stacy, G. P., Jr., Jobe, R. L., Taylor, L. K., & Hansen, D. E. (1992). Stretch-induced depolarizations as a trigger of arrhythmias in isolated canine left ventricles. *Am J Physiol, 263*(2 Pt 2), pp. H613-621.

Suchyna, T. M., Johnson, J. H., Hamer, K., Leykam, J. F., Gage, D. A., Clemo, H. F., et al. (2000). Identification of a peptide toxin from Grammostola spatulata spider venom that blocks cation-selective stretch-activated channels. *J Gen Physiol, 115*(5), pp. 583-598.

Swynghedauw, B. (1999). Molecular mechanisms of myocardial remodeling. *Physiol Rev, 79*(1), pp. 215-262.

Szallasi, A., Cortright, D. N., Blum, C. A., & Eid, S. R. (2007). The vanilloid receptor TRPV1: 10 years from channel cloning to antagonist proof-of-concept. *Nat Rev Drug Discov, 6*(5), pp. 357-372.

Takahashi, N., Kozai, D., Kobayashi, R., Ebert, M., & Mori, Y. (2011). Roles of TRPM2 in oxidative stress. *Cell Calcium*, pp.

Ter Keurs, H. E., & Boyden, P. A. (2007). Calcium and arrhythmogenesis. *Physiol Rev, 87*(2), pp. 457-506.

Towbin, J. A., & Vatta, M. (2001). Molecular biology and the prolonged QT syndromes. *Am J Med, 110*(5), pp. 385-398.

Tsai, E. J., & Kass, D. A. (2009). Cyclic GMP signaling in cardiovascular pathophysiology and therapeutics. *Pharmacol Ther, 122*(3), pp. 216-238.

Vassort, G., Bideaux, P., & Alvarez, J. (2010). Could early ischemic arrhythmia triggered by purinergic activation of the transient receptor potential channels be prevented by creatine? *Exp Clin Cardiol, 15*(4), pp. e104-108.

Vay, L., Gu, C., & McNaughton, P. A. (2011). The thermo-TRP ion channel family: properties and therapeutic implications. *Br J Pharmacol*, pp.

Venetucci, L. A., Trafford, A. W., O'Neill, S. C., & Eisner, D. A. (2008). The sarcoplasmic reticulum and arrhythmogenic calcium release. *Cardiovasc Res, 77*(2), pp. 285-292.

Ward, M. L., Williams, I. A., Chu, Y., Cooper, P. J., Ju, Y. K., & Allen, D. G. (2008). Stretch-activated channels in the heart: contributions to length-dependence and to cardiomyopathy. *Prog Biophys Mol Biol, 97*(2-3), pp. 232-249.

Watanabe, H., Murakami, M., Ohba, T., Takahashi, Y., & Ito, H. (2008). TRP channel and cardiovascular disease. *Pharmacol Ther, 118*(3), pp. 337-351.

Wehrens, X. H., Lehnart, S. E., Huang, F., Vest, J. A., Reiken, S. R., Mohler, P. J., et al. (2003). FKBP12.6 deficiency and defective calcium release channel (ryanodine receptor) function linked to exercise-induced sudden cardiac death. *Cell, 113*(7), pp. 829-840.

Wijffels, M. C., Kirchhof, C. J., Dorland, R., & Allessie, M. A. (1995). Atrial fibrillation begets atrial fibrillation. A study in awake chronically instrumented goats. *Circulation, 92*(7), pp. 1954-1968.

Wu, L. J., Sweet, T. B., & Clapham, D. E. (2010). International Union of Basic and Clinical Pharmacology. LXXVI. Current progress in the mammalian TRP ion channel family. *Pharmacol Rev, 62*(3), pp. 381-404.

Wu, Y., & Anderson, M. E. (2000). Ca^{2+}-activated non-selective cation current in rabbit ventricular myocytes. *J Physiol, 522 Pt 1*, pp. 51-57.

Yamamoto, S., Shimizu, S., Kiyonaka, S., Takahashi, N., Wajima, T., Hara, Y., et al. (2008). TRPM2-mediated Ca2+influx induces chemokine production in monocytes that aggravates inflammatory neutrophil infiltration. *Nat Med, 14*(7), pp. 738-747.

Yang, K. T., Chang, W. L., Yang, P. C., Chien, C. L., Lai, M. S., Su, M. J., et al. (2006). Activation of the transient receptor potential M2 channel and poly(ADP-ribose) polymerase is involved in oxidative stress-induced cardiomyocyte death. *Cell Death Differ, 13*(10), pp. 1815-1826.

Yasuda, N., Miura, S., Akazawa, H., Tanaka, T., Qin, Y., Kiya, Y., et al. (2008). Conformational switch of angiotensin II type 1 receptor underlying mechanical stress-induced activation. *EMBO Rep, 9*(2), pp. 179-186.

Yu, Y., Sweeney, M., Zhang, S., Platoshyn, O., Landsberg, J., Rothman, A., et al. (2003). PDGF stimulates pulmonary vascular smooth muscle cell proliferation by upregulating TRPC6 expression. *Am J Physiol Cell Physiol, 284*(2), pp. C316-330.

Yue, L., Xie, J., & Nattel, S. Molecular determinants of cardiac fibroblast electrical function and therapeutic implications for atrial fibrillation. (2011). *Cardiovasc Res, 89*(4), pp. 744-753.

Zareba, W., Moss, A. J., Locati, E. H., Lehmann, M. H., Peterson, D. R., Hall, W. J., et al. (2003). Modulating effects of age and gender on the clinical course of long QT syndrome by genotype. *J Am Coll Cardiol, 42*(1), pp. 103-109.

Zhu, J., Liu, M., Kennedy, R. H., & Liu, S. J. (2006). TNF-alpha-induced impairment of mitochondrial integrity and apoptosis mediated by caspase-8 in adult ventricular myocytes. *Cytokine, 34*(1-2), pp. 96-105.

Zima, A. V., & Blatter, L. A. (2006). Redox regulation of cardiac calcium channels and transporters. *Cardiovasc Res, 71*(2), pp. 310-321.

5

Contributions of Ion Channels in Cardiac Arrhythmias

Jing Hongjuan and Zhang Lu
Henan University of Technology, College of Biological Engineering, Zhengzhou, China

1. Introduction

The cardiac action potential is arised by the highly orchestrated activity of dozens of ion channel proteins. These transmembrane proteins govern the influx of ion across the sarcolemma of cardiomyocytes generating the ionic currents responsible for excitation. In order to myocardium contract and ensure rhythmic pump function, the long-lasting action potential of the working myocardium maintains a refractory state. Because some channels must recover from inactivation after-repolarization before they have ability of re-opening, and during this time, the myocardial cells remain refractory for re-excitation.

Typical normal action potentials consist of five distinct phases (Figure 1). Na^+ influx triggers a rapid depolarization (phase 0) followed by an early fast repolarization phase (phase 1) and

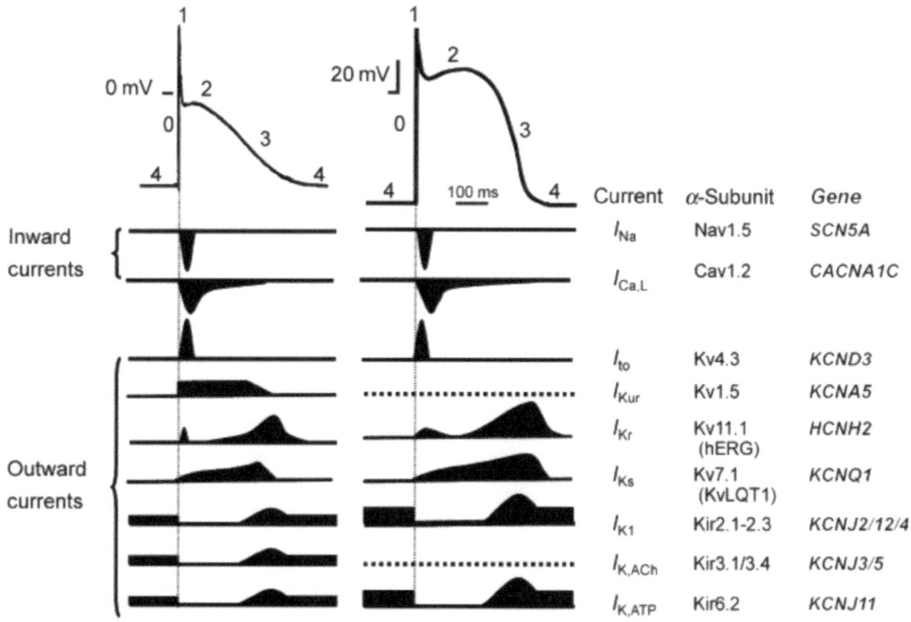

Fig. 1. (cited from The Sicilian gambit, 2008). Currents of sodium, calcium and potassium channels underlie the atrial and ventricular action potential.

a plateau phase (phase 2), in which repolarization is slowed due to the activation of inward Ca^{2+} current. During the final rapid repolarization phase (phase 3), membrane potential returns to the resting level (phase 4). Therefore, normal action potentials attributed to the normal function of ion channel participated to formation of action potentials.

1.1 Ion channels in human heart disease

Regular excitation is formed by normal AP which generated in the sino-atrial node and spreads throughout the heart in an orderly manner. Oppositely, disorganization of electrical activity is the basis of cardiac arrhythmias. Arrhythmias are caused by the perturbation of physiological impulse formation, impaired impulse conduction, or disturbed electrical recovery. Abnormal excitability of myocardial cells may give rise to kinds of cardiac diseases.

The most ordinary cardiac arrhythmia diseases was inherited long QT syndrome (LQTS) which was recognized 40 years ago as 2 distinct clinical phenotypes, such as the Romano-Ward and the Jervell and Lange-Nielsen syndromes. Interestingly, while LQTS was initially thought to be a pure cardiac channelopathy, it is now clear that non-ion-channel encoding genes may also cause the desease. Nevertheless, LQTs attributed to dysfunctions of ionic currents, either directly (ion channel) or indirectly (chaperones and/or other modulators).

To date, 12 forms of inherited LQTS described because LQTS arise from polygenic causes and 9 of them directly combine with ion channels (Table 1). LQT1, 2, 5, and 6 are referred to prolong the plateau of cardiac APs (phase 2) by reducing K^+ channel currents activated during depolarization. LQT1 and 5 are caused by mutations in KCNQ1 (KvLQT1) and KCNE1 (MinK), which encode the α and ancillary β subunits, respectively and together form the slowly activating delayed rectifier K^+ current (I_{Ks}). LQT2 and 6 are caused by mutations in KCNH2 (human-ether a-go-go-related gene; HERG) and KCNE2 (MiRP1), which encode the α and putative β subunits, respectively and together form the rapidly activating delayed rectifier K^+ current (I_{Kr}). LQT7 is characterized by mutations in KCNJ2 (Kir2.1), which reduces the inward rectifier K^+ channel current (I_{K1}) to slow the return of the membrane to the resting potential. These cause failure of normal inactivation to decrease of K^+ current (loss of function) and abbreviate action potentials. Besides potassium channel, LQT3, 10 attributed to mutations in hNaV1.5 (SCN5a), and SCNb4, which encode α and ancillary β subunits of Na^+ channel. LQT8 are determined by mutation in CACNA1c, which encode alpha subunit of calcium channel. LOT3,10 and LQT8 arise from the increase of Na^+ currents and Ca^{2+} currents, respectively, for prolong action potential. Therefore, "loss of function" or "gain of function" mutations in the affected ion channels are often formed different phenotypes of cardiac arrhythmia desease.

Except the mentioned above, LQT4,9,11,12 are determined by mutation in ANK2, Cav3, AKAP9 and SNTA1, which encode ankyrin B, caveolin, A-kinase-anchoring protein and alphal1-syntrophin, respectively. All proteins increase or decrease the ironic currents (loss of function or gain of function). Although the remarkable genetic heterogeneity in LQT, three genes, such as KCNQ1 (LQT1), KCNH2 (LQT2) and SCN5A (LQT3), are dominant and cover more than 90 percentage of LQTS patients with identified mutations.

With exception of LQTS, some of these involve gain of function mutations in K^+ channels (short QT syndrome) and loss of function mutations in and Ca channel and Na^+ channels (Brugada syndrome, cardiac conduction disease, etc). Additional congenital arrhythmia syndromes continue to be described, and these are summarized in Table 1.

current	disease	gene name	chromosomal locus	Protein	functional effect	inheritance
I_{Na}	LQT3	SCN5A	3p21	sodium channel alpha subunit (Nav1.5)	gain of function	AD
	BrS1	SCN5A	3p21	sodium channel alpha subunit (Nav1.5)	loss of function	AD
	AF3	SCN5A	3p21	sodium channel alpha subunit (Nav1.5)	loss of function	AD
	PCCD	SCN5A	3p21	sodium channel alpha subunit (Nav1.5)	loss of function	AD
	SSS	SCN5A	3p21	sodium channel alpha subunit (Nav1.5)	loss of function	AD
	LQT10	SCNb4	11q23.3	sodium channel beta subunit	increas sodium channel	AD
$I_{Ca,L}$	TS/LQT8	CACNA1C	12p13.3	calcium channel alpha subunit	gain of function	AD/mosaicism
	BrS3	CACNA1C	12p13.3	calcium channel alpha subunit	loss of function	AD
	BrS4	CACNB2b	10p12	calcium channel alpha subunit		AD
I_{KS}	LQT1	KCNQ1	11p15.5	I_{Ks} potassium channel alpha subunit (KvLQT1)	loss of function	AD
	JLN1	KCNQ1	11p15.5	I_{Ks} potassium channel alpha subunit (KvLQT1)	gain of function	AR
	AQT2	KCNQ1	11p15.5	I_{Ks} potassium channel alpha subunit (KvLQT1)	gain of function	AD
	AF1	KCNQ1	11p15.5	I_{Ks} potassium channel alpha subunit (KvLQT1)	gain of function	AD
	LQT5	KCNE1	21q21.1-q22.2	I_{Ks} potassium channel beta subunit (Mink)	loss of function	AD
	JLN2	KCNE1	21q21.1-q22.2	I_{Ks} potassium channel beta subunit (Mink)	gain of function	AR
	AF5	KCNE1	21q21.1-q22.2	I_{Ks} potassium channel beta subunit (Mink)	gain of function	AD

current	disease	gene name	chromosomal locus	Protein	functional effect	inheritance
I_{Kr}	LQT2	KCNH2	7q35-q36	I_{Kr} potassium channel alpha subunit (hERG)	loss of function	AD
	SQT1	KCNH2	7q35-q36	I_{Kr} potassium channel alpha subunit (hERG)	gain of function	AD
	AF2	KCNH2	7q35-q36	I_{Kr} potassium channel alpha subunit (hERG)	gain of function	AD
	LQT6	KCNE2	21q21.1-q22.2	I_{Kr} potassium channel beta subunit (MiRP)	loss of function	AD
	AF6	KCNE2	21q21.1-q22.2	I_{Kr} potassium channel beta subunit (MiRP)	gain of function	AD
I_{K1}	AND/LQT&	KCNJ2	17q23.2-q24.2	I_{K1} potassium channel (Kir2.1)	loss of function	AD
	SQT3	KCNJ2	17q23.2-q24.2	I_{K1} potassium channel (Kir2.1)	gain of function	AD
	AF4	KCNJ2	17q23.2-q24.2	I_{K1} potassium channel (Kir2.1)	gain of function	AD

Table 1. Mutations of ion channels

1.2 Mechanism of ion channels dysfunction

Based on the discussion mentioned above we can easy to understand the mutation how reduce or increase the currents and lead the kinds of cardiac arrhythmia. The change of the magnitude of currents in cardiac is based on the below three factors. For instance, the total number of channels on the membrane (N), the open probability of the channel (P_0) and the conductance of single channel (i). Gain of function or loss of function mutations of ion channel through changing of N, Po and I alone or all contribute to kinds of congenital cardiac arrhythmia.

1.2.1 Change of the channel number

There are two distinct process in which can change the number of channel in the plasma membrane, one is in the synthesis channel process and another is during the channel trafficking.

About defective synthesis of mutations contained the premature termination codons is maybe the most mutations of ion channel. For example, there are one fourths of all mutations of hERG channel (http: //www. fsm. it/cardmoc). The protein encoded by the mutation with premature termination codon is a truncated one which can be eliminated by nonsense-mediated mRNA decay. And the hERG truncation mutation is proved to be clear by the nonsense-mediated mRNA decay in recently.

Exception of the nonsense-mediated mRNA decay, another important clear mechanism is at mRNA level by microRNA (miRNA) mediated mRNA silencing. The degradation of the target

mRNA is through partial complementary combination with the miRNA followed binding with kinds of protein or nucleotide to form a huge ribosome. To date, many miRNA are detected in heart and decrease of ion channel protein at translaton or/and transcript levels.
There are three steps during the process of ion channel synthesis: i) the formation of core-glycoslyted monomer in ER followed the correct to the tetramer ii), iii) then complex glycaslytaton to form the mature subunit in Gorgi. Accordingly, Western blot check can be utend to detect weather composition of the channel protein is complete. The primarychannel protein is common synthesized in ER.
In order to export completely from the synthesis location (ER), each channel subunit protein contained more than one of the ER exit signal (D/E-X-D/E) motif which can guide the protein correctly from ER to Golgi, where X represens any kinds of amino acid. To ensure the channel deviated from ER, channel form a tetramer in ER by masking or shielding the ER retention signal. Therefore, mutations in ER exit signal or with correlation of the assembly of channel maybe lead to the retention in ER then decrease the number of channel in the membrane.

1.2.2 Change of channel open probability

Change of activation and inactivation maybe are two ways of altering of channel open probability. In *Xenopus laevis* oocytes system, to date many mutations have been detected to alter the channel gated. But there are much difference between the oocytes system and the mammalian system. In addition, there are many mutations that have been expressed in mammalian and shown to result in gating defects.

1.2.3 Change of single channel conductance

To alter the conductance of single channel, the mutation sites of ion channel exits in the vicinity of the selective filter. Owing to the selective filter of ion channel is determined the kinds of ions across the channel. Accordingly, the single channel conductance change may be attributed to the conformation altering of the selective filter.

2. Sodium channel

Cardiac voltage-gated sodium channel has critical role in excitability of myocardial cells and proper conduction of the electrical impulse within the heart. Infux of Na^+ across sodium channel is responsible for the initial fast upstroke of the cardiac action potential. Therefore, this inward sodium channel triggers the initiation and propagation of action potential throughout the myocardium. The gene of *SCN5A* encodes the major sodium channel in heart.

2.1 Structure of sodium channel

The voltage-gated sodium channel is composed by a pore-forming α subunit and an ancillary β subunit. Nav1.5 encoded by *SCN5A* consists of four homologous domains (D I - D II) and each domain has six transmembrane segments (S1-S6). Similar to other voltage-gated ion channel, the S4 contained many positive residues in each domain forms the voltage sensor and the S4 and S5 in all domains together make up ion-conductance pore including the selectivity filter. When sodium channel is activated, influx of Na^+ begin, thereby the depolarizing of the membrane until the activation of L-calcium channel, at last forming the upstroke of action potential. Continue to depolarization, the fast and low inactivation happen causing the sodium channel close. Sodium channel gating properties and current kinetics may be altered when channel is dysfunction.

Cardiac sodium channel function can be regulated by a vast number of proteins. The single tansmembrane β-subunit consists of a small C-terminal cytoplasmic domain and a large glycosylated N-terminal extracellular domain. The ancillary subunit alters the currents density and kinetics by physical interaction with the α subunit. Other proteins regulating Nav1.5 by directly binding include ankyrins, fibroblast growth factor homologous factor 1B, calmodulin, caveolin-3, Nedd4-like ubiquitin-protein ligases, dystrophin, and syntrophin, as well as glycerol-3-phosphate dehydrogenase 1-like protein and MOG1. In addition, sodium channel density and kinetics are furthermore also regulated by phosporylation and glycosylation, even by changes in temperature.

2.2 Functions of sodium channel in heart

During myocardial ischemia, the mechanisms involved in arrhythmogenesis are complex, but excitability and conduction are considered as the major determinants. During ischemia, local metabolic changes within the myocardium lead to inactivation of the sodium current and consequent repression of cardiac excitability and slowing of conduction. In clinical, slowing conduction produced by sodium channel blockers application has been shown to be proarrhythmic. Some papers have reported an association between *SCN5A* loss-of-function mutations and the occurrence of ischemia-induced severe episodes of ventricular tachyarrhythmias. It is as yet unknown whether SCN5A mutations and/or polymorphisms play a substantial role in the prevalence of sudden arrhythmic death in the setting of myocardial infarction,

2.3 Cardiac sodium channelopathies

To date, more than 150 mutations in *SCN5A* have been reported, the vast majority of them caused either LQTS3 and Brugada syndrome. Some patients with LQTS can be healing well whereas most of them may increase risk for sudden death due to ventricular tachyarrhythmias, in particular torsades de pointes. The character of LQTS3 is that display arrhythmias predominantly during rest or sleep videlicet at slow heart rate. Therefore, the first clinical event of the patient with LQTS3 often is cardiac arrest rather than syncope. About the molecualr mechanism of LQTS, vast majority of mutations in *SCN5A* produced the disruption of the fast inactivation but not the slow inactivation. The disruption allows the sodium channel reopen and produces the persistent inward current during the action potential plateau phase. Gain of function mutations in sodium channel delays the depolarization of the action potential and causes the prolongation of the action potential.

Brugada syndrome, a familial disease which charactered by ventricular arrhythmia and sudden cardia death even occuring in healthy person at relatively young age (mainly between 30 to 40) and more in male, is first raised by brothers of Brugada in 1992. the features on ECG show the elevation of ST segments in the precordial line. Mutation in *SCN5A* is acquired as original of the SQTS3 in a familial disorder in 1998. More than 100 mutations in *SCN5A* is related the Brugada syndrome. Besides the mutation in *SCN5A*, mutations in the β-subunits *SCN1B* and *SCN3B*, and the regulatory protein GPD1-L have been described in some Brugada syndrome patients. In a word, mutations in *SCN5A* or ancillary subunit caused to Brugada syndrome becausing of the reduction of sodium channel availabality, loss of function. Some factors cause loss of function in ion channel. For example the decreased trafficking will degrade the number of sodium channel (N) in membrane surface, or disruption of activation, accelerated inactivation, and impaired recovery from inactivation will alter channel gating properties (the open probability and the single channel conductance).

Loss of mutations in *SCN5A* underlies the mechanism of progressive cardiac conduntance defect (PCCD) due to reduction the sodium channel availability. PCCD is charactered by progressive conduction slowing through the His-Purkinje system, leading to the complete AV block, syncope and sudden death. Same to PCCD, Sick Sinus Syndrome is also caused by the mutations in *SCN5A* by decreasing the current of inward sodium currents. Sodium channel contribute to the cardiac automaticity owe to the inward sodium currents in depolarizing progress. Therefore, automaticity of sinoatrial pacemake can also be regulated by the sodium channel. Atrial fibrillation is often happened in elderly person with the abnormal heart and younger person with normal structure. In recent, both loss of function and gain of function mutations in *SCN5A* have been identified as atrial fibrillation due to decrease atrial conductance velocity attributed to the degrade of sodium inward currents and increase atrial action potential duration and excitability owe to the raise of sodium channel avaibality, respectively. In addition, the patients with dilated cardiomyopathy are evoked by the mutations in *SCN5A*.

In recent years, "overlap syndrome" of cardiac sodium channel deseases have known to exit. The term of "overlap syndrome" is refered to extensive clinical and biophysical overlap. For example, the patients with the mutation *SCN5A*-1795insD$^{+/-}$ shows extensive variability in type and severity of symptoms of sodium channel disease. Otherwise, the single mutation in *SCN5A* alone but express pleiotropic effects make further verified through a transgenic mice *SCN5A*-1798insD+/- (equal to human *SCN5A*-1795insD$^{+/-}$). It is further confirmed that a single *SCN5A*-1795insD$^{+/-}$ mutation is sufficient to express the overlap syndrome of the sodium channel. Heterogenous biophysical properties of ion channel mutations causing the mixed disease expressively are now increasing recognized. Therefore, it is necessary that improve diagnosis for the sodium channelopathies.

3. Calcium channel

Voltage gated calcium channel is the main channel across by Ca^{2+} into the intracellular in many excited cell. L-type Cav1.2 channel is an important voltage gated calcium channel and have been detected in many organs. Notwithstanding the widespread important function of the L-type calcium channel, the mutations have been identified is very rare. Mutations of deletion of the pore forming part in Cav1.2 channel change significantly the properties of the channel leading to the embryonically lethal. On the contrary, mutations associated with mold effects on $I_{Ca,L}$ kinetics is well adapted and the patients with no obvious symptoms.

3.1 Structure of L-type Ca_V1.2 channel

Similar to the voltage-gated sodium channel, structure of L-type Ca_V1.2 channel is formed by a pore-forming subunit divided for four dormains (from I to II). Each domain consists of six transmembrane segments (S1 to S6). As the common to other voltage gated channel, the S4 of each domain is the voltage sensor moving across the membrane corresponding to the depolarization of the membrane potential. The part of S5, S6 and the linker S5-6 in each domain are composed to the ion conduction pathway.

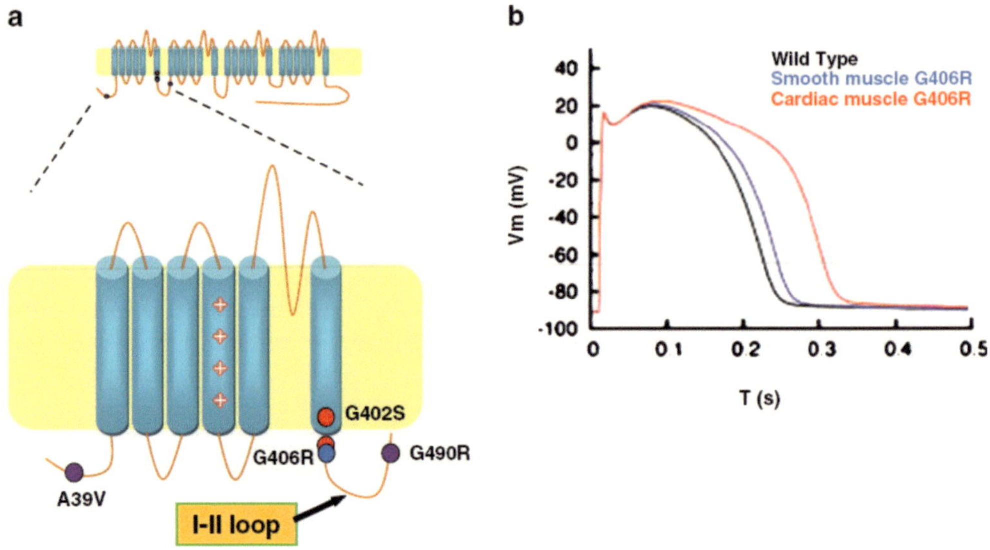

Fig. 2. a (cited from Liao and Soong, 2010). Location of the mutations identified in $Ca_V1.2$ pore-forming α 1 subunit. Red circles (G402S and G406R) reprents spliced cardiac exon. Blue circle (G406R) is located in smooth muscle exon. Purple circles (A39V and G490R) represents constitutive exons. b Computer modeling revealed cardiac action potential when the mutation in smooth muscle exon and in cardiac exon.

3.2 Ancillary subunits

To date, four β subunits of calcium channel genes are expressed in the heart. The ancillary subunits can in theory bind to the Cav1.2 subunit at the α1 interaction domain (AID). The domain is highly conserved binding motif of 18 amino acid residues present in the cytoplasmic linker between repeat I and II of α1 subunits. The β2 subunit is generally believed to constitute the intracellular, accessory subunit of the Cav1.2 channel in adult mammalian myocardium.

There are two distinct function of β subunit binding with the pore-forming subunit: before binding as a chaperone helping α subunit correct location at the membrane, after binding as an allosteric modulator to regulate the kinetic of the currents. Otherwise, different β subunit increase the currents of $I_{Ca,L}$ at different levels by increasing the the channel opening probability, produce distinctive effects on channel inactivation kinetics and induce hyperpolarizing shifts in the voltage-dependence of channel activation.

Recent studies have shown that the ancillary subunits are members of the membrane-associated guanylate kinase (MAGUK) family of proteins by crystallographic information. Therefore, the ancillary subunits, as a ideal targets, interact with other protein such as ahnak or various members of the Gem/kir family of small Ras-like GTPase.

3.3 Functions of L-type Cav1.2 in heart

The L-type Cav1.2 channel plays a critical and dominant role in triggering excitation-contraction coupling in cardiomycytes through the influx of the calcium ions to form the plateau of the ventricular action potential. Otherwise, the L-type Cav1.2 channel contribute to the trigger of the contraction when initiate the Ca^{2+} from the sarcoplasmic reticulum.

LQTS8 (also called Timothy syndrome) is first reported in 1990s with the symptoms of syndactyly. The molecular basis of Timothy Sydrome is the mutations in L-type Cav1.2 at IS6 segment encoded by the two mutually exclusive exons 8/8a. Timothy syndrome is several features. Firstly, mutations are common caused by the deamination of a methylated cytosine to a thymine at de nove. Secondly, gain of function of L-type Cav1.2 lead to the increase of current density of $I_{Ca,L}$ through slowing the inactivation of the channel. The net effects of the mutations increase of intracellular calcium ion. Thirdly, mutations are common in the mutually exclusive exons. The mutation of exons alters dramatically channel properties and the unaffected exon function normally. Lastly, mutation in Cav1.2 is also related to normal function of immune system.

Different Cav1.2.variants are formed by the extensive alternative splicing by changing the pattern of splicing causing a series of disease. Among of them, only a few major splicing site can be divided to the cardiac and smooth muscle subfamily. In human heart, Cav1.2 channel contained cardiac exon may be 77 percent of all Cav1.2 channel. The first Timothy Syndrome mutation G406R is at the smooth muscle exon whereas other mutation G406R and F402s is at the cardiac exon. The latter can be named as TS2 and the cardiac arrhythmia of what is more serous than TS.

TS2 mutant Cav1.2 belong to gain of function mutation leading to more calcium ion into the cytoplasm. Therefore, the action potential duration are be prolonged and a longer QT interval on ECG is shown. Comparision with TS (mutaions at smooth muscle exon), TS2 (mutations at cardiac exon) produces more effects on action potential duration and excitability. For example, the prolongation of action potential duration by mutation at cardiac exon and smooth muscle exon is 30% and 8% by computer analysis, respectively. Therefore, symptom of patient with TS is molder than one with TS2.

Otherwise, loss of function mutation in Cav1.2 or ancillary subunit cause to Brugada syndrome charactered by the elevating QT segments and shortening QT interval on ECG. The ages of the patients with Brugada syndrome is ranging from 21 to 44 years old which is elder than TS patients. Besides the dysfunction in cardiac tissues, other organs are nearly normal in patient with Brugada syndrome.

4. Potassium channel

Potassium channel is the largest family of ion channel protein and divided into voltage- and ligand- potassium channel owing to activating by voltage and ligand, respectively. Most of potassium channel are determined and depended by membrane potential. The ion-conducting pore of a K^+ channel is formed by four α-subunits that co-assemble as homo- or hetero-tetramers with different biophysical properties. Their gating characteristics can also be modulated by ancillary subunits or all kinds of blocker or activator.

4.1 Classification of the cardiac potassium channel

On the basis of their function, cardiac K^+ channels are further classified into the transient outward channels, the delayed rectifier channels and the inward rectifier channels (*Figure 1*). Firstly, the transient outward current (I_{to}) formed by Kv4.3 manifests rapid activation and subsequent inactivation during the early repolarization phase (at phase 1). (ii) The delayed rectifier channels consist of at least three members Kv1.5, Kv11.1 and Kv7.1, for three different currents I_{Kur}, I_{Kr}, and I_{Ks}, respectively. All three channels activate at positive potentials but with distinct time courses, for example ultrarapid, rapid, and slow, respectively. Inactivation of I_{Kur} and I_{Ks} is slow, on the contrary that of I_{Kr} is extremely fast. (iii) The cardiac inward rectifier potassium channels have more than three components. The major classical of one is Kir2,1-2.3 which form I_{K1} currents. This channel is always open and conducts K^+ better into than out of the cell. Another channel expressed in atrial myocytes is an acetylcholine-dependent channel whicn conducts $I_{K,Ach}$ corresponding with the stimulation of G-protein-coupled muscarinic (M2) and adenosine (A1) receptors. The activation of $I_{K,ACh}$ shortens the active potential duration (APD). The third one in cardiomyocytes is ordinary closed under physiological metabolic conditions and is activated when the cells are deprived of intra-cellular adenosine triphosphate (ATP). Similar to $I_{K,ACh}$, $I_{K,ATP}$ causes profound APD shortening.

Notwithstanding general similarity in the mechanism of action potential arised, the distribution of potassium channel in cardiac ventricular myocardium and cardiac atrium is the most striking difference. For example, I_{Kur} and $I_{K,Ach}$ currents are both detected just in atrial but not in ventricular. Under the positive potential I_{Kur} is activated rapidly followed by $I_{Ca,L}$ activation and therefore lead to less positive plateau phase in atrial than ventricular cells.

4.2 Structure of potassium channel

Remarkable advances about the structure-function relationship in ion channel have great progress in over past 30 years. Especially the progress in two experimental techniques, one is the single channel conductance recorded limpidly and plainly by patch clamp and another is the first determination at atomic-resolution of the structure of potassium channel protein. By means of these techniques, we can monitor real-time behaviour of single macromolecule in cell membrane and associate the behaviour with the molecular architecture of the protein

4.2.1 Structures of voltage gated potassium channel

Voltage-gated potassium channel is a homotetramer formed by each subunit containing six transmembrane domains (S1-S6). The pore domain comprise of the S5, the pore helix and S6 segment. The S1-S4 segments of each subunit form the voltage sensor domains (VSD). The part of VCD regulates the open and close of the pore domain through moving across membrane in response to change of membrane potential. The channel pore is anisomerous and its dimensions change when the transition of channel gates from a closed to an open state. The K^+-selectivity filter, a narrow cylinder, exists in the extracellular end of the pore that optimally utilize for conduction of K^+ ions. The difference of the selectivity filter of Kv channels with other channel is charactered by the highly conserved sequence Thr-Val-Gly-Tyr-Gly (the K^+ signature sequence), located at the carboxy-terminal end of the pore helix. In hERG channel, the Thr and Tyr residues are substituted with Ser and Phe. The hydroxyl group of Thr in side-chain and the carbonyl oxygen atoms of the other four residues in each subunit all expose to the narrow K^+ selectivity filter. These atoms mentioned above (OH^- and O) encircle several octahedral binding sites that compete with the single water molecule of hydrated K^+ ions and make a single water molecule alone arranged in a single line pass across the filter.

The central cavity under the selectivity filter is much more widen and is a filled water region boundary by the S6 α-helices. In the closed state, the four S6 domains criss-cross near the cytoplasmic interface to form a narrow aperture that is too small to permit entry of ions from the cytoplasm. In response to membrane depolarization, the S6 α-helices splay outwards and increase the diameter of the aperture to allow passage of ions.

4.2.2 Structures of Kir channel

Inward rectifier K^+ channels (Kirs) consist of two transmembrane domains (M1 and M2). M1 and M2, equal to the S5 and S6 part of voltage-gated potassium channel, is connected by a pore containing the G(Y/F)G sequence. In addition, the Kirs channels comprise of intracellular N- and C-termini. This architecture is typical structure of K_{ATP} and K_{ir}channels. They conduct K^+ currents more in the inward direction than the outward and play an important role in setting the resting potential close to the equilibrium potential for K^+ (E_K, approximately -90 mV for $[K^+]_o$ = 5 mM) and in repolarization. Kir channels form either homo- or heterotetramers.

About the essential properties of rectification which attributed to blocking of Kir2 channels by intracellular organic cations called polyamines response to potent and strongly voltage-dependent. Of the polyamines, free spermine in cell is the most potent inducer of inward rectification, followed by spermidine, putrescine, and then Mg^{2+}. Accordingly, the "activation" of inward rectifiers upon membrane hyperpolarization is essentially uncoupling of polyamines or Mg^{2+} from the Kir channel pore.

The general architecture of the Kir channels and the key structures involved in permeation and block is well established. Similar to bacterial homologs, the Kir channel in mammalian has a selective filter at the extracellular of the membrane with a signature sequence GYG. Under the filter there are a widen water cavity towards the intracellular of the membrane. There are a number of residues in Kir2 critical for inward rectification. For example, Mutations of D172 located at the level of the water cavity is firstly identified, a 'rectification controller'. Spermine has high affinity with D172 in the vincity of the filter and unbinding from the residues highly voltage-dependent. Another important residue in rectification is E224 and E299 in the cytoplasmic region which form a ring of acidic. Contrast to D172, spermine has a low-affinity binding with E224 and E299 and low voltage-dependent. Spermine, as the largest (~16–18 Å) polyamine, the pore of the Kir2 is long enough to easily accommodate two or more spermine.

In native $I_{K,ACh}$ channels, spermine can also induce strong inward rectification. There are half of the residues in underlying Kir3.1/Kir3.4 channels equal to D172 and E224 in Kir2.1. The negative residues in Kir3.1/Kir3.4 channels have important role causing strong inward rectification. Although Kir2 and Kir3 have many common similarities there are lots of differences in the kinetical properties between both of them (Anumonwo and Lopatin, 2011).

5. Kv11.1

Kv11.1 formed a kind of the delayed rectifier currents I_{Kr} encoded by *KCNH2* which is identified as the molecular basis of LQT2 in 1995. To date, nearly 300 different mutations of Kv11.1 is the direct reason of congenital LQTs (http://www.fsm.it/cardmoc/; see Table 1) and almost all drugs induced acquired LQTS do so through interaction with the hERG channel. Besides that, dysfunction of Kv11.1 may cause short QT syndrome and artrial fibrillation. Therefore, Kv11.1 has vital role in excitability and action potential conductance in heart

5.1 The features of the structure

Differences from other Kv potassium channel, hERG channel has a unique extracellular part between S5 and the "pore", so called "S5P linker" that contained an amphipathic helix. With exception of transmembrane segment, hERG has intracellular N-terminal and C-terminal. The N-terminal has a Per-Arnt-Sim (PAS) domain which is unique to hERG channe in mammalian ion channel and play a role in deactivation of the channel. The C-terminal has a cyclic nucleotide binding domain (CNBD) which has relatively little effect on gating by binding with cAMP. However, mutation of the domain cause trafficking defects followed by loss of function of hERG channel and the last lead to cardiac arrhythmia.

5.2 Kinetic characters of Kv11.1

Similar to other Kv potassium channel, hERG channel exits at least three distinct conformational states: closed, open and inactivated. Transition from closed to open states or from open to inactivated state of channel attributed to the activation or inactivation which evokes the constrain of the conduction pathway and disrupted ion translocation. hERG channel have significant homology to other Kv family members by sequence analysis. However, kinetics characters of hERG channel activation and inactivation is distinct with other Kv channel. Contrast with other Kv channel, activation of hERG channel is much slower (ι_{on} ranging from 100s of ms to many second) and inactivation is more rapid (ι_{off} ranging from 1 to 10 ms) and voltage-dependent. Because of the slow activation of hERG at depolarized potentials, little outward currents produced by the channel flows through the phase 1 and 2 of cardiac action potential. Reduced outward currents conduce to the maintenance of the plateau of cardiac action potential by allowing Ca^{2+} entry and avoid the cell refractory to premature excitation. In addition, the increase outward currents, due to the much faster recovering from inactivation, is the most important determination of the plateau of cardiac action potential. Besides that the distinct gating kinetics of hERG channel leads to form the character I_{Kur} currents which is help for suppression of propagation of premature beats. Therefore, hERG channel has crucial role in normal or abnormal cardiac action potential.

5.2.1 Activation

The gate of potassium channel is the bundle crossing formed by four the intracellular parts of S6 transmembrane helices of each subunit. The gate at closed state is too narrow to allow transverse of K^+ ions. Transition to open state attribute to these helices which kink at a gate hinge revoking to enlargement of the pore and allow potassium ion pass it. In the bacterial KcsA, MthK and KvAP channels, a conserved Gly residue in S6 is proposed to serve as the hinge for the activation gate. Mutation of the putative Gly hinge in hERG alters gating but does not prevent channel opening. Although Kv1–Kv4 channels also have a Gly in the same location, a different molecular hinge may mediate channel activation. Therefore, the gating hinge, common formed by PVP motif in Kv1-Kv4, has vital roles in change of channel gate whereas the second proline of PVP motif was replaced by glycine in hERG channel.

The S1-S4 VSDs also have important role in regulating the transition from closed to open state in voltage-gated potassium channel. The voltage sensor in hERG channel which is the six basic positive amino acid every 3 residues localized in the position between 525 and 538 of the S4 domain Especially, the most important amino acid is the K525, R528 and K538 conducing to voltage sensing for slow activation. With exception of the positive residues, the acidic amino acid in S1-S4 stablize the VSD at open and closed conformation through forming salt bridge with S4 residues.

It is well known that the voltage sensing regulating the channel open or closed by voltage sensor domain (VSDs) up or down across the transmembranes. However, to date the exact rearrangement of the structure between up or down and the exact magnitude of movement of VSD is still debated. For instance, although the structure of mammalian Kv1.2 channel at open state, especially the location of VSD up relative to the membrane have revealed. But crystal structure of the channel at closed state scilicet the down relative to the membrane do not still detected. Another meaning thing is about the distinct kinetics of the hERG channel because the overall of SVD is high homology with other members of Kv channel family by analysis sequence and hydropathy plots.

To find the reason that the kinetics of hERG is so different, many scientists are attracted in the field and find several key pieces of evidence. When the gating currents corresponding to the movement of voltage sensor domain are measured at the same time the results show that a slow time course corresponding with the slow the activation. From the results we can conclude that the slow activation of hERG attribute to the slow movements of VSDs

5.2.2 Inactivation

About the hERG channel, the mechanism of the inactivation is the C-type at original stage. However, hERG inactivation is orders of magnitude faster than C-type inactivation and its intrinsically voltage-dependent. Many papers pay attention to the molecular basis of the voltage-sensitive of channel inactivation and the relationship between activation and inactivation gating, whether the process are couple or completely separate. Some data indicate that other part but not the S4 contribute to regulate the hERG inactivation. Ser620 and Ser 631 in the P-domain are vital for inactivation. In addition, the charge change of S5P can markedly alter the inactivation of hERG. Therefore, Perrin conclude that different parts of voltage sensor domain participate in regulate the channel activation and inactivation. The amphipathic α-helix of S5P contain in the regulation of hERG inactivaon, due to the relative movements between the α-helix of S5P and the pore domain.

5.2.3 The regulation of KCNE2

It is well known that KCNE2 (Mirp1) was described as a modulator of the ether-à-go-go-related gene 1 (ERG1) potassium current. The protein of KCNE2 is a single transmembrane peptide with an intracellular C-terminal and an extracellular N-terminal. Coexpression with Kv11.1 increase the currents of I_{Kr} owing to increasing the single conductance, altering the kinetic characters of inactivation and inactivation. Later KCNE2 was found to also change the KCNQ1 potassium current by drastically changing the gating properties. Mutations in KCNE2 are associated with long QT syndrome (LQT6) (http://www.fsm.it/cardmoc/) because of a decreasing influence on both ERG1 and KCNQ1 currents by KCNE2 mutation. Accordingly, both types of complexes KCNQ1/KCNE1 and KCNH2/KCNE2 could play a functional role in the heart.

5.3 Functions of Kv11.1 in heart

Loss of function and gain of function mutations in Kv11.1 produce to the formation and conductance of action potential in cardiac tissues. Loss of function mutations decreases the currents of I_{Kr} due to decrease of channel number, channel open probability and single channel conductance as mentioned above.

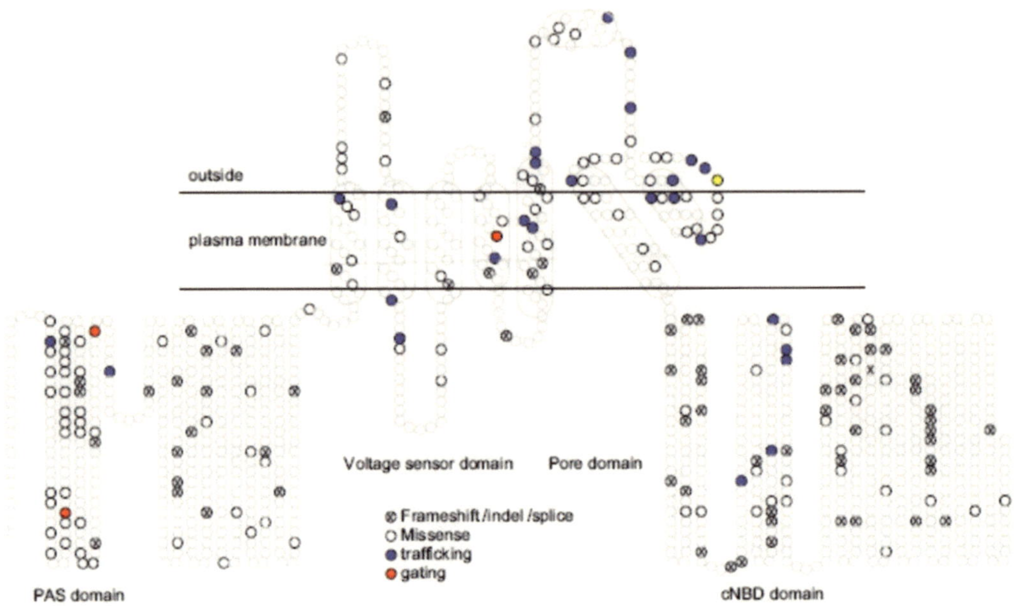

Fig. 3. (adapted from Perrin et al, 2008) Topological map of position of nearly 300 different mutations in hERG in LQTS2.

5.3.1 Congenital cardiac arrhythmia

LQTs is charactered by the prolongation of QT interval on ECG of the patients. Loss of function in Kv11.1 caused LQT2. Defective synthesis of mutations contained the premature termination codons is maybe the one fourths of all mutations of hERG channel (http: //www. fsm. it/cardmoc). Otherwise, hERG mutation of R534C display an increased open probability expressed in *Xenopus laevis* oocytes whereas in clinically the mutant induces the gain of function. Therefore, it is importance of detecting the mutations in mammalian system.

Gain of function mutation in KCNH2 cause increasing of currents amplitude I_{Kr} which lead to shorten the action potential duration and in final to decurtate the QT interval on ECG. Some patients with SQT will be healing well in the future through the regulation of themselves. However, if the cardiac action potential is persistent shorten and produce diminishing of refractory period between the continual bisaction potential. At last, SQT may be get worse the atrial fibrillation and sudden death or syncop.

5.3.2 Acquired LQTS

Comparision with congenital LQTS, acquired LQTS is more common cause of TdP. Lots of factors can induce to form acquired LQTS, such as myocardial ischemia, electrolyte disturbances, bradycardia and so on. Of the most important factors is drug. Accordingly, the drug-induced LQTS is equal to the acquired LQTS in most case. However, acquired LQTS and drug-induced LQTS is essential two different concepts.

Many kinds of drug can induce the acquired LQTS, for instance antiarrhythmia drug, antibiotic, antihistamine and so on. Atiarrhythmia drug quinidine is a relatively frequent side effects, caused 2-9% of treated patient induced RdP. Other drugs induced TdP is less than antiarrhythmia drugs. The compounds (dofetilide, sotalol and ibutilide), predictable designed to block cardiac repolarizing currents, can induce the prolongation of the OT interval which unfortunately arises as a side effect of the compound treated for non-cardiac diseases. Therefore, the compound in already marketed drugs will be withdrawal or restriction. In order to the expenses of the pharmaceutical companies, it is now common practice to screen for compound for hERG-channel activity early during preclinical safety assessment. However, in clinical the blockage of hERG can counteract by blocking of L-type of calcium channel.

Most of drugs which can induce acquired LQTS can also block of hERG channel. Contrast to other Kv channel, the hERG is unusually susceptible to blockage by drugs is unknown, suggesting that it has a unique binding site. In order to find the interact sites hERG with the blockers, an ala-scanning mutagenesis approach is used. Mutations of two polar residues (Thr 623 and Ser 624) located at the base of the pore helix and mutations two aromatic residues Tyr652 and Phe656 located in the S6 domain of hERG has vital roles in combination with the compounds. The side chains of all four residues are oriented toward the large central cavity of the channel and can block the transmembrane pass of potassium ions by combining with the blocker.

5.4 Future perspectives

Over the past 16 years a great deal of discovery of hERG channel has been detected but there is still much to explore about the channel.

6. Kv7.1

Kv7.1 (also known as KCNQ1, KvLQT1) is the α-subunit of a voltage-gated potassium channel cloned in 1996 by Wang and co-workers using linkage analyses of LQTS1 patients and expressed in several tissues including cardiac myocytes and epithelial cells. The most important roles of KCNQ1 channels are repolarization of the cardiac tissue following an action potential. In cardiac myocytes, the KCNQ1 subunit assembles with the KCNE1 β-subunit (minK) to form a channel complex. The channel complex of KCNQ1/KCNE1 produce the delayed rectifier current I_{Ks}, which is partly responsible for terminating the cardiac action potential during phase 2. Up to now, there are nearly three hundred mutation of KCNQ1 have been detected. Most of the mutations produce the loss of function of KCNQ1, lead to the LQTS (http://www.fsm.it/cardmoc/), a most kind of cardiac arrhythmia characterized by prolongation of QT interval in electrocardiogram, syncope and sudden death. Only a few gain-of function mutations have been verified and have correlate with the atrial fibrillation or the short QT syndrome (SQTs).

Based on the molecular mechanism of altering of KCNQ1 currents, mutations of the channel are divided into impaired trafficking, impaired voltage dependence, impaired selectivity and impaired tetramerization. For the majority of these three hundred KCNQ1 mutations, little is known about the molecular mechanism producing to the pathologies or limited to which of the categories. Therefore, there are many unknown knowledge about the three hundred KCNQ1 mutaions and make further progress in the future with the application of new technology of structure prediction in study.

6.1 Structure and electrophysiological characters of KCNQ1

As a member of Kv potassium channel, KCNQ1 channel show a high similarity to voltage-gated potassium channels of the Kv type which assemble a tetramer, with each subunit of

KCNQ1 contained S1-S6 trans-membrane. Different from other Kv members, KCNQ1 often form heterotetramer with auxiliary subunits contained one-transmembrane in vivo. To date, there are five member of KCNE family have been detected and in *Xenopus laevis* oocytes or mammalian system the α subunit of KCNQ1 channel can combinate with any one of them to form miscellaneous kinds heterotetramer with distinct kinetic characters of channel such as activation, inactivation or deactivation and so on. Accordingly, α subunit of KCNQ1 channel has been check in lots of tissues in the body and with different physiological characters.

In the full-length human KCNQ1 gene, 16 exons constitute of KCNQ1 with the very GC-rich 5′-end. The translated protein is composed of 676 residues and has six transmembrane domains S1-S6, a pore loop with a typical potassium-channel pore signature sequence (GYGD), and intracellular NH_2 and COOH terminals covering 122 and 322 residues, respectively. To date, with the exception of KCNQ1, there are other four members in the KCNQ family have been detected, such as KCNQ2-5. Comparision with other members of KCNQ family, KCNQ can not assemble a hetertetramer with other members and just forming a homotetramer only with themselves.

As a voltage-gated potassium channel, KCNQ1 was activated by decreasing of depolarization. And similar the other voltage-gated potassium channel, the voltage sensor is located in the S4. However, mutations in the linker of between S4 and S5 still have effect on activation of the KCNQ1 channel. When KCNQ1 channel are fully open at the positive potential followed by a strikingly repolarization produces a hook currents which represent a fraction of KCNQ1 channel inactivation. Because the channel will be open again from the closed state. Researches show that the five transmembrane and the pore part of each subunit have vital roles in the inactivation of KCNQ1 channel.

6.2 Regulation of KCNQ1 channel activation and inactivation

As mentioned above, the KCNQ1 subunit and the ancillary subunit KCNE1 collect together to form the currents of I_{Ks} in cardiac tissues. The KCNE1 subunit has important roles in regulation of kinetical properties of KCNQ1 channel. For example, the currents formed by KCNQ1 subunit alone is activated rapidly whereas ones formed by coexpressed of KCNQ1 and KCNE1 is activated very slowly. In addition, the presence of KCNE1 produce a large increase in the macroscopic KCNQ1 currents, a positive shift of voltage-dependence curves, slowing of the activation and deactivation and almost of absent of inactivation. Some researches have shown that the distinguished increase of the magnitude of currents of KCNQ1/KCNQ1 complex is owing to increase the single channel conductance for four to sevenfold and almost eliminate the inactivation the channel by KCNE1 subunit. As for the exact combination of KCNQ1 and KCNE1 subunit, there are distinct views about it. Some results display that KCNE1 lines to the conductance pathway. On the contrary other results show the combination site is out of the conductance pathway. Van Horn proposes a Q1/E1-TMD model, a new model to elucidate the interaction of protein-protein about KCNQ1 and KCNE1 in recent researches. The emphasis of the new model is on the KCNE1 transmembrane domain (also called TMD). It is generally accepted that in closed state the S4-S5 linker interact with the C-end of S6 from another subunit to lock it in the closed configuration. In response to depolarization, the change of conformation of S4 voltage sensor, the S4-S5 linker pull off and deviate from the S6 inducing the channel open. The Q1/E1-TMD model consider that the C-terminal end of KCNE sits on the end of the S4–S5 linker while simultaneously N-terminal end makes extensive (and presumably adhesive) contacts in the cleft between the voltage sensor and pore domains of the channel. Therefore, during the transition of the channel from closed to open state, the presence of KCNE1 TMD will interfere with the S4-S5 linker deviating from the S6. Uniformly, because of the KCNE1 presence, transition state open to close become very slow and is help for maintenance of the open state of the channel.

Besides the ancillary subunit of KCNE1, there are other members (KCNE2-5) in the family. It is interesting that all ancillary subunits can co-assemble with KCNQ1 channel in different tissue and alter the kinetic characters of KCNQ1 channel. In cardiac tissue, besides of KCNE2, KCNE2 is another important ancillary subunit. KCNE2 (also named Mirp1), originally described as a ancillary of the ether-à-go-go-related gene 1 (ERG1) potassium current, was later found to change the KCNQ1 potassium current though drastically changing the gating properties. Otherwise, in organs such as stomach and intestine, Moreover, the mRNA of KCNE4 and KCNE5 has been detected in the heart. They may be has vital roles in maintaneine of the ordinary function of the heart. However, there is no relative report about it.

6.3 Functions of KCNQ1 channel in heart

Currents of I_{Ks} formed by KCNQ1/KCNE1 have slow activation, whereas I_{Kur} and I_{K1} constituted by ERG1 and Kir2.x, respectively, have rapide activation kinetics. The three repolarizing potassium currents together have been called the repolarization reserve because to some extent they can substitute for each other. However, in the fast heart beat, only I_{Ks} currents are upregulated by phosphorylation and by current accumulation due to slow deactivation. In addition, In heart tissue, distribution of KCNQ1 through the cardiac wall is also inhomogeneous and the expression of KCNQ1 is less in medmyocardium than epi- and endomyocardium.

The cardiac function of KCNQ1 and its accessory subunits is emphasized by the functional impact of numerous mutations in these proteins (http://www.fsm.it/cardmoc/). Mutations in KCNQ1 causing loss of function by trafficking defective, assembly defective, or single channel conductance lead to prolonged action potentials and LQTS. A domain located near the COOH terminal (residues 589–620) is responsible for this assembly specificity, and deletion of a part of this domain leads to an impaired assembly of the channel complexes followed by mistrafficking. Mutations in ancillary subunits such as KCNE1 and KCNE1 also cause LQTS4 and LQTS5, respectively.

KCNQ1 mutation (S140G), as a gain of function mutation, is detected in a family with arterial fibrillation inherited as an autosomal dominant way through four generations. The mutation shortens the action potential through increasing the currents of $I_{Ks.}$ Similarly, a gain-of-function mutation in KCNE2 (R27C) increasing the activity of the KCNQ1/KCNE2 channel has also been implicated in atrial fibrillation.

Acquired LQTS is predominantly found when the patients take the blocker of hERG channel as medicine. Because the currents of I_{Kr} are blocked, the repolarization reserve is decreased and the disperation of repolarization is leaded to a further increase due to the inhomogeneous distribution of KCNQ1 in heart wall.

7. Kv4.3

Kv4.3 is formed the rapid activated currents I_{to} (encoded by *KCND3*) which is a voltage-dependent, 4-aminopyridine (4-AP) sensitive, calcium-independent K^+ current (I_{to}). I_{to} have been detected in human artial and ventricular myocytes and is responsible for the early rapid depolarization (at phase 1) so determining the height of plateau. Therefore, I_{to} will influence of other ion channel activation such as the L-type calcium channel and the delayed rectifier channel (KCNQ1). Distribution of Kv4.3 is heterogeneous through the cardiac tissue. For example, I_{to} density in atrial tissue, Purkinje fibers, epicardial and midmyocardial (M) cells is higher than in the endocardial cells. The prominent epicardial I_{to} conduce to the depression of epicardial in ischemia and to the progress of a significant dispersion of repolarization between normal and ischemic epicardium, between epicardium and endocardium.

7.1 Regulation of Kv4.3

Kv4.3 can be blocked by many compounds but which bind with the channel either at open state or at close state. It has been raised that blocker of I_{to} prolong the action potential duration in atria or in ischemic ventricular tissues. However, blockage of I_{to} subsequently changes the other potassium channel underlying during repolariztion of cardiac action potential. Reduction of I_{to} magnitude can shorten the duration of ventricular action potential. Therefore, it is still unclear that the exact role in control human cardiac action potential.

Channel properties of Kv4.3 is modified by the phosphorylation, mediated by protein kinase A (PKA) and C (PKC) through altering the channel kinetic (activation, inactivation or single channel conductance) and the expression of active channel in the membrane. Decrease in I_{to} by PKC attributed to enhance the inactivation and step down the time of deactivate of the channel Kv4.3. a-adrenergic agonists reduce I_{to} magnitude in rat ventricular myocytes and oppositely the β-adrenergic agonists has no effect on I_{to} currents.

7.2 Functions of Kv4,3 in heart

Heart failure, cardiac hypertrophy and myocardial ischemia and infarction decrease the magnitude of Ito resulting in the prolongation of action potential. The degrade in I_{to} in heart failure may be adaptive in the short-term because increased depolarization during the cardiac cycle means that more time is available for excitation–contraction coupling, which moderate the decrease in cardiac output, however it becomes maladaptive in the long-term, because a prolongation of the APD may contribute to arrhythmogenesis, either by causing inhomogeneous repolarization or by increasing the likelihood of early afterdepolarizations. On the contrary, it is proved that up-regulation of I_{to} in cardiac hypertrophy and in cardiac myocytes after induced myocardial infarction. Increase in Ito presents as a protector moderating the excessive prolongation of action potential duration and Ca^{2+} inflow to minimize the incidence of ventricular arrhythmia. In addition, the patients with chronic atrial fibrillation decrease the currents of I_{to} and downregulate the mRNA.

8. Kv1.5

I_{kur} currents in human atrium are formed by the α subunit (Kv1.5) and β ancillary subunit (Kvβ1.2). The features of I_{Kur}, as outward rectifired currents, are activated rapidly in the plateau range and inactivation slowly. Interestingly, currents of I_{Kur} just have been detected in human atria rather than cardiac ventricle. Therefore, currents of I_{Kur} have vital roles during the atrial repolarization. There is a huge difference of Kv1.5 from other ion cardiac channel. Distribution of Kv1.5 is homogeneous across the atrial wall.

8.1 Regulations of Kv1.5

hKv1.5 can be regulated by both PKA and PKC. One consensus site in Kv1.5 for phphosphorylation by PKC is located on the extracellular S4–S5 linker and 4 consensus sites for PKA is located in the N- and C-terminal domains. Isoproterenol and adenylate cyclase both increase the magnitude of I_{Kur} and the increase can be counteract by PKA inhibitor. Otherwise, propranolol and phenylephrine decrease the amplitude of I_{Kur} moderating by the PKC inhibitor. Accordingly, β-adrenergic stimulation enhances the currents of I_{Kur} by PKA. Oppositely, α-adrenergic stimulation inhibits I_{Kur} currents by PKC. Human thrombin or rat 5-HT1c receptors inhibits the currents of IKur by increasing phospholipase C (PLC). Moreover, the Scr tyrosing kinase inhibits the hKv1.5 by phosphorylation of the N-terminus proline-rich sequences mediated by SH3 domain of the tyrosine kinase.

8.2 Functions of I_{Kur} in heart

I_{Kur} is relatively insensitive to TEA, Ba^{2+} and class III antiarrhythmics of the methanesulfonanilide group. Antiarrhythmia drug is often weak bases that predominant cationic ion at pH7. At the channel open state, the cationic ion can bind with the pore and/or selective filter domain of the channel leading to the blockage of the channel. The binding site for some drugs is existed at the external mouth of the channel pore formed by the P loop and adjacent S5–S6 segments.

Because of the Kv1.5 just located in atria, the channel is a promising target for the development of new safe antiarrhythmic drugs to prevent atrial fibrillation and without a risk of ventricular proarrhythmia. However, In patients in chronic artrial fibrillation, the action potential duration in atria is significantly prolongated due to both blockage of $I_{ca,L}$ and I_{Kur}. Accordingly, it is not expected what will be happened by use of I_{Kur} blocker to treat the patient with chronic AF. In a rat, rapid atrial pacing just immediately and transiently increases the mRNA of Kv1.5 rather than the ones of KCNQ1 and hERG. It shows that Kv4.3 at least in part contribute to the rapid shortening of the atrial refractoriness at the onset of AF. Therefore, the selective blockers of I_{Kur} counteract the shortening of atrial action potential duration at rapid rate state. From mentioned above, application of I_{Kur} selective blocker in clinical is a challege job in the future.

9. Kir2.1 and Kir3

Inward rectifiers (Kir) is composed of a large family of potassium channel. Among them, only two subfamilies (Kir2 and Kir3) share great structural similarity and underlie classical 'strong inwardly rectifying currents' originally observed in skeletal and cardiac muscle. In cardiac tissue, there are only two similar types of these currents: (1) I_{K1}, as a constitutively active Kir current, is more prominent in ventricular tissue, and (2) $I_{K,Ach}$, as a receptor-activated Kir current, is more prominent in atrial tissue, as well as in SA node and AV node. There are two common features of the kir2 and Kir3. one is a strongly voltage-dependent decline of potassium conductance upon membrane depolarization producing a characteristic region of so-called 'negative slope' conductance. Another unique property of Kir currents is the unusual dependence of rectification on extracellular K^+. In order to comprehend the two characters of Kir channel, firstly to fully the molecular basis of the channels.

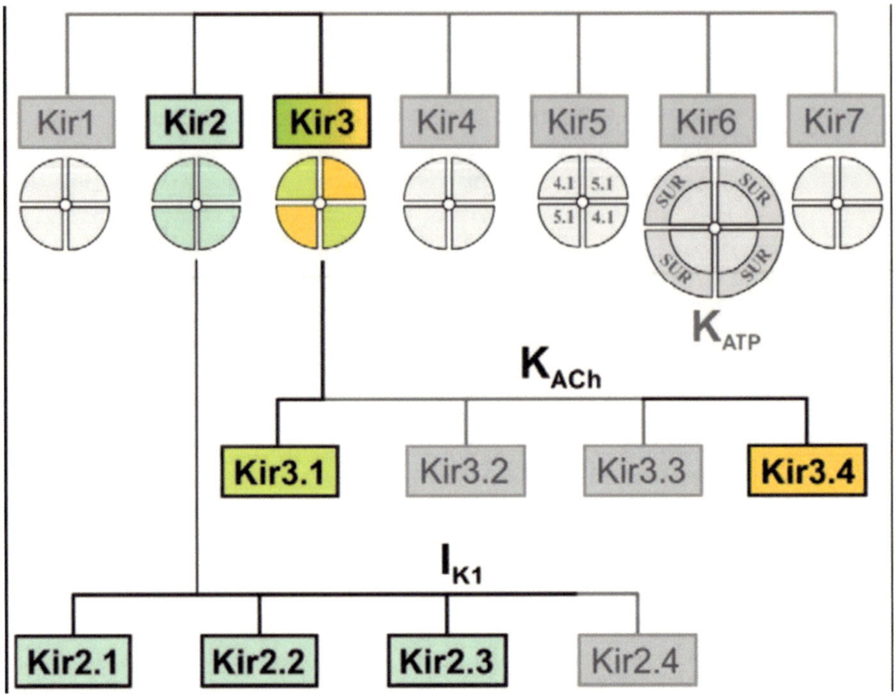

Fig. 4. (cited from Anumonwo et al, 2009). The family of inward rectifier potassium channels. All members of this family share significant structural similarity, but only Kir2 and Kir3 subfamilies represent channels carrying classical strongly rectifying currents.

In human heart, the distribution of I_{K1} and $I_{K,Ach}$ has distinct region. I_{K1} is more prominent in the ventricles, including Purkinje myocytes. $I_{K,Ach}$ has generally an opposite distribution to that of I_{K1}. It is more prominent in the atria than in ventricles. Similarity, the current density of I_{K1} and $I_{K,Ach}$ may vary across the ventricular or atrial tissues, distinctively. About the subunit composition of $I_{K,Ach}$, under normal conditions native $I_{K,Ach}$ channels are heteromers of Kir3.1/ Kir3.4 subunits. However, recent data suggest that Kir3.4 subunit alone has similar function with the native $I_{K,Ach}$. Comparision with $I_{K,Ach}$, I_{K1} is formed by coassembly of the Kir2.1.x subfamily of proteins (Kir 2.1, 2.2, and 2.3) with Kir2.1 the most abundant subtype in ventricular tissue.

9.1 Functions of Kir2 and Kir3 in heart

To date, I_{K1}, formed by coassembly of the Kir2.1.x subfamily of proteins (Kir 2.1, 2.2, and 2.3) In cardiac tissue, is the major component of inward rectifier potassium current and have a vital role in determinant of the resting membrane potential and conduces to the terminal phase of repolarization (phase 3). Loss of function of Kir2 channel ≥ 90%, the heart of transgene (TG) mice led to prolongation of QRS and QT intervals as well as expected prolongation of action potential. Surprisingly, resting membrane potential in TG ventricular myocytes was nearly unaffected. It is unexpectedly that upregulation of I_{K1} in TG mice expressing Kir2.1 subunits, gain of function, cause to multiple abnormalities of cardiac excitability contained significant AP shortening and various types of atrial and ventricular arrhythmias.

In heart, another contribution of I_{K1} to excitability is through an unusual and strong dependence on extracellular K^+. During repetitive firing, cardiac activity is followed by markedly changes in the concentration of K^+ in the restricted (0.01–5 µM) intercellular space, even more accumulation in the t-tubules. Increase of extracellular K^+ should be accompanied by the increase of I_{K1} conductance with results on electrical activity, e.g., AP duration and propagation

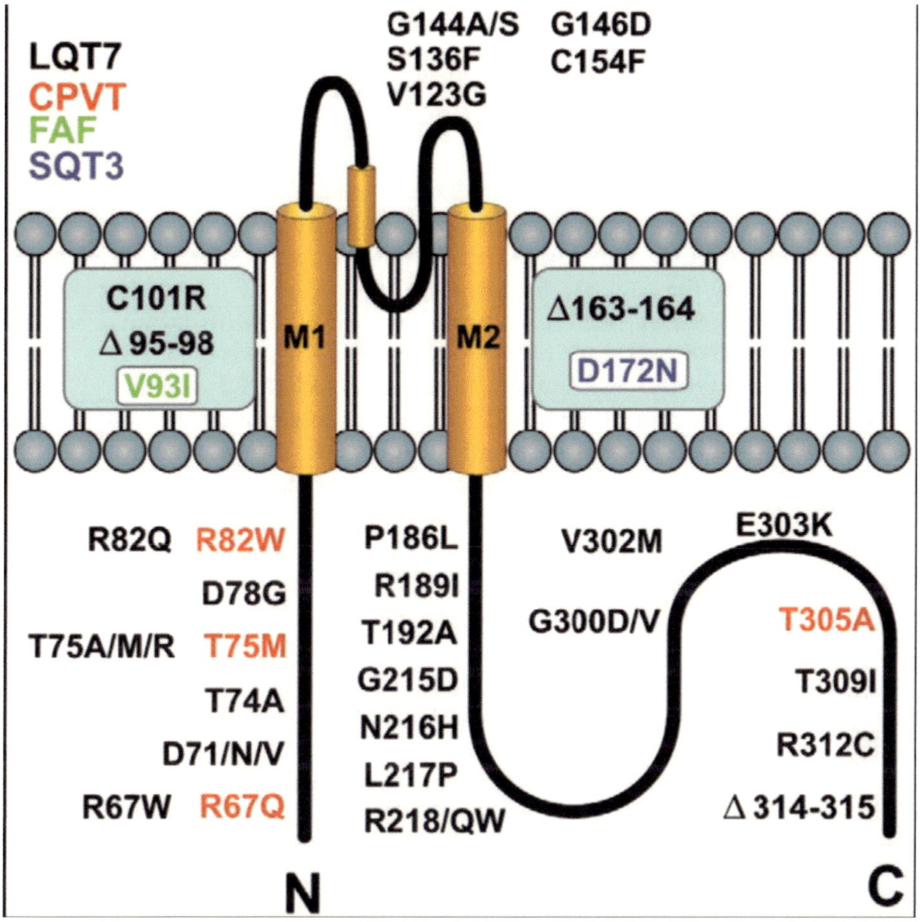

Fig. 5. (cited from Anumonwo et al, 2009). Mutations on Kir2.1 protein associated with channelopathies of the classical inward rectifier channel. Mutant residues are color coded to represent the long QT7 (LQT7; black), catecholaminergic polymorphic ventricular tachycardia (CPVT; red), familial atrial fibrillation (FAF; green), and short QT3 (SQT3; blue).

To date, four channelopathies related with inward rectifier currents have been detected, all due to loss of function or gain of function of I_{K1} currents (encoded by KCNJ2), LQT7, catecholaminergic polymorphic ventricular tachycardia (CPVT), familial atrial fibrillation (FAF), and short QT3. LQT7 at early is also called Andersen syndrome (AS) or Andersen-Tawil syndrome (ATS). Symptoms of the disease are characterized by a triad of clinical phenotypes affecting morphogenesis as well as the functioning of skeletal and cardiac muscles. ATS patients are often companied by features that include scoliosis, cleft palate, and short stature and display skeletal muscle weakness. Besides that, cardiac electrical abnormalities include prolongation of the QT interval, short runs of ventricular tachycardia, ventricular bigeminy and multi-focal ventricular ectopy mediated by adrenergic stimulation. However, recent works suggest that classification of ATS into LQTS is incorrect because of the former largely related to the abnormalities of the T–U complex. Because more than half of ATS is the mutations in KCNJ2 the term AST1 is reffered to the disease of I_{Kir2}. To date, more than 33 mutation in KCNJ2 is related to AST1 and the mutations have been identified as the autosomal-dominant. Some of mutations, such as D71V in AST1 patients, can decrease by ~94% of the magnitude of wild type currents I_{Kir2}. Several of ATS1 mutations, such as R21Q/W mutations, result in a loss-of function in the $K_{ir2.1}$ channels due to reduced interaction with membrane PIP_2.

Short QT syndrome (SQTS) is charactered by the shorten of QT interval on ECG. SQTS is an inherited abnormality that predisposes afflicted individuals to a high risk of having fibrillation (atrial/ventricular) and sudden death. Three forms of SQTS have been identified and SQTS3 is caused by the gain of function of mutations in inward rectifier channel gene, KCNJ2. SQTS3, charactered by electrocardiographic phenotype with asymmetrical T waves, is distinguished with other two kinds of SQTS. The molecular basis of SQTS3 is the mutation D172N at a position critical for inward rectification of Kir2.1 channel. Heterologous coexpression of wild type and mutant Kir2.1 subunits showed increased outward currents in mutant channels which account for the tall, asymmetrical T waves on the ECG of LQTS3 patients. Researches by computer simulations suggest that mutations in SQT3 might predispose patients to a higher risk of reentrant arrhythmias.

Mutation of V93I in Kir2.1 is associated with familial atrial fibrillation, thereby implicating I_{K1} in this disease. In addition, the mutant channels have larger outward currents by whole-cell patch-clamp studies, however the underlying mechanism(s) responsible for the increase remains unknown.

In a recent study, three novel (R67Q, R85W, and T305A) mutations belonged to CPVT3 and one previously described (T75M) mutations in KCNJ2 are identified. ECG analysis reveals prominent U-waves, ventricular ectopy, and polymorphic ventricular tachycardia. It is interestingly that there were no dysmorphic features or skeletal muscle abnormalities in the patients. Whole-cell patch-clamp experiments revealed that mutant channels had significantly reduced by ≥ 95 % amplitude of wild type outward current and that T75M and R67Q mutations had dominant negative effects when co-expressed with wild type channels. Importantly, the study showed that the T305A mutation selectively affected channel rectification properties.

Cardiac strong inward rectifier potassium channels continue to surprise researchers with their novel roles in cardiac excitability, complex structure, function, and regulation. While significant progress has been made in recent years, clearly, many questions still remain to be answered and we certainly will soon witness new, and likely unexpected, discoveries in this field.

10. $K_{ir6.2}$

ATP-sensitive potassium (K_{ATP}) channels (encoded by KCNJ11) are evolutionarily conserved and are first discovered in the cardiac sarcolemma where they are expressed in high density.

I_{KATP} is formed by the complex protein composed by the pore-forming subunit and the regulatory sulfonylurea receptor which is an ATPase-harboring ATP-binding cassette protein. To date, members of the inwardly rectifying K^+ channel family (Kir6.1 and Kir6.2) and the sulfonylurea receptor isoforms (SUR1, SUR2A and SUR2B) have been identified. In cardiac tissue, K_{ATP} channel is a hetero-octameric complex composed of four pairs of these two distinct subunits Kir6.2 and SUR2A. The structure of K_{ATP} channel is very similar to Kir3 and Kir2. Therefore, there is no redundant description in this part.

10.1 Functions of K_{ATP} channels in heart

K_{ATP} channels, as a cardio-protective role, were recognized early in ischemia heart. The channel can mediate shortening of the cardiac action potential by increase of the I_{KATP} currents then control calcium influx into the cytosol. Moreover, when the heart expose to a brief periods of ischemia causing a sustained ischemic insult K_{ATP} channel activity can depress significantly the injury produced by ischemia such as infarct size, coined ischemic preconditioning. Therefore, in ischemia heart, K_{ATP} channel can degrade markedly heart injure caused by ischemia.

Another important function of K_{ATP} channel is during the process of stress without distress in heart. The concept of "stress without distress" is referred to describe the ability of an organism to confront and/or escape imposed threat. The concept is very likewise to the "flight-or-fight" response, through the general adaptation syndrome. For example, acute exercise-stress causes a systemic sympathetic stimulation that raises cardiac contractility, heart rate and thereby provides the necessary higher cardiac output. How huge change of the heart excitability has happened after acute exercise. Many researches suggest that stress without distress is dependent in the K_{ATP} channel in heart. The change of this enhanced cardiac output imposes a significant metabolic in large part of the heart due to the highly energy consuming calcium handling machinery. A compensatory increase in outward potassium current formed by K_{ATP} channel is normally activated to offset the resulting calcium influx in order to reducing energy-demanding myocardial calcium overload.

K_{ATP} channel also has important roles in heart failure. Heart failure has no effect on the intrinsic biophysical properties of the cardiac K_{ATP} channel whereas the structural remodeling disrupts communication of energetic signal and channel. Then the disruption leads to interfere markedly the metabolic regulation of the channel at last. Accordingly, metabolic dysregulation of K_{ATP} channels created by the disease-induced structural remodeling appears to contribute to the dysfunction of heart failure.

11. Acknowledgment

The paper is supported by a start-up grant from Henan University of Technology (2009BS006).

12. References

Anumonwo JMB, Lopatin AN. 2010. Cardiac strong inward rectifier potassium channels. *J Mol Cell Cardiol* 48: 45–54

Delisle BP, Anson BD, Rajamani S, January CT. 2004. Biology of cardiac arrhythmias ion channel protein trafficking. *Circ. Res* 94: 1418-1428

Fowler SJ, Cerrone M, Napolitano C, Priori SG. 2010. Genetic testing for inherited cardiac arrhythmias. *Hellenic J Cardiol* 51:92-103

Haase H. 2007. Ahnak, a new player in β-adrenergic regulation of the cardiac L-type Ca^{2+} channel. *Cardiovasc Res* 73: 19–25.

Jespersen T, Grunnet M, Olesen SP. 2005. The KCNQ1 Potassium Channel: From Gene to Physiological Function. *Physiology* 20:408-416.

Jeyaraj D, Ashwath M, and Rosenbaum DS. 2010. Pathophysiology and clinical implications of cardiac memory. *Pacing Clin Electrophysiol* 33(3): 346–352.

Liao P, Soong TW. 2010. $Ca_V1.2$ channelopathies: from arrhythmias to autism, bipolar disorder, and immunodeficiency. *Eur J Physiol* 460:353–359

Pero D, Rodriguez N, Choveau F, Baró I, Mérot J, Loussouarn G. 2008. Kv7.1 (KCNQ1) properties and channelopathies. *J Physiol* 586.7: 1785-1789

Perrin MJ, Subbiah RN, Vandenberg JI, Hill AP. 2008. Human ether-a-go-go related gene (hERG) K^+ channels: function and disfunction. *Prog biophy molr bio* 98: 137-148

Ravens U, Cerbai E. 2008. Role of potassium currents in cardiac arrhythmias. *Europace* 10: 1133–1137

Remme CA, Bezzina CR. 2010. Sodium channel (Dys) Ffunction and cardiac arrhythmia. *Cardiovasc ther* 28: 287-294.

Sanguinetti MC, Tritani-Firouzi M. 2006. hERG potassium channels and cardiac arrhythmia. *Nature* 466: 463-469

Sicilian G. 1991. A new approach to the classification of antiarrhythmic drugs based on their actions on arrhythmogenic mechanisms. Task Force of the Working Group on Arrhythmias of the European Society of Cardiology. *Circulation* 84:1831–51.

Sung RJ, Wu YH, Lai NHJ, Teng CH, Luo CH, Tien HC, Lo CP, Wu SN. 2010. β-Adrenergic modulation of arrhythmogenesis and identification of targeted sites of antiarrhythmic therapy in Timothy (LQT8) syndrome: a theoretical study. *Am J Physiol Heart Circ Physiol* 298: H33–H44,

Tristani-Firouzi M, Etheridge SP. 2010. Kir 2.1 channelopathies: the Andersen–Tawil syndrome. *Eur J Physiol* 460:289–294

Ufret-Vincenty CA, Baro DJ, Lederer WJ , Rockman HA,. Quiňones LE, and Santana LF. 2001. Role of sodium channel deglycosylation in the genesis of cardiac arrhythmias in heart failure. *J Biol Chem* 276 (30): 28197–28203

Van Horn WD, Vanoye CG, Sanders CR. 2011. Working model for the structural basis for KCNE1 modulation of the KCNQ1 potassium channel. *Currt Opin Struc Biol* 21:283–291

6

L-Type Ca^{2+} Current in Cardiac Arrhythmias

Gema Ruiz-Hurtado[1], Julio L. Alvarez[2] and Jean-Pierre Benitah[1]
[1]*Signalisation et Physiopathologie Cardiaque, Inserm U769 - LabEx LERMIT, Faculty of Pharmacy - IFR141, University of Paris-Sud, F-92296 Chatenay-Malabry*
[2]*Laboratorio de Electrofisiología, Instituto de Cardiología y Cirugía Cardiovascular, La Habana,*
[1]*France*
[2]*Cuba*

1. Introduction

Cardiac arrhythmias result from the confluence of structural and functional changes in the heart and genetic predisposition, reflecting an interaction between a susceptible substrate (e.g. an anatomically defined circuit, a myocardial scar, fibrosis or a monogenic arrhythmia syndrome) and a specific electrophysiological triggering event. Such triggered activities arises from delayed afterdepolarizations (DADs) or early afterdepolarizations (EADs), in which action potential prolongation and aberrant Ca^{2+} fluxes are a recurrent theme.

Ca^{2+} channels in cardiomyocytes provide the main influx pathway for Ca^{2+}. Three types of high threshold Ca^{2+} channels are expressed in heart: two L-type channels, $Ca_v1.2$ and $Ca_v1.3$ and a P-type channel, $Ca_v2.1$. The $Ca_v2.1$ channel protein is expressed at a very low level the in heart (Starr et al., 1991) while $Ca_v1.3$ is mainly expressed in fetal hearts and only in adult sinoatrial and atrioventricular nodes and atrial tissues of adult (Lipscombe et al., 2004; Qu et al., 2005). We will focus attention on the $Ca_v1.2$ L-type Ca^{2+} channel (LTCC) which is the main player in electrical activity and excitation-contraction coupling (EC coupling) in the ventricular cardiomyocyte.

The LTCC of cardiomyocytes is a complex multimeric molecular sarcolemmal ensemble that during an action potential (AP) allows Ca^{2+} to flow down its electrochemical gradient into the cardiac cell. LTCCs are mostly localized in the transverse tubular system of cardiomyocytes (Wibo et al., 1991; Kawai et al., 1999; Brette et al., 2004). Activation of LTCC generates a Ca^{2+} current (I_{CaL}) through the sarcolemma large enough to be involved in AP overshoot and in the control of AP duration (APD) in different cardiac cells types (Bers, 2001). I_{CaL} serves as a trigger for Ca^{2+} release from the sarcoplasmic reticulum (SR) during the excitation-contraction coupling by a mechanism known as calcium-induced calcium release (CICR, Fabiato & Fabiato, 1975; Bers, 2001). LTCC activation can also play a role in transcription mechanisms in cardiomyocytes (Atar et al., 1995; Brette et al., 2006). Several hormones and neuromediators modulate the activity of LTCC via complex intracellular signaling pathways and, as well, several intracellular molecules and the cytoskeleton can influence LTCC activity (Benitah et al., 2010). However, intracellular Ca^{2+} concentration is strictly controlled in normal cells by different mechanisms (Bers, 2001) since a Ca^{2+} overload can have deleterious effects including arrhythmias and myocardial remodeling via a genetic reprogramming of the cardiac cell (Benitah et al., 2003).

2. Macromolecular structure

The typical structure of LTCC in ventricular cardiomyocytes is a macromolecular multimeric complex consisting of a ~240 kDa pore-forming unit α_1C (encoded by the CACNA1C gene) and two auxiliary (modulator) subunits: an intracellular β subunit (mainly β_{2A}, encoded by the CACNB2A gene) and the dimer $\alpha_2\delta$ subunit (mainly $\alpha_2\delta$-1, encoded by the CACNA2D1 gene) in a 1:1:1 ratio (Catterall et al., 2005). The α_1C subunit consists of four homologous repeating motifs (I–IV), each one composed of six membrane-spanning α-helices (S1 to S6) linked by variable extracellular and cytoplasmic loops (linkers). This subunit contains all the necessary structures to allow the channel to gate (activation and inactivation) and confers the Ca^{2+} selectivity as well as the electrophysiological and pharmacological properties of the LTCC (Takahashi & Catterall, 1987; Catterall, 2000; Carafoli et al., 2001; Lacinová & Hoffmann, 2001; Bodi et al., 2005; Lacinova & Hofmann, 2005; Brette et al., 2006; Benitah et al., 2010). However, more native LTCC properties can be achieved when all three subunits are present (Lacinová & Hoffmann, 2001; Lacinova & Hofmann, 2005; Benitah et al., 2010). The β_{2A} subunit seems to be involved in membrane targeting of α_1C and influence LTCC inactivation (Bodi et al., 2005; Lacinova & Hofmann, 2005; Brette et al., 2006). Its structure reveals a module of two interacting domains, a Src homology 3 (SH3) domain and a Guanylate Kinase (GK) domain (Chen et al., 2004; Bodi et al., 2005). It was initially believed that its conserved sequence, BID (Beta Interaction Domain), interacted directly with the Alpha Interaction Domain (AID) within the intracellular loop between domains I and II of the α_1C subunit (De Waard et al., 1996; Arikkath & Campbell, 2003). However, recent data indicate that BID is largely buried in the $Ca_v\beta$ core and is unavailable for protein-protein interactions (Chen et al., 2004; Van Petegem et al., 2004). The AID is bound in a hydrophobic groove (α-binding pocket, ABP) in the GK domain and positions the β-subunit near the intracellular pore-lining segment I6 (which is important in Ca^{2+} channel inactivation) thus providing evidence that $Ca_v\beta$ influence Ca^{2+} channel gating by direct modulation of this segment (Van Petegem et al., 2004). Although the BID does not participate directly in binding the α_1C subunit, structural integrity and bridging of the SH3 and GK domains are greatly influenced by BID. The $\alpha_2\delta$-1 subunit seems to be involved in targeting (or stabilization) of the α_1C to the sarcolemma (Lacinová & Hoffmann, 2001; Lacinova & Hofmann, 2005; Brette et al., 2006; Benitah et al., 2010) and could confer more native LTCC properties. The δ subunit is composed of a single transmembrane segment with a very short intracellular C-term and links by disulphide bonds the α_2 subunit that is entirely extracellular (Davies et al., 2007). The α_2 subunit contains a Von Willebrand factor A domain (VWA) that has a metal-ion-dependent adhesion site that seems to be key in trafficking the α_1C subunit to the membrane (Canti et al., 2005).

3. Biophysics of the cardiac L-type Ca^{2+} channel

3.1 Selectivity and permeation

The cardiac LTCC is a multi-ion pore in which a Ca^{2+} ion bound to a high affinity site can be repelled by a second Ca^{2+} ion entering the pore thus allowing selectivity with high ionic flux (Hess & Tsien, 1984). The LTCC pore exhibits two different affinities for Ca^{2+}: a K_D ~ 1 μM for Ca^{2+} block of monovalent current through the channel and a K_D ~ 10-14 mM for saturation of divalent current (which can be lower if surface charge screening is taken into account at high divalent concentrations), suggesting the existence of two Ca^{2+} binding sites within the channel's pore (Almers & McCleskey, 1984; Hess & Tsien, 1984). In the absence of Ca^{2+} other ions can pass the channel and unitary conductance measurements gave the following sequence $Ca^{2+} < Ba^{2+} < Li^{+} < Na^{+} < K^{+} < Cs^{+}$ (Hess et al., 1986). Four glutamate residues, one in each of the four P-loops of the LTCC (the EEEE locus), are important for channel selectivity (Tang et al., 1993; Yang et al., 1993). The current view of the selectivity filter considers that the EEEE locus is physically flexible (Sather & McCleskey, 2003). Some recent results suggest that an EEEE locus is not enough to explain selectivity and permeation in LTCC and other high voltage activated Ca^{2+} channels. A set of non conserved (channel specific) charged residues (Divalent Cation Selection or DCS locus) located in the upper half of the channel (pointing toward the pore) could form a second Ca^{2+} binding site important in defining a Ca^{2+} permeability profile. It was proposed that the number of charged residues in the DCS locus is critical for Ca^{2+} binding. In the cardiac LTCC the DCS locus contains three negative charges (DSED) that seem to be important for the high Ba^{2+} conductance (Cens et al., 2007).

3.2 Activation, inactivation and reactivation of LTCC

In a ventricular cardiomyocyte at rest (resting potential ~ -80 mV) there is a transmembrane Ca^{2+} concentration gradient (~ 2 mM outside, ~ 100 nM inside) that generates a huge driving force (electrochemical gradient) for Ca^{2+} that tends to move it into the cell. Activation of LTCC allows Ca^{2+} to enter the cardiomyocyte during the AP and constitutes the major Ca^{2+} entry pathway. With a threshold at -40 mV (or slightly positive to), activation of I_{CaL} is fast with a time constant of 2-3 ms and time-to peak inward current ranging around 4-5 ms or less at the membrane potentials at which maximal inward current occurs (0 to +10 mV), and even faster at higher depolarizations (McDonald et al., 1994; Bers, 2001). Similar to Na^{+} channels, LTCC inactivate but with a much slower inactivation time course. With Ca^{2+} as charge carrier, I_{CaL} inactivation is usually a biexponential process with an "U-shaped" voltage-dependence. Minimal values for time constants of 4 to 10 ms (τ_{fast}) and 40 to 60 ms (τ_{slow}) occur at around 0 and +10 mV depending on cardiomyocyte type (McDonald et al., 1994; Bers, 2001). Deactivation of peak I_{CaL} after a short depolarizing pulse and repolarization to a negative holding potential is fast with a time constant ranging between 0.2 and 0.5 ms (Josephson et al., 1984; Cohen et al., 1992). However, it can be slower in rat cardiomyocytes (~1 ms) (Richard et al., 1993).

3.2.1 Current-to-Voltage relationship

Current-to-voltage relationship for I_{CaL} is bell-shaped with a threshold around -40 or -30 mV and a peak inward current at 0 (or +10 mV); it is almost linear at positive potentials and reverses around +60 to +70 mV at normal Ca^{2+} concentrations. At potentials beyond its reversal, I_{CaL} exhibits some inward going rectification (McDonald et al., 1994; Bers, 2001). Whole cell I_{CaL} can be roughly described by a Hodgkin-Huxley formalism considering that

$$I_{CaL} = G_{CaL} \cdot d_{\infty}\, f_{\infty}\, (V_m - V_{Ca})$$

where G_{CaL} is the maximal Ca^{2+} conductance, d_{∞} is the activation gate variable, f_{∞} the inactivation gate variable, V_m is the membrane potential and V_{Ca} is the Ca^{2+} reversal potential (Luo & Rudy, 1994). Since I_{CaL} inactivation is both voltage- and Ca^{2+}-dependent (see below), the formalism can be more complex and could include a variable related to the Ca^{2+}-dependent inactivation (CDI) process (Hirano & Hiraoka, 2003; Findlay et al., 2008). However, since the Hodgkin-Huxley formalism does not represent kinetic states of the ion channel, single channel-based Markov models could be more useful to fully describe coupling between kinetic gating transitions and molecular interactions in LTCC (Faber et al., 2007). At the single channel level, current-to-voltage relationship for LTCC is essentially ohmic over the whole potential range with some inward rectification near the reversal potential (McDonald et al., 1994). Since the single channel current i_{CaL} can be described as

$$i_{CaL} = \gamma_{Ca} (V_m - V_{Ca})$$

where γ_{Ca} is the unitary conductance, the relationship between whole cell I_{CaL} and i_{CaL} is

$$I_{CaL} = NP_o\, i_{CaL} = NP_o\, \gamma_{Ca} (V_m - V_{Ca})$$

where N is the total number of functional channels and P_o the probability that a channel is open.
Unitary conductance of LTCC is 3-5 pS when Ca^{2+} is the charge carrier and 15 - 25 pS with Ba^{2+} as charge carrier (McDonald et al., 1994; Bers, 2001; Guia et al., 2001). However, subconductance levels of 50% to 70% of the major conductance have been also demonstrated (McDonald et al., 1994). On depolarization LTCC activity can vary between different modes: gating mode 0 (or "null mode") in which the channel is not available to open; gating mode 1 (or "normal") consisting of short bursts of brief openings and closings and gating mode 2 (with high P_o) in which the channel show long openings interrupted by short closings. This gating mode 2 is induced by phosphorylation, "Ca^{2+} channel agonists" (such as BAY K 8644) or strong depolarizations (Pietrobon & Hess, 1990; McDonald et al., 1994).

3.2.2 Voltage-dependence of activation and inactivation

Steady-state activation of I_{CaL} (d_∞) has a sigmoidal relationship with the membrane potential with a half-activation potential around -15 mV. The relationship for the inactivation variable (f_∞; availability) is more complex since for potentials from -80 to 0 mV it is sigmoidal with a half-inactivation potential around -35 mV; however an "overshoot" can often be seen at potentials negative to -50 mV in cells clamped at negative holding potentials (> -80 mV). Other singularities of the availability curve of I_{CaL} are that f_∞ rarely attains a zero value but a minimum between 0 and +10 mV and that the curve bends up at potentials positive to +10 mV, a phenomenon that is related to the CDI of I_{CaL} (Mentrard et al., 1984). These characteristics d_∞ and f_∞ are consistently seen in cardiomyocytes from different species including humans (McDonald et al., 1994; Bers, 2001; Treinys & Jurevicius, 2008; Benitah et al., 2010).

3.2.3 Voltage- and Ca^{2+}-dependent inactivation of LTCC

Time-dependent inactivation of I_{CaL} during depolarization is both voltage- and Ca^{2+}-dependent (Kass & Sanguinetti, 1984; Mentrard et al., 1984; Lee et al., 1985; Hadley & Hume, 1987). A very slow inactivation has also been described in the heart including human ventricular myocytes (Schouten & Morad, 1989; Benitah et al., 1992). CDI can be considered as the result of a two-component process, one due to Ca^{2+} ions passing through the channel and another due to Ca^{2+} release from the SR in the vicinity of the LTCC (Imredy & Yue, 1992; Richard et al., 2006; Faber et al., 2007). CDI can be easily shown up by using Ba^{2+} instead of Ca^{2+} as charge carrier which markedly prolonged LTCC inactivation time course. An increase in current amplitude is also seen since the LTCC has less affinity for Ba^{2+} than for Ca^{2+} (Hess et al., 1986). It is generally believed that under this condition, LTCC inactivation is essentially controlled by a voltage-dependent inactivation mechanism (VDI). However, this paradigm has been called into question since it has been well demonstrated that Ba^{2+} can induce ion (or current) -dependent inactivation (Markwardt & Nilius, 1988; Ferreira et al., 1997; Ferreira et al., 2003) and thus the "apparent VDI" with Ba^{2+} as charge carrier also shows fast and slow components. Evidences exist that VDI can also have fast and slow components (Hering et al., 2000; Ferreira et al., 2003; Findlay, 2004). The situation could be even more complicated since, at least for N-type Ca^{2+} channels, the permeant ion could interact in a complex way with the voltage sensor (Shirokov, 1999).

The relative contribution of CDI to total inactivation of I_{CaL} is still under dispute. It is commonly accepted that the fast inactivation phase of I_{CaL} represents the CDI component (Findlay, 2004). However, it has been shown that the fast inactivation time constant of I_{CaL} of rat ventricular cardiomyocytes was "unexpectedly" slowed down after I_{CaL} was increased by β-adrenergic stimulation, as well as after manipulations not involving CDI (Alvarez et al., 2004; Haase et al., 2005; Alvarez et al., 2010). This makes difficult to ascertain which one of CDI or fast VDI predominates in the fast inactivation phase of I_{CaL} with Ca^{2+} as charge carrier. Nevertheless, it has been suggested that VDI could be more important under control conditions and that after β-adrenergic stimulation, CDI becomes the main inactivation mechanism due to a slow down of VDI (Findlay, 2004). It should be noted that CDI could be visualized as a "Ca^{2+}-dependent brake for a pre-existing voltage-dependent inactivation" based on the conserved regulation of both VDI and CDI by the auxiliary β-subunit, and that the I-II intracellular loop, essential for VDI, could also play a role in CDI (Cens et al., 1999; Cens et al., 2006). The precise mechanisms underlying CDI are not completely well defined. However, a general picture emerged in which in the presence of Ca^{2+} (entering through the LTCC or released from the SR) a calmodulin (CaM) molecule binds to the C-terminal tail of the α_1C subunit to promote CDI. CaM binds to two segments (LA and IQ), in a Ca^{2+}-dependent manner (Xiong et al., 2005) and it has been shown that the amino acid sequence of the IQ region in the α_1C subunit is critical for CaM binding and CDI (Ohrtman et al., 2008). Several other structures seem to be involved in CDI such as an EF-hand locus in the C-terminus of α_1C subunit (Peterson et al., 2000), the $Ca_v\beta$ subunit (Zhang et al., 2005), the N-terminus of the α_1C subunit, the I-II intracellular linker (Pitt et al., 2001; Erickson et al., 2003; Kobrinsky et al., 2005) and the pore region involved in slow inactivation (Shi & Soldatov, 2002).

3.2.4 Reactivation

Reactivation (removal of inactivation) of LTCC has been described as a mono or biexponential process, however, the time for half reactivation (t_{50}) can be considered as a reliable parameter and has been reported to be in the range of 70-100 ms in cardiomyocytes clamped at negative holding potentials (-80 mV or more negative) and an overshoot at short coupling intervals is often seen. At more depolarized holding potentials, t_{50} can be notably increased and the overshoot disappears (Argibay et al., 1988; Tseng, 1988; Schouten & Morad, 1989; Alvarez & Vassort, 1992). A voltage-dependent transition into a closed available state and/or reopenings from the inactivated state could explain in part the reactivation of LTCC (Jones, 1991; Slesinger & Lansman, 1991). However, reactivation of LTCC is a more complex phenomenon since it is Ca^{2+}-dependent (Argibay et al., 1988; Tseng, 1988) and thus related to CDI. The overshoot in I_{CaL} reactivation could be of physiological relevance since it is, at least in part, related to the well-known increase in premature (extrasystolic) APD in well polarized cardiomyocytes but not in partially depolarized ones (Hiraoka & Sano, 1976).

3.3 Facilitation of LTCC

The overshoots seen in the availability and reactivation curves of I_{CaL} are both a manifestation of a "facilitation" phenomenon of LTCC. In both cases an increase in τ_{fast} is commonly observed and both seem to be related to the pacing-dependent (staircase) facilitation of I_{CaL} (Lee, 1987). However, the "overshoots" and the staircase phenomena could be dependent on the basal I_{CaL} density disappearing at higher current densities (Argibay et al., 1988; Alvarez & Vassort, 1992; Piot et al., 1996). Facilitation of LTCC has been more extensively studied by stimulating cardiomyocytes at high rates after a rest period or by applying prepulses of moderate and high amplitude (Richard et al., 2006). At negative holding potentials (> -80 mV) the frequency-dependent changes in I_{CaL} amplitude upon stimulation can be variable: significant (Lee, 1987), modest or absent (Piot et al., 1996; Delgado et al., 1999) and even modestly decrease (Argibay et al., 1988; Alvarez & Vassort, 1992; Alvarez et al., 2004). However, an increase in τ_{fast} has been consistently reported in these conditions, resulting, independently of what happens with I_{CaL} amplitude, in a significant increase in Ca^{2+} influx (Delgado et al., 1999). The mechanism of this "Ca^{2+}-dependent facilitation" (CDF) or potentiation seems to be related to a negative feedback involving less CDI at frequencies at which Ca^{2+} load and release from the SR are decreased (Delgado et al., 1999). This phenomenon has often been related to phosphorylation by cyclic AMP-dependent protein kinase (Tiaho et al., 1994; Piot et al., 1996) although there are also reports that β-adrenergic stimulation significantly diminished I_{CaL} facilitation (Zygmunt & Maylie, 1990; Delgado et al., 1999; Alvarez et al., 2004). Disruption of the interaction between α_1C and β_{2A} subunits also abolished CDF (Alvarez et al., 2004). In this sense, this phenomenon is still far to be completely understood. CDF also involves CaM and the Ca^{2+}/CaM kinase II (CaMKII). Similar to CDI, the CDF requires the binding of CaM to the IQ motif located in the α_1C C-terminus but to a structural frame different to that involved in CDI (Zuhlke et al., 1999). Activation of CaMKII by Ca^{2+} entry or release from the SR is also involved in I_{CaL} facilitation (Anderson et al., 1994; Yuan & Bers, 1994; Anderson, 2004). More recently phosphorylation of β_{2A} has been reported to be critical for CaMKII-dependent I_{CaL} facilitation (Grueter et al., 2006).

Similar to frequency-dependent facilitation, prepulse-induced facilitation of I_{CaL} is characterized by an increase in τ_{fast} (Barrere-Lemaire et al., 2000) and its underlying mechanism seems to involve a negative feedback on LTCC related to CDI as discussed above (Guo & Duff, 2003) and a positive feedback on LTCC following CaMKII activation by membrane potential and Ca^{2+} entry (Xiao et al., 1994).

3.4 LTCC "window" current

Activation and inactivation (availability) curves overlap at membrane potentials between the threshold for I_{CaL} at -40 to potentials of 0 or +10 mV thus defining a "window" Ca^{2+} current ($d_\infty . f_\infty > 0$) in the plateau range of the cardiac AP. The peak window current (which is proportional to $d_\infty . f_\infty$) is between -25 and -20 mV and could be as large as 10% of maximal I_{CaL} (McDonald et al., 1994). Its existence has been verified in whole cell recordings (Hirano et al., 1992; McDonald et al., 1994). Within this window LTCC channels can cycle between closed, open and inactivated states but a transition again to the closed state and reopenings are possible before inactivating again (Shorofsky & January, 1992). Such reopenings have been clearly demonstrated in single channel recordings (Shorofsky & January, 1992; McDonald et al., 1994) and constitute the underlying mechanism for the EAD (January et al., 1988). EADs are more frequently observed at low rates when the APD is increased and during interventions that increase I_{CaL} (e.g. after activation of β-adrenergic receptors). They are supposed to underlie the cellular mechanism of "Torsades de Pointes" (TdP) in long QT syndromes (Napolitano & Antzelevitch, 2011). Transient K^+ outward current (I_{to}) reactivation at low rates could contribute to generation of EADs since it drives the membrane (plateau) potential to more negative "take off" potentials and warrants higher peak amplitude of EADs (January et al., 1988). β-adrenergic stimulation increases I_{CaL} and shifts the window current to more negative potentials due to an increase in channel's P_o at more negative potentials (hyperpolarizing shifts in d_∞) and a shift of f_∞ to more hyperpolarized potentials (McDonald et al., 1994) thus favoring the appearance of EADs. It is to be noted that, at these membrane potentials, the fast Na^+ current (I_{Na}) and I_{to} are inactivated, the inward rectifier current I_{K1} is decreased and outward rectifier currents are just activating. As a result the total membrane resistance is increased (Weidmann, 1951) thus making the membrane space constant high enough to guarantee a rather high safety margin for the slow response to be conducted for a given I_{CaL} density.

3.4.1 A note on "EADs" recorded in multicellular cardiac preparations

It is possible that in some cases EADs recorded in multicellular cardiac preparations represent a reentry from a distant site rather than a true EAD arising from the recording site. In any case, the mechanism underlying this activity is the same as the previously described for EAD. This reentry mechanism, at these short coupling intervals (during the AP plateau) is due to "slow response" APs that can be conducted with a large enough safety margin and are due to the activation of LTCC (Cranefield, 1975). The biophysical properties of LTCC described above, can fully account for the conducted slow response APs in partially depolarized cells. Under several pathological conditions these slow responses can be conducted and are at the origin of reentry, for example in depressed fibres in ischemia (Cranefield, 1975) since the slow response APs are rather resistant to hypoxia (Alvarez et al., 1981), in TdP associated to long QT syndromes (Antzelevitch & Burashnikov, 2001) (see below) or during the verapamil-sensitive reentrant intranodal tachycardia involving the AV node (Wellens et al., 1977).

3.4.2 A role for a second window current?

The characteristics of the activation and inactivation curves of I_{CaL} could predict the existence of a "second window" current at potentials positive to +10 mV since at these values, the product $d_\infty.f_\infty$ is > 0. Whether the overlap between d_∞ (=1) and the increasing f_∞ at positive prepulse potentials could represent a true "secondary" window current or not is debatable, but it is clear that after these prepulse potentials LTCCs recover from inactivation and reopen in a sort of "facilitation" (Pietrobon & Hess, 1990). Nonetheless, the physiological (or physiopathological) relevance of this window current is uncertain since at these membrane potentials the fast I_{Na} is the main depolarizing current and physiologically membrane potentials over +40 mV never exist. This property, however, has been important for the characterization of the CDI of LTCC in cardiac cells (Mentrard et al., 1984).

4. Role of I_{CaL} in the cardiac arrythmogenesis associated to acquired pathophysiological states

4.1 Myocardial ischemia and ventricular fibrillation

Ventricular fibrillation (VF) and myocardial ischemia are inseparable. In general terms, myocardial ischemia is defined as disequilibrium between myocardial oxygen demand versus supply, which episodes can trigger serious and fatal arrhythmic events. Thus, in the clinical setting around 80% of all sudden cardiac deaths (SCD) are due to myocardial ischemia. The most common sequence of events leading SCD appears to be the degeneration of ventricular tachycardia (VT) into ventricular fibrillation (VF) (Rubart & Zipes, 2005). VF is thought as a disorganized cardiac activation in which electrical waves propagate through the ventricles haphazardly and unpredictably (Jalife, 2000). The last consequence of this disorganized process is strong alteration in the adequate contractions of the ventricles that fail to eject blood effectively as a consequence of a strong electrical dysfunction, which is detected in the heart even during the first minutes after acute myocardial ischemia (usually lasting for 30 min) where abundant arrhythmogenesis is detected. During acute ischemia, in the border zone between the ischemic and normal tissue the excitability is increased resulting in spontaneous activation of Purkinje fibers initiating VT. During reperfusion the rapid inhomogeneous improvement in tissue excitability contributes to arrhythmogenesis again (Opthof et al., 1993; Luqman et al., 2007).

At intracellular level, an important ionic imbalance occurs during myocardial ischemia. This electrophysiological imbalance is characterized by the opening of ATP-sensitive potassium channels (I_{KATP}) and causes acidosis and hypoxia of myocardial cells together with an aberrant intracellular Ca^{2+} handling that is determinant to trigger arrhythmias. Because I_{CaL} constitutes the first trigger for the EC coupling necessary for each beat in the heart, a lot of attention has been focused in the involvement of I_{CaL} in the conversion of VT to VF. With myocardial ischemia, the abrupt cessation of blood flow provokes a new distribution of a number of ions. The abnormal increase in the intracellular Na^+ concentration ($[Na^+]_i$) consequently results in an increase in the intracellular Ca^{2+} concentration ($[Ca^{2+}]_i$) due to an increase in the Ca^{2+} influx via the Na^+/Ca^{2+} exchanger (NCX) working in the reverse manner and also via depolarization-activated LTCCs. These events induce cellular Ca^{2+} overload (as a consequence of cellular Na^+ overload) favoring the presence of spontaneous (non-voltage dependent) diastolic Ca^{2+} release as Ca^{2+} waves that induce depolarization of myocyte membrane triggering DAD and finally DAD-related arrhythmias (Schlotthauer & Bers, 2000). The presence of DADs also can trigger abnormal electrical activity with the wavebreak causing VF (Koretsune & Marban, 1989; Lakatta & Guarnieri, 1993).

It is important to point out that cardiac ischemia is also characterized by a significant increase in circulating and tissue cathecholamine levels, which increase the probability of VT and SCD (Dorian, 2005). In the presence of β-adrenergic receptor (β-AR) stimulation and hypoxic conditions, a significant increase in Ca^{2+} influx through I_{CaL} is able to prolong APD and also triggers EADs (Gaur et al., 2009), which in ventricular myocytes appear not to be due to spontaneous regional increase in $[Ca^{2+}]_i$ or propagating Ca^{2+} waves. These results can be explained by the increase in the sensitivity of LTCC due to changes in gating properties by the modification of the phosphorylated state or by the modification of thiol groups of the channel, since the presence of dithiothreitol or catalase mimics the effect of acute hypoxia on I_{CaL} (Hool, 2000; Hool & Arthur, 2002; Tanskanen et al., 2005). Alterations in I_{CaL} have been also detected in simulated experimental ischemic-like conditions in single pacemaker cells isolated from the rabbit sinoatrial node (SAN). In contrast to ventricular myocytes, I_{CaL} is declined under metabolic inhibition or ischemic conditions in SAN cells (Vinogradova et al., 2000; Ju & Allen, 2003). However, it has been reported that *in vitro* ischemic conditions enhanced I_{CaL} significantly at potentials between -30 and +30 mV suggesting that the greater I_{CaL} could account for a 6 mV increase in the AP overshoot (Du & Nathan, 2007a). This is related to an increase in the G_{CaL} and a positive shift of the f_∞ curve and reduction of inactivation, likely due to a H^+- increased of I_{CaL} (Du & Nathan, 2007b).

Torsades de Pointes (TdP) is a polymorphic type of VT also associated to acquired QT prolongation and maintained bradycardia that potentially leads to SCD (Jackman et al., 1988). Several studies carried out in rabbits and dogs prone to spontaneous TdP as a consequence of the chronic atrioventricular block (AVB) showed important alterations in the control of Ca^{2+} (Sipido et al., 2000; Antoons et al., 2007; Qi et al., 2009). For example, AVB in dogs resulted in an increase in the SR Ca^{2+} content which improved Ca^{2+} release from SR as Ca^{2+} transients (Sipido et al., 2000). Although, the overall density-voltage relationship of I_{CaL} is unchanged, a depolarizing shift in the f_{∞} curve resulted in an increased window current (Antoons et al., 2007). The CaM activation of CaMKII has been proposed to underlie this effect, as well the induced EADs (Qi et al., 2009).

4.2 Atrial fibrillation

Among supraventricular tachyarrhythmias, atrial fibrillation (AF) is the most common. Its prevalence is considerably increased with age, and thus AF is now classified as an epidemic (Lip et al., 2007). The cellular and molecular bases of AF electrophysiology and the underlying mechanisms have been extensively investigated (Hatem et al., 2010). The definition of the latest report of the American College of Cardiology/American Heart Association/European Society of Cardiology (ACC/AHA/ESC) guidelines for AF is limited to a description of the pattern of irregular atrial waveforms on the electrocardiogram (ECG) as a supraventricular tachyarrhythmia characterized by uncoordinated atrial activation with a replacement of consistent P waves by rapid oscillations or fibrillatory waves (Fuster et al., 2011). At the cellular level, AF is characterized by strong alterations in the cardiac electrophysiology. The repolarizing currents such as I_{to} is almost suppressed and the voltage-gated K^+ current (I_{Kur}) is decreased by around 50% (Le Grand et al., 1994; Van Wagoner et al., 1997). While upon the onset of AF, an increase in the intracellular Ca^{2+} load is observed, in persistent AF the intracellular Ca^{2+} load is restored to normal levels. There is a consensus in the drastic reduction in I_{CaL} (around 70%) that is observed during experimental and clinical AF. Because this current is the main depolarizing current that activates during plateau phase of the AP, its reduction contributes greatly to the shortening of the AP, reducing atrial effective refractory period with a loss of physiological rate adaptation and finally favouring the formation of re-entrant circuits during AF (Le Grand et al., 1994; Van Wagoner et al., 1997; Yue et al., 1997). Several authors have postulated a significant decrease in the number of Ca^{2+} channels subunits $Ca_v1.2$ associated with AF (Brundel et al., 2001; Shinagawa et al., 2003). In fact, experiments carried out in cultured adult canine atrial myocytes subjected to *in vitro* model of atrial tachycardia by continuous tachypacing have demonstrated that during the first hours of pacing exist a Ca^{2+} overload involved in the activation of the phosphatase (PP) calcineurin (Cn) that allows the translocation of the transcriptor factor NFAT into the nucleus. This rapid Ca^{2+} overload induces the activation of the Ca^{2+}-dependent CaM-Cn-NFAT system to cause the transcriptional downregulation of α_1C subunit mRNA expression and also in the levels of $Ca_v1.2$ protein expression that is observed from 8 hours of pacing (Qi et al., 2008). These results are in conflict with others demonstrating no changes in mRNA and protein levels of the pore-forming α_1C and the regulatory β_{2A} subunits in atrial myocardium from patients with chronic AF (Schotten et al., 2003). Nevertheless, the reduction of I_{CaL} can also be the result of changes in gating properties of the channel (Bodi et al., 2005), due to alterations in the phosphorylation state of the LTCC. Indeed, it has been observed that the maximum of the current-voltage relationship of I_{CaL} is rightward shifted to more positive potentials in AF, suggesting phosphorylation-dependent changes in the channel regulation more than changes in its expression (Christ et al., 2004). In addition, it has been also described a high sensitivity of I_{CaL} to β-adrenergic agonists during AF, suggesting that LTCCs are in a dephosphorylated and silent state (Boixel et al., 2001; Schotten et al., 2003; Dinanian et al., 2008; Hatem et al., 2010). Moreover, the activity of CaMKII is increased in AF (Neef et al., 2010). However, increased CaMKII activity in AF seems to be offset by an increased PP activity, because CaMKII inhibitor KN-93 reduce I_{CaL} in control cells, while it did not affect I_{CaL} in AF cells (Greiser et al., 2007; Greiser et al., 2011). Moreover, the PP inhibitor, okadaic acid, increased I_{CaL} to almost normal levels in human atrial myocytes from AF patients (Christ et al., 2004; Greiser et al., 2011). In conclusion, in AF the ratio between protein kinase/phosphatase is altered in favor of increased PP activity, suggesting that the basal phosphorylation of the Ca^{2+} channel is reduced which induces lower basal I_{CaL} activity.

It seems clear that the abnormal atrial electrical remodeling associated to AF contributes to perpetuation of the arrhythmia and has profound effects on intracellular Ca^{2+} handling (Greiser et al., 2011). Contractile force of atrial tissue strips from patients with AF is also reduced around 75% and exposure to high extracellular Ca^{2+} concentration is able to restore atrial functions (Schotten et al., 2001; Schotten et al., 2004). In a sheep model of persistent AF, even with only a slight reduction in I_{CaL} (around 24%), its efficiency to highly reduced CICR (Lenaerts et al., 2009). In the presence of Ca^{2+} chelators, I_{CaL} was unchanged in AF conditions while it is increased in control cells. These results are well-matched with a possible reduction in the CDI of I_{CaL}.

4.3 Cardiac hypertrophy and heart failure

Following a pathological stress, the heart can adapt by developing cardiac hypertrophy, which improves contractile force as an adaptative mechanism to meet the new body demands. In this case, the cardiac hypertrophy is "compensated", as in physiologic cardiac hypertrophy by exercise or during the pregnancy. When the stimulus is prolonged, cardiac hypertrophy can "decompensate" toward heart failure (HF) with compromised pump function (Benitah et al., 2010). One of the best documented changes in hypertrophy and HF, both in animal models and in humans, is the prolongation of the AP, which is highly significant in the production of ventricular arrhythmias. Important abnormalities of intracellular Ca^{2+} handling has been showed in the hypertrophic and failing myocytes: reduced SERCA function, enhanced NCX function and enhanced SR Ca^{2+} leak contributing to the reduced SR Ca^{2+} load (Bers et al., 2003). It is also well known that changes in I_{CaL} in the hypertrophic and failing heart can also contribute to the electrical instability. Although the different degrees in the severity of pathological stresses as well as the variability among different models appear to influence the regulation of I_{CaL}, the amplitude of I_{CaL} is increased in hypertrophied and failing myocytes while its density (normalized to cell capacitance, as an indirect measure of cell surface) is unchanged (Benitah et al., 2002a; Benitah et al., 2003; Song et al., 2005; Loyer et al., 2008). In an early analysis of a pressure-overloaded cardiac hypertrophy model, I_{CaL} was augmented in non-hypertrophic cells (Keung, 1989). It was thus suggested that I_{CaL} could be increased before the cellular hypertrophy and then, as the cell grows, I_{CaL} density would regain control values and even decrease in models of overt HF (Aimond et al., 1999; Benitah et al., 2002b). This process involves, at least partly, the cardiac mineralocorticoid pathway (Perrier et al., 2004; Benitah et al., 2010). Although most reports agree with the idea that I_{CaL} density is normal in failing hearts, its kinetic seems to be significantly altered (Ryder et al., 1993; Bito et al., 2008). Thus, the decay of the whole-cell

I_{CaL} and its CDI have been found to be slowed, causing a reduction in the peak of the $[Ca^{2+}]_i$ transients producing less Ca^{2+}-induced inactivation of I_{CaL}. Thus, the maintained I_{CaL} density together with a slowing of its inactivation would at the end increase the total account of Ca^{2+} entry through the channel (Aimond et al., 1999; Benitah et al., 2010). Such slowing of the decay of the current has a direct effect on the EC-coupling and is involved in the prolongation of APD favoring EADs observed in failing conditions (Tomaselli & Rose, 2000). An increase in P_o and availability of LTCCs in human failing myocardium have been reported (Schröder et al., 1998), suggesting that the failing myocytes has fewer but more active channels. Hence, the response of I_{CaL} to cAMP is reduced in ventricular myocytes from failing hearts (Chen et al., 2002). The attenuated increase of I_{CaL} by β-adrenergic stimulation is consistent with a reduction in the maximal number of channels, which have a higher activity (Bito et al., 2008). This is related to the concept of "defective EC coupling" in HF (Gómez et al., 1997): The failing myocytes had a significant reduction in triggered Ca^{2+} release from the SR despite unaltered I_{CaL}, which could be due to structural alteration in the relation between LTCCs and ryanodine receptors, related to important structural changes as a loss of T-tubules density in human and experimental HF (He et al., 2001; Balijepalli et al., 2003; Louch et al., 2004; Lyon et al., 2009; Horiuchi-Hirose et al., 2011). The increased basal activity at the single Ca^{2+} channel levels is also consistent with changes in the phosphorylation state of the channel. Thus, both increases in PKA and CaMKII-dependent phosphorylation of LTCC have been described in failing myocytes (Schröder et al., 1998; Chen et al., 2008; Wang et al., 2008). PKA activation through β-adrenergic stimulation leads to increase I_{CaL}, as well as the CaMKII-dependent phosphorylation of both pore-forming α_1C and β_2 subunits, which also increased I_{CaL} CDF (Yuan & Bers, 1994; Hudmon et al., 2005; Grueter et al., 2006). In cardiac hypertrophy with prolongation of APD, these features are important since I_{CaL} can be inappropriately reactivated and contribute to EADs triggered arrhythmia (Wu et al., 2002; Anderson et al., 2011). Moreover, $Ca_v\beta_2$ expression is downregulated in the compensated phase of cardiac hypertrophy, while an upregulation is observed in failing states, which could explain the increase in the activity of LTCCs observed in single channel studies (Hullin et al., 2007).

5. Inherited channelopathies or genetically determined ion-channel disorder

The critical role of LTCCs in cardiac cells has led many to suggest that inherited defects of LTCCs could be incompatible with life. This view dramatically changed in the 2004 when the CaCNA1C gene was found to show genetic linkage to life-threatening arrhythmias associated with Timothy syndrome (Splawski et al., 2004). Since, we witnessed an explosion of information linking LTCC genes mutations (more than 25 mutations identified in the past decade) with a wide variety of inherited arrhythmia syndromes (Napolitano & Antzelevitch, 2011).

5.1 LQT8 or Timothy syndrome

Identified in the 1990s (Marks et al., 1995), Timothy syndrome, or syndactyly-associated LQTS or LQT8, is a dominantly inherited genetic condition characterized by multisystem dysfunction, with severe arrhythmic disorders including: QT prolongation; 2:1 atrioventricular block (due to delayed ventricular repolarisation); T-wave alternans, polymorphic VT, and TdP; and abnormal changes in multiple organs (heart, skin, eyes, teeth, immune system, brain, and dysmorphism, such as syndactyly). Patients with LQT8 may also have episodic hypoglycaemia, which can trigger arrhythmias, and structural heart anomalies, including patent ductus arteriosus, patent foramen ovale, ventricular septum defect, and tetralogy of Fallot. Prognosis is very poor and SCD often occurs during childhood.

Gain-of-function mutations in CACNA1C, localized at the end of IS6 segment that is important for the regulation of channel inactivation and the binding of the $Ca_v\beta$ subunit, have been associated with Timothy syndrome (Splawski et al., 2004; Splawski et al., 2005). A missense mutation G406R in the minor alternatively splice exon 8 of CACNA1C gene, as been first identified in all probands analysed (Splawski et al., 2004). Later, two other Gly mutations in the mutually exclusive major spliced exon 8a (G402S and G406R) were shown to cause a very similar syndrome but without the syndactyly (Splawski et al., 2005). These mutations exert powerful effect on inactivation, slowing the VDI irrespective of auxiliary β subunits, while through a proposed low-P_o gating shift speeding the kinetics of CDI (Barrett & Tsien, 2008), which was previously reported unchanged (Splawski et al., 2005). Moreover, the mutation did not affect closed-state VDI, which might explain absence of hypertension associated with LQT8, and along with impaired open-state VDI, slowed activation and deactivation (Yarotskyy et al., 2009). The later is in part consistent with spontaneous increased occurrence of mode 2 gating at single channel level, which has been associated with the generation of a consensus phosphorylation site for CaMKII (Erxleben et al., 2006). Indeed, on isolated rat cardiomyocytes infected with dihydropyridine-resistant G406R $Ca_v1.2$ channel, CaMKII autophosphorylation is increased, which mediated enhanced I_{CaL} facilitation, AP prolongation, increased Ca^{2+} spark frequency and afterdepolarizations (Thiel et al., 2008). The impaired inactivation of LTCC leads to sustained Ca^{2+} influx, AP prolongation, and Ca^{2+} overload, which promotes EADs and DADs (Jacobs et al., 2006; Sicouri et al., 2007). Roscovitine, a compound that increases the VDI, rescues the electrophysiological and Ca^{2+} homeostasis properties of Timothy syndrome cardiomyocytes (Yazawa et al.). Ca^{2+} channel blockade (eg, by verapamil and diltiazem) can control arrhythmias without affecting the QT interval, and is a possible treatment (Napolitano et al., 2006).

5.2 I_{CaL} and LQT syndrome

The QT interval is an electrocardiographic index of ventricular repolarization and a measure of the duration of the ventricular AP. Ca^{2+} influx through LTCC plays a significant role in maintaining the plateau phase of AP and hence contributes importantly to APD and QT interval. Therefore, administration of CCB is a logical strategy in all types of LQTS. In the clinical study involving recording of monophasic AP (MAP) in eight patients with LQTS, verapamil effectively abbreviated MAP duration and suppressed epinephrine-induced EADs (Shimizu et al., 1995). At the bench side, verapamil effectively abbreviates QT interval and suppresses TdP in models of congenital and acquired LQTS (LQT1+ LQT2) (Aiba et al., 2005). In a rabbit model of drug-induced LQT2, the increased I_{CaL} at the base of hearts, attributable to gender and regional difference in $Ca_v1.2$ expression, is an important determinant of the arrhythmia phenotype (Sims et al., 2008). This echoes clinical reports suggesting that Ca^{2+} channel antagonists might be appropriate as adjunctive therapy for arrhythmia suppression in LQT1, LQT2 and even LQT3 (Shimizu et al., 2005). Hence, an anti-arrhythmic effect of the specific LTCC antagonist nifedipine has been reported in mice with targeted disruption of the Na^+ channel gene (Thomas et al., 2007), as well as in intact hearts from LQT5 mice model (Balasubramaniam et al., 2003).

5.3 J wave syndromes

Because they share a common arrhythmic platform and similarities in ECG characteristics, clinical outcomes and risk factors, congenital and acquired forms of Brugada (BrS) and early repolarization (ERS) syndromes have been grouped together under the heading of J wave syndromes (Antzelevitch & Yan, 2010). Recent studies have implicated loss of function mutations in all 3 subunits of the cardiac LTCC in the generation and accentuation of electrocardiographic J waves associated with these syndromes (Antzelevitch et al., 2007; Cordeiro et al., 2009); (Burashnikov et al.).

5.3.1 Short QT syndrome

Although QT prolongation has long been known to increase the risk of SCD and overall cardiac mortality among patients with a variety of underlying etiologies, a shorter than normal QT interval could also be detrimental leading to the concept of a new clinical entity, the short QT syndrome, associated with AF and SCD (Gussak et al., 2000). Since more than 30 patients with SQTS have been reported (Schulze-Bahr et al., 1997; Gaita et al., 2003; Schimpf et al., 2005; Giustetto et al., 2006).

SQT4 and SQT5 are associated with mutations in CACNA1C and CACNB2B (Antzelevitch et al., 2007). These mutations reduce I_{CaL}, shorten QT, and are associated with asymmetrical T waves, attenuated QT-heart rate relations, and AF. More recently, a new variant of SQTS at a heterozygous state caused by a mutation in the CACNA2D1 gene has been reported (Templin et al., 2011). This mutation leads also to a decreased I_{CaL}, without modification in the $Ca_v1.2$ expression suggesting alteration of some of the biophysical single channel properties of channel.

5.3.2 Brugada syndrome

Brugada syndrome (BrS), an inherited cardiac arrhythmia syndrome associated with a relatively high risk of VF, was first described as a new clinical entity in 1992 (Brugada & Brugada, 1992). The ECG features of the Brugada patient includes an accentuated J wave displaying a real or apparent right branch bundle block and ST segment elevation in the right precordial leads. Although the BrS has thus far been linked to mutations that impede Na^+ channel expression or function, alterations in I_{CaL} current with CCBs have been implicated in the development of BrS both clinically (Shimizu, 2005) and experimentally (Fish & Antzelevitch, 2004).

Recently, novel mutations of the cardiac LTCC genes responsible for shortening of the QT interval in families characterized by SCD, AF and a BrS type I ECG pattern have been reported (Antzelevitch et al., 2007). Functional analyses revealed loss-of-function missense mutations of the CACNA1C (A39V in the N-terminus and G490R in the I-II domain linker) and CACNB2 (S481L). These mutations reduce I_{CaL} amplitude (due to trafficking defect for A39V), shorten QT, and are associated with asymmetrical T waves, attenuated QT-heart rate relations, and AF. Some patients also have tall, peaked T waves. These patients can also have BrS-type ST elevation in the right precordial leads with or without drug provocation, suggesting that the same reduction in I_{CaL} underlies both SQTs and BrS. More recently, a novel missense mutation (T11L) in CACNB2B has been associated with BrS (Cordeiro et al., 2009). Characterized in heterologous expression system, this mutation induced faster inactivation kinetics and hyperpolarized shift in the steady-state inactivation without any other alteration in I_{CaL}, resulting in a reduced depolarizing current in response to epicardial AP waveform.

6. Current antiarrhythmic strategies and I_{CaL}

Current therapy to prevent cardiac arrhythmia is multidimensional and complicated. The conventional antiarrhythmic drugs have limited efficacy and safety. In the case of the most common cardiac arrhythmia, AF, treatment strategies can be pharmacological or interventional (e.g. catheter ablation techniques) but are also complicated by the presence of co-morbidities such as hypertension, diabetes, and/or pre-existing cardiovascular diseases (HF or coronary artery disease) (Prystowsky et al., 2010). Within the pharmacological strategies there are several groups of drugs including β-blockers, angiotensin-converting enzyme (ACE) inhibitors, angiotensin II receptor blockers (ARBs), lipid-lowering and antithrombotic agents, spironolactone, among others, which have also demonstrated its efficacy in the prevention of SDC (Alberte & Zipes, 2003). From among all of them, the greatest reduction in cardiovascular mortality has been demonstrated with the treatment of β-blockers (Dorian, 2005). However, these drugs most likely exert their antiarrhythmic potential indirectly by affecting "upstream events" that contribute to the development of electrophysiological instability (Rubart & Zipes, 2005).

It has been demonstrated that the direct blockade of I_{CaL} with dihydropyridine Ca^{2+} channel blockers (CCBs) produces a strong shortening in the APD. So, blocking I_{CaL} is a potent means of suppressing VF. In Langendorff-perfused rabbit hearts, verapamil decreased the frequency of arrhythmia and changed it from disorganized VF into more organized VT (Samie et al., 2000). Similar results were also obtained using nifedipine (Choi et al., 2002). Therefore, CCBs could be considered promising antiarrhythmic drugs. However, the effects of these drugs have not emerged as unequivocally favorable in all clinical studies. Thus, verapamil and diltiazem can, in some cases, prevent episodes of acute ischemia VF in human, but they do not demonstrated to have as much of a beneficial effect on overall mortality as β-blockers or angiotensin-converting enzyme (ACE) inhibitors (Bodi et al., 2005). The problem observed with the direct blockade of I_{CaL} using CBBs is that, at the same time that VT is prevented, the contractility could be suppressed, precluding their clinical usefulness as antifibrillatory drugs. Therefore, in the last years it has been proposed that only modifying I_{CaL} kinetic properties, instead of blocking I_{CaL}, could produce equivalent anti-fibrillatory effects without impairing EC coupling (Mahajan et al., 2008).

In the clinical setting it is well established that the improvement in the current approach to treat AF is completely necessary. Amiodarone is the most effective antiarrhythmic drug for maintaining sinus rhythm in patients with AF. However, the extra-cardiac side effects have been a limiting factor, especially during chronic use, and may offset its benefits. Dronedarone is a new antiarrhythmic drug similar to amidarone that has been developed to provide rhythm and rate control in AF patients with fewer side effects. Dronedarone is considered as a potent blocker of multiple ion currents, including I_{CaL}, and also exhibits antiadrenergic effects. In myocytes from several experimental animals, it has been demonstrated that the effect of dronedarone on I_{CaL} consists in 76% block at dose of 10 μM with IC_{50}=0.18 μM (Varró et al., 2001; Gautier et al., 2003). Dronedarone has also important antiarrhythmic effects. Intravenous administration of dronedarone shortened ventricular APD, suppressed EADs, ectopic beats and also TdP (Verduyn et al., 1999). Moreover, intravenous dronedarone was able to prevent VF in a rat model of ischemia and reperfusion-induced arrhythmias (Manning et al., 1995). Similarly, several clinical trials have demonstrated that dronedarone is able to maintain sinus rhythm and control ventricular rate in AF, reducing the number of cardiovascular hospitalizations and mortality in patients with high-risk of AF (Singh et al., 2007; Davy et al., 2008; Hohnloser et al., 2009). The current DIONYSOS clinical trial has demonstrated that in a short-term, dronedarone was less effective than amiodarone in decreasing AF recurrence and maintaining normal sinus rhythm, but had a better safety profile, specifically with regard to thyroid and neurologic events and a lack of interaction with oral anticoagulants (Le Heuzey et al., 2010). However, the ANDROMEDA clinical trial has showed that dronedarone is also contraindicated in severe or deteriorating HF (Køber et al., 2008). The reason of that is because of a negative inotropic effect of dronedarone resulting from inhibition of I_{CaL} that could have contributed to worsening of severe HF, increasing its mortality (Gautier et al., 2003; Zimetbaum, 2009). Therefore, dronedarone is still under clinical studies and has to demonstrate its real antiarrhythmic potency and effectiveness over other antiarrhythmic as well as its possible effects in the management of additional arrhythmias, e.g. VT.

7. References

Aiba, T., Shimizu, W., Inagaki, M., Noda, T., Miyoshi, S., Ding, W.G., Zankov, D.P., Toyoda, F., Matsuura, H., Horie, M. & Sunagawa, K. (2005). Cellular and ionic mechanism for drug-induced long QT syndrome and effectiveness of verapamil. *J Am Coll Cardiol.* 45, 2, 300-307.

Aimond, F., Alvarez, J.L., Rauzier, J.M., Lorente, P. & Vassort, G. (1999). Ionic basis of ventricular arrhythmias in remodeled rat heart during long-term myocardial infarction. *Cardiovasc Res.* 42, 2, 402-415.

Alberte, C. & Zipes, D.P. (2003). Use of nonantiarrhythmic drugs for prevention of sudden cardiac death. *J Cardiovasc Electrophysiol.* 14, 9 Suppl, S87-95.

Almers, W. & McCleskey, E.W. (1984). Non-selective conductance in calcium channels of frog muscle: calcium selectivity in a single-file pore. *J Physiol.* 353, 585-608.

Alvarez, J., Dorticos, F. & Morlans, J. (1981). Changes in electrical and mechanical activities of rabbit papillary muscle during hypoxic perfusion. *J Physiol (Paris).* 77, 8, 807-812.

Alvarez, J., Hamplova, J., Hohaus, A., Morano, I., Haase, H. & Vassort, G. (2004). Calcium current in rat cardiomyocytes is modulated by the carboxyl-terminal ahnak domain. *J Biol Chem.* 279, 13, 12456-12461.

Alvarez, J.L., Petzhold, D., Pankonien, I., Behlke, J., Kouno, M., Vassort, G., Morano, I. & Haase, H. (2010). Ahnak1 modulates L-type Ca(2+) channel inactivation of rodent cardiomyocytes. *Pflugers Arch.* 460, 4, 719-730.

Alvarez, J.L. & Vassort, G. (1992). Properties of the low threshold Ca current in single frog atrial cardiomyocytes. A comparison with the high threshold Ca current. *J Gen Physiol.* 100, 3, 519-545.

Anderson, M.E. (2004). Calmodulin kinase and L-type calcium channels; a recipe for arrhythmias? *Trends Cardiovasc Med.* 14, 4, 152-161.

Anderson, M.E., Braun, A.P., Schulman, H. & Premack, B.A. (1994). Multifunctional Ca2+/calmodulin-dependent protein kinase mediates Ca(2+)-induced enhancement of the L-type Ca2+ current in rabbit ventricular myocytes. *Circ Res.* 75, 5, 854-861.

Anderson, M.E., Brown, J.H. & Bers, D.M. (2011). CaMKII in myocardial hypertrophy and heart failure. *J Mol Cell Cardiol.*

Antoons, G., Volders, P.G., Stankovicova, T., Bito, V., Stengl, M., Vos, M.A. & Sipido, K.R. (2007). Window Ca2+ current and its modulation by Ca2+ release in hypertrophied cardiac myocytes from dogs with chronic atrioventricular block. *J Physiol*. 579, Pt 1, 147-160.

Antzelevitch, C. & Burashnikov, A. 2001. Mechanisms of arrhythmogenesis. Vol. 2nd edition. 51-79 pp.

Antzelevitch, C., Pollevick, G.D., Cordeiro, J.M., Casis, O., Sanguinetti, M.C., Aizawa, Y., Guerchicoff, A., Pfeiffer, R., Oliva, A., Wollnik, B., Gelber, P., Bonaros, E.P., Jr., Burashnikov, E., Wu, Y., Sargent, J.D., Schickel, S., Oberheiden, R., Bhatia, A., Hsu, L.F., Haissaguerre, M., Schimpf, R., Borggrefe, M. & Wolpert, C. (2007). Loss-of-function mutations in the cardiac calcium channel underlie a new clinical entity characterized by ST-segment elevation, short QT intervals, and sudden cardiac death. *Circulation*. 115, 4, 442-449.

Antzelevitch, C. & Yan, G.X. (2010). J wave syndromes. *Heart Rhythm*. 7, 4, 549-558.

Argibay, J.A., Fischmeister, R. & Hartzell, H.C. (1988). Inactivation, reactivation and pacing dependence of calcium current in frog cardiocytes: correlation with current density. *J Physiol*. 401, 201-226.

Arikkath, J. & Campbell, K.P. (2003). Auxiliary subunits: essential components of the voltage-gated calcium channel complex. *Curr Opin Neurobiol*. 13, 3, 298-307.

Atar, D., Backx, P.H., Appel, M.M., Gao, W.D. & Marban, E. (1995). Excitation-transcription coupling mediated by zinc influx through voltage-dependent calcium channels. *J Biol Chem*. 270, 6, 2473-2477.

Balasubramaniam, R., Grace, A.A., Saumarez, R.C., Vandenberg, J.I. & Huang, C.L. (2003). Electrogram prolongation and nifedipine-suppressible ventricular arrhythmias in mice following targeted disruption of KCNE1. *J Physiol*. 552, Pt 2, 535-546.

Balijepalli, R.C., Lokuta, A.J., Maertz, N.A., Buck, J.M., Haworth, R.A., Valdivia, H.H. & Kamp, T.J. (2003). Depletion of T-tubules and specific subcellular changes in sarcolemmal proteins in tachycardia-induced heart failure. *Cardiovasc Res*. 59, 1, 67-77.

Barrere-Lemaire, S., Piot, C., Leclercq, F., Nargeot, J. & Richard, S. (2000). Facilitation of L-type calcium currents by diastolic depolarization in cardiac cells: impairment in heart failure. *Cardiovasc Res*. 47, 2, 336-349.

Barrett, C.F. & Tsien, R.W. (2008). The Timothy syndrome mutation differentially affects voltage- and calcium-dependent inactivation of CaV1.2 L-type calcium channels. *Proc Natl Acad Sci U S A*. 105, 6, 2157-2162.

Benitah, J.P., Alvarez, J.L. & Gómez, A.M. (2010). L-type Ca(2+) current in ventricular cardiomyocytes. *J Mol Cell Cardiol*. 48, 1, 26-36.

Benitah, J.P., Bailly, P., D'Agrosa, M.C., Da Ponte, J.P., Delgado, C. & Lorente, P. (1992). Slow inward current in single cells isolated from adult human ventricles. *Pflugers Arch*. 421, 2-3, 176-187.

Benitah, J.P., Gómez, A.M., Fauconnier, J., Kerfant, B.G., Perrier, E., Vassort, G. & Richard, S. (2002a). Voltage-gated Ca2+ currents in the human pathophysiologic heart: a review. *Basic Res Cardiol*. 97 Suppl 1, I11-18.

Benitah, J.P., Gomez, A.M., Virsolvy, A. & Richard, S. (2003). New perspectives on the key role of calcium in the progression of heart disease. *J Muscle Res Cell Motil*. 24, 4-6, 275-283.

Benitah, J.P., Kerfant, B.G., Vassort, G., Richard, S. & Gomez, A.M. (2002b). Altered communication between L-type calcium channels and ryanodine receptors in heart failure. *Front Biosci*. 7, e263-275.

Bers, D.M. 2001. Excitation-Contraction Coupling and Cardiac Contractile Force, 2nd ed. edition. Kluwer,, Dordrecht, The Netherlands.
Bers, D.M., Eisner, D.A. & Valdivia, H.H. (2003). Sarcoplasmic reticulum Ca2+ and heart failure: roles of diastolic leak and Ca2+ transport. *Circ Res*. 93, 6, 487-490.
Bito, V., Heinzel, F.R., Biesmans, L., Antoons, G. & Sipido, K.R. (2008). Crosstalk between L-type Ca2+ channels and the sarcoplasmic reticulum: alterations during cardiac remodelling. *Cardiovasc Res*. 77, 2, 315-324.
Bodi, I., Mikala, G., Koch, S.E., Akhter, S.A. & Schwartz, A. (2005). The L-type calcium channel in the heart: the beat goes on. *J Clin Invest*. 115, 12, 3306-3317.
Boixel, C., Gonzalez, W., Louedec, L. & Hatem, S.N. (2001). Mechanisms of L-type Ca(2+) current downregulation in rat atrial myocytes during heart failure. *Circ Res*. 89, 7, 607-613.
Brette, F., Leroy, J., Le Guennec, J.Y. & Salle, L. (2006). Ca2+ currents in cardiac myocytes: Old story, new insights. *Prog Biophys Mol Biol*. 91, 1-2, 1-82.
Brette, F., Salle, L. & Orchard, C.H. (2004). Differential modulation of L-type Ca2+ current by SR Ca2+ release at the T-tubules and surface membrane of rat ventricular myocytes. *Circ Res*. 95, 1, e1-7.
Brugada, P. & Brugada, J. (1992). Right bundle branch block, persistent ST segment elevation and sudden cardiac death: a distinct clinical and electrocardiographic syndrome. A multicenter report. *J Am Coll Cardiol*. 20, 6, 1391-1396.
Brundel, B.J., Van Gelder , I.C., Henning, R.H., Tieleman, R.G., Tuinenburg, A.E., Wietses, M., Grandjean, J.G., Van Gilst , W.H. & Crijns, H.J. (2001). Ion channel remodeling is related to intraoperative atrial effective refractory periods in patients with paroxysmal and persistent atrial fibrillation. *Circulation*. 103, 5, 684-690.
Burashnikov, E., Pfeiffer, R., Barajas-Martinez, H., Delpon, E., Hu, D., Desai, M., Borggrefe, M., Haissaguerre, M., Kanter, R., Pollevick, G.D., Guerchicoff, A., Laino, R., Marieb, M., Nademanee, K., Nam, G.B., Robles, R., Schimpf, R., Stapleton, D.D., Viskin, S., Winters, S., Wolpert, C., Zimmern, S., Veltmann, C. & Antzelevitch, C. Mutations in the cardiac L-type calcium channel associated with inherited J-wave syndromes and sudden cardiac death. *Heart Rhythm*. 7, 12, 1872-1882.
Canti, C., Nieto-Rostro, M., Foucault, I., Heblich, F., Wratten, J., Richards, M.W., Hendrich, J., Douglas, L., Page, K.M., Davies, A. & Dolphin, A.C. (2005). The metal-ion-dependent adhesion site in the Von Willebrand factor-A domain of alpha2delta subunits is key to trafficking voltage-gated Ca2+ channels. *Proc Natl Acad Sci U S A*. 102, 32, 11230-11235.
Carafoli, E., Santella, L., Branca, D. & Brini, M. (2001). Generation, control, and processing of cellular calcium signals. *Crit Rev Biochem Mol Biol*. 36, 2, 107-260.
Catterall, W.A. (2000). Structure and regulation of voltage-gated Ca2+ channels. *Annu Rev Cell Dev Biol*. 16, 521-555.
Catterall, W.A., Perez-Reyes, E., Snutch, T.P. & Striessnig, J. (2005). International Union of Pharmacology. XLVIII. Nomenclature and structure-function relationships of voltage-gated calcium channels. *Pharmacol Rev*. 57, 4, 411-425.
Cens, T., Restituito, S., Galas, S. & Charnet, P. (1999). Voltage and calcium use the same molecular determinants to inactivate calcium channels. *J Biol Chem*. 274, 9, 5483-5490.

Cens, T., Rousset, M., Kajava, A. & Charnet, P. (2007). Molecular determinant for specific Ca/Ba selectivity profiles of low and high threshold Ca2+ channels. *J Gen Physiol.* 130, 4, 415-425.

Cens, T., Rousset, M., Leyris, J.P., Fesquet, P. & Charnet, P. (2006). Voltage- and calcium-dependent inactivation in high voltage-gated Ca(2+) channels. *Prog Biophys Mol Biol.* 90, 1-3, 104-117.

Chen, X., Piacentino, V., 3rd, Furukawa, S., Goldman, B., Margulies, K.B. & Houser, S.R. (2002). L-type Ca2+ channel density and regulation are altered in failing human ventricular myocytes and recover after support with mechanical assist devices. *Circ Res.* 91, 6, 517-524.

Chen, X., Zhang, X., Harris, D.M., Piacentino, V., 3rd, Berretta, R.M., Margulies, K.B. & Houser, S.R. (2008). Reduced effects of BAY K 8644 on L-type Ca2+ current in failing human cardiac myocytes are related to abnormal adrenergic regulation. *Am J Physiol Heart Circ Physiol.* 294, 5, H2257-2267.

Chen, Y.H., Li, M.H., Zhang, Y., He, L.L., Yamada, Y., Fitzmaurice, A., Shen, Y., Zhang, H., Tong, L. & Yang, J. (2004). Structural basis of the alpha1-beta subunit interaction of voltage-gated Ca2+ channels. *Nature.* 429, 6992, 675-680.

Choi, B.R., Nho, W., Liu, T. & Salama, G. (2002). Life span of ventricular fibrillation frequencies. *Circ Res.* 91, 4, 339-345.

Christ, T., Boknik, P., Wöhrl, S., Wettwer, E., Graf, E.M., Bosch, R.F., Knaut, M., Schmitz, W., Ravens, U. & Dobrev, D. (2004). L-type Ca2+ current downregulation in chronic human atrial fibrillation is associated with increased activity of protein phosphatases. *Circulation.* 110, 17, 2651-2657.

Cohen, C.J., Spires, S. & Van Skiver, D. (1992). Block of T-type Ca channels in guinea pig atrial cells by antiarrhythmic agents and Ca channel antagonists. *J Gen Physiol.* 100, 4, 703-728.

Cordeiro, J.M., Marieb, M., Pfeiffer, R., Calloe, K., Burashnikov, E. & Antzelevitch, C. (2009). Accelerated inactivation of the L-type calcium current due to a mutation in CACNB2b underlies Brugada syndrome. *J Mol Cell Cardiol.* 46, 5, 695-703.

Cranefield, P.F. 1975. The conduction of the slow response. Futura Publishing Co.

Davies, A., Hendrich, J., Van Minh, A.T., Wratten, J., Douglas, L. & Dolphin, A.C. (2007). Functional biology of the alpha(2)delta subunits of voltage-gated calcium channels. *Trends Pharmacol Sci.* 28, 5, 220-228.

Davy, J.M., Herold, M., Hoglund, C., Timmermans, A., Alings, A., Radzik, D., Van Kempen, L. & Investigators, E.S. (2008). Dronedarone for the control of ventricular rate in permanent atrial fibrillation: the Efficacy and safety of dRonedArone for the cOntrol of ventricular rate during atrial fibrillation (ERATO) study. *Am Heart J.* 156, 3, 527.e521-529.

De Waard, M., Scott, V.E., Pragnell, M. & Campbell, K.P. (1996). Identification of critical amino acids involved in alpha1-beta interaction in voltage-dependent Ca2+ channels. *FEBS Lett.* 380, 3, 272-276.

Delgado, C., Artiles, A., Gomez, A.M. & Vassort, G. (1999). Frequency-dependent increase in cardiac Ca2+ current is due to reduced Ca2+ release by the sarcoplasmic reticulum. *J Mol Cell Cardiol.* 31, 10, 1783-1793.

Dinanian, S., Boixel, C., Juin, C., Hulot, J.S., Coulombe, A., Rücker-Martin, C., Bonnet, N., Le Grand, B., Slama, M., Mercadier, J.J. & Hatem, S.N. (2008). Downregulation of the calcium current in human right atrial myocytes from patients in sinus rhythm but with a high risk of atrial fibrillation. *Eur Heart J*. 29, 9, 1190-1197.

Dorian, P. (2005). Antiarrhythmic action of beta-blockers: potential mechanisms. *J Cardiovasc Pharmacol Ther*. 10 Suppl 1, S15-22.

Du, Y.M. & Nathan, R.D. (2007a). Ionic basis of ischemia-induced bradycardia in the rabbit sinoatrial node. *J Mol Cell Cardiol*. 42, 2, 315-325.

Du, Y.M. & Nathan, R.D. (2007b). Simulated ischemia enhances L-type calcium current in pacemaker cells isolated from the rabbit sinoatrial node. *Am J Physiol Heart Circ Physiol*. 293, 5, H2986-2994.

Erickson, M.G., Liang, H., Mori, M.X. & Yue, D.T. (2003). FRET two-hybrid mapping reveals function and location of L-type Ca2+ channel CaM preassociation. *Neuron*. 39, 1, 97-107.

Erxleben, C., Liao, Y., Gentile, S., Chin, D., Gomez-Alegria, C., Mori, Y., Birnbaumer, L. & Armstrong, D.L. (2006). Cyclosporin and Timothy syndrome increase mode 2 gating of CaV1.2 calcium channels through aberrant phosphorylation of S6 helices. *Proc Natl Acad Sci U S A*. 103, 10, 3932-3937.

Faber, G.M., Silva, J., Livshitz, L. & Rudy, Y. (2007). Kinetic properties of the cardiac L-type Ca2+ channel and its role in myocyte electrophysiology: a theoretical investigation. *Biophys J*. 92, 5, 1522-1543.

Fabiato, A. & Fabiato, F. (1975). Contractions induced by a calcium-triggered release of calcium from the sarcoplasmic reticulum of single skinned cardiac cells. *J Physiol*. 249, 3, 469-495.

Ferreira, G., Rios, E. & Reyes, N. (2003). Two components of voltage-dependent inactivation in Ca(v)1.2 channels revealed by its gating currents. *Biophys J*. 84, 6, 3662-3678.

Ferreira, G., Yi, J., Rios, E. & Shirokov, R. (1997). Ion-dependent inactivation of barium current through L-type calcium channels. *J Gen Physiol*. 109, 4, 449-461.

Findlay, I. (2004). Physiological modulation of inactivation in L-type Ca2+ channels: one switch. *J Physiol*. 554, Pt 2, 275-283.

Findlay, I., Suzuki, S., Murakami, S. & Kurachi, Y. (2008). Physiological modulation of voltage-dependent inactivation in the cardiac muscle L-type calcium channel: a modelling study. *Prog Biophys Mol Biol*. 96, 1-3, 482-498.

Fish, J.M. & Antzelevitch, C. (2004). Role of sodium and calcium channel block in unmasking the Brugada syndrome. *Heart Rhythm*. 1, 2, 210-217.

Fuster, V., Rydén, L.E., Cannom, D.S., Crijns, H.J., Curtis, A.B., Ellenbogen, K.A., Halperin, J.L., Kay, G.N., Le Huezey, J.Y., Lowe, J.E., Olsson, S.B., Prystowsky, E.N., Tamargo, J.L. & Wann, L.S. (2011). 2011 ACCF/AHA/HRS focused updates incorporated into the ACC/AHA/ESC 2006 Guidelines for the management of patients with atrial fibrillation: a report of the American College of Cardiology Foundation/American Heart Association Task Force on Practice Guidelines developed in partnership with the European Society of Cardiology and in collaboration with the European Heart Rhythm Association and the Heart Rhythm Society. *J Am Coll Cardiol*. 57, 11, e101-198.

Gaita, F., Giustetto, C., Bianchi, F., Wolpert, C., Schimpf, R., Riccardi, R., Grossi, S., Richiardi, E. & Borggrefe, M. (2003). Short QT Syndrome: a familial cause of sudden death. *Circulation*. 108, 8, 965-970.

Gaur, N., Rudy, Y. & Hool, L. (2009). Contributions of ion channel currents to ventricular action potential changes and induction of early afterdepolarizations during acute hypoxia. *Circ Res*. 105, 12, 1196-1203.

Gautier, P., Guillemare, E., Marion, A., Bertrand, J.P., Tourneur, Y. & Nisato, D. (2003). Electrophysiologic characterization of dronedarone in guinea pig ventricular cells. *J Cardiovasc Pharmacol*. 41, 2, 191-202.

Giustetto, C., Di Monte, F., Wolpert, C., Borggrefe, M., Schimpf, R., Sbragia, P., Leone, G., Maury, P., Anttonen, O., Haissaguerre, M. & Gaita, F. (2006). Short QT syndrome: clinical findings and diagnostic-therapeutic implications. *Eur Heart J*. 27, 20, 2440-2447.

Gómez, A.M., Valdivia, H.H., Cheng, H., Lederer, M.R., Santana, L.F., Cannell, M.B., McCune, S.A., Altschuld, R.A. & Lederer, W.J. (1997). Defective excitation-contraction coupling in experimental cardiac hypertrophy and heart failure. *Science*. 276, 5313, 800-806.

Greiser, M., Halaszovich, C.R., Frechen, D., Boknik, P., Ravens, U., Dobrev, D., Lückhoff, A. & Schotten, U. (2007). Pharmacological evidence for altered src kinase regulation of I (Ca,L) in patients with chronic atrial fibrillation. *Naunyn Schmiedebergs Arch Pharmacol*. 375, 6, 383-392.

Greiser, M., Lederer, W.J. & Schotten, U. (2011). Alterations of atrial Ca(2+) handling as cause and consequence of atrial fibrillation. *Cardiovasc Res*. 89, 4, 722-733.

Grueter, C.E., Abiria, S.A., Dzhura, I., Wu, Y., Ham, A.J., Mohler, P.J., Anderson, M.E. & Colbran, R.J. (2006). L-type Ca2+ channel facilitation mediated by phosphorylation of the beta subunit by CaMKII. *Mol Cell*. 23, 5, 641-650.

Guia, A., Stern, M.D., Lakatta, E.G. & Josephson, I.R. (2001). Ion concentration-dependence of rat cardiac unitary L-type calcium channel conductance. *Biophys J*. 80, 6, 2742-2750.

Guo, J. & Duff, H.J. (2003). Inactivation of ICa-L is the major determinant of use-dependent facilitation in rat cardiomyocytes. *J Physiol*. 547, Pt 3, 797-805.

Gussak, I., Brugada, P., Brugada, J., Wright, R.S., Kopecky, S.L., Chaitman, B.R. & Bjerregaard, P. (2000). Idiopathic short QT interval: a new clinical syndrome? *Cardiology*. 94, 2, 99-102.

Haase, H., Alvarez, J., Petzhold, D., Doller, A., Behlke, J., Erdmann, J., Hetzer, R., Regitz-Zagrosek, V., Vassort, G. & Morano, I. (2005). Ahnak is critical for cardiac Ca(V)1.2 calcium channel function and its beta-adrenergic regulation. *Faseb J*. 19, 14, 1969-1977.

Hadley, R.W. & Hume, J.R. (1987). An intrinsic potential-dependent inactivation mechanism associated with calcium channels in guinea-pig myocytes. *J Physiol*. 389, 205-222.

Hatem, S.N., Coulombe, A. & Balse, E. (2010). Specificities of atrial electrophysiology: Clues to a better understanding of cardiac function and the mechanisms of arrhythmias. *J Mol Cell Cardiol*. 48, 1, 90-95.

He, J., Conklin, M.W., Foell, J.D., Wolff, M.R., Haworth, R.A., Coronado, R. & Kamp, T.J. (2001). Reduction in density of transverse tubules and L-type Ca(2+) channels in canine tachycardia-induced heart failure. *Cardiovasc Res*. 49, 2, 298-307.

Hering, S., Berjukow, S., Sokolov, S., Marksteiner, R., Weiss, R.G., Kraus, R. & Timin, E.N. (2000). Molecular determinants of inactivation in voltage-gated Ca2+ channels. *J Physiol*. 528 Pt 2, 237-249.

Hess, P., Lansman, J.B. & Tsien, R.W. (1986). Calcium channel selectivity for divalent and monovalent cations. Voltage and concentration dependence of single channel current in ventricular heart cells. *J Gen Physiol*. 88, 3, 293-319.

Hess, P. & Tsien, R.W. (1984). Mechanism of ion permeation through calcium channels. *Nature*. 309, 5967, 453-456.

Hirano, Y. & Hiraoka, M. (2003). Ca2+ entry-dependent inactivation of L-type Ca current: a novel formulation for cardiac action potential models. *Biophys J*. 84, 1, 696-708.

Hirano, Y., Moscucci, A. & January, C.T. (1992). Direct measurement of L-type Ca2+ window current in heart cells. *Circ Res*. 70, 3, 445-455.

Hiraoka, M. & Sano, T. (1976). Role of slow inward current in the genesis of ventricular arrhythmia. *Jpn Circ J*. 40, 12, 1419-1427.

Hohnloser, S.H., Crijns, H.J., van Eickels, M., Gaudin, C., Page, R.L., Torp-Pedersen, C., Connolly, S.J. & Investigators, A. (2009). Effect of dronedarone on cardiovascular events in atrial fibrillation. *N Engl J Med*. 360, 7, 668-678.

Hool, L.C. (2000). Hypoxia increases the sensitivity of the L-type Ca(2+) current to beta-adrenergic receptor stimulation via a C2 region-containing protein kinase C isoform. *Circ Res*. 87, 12, 1164-1171.

Hool, L.C. & Arthur, P.G. (2002). Decreasing cellular hydrogen peroxide with catalase mimics the effects of hypoxia on the sensitivity of the L-type Ca2+ channel to beta-adrenergic receptor stimulation in cardiac myocytes. *Circ Res*. 91, 7, 601-609.

Horiuchi-Hirose, M., Kashihara, T., Nakada, T., Kurebayashi, N., Shimojo, H., Shibazaki, T., Sheng, X., Yano, S., Hirose, M., Hongo, M., Sakurai, T., Moriizumi, T., Ueda, H. & Yamada, M. (2011). Decrease in the density of t-tubular L-type Ca2+ channel currents in failing ventricular myocytes. *Am J Physiol Heart Circ Physiol*. 300, 3, H978-988.

Hudmon, A., Schulman, H., Kim, J., Maltez, J.M., Tsien, R.W. & Pitt, G.S. (2005). CaMKII tethers to L-type Ca2+ channels, establishing a local and dedicated integrator of Ca2+ signals for facilitation. *J Cell Biol*. 171, 3, 537-547.

Hullin, R., Matthes, J., von Vietinghoff, S., Bodi, I., Rubio, M., D'Souza, K., Friedrich Khan, I., Rottlander, D., Hoppe, U.C., Mohacsi, P., Schmitteckert, E., Gilsbach, R., Bunemann, M., Hein, L., Schwartz, A. & Herzig, S. (2007). Increased expression of the auxiliary beta2-subunit of ventricular L-type Ca2+ channels leads to single-channel activity characteristic of heart failure. *PLoS ONE*. 2, 3, e292.

Imredy, J.P. & Yue, D.T. (1992). Submicroscopic Ca2+ diffusion mediates inhibitory coupling between individual Ca2+ channels. *Neuron*. 9, 2, 197-207.

Jackman, W.M., Friday, K.J., Anderson, J.L., Aliot, E.M., Clark, M. & Lazzara, R. (1988). The long QT syndromes: a critical review, new clinical observations and a unifying hypothesis. *Prog Cardiovasc Dis*. 31, 2, 115-172.

Jacobs, A., Knight, B.P., McDonald, K.T. & Burke, M.C. (2006). Verapamil decreases ventricular tachyarrhythmias in a patient with Timothy syndrome (LQT8). *Heart Rhythm*. 3, 8, 967-970.

Jalife, J. (2000). Ventricular fibrillation: mechanisms of initiation and maintenance. *Annu Rev Physiol*. 62, 25-50.

January, C.T., Riddle, J.M. & Salata, J.J. (1988). A model for early afterdepolarizations: induction with the Ca2+ channel agonist Bay K 8644. *Circ Res*. 62, 3, 563-571.

Jones, S.W. (1991). Ion channels. Not an open-and-shut case. *Nature*. 353, 6345, 603-604.

Josephson, I.R., Sanchez-Chapula, J. & Brown, A.M. (1984). A comparison of calcium currents in rat and guinea pig single ventricular cells. *Circ Res*. 54, 2, 144-156.

Ju, Y.K. & Allen, D.G. (2003). Early effects of metabolic inhibition on intracellular Ca2+ in toad pacemaker cells: involvement of Ca2+ stores. *Am J Physiol Heart Circ Physiol*. 284, 4, H1087-1094.

Kass, R.S. & Sanguinetti, M.C. (1984). Inactivation of calcium channel current in the calf cardiac Purkinje fiber. Evidence for voltage- and calcium-mediated mechanisms. *J Gen Physiol*. 84, 5, 705-726.

Kawai, M., Hussain, M. & Orchard, C.H. (1999). Excitation-contraction coupling in rat ventricular myocytes after formamide-induced detubulation. *Am J Physiol*. 277, 2 Pt 2, H603-609.

Keung, E.C. (1989). Calcium current is increased in isolated adult myocytes from hypertrophied rat myocardium. *Circ Res*. 64, 4, 753-763.

Køber, L., Torp-Pedersen, C., McMurray, J.J., Gøtzsche, O., Lévy, S., Crijns, H., Amlie, J., Carlsen, J. & Group, D.S. (2008). Increased mortality after dronedarone therapy for severe heart failure. *N Engl J Med*. 358, 25, 2678-2687.

Kobrinsky, E., Tiwari, S., Maltsev, V.A., Harry, J.B., Lakatta, E., Abernethy, D.R. & Soldatov, N.M. (2005). Differential role of the alpha1C subunit tails in regulation of the Cav1.2 channel by membrane potential, beta subunits, and Ca2+ ions. *J Biol Chem*. 280, 13, 12474-12485.

Koretsune, Y. & Marban, E. (1989). Cell calcium in the pathophysiology of ventricular fibrillation and in the pathogenesis of postarrhythmic contractile dysfunction. *Circulation*. 80, 2, 369-379.

Lacinová, L. & Hoffmann, F. 2001. Voltage-dependent calcium channels. Vol. 4th ed. . Academic Press. 247-257 pp.

Lacinova, L. & Hofmann, F. (2005). Ca2+- and voltage-dependent inactivation of the expressed L-type Ca(v)1.2 calcium channel. *Arch Biochem Biophys*. 437, 1, 42-50.

Lakatta, E.G. & Guarnieri, T. (1993). Spontaneous myocardial calcium oscillations: are they linked to ventricular fibrillation? *J Cardiovasc Electrophysiol*. 4, 4, 473-489.

Le Grand, B.L., Hatem, S., Deroubaix, E., Couétil, J.P. & Coraboeuf, E. (1994). Depressed transient outward and calcium currents in dilated human atria. *Cardiovasc Res*. 28, 4, 548-556.

Le Heuzey, J.Y., De Ferrari, G.M., Radzik, D., Santini, M., Zhu, J. & Davy, J.M. (2010). A short-term, randomized, double-blind, parallel-group study to evaluate the efficacy and safety of dronedarone versus amiodarone in patients with persistent atrial fibrillation: the DIONYSOS study. *J Cardiovasc Electrophysiol*. 21, 6, 597-605.

Lee, K.S. (1987). Potentiation of the calcium-channel currents of internally perfused mammalian heart cells by repetitive depolarization. *Proc Natl Acad Sci U S A*. 84, 11, 3941-3945.

Lee, K.S., Marban, E. & Tsien, R.W. (1985). Inactivation of calcium channels in mammalian heart cells: joint dependence on membrane potential and intracellular calcium. *J Physiol*. 364, 395-411.

Lenaerts, I., Bito, V., Heinzel, F.R., Driesen, R.B., Holemans, P., D'hooge, J., Heidbüchel, H., Sipido, K.R. & Willems, R. (2009). Ultrastructural and functional remodeling of the coupling between Ca2+ influx and sarcoplasmic reticulum Ca2+ release in right atrial myocytes from experimental persistent atrial fibrillation. *Circ Res*. 105, 9, 876-885.

Lip, G.Y., Kakar, P. & Watson, T. (2007). Atrial fibrillation--the growing epidemic. *Heart*. 93, 5, 542-543.
Lipscombe, D., Helton, T.D. & Xu, W. (2004). L-type calcium channels: the low down. *J Neurophysiol*. 92, 5, 2633-2641.
Louch, W.E., Bito, V., Heinzel, F.R., Macianskiene, R., Vanhaecke, J., Flameng, W., Mubagwa, K. & Sipido, K.R. (2004). Reduced synchrony of Ca2+ release with loss of T-tubules-a comparison to Ca2+ release in human failing cardiomyocytes. *Cardiovasc Res*. 62, 1, 63-73.
Loyer, X., Gomez, A.M., Milliez, P., Fernandez-Velasco, M., Vangheluwe, P., Vinet, L., Charue, D., Vaudin, E., Zhang, W., Sainte-Marie, Y., Robidel, E., Marty, I., Mayer, B., Jaisser, F., Mercadier, J.J., Richard, S., Shah, A.M., Benitah, J.P., Samuel, J.L. & Heymes, C. (2008). Cardiomyocyte overexpression of neuronal nitric oxide synthase delays transition toward heart failure in response to pressure overload by preserving calcium cycling. *Circulation*. 117, 25, 3187-3198.
Luo, C.H. & Rudy, Y. (1994). A dynamic model of the cardiac ventricular action potential. I. Simulations of ionic currents and concentration changes. *Circ Res*. 74, 6, 1071-1096.
Luqman, N., Sung, R.J., Wang, C.L. & Kuo, C.T. (2007). Myocardial ischemia and ventricular fibrillation: pathophysiology and clinical implications. *Int J Cardiol*. 119, 3, 283-290.
Lyon, A.R., Macleod, K.T., Zhang, Y., Garcia, E., Kanda, G.K., Lab, M.J., Korchev, Y.E., Harding, S.E. & Gorelik, J. (2009). Loss of T-tubules and other changes to surface topography in ventricular myocytes from failing human and rat heart. *Proc Natl Acad Sci U S A*.
Mahajan, A., Sato, D., Shiferaw, Y., Baher, A., Xie, L.H., Peralta, R., Olcese, R., Garfinkel, A., Qu, Z. & Weiss, J.N. (2008). Modifying L-type calcium current kinetics: consequences for cardiac excitation and arrhythmia dynamics. *Biophys J*. 94, 2, 411-423.
Manning, A.S., Bruyninckx, C., Ramboux, J. & Chatelain, P. (1995). SR 33589, a new amiodarone-like agent: effect on ischemia- and reperfusion-induced arrhythmias in anesthetized rats. *J Cardiovasc Pharmacol*. 26, 3, 453-461.
Marks, M.L., Trippel, D.L. & Keating, M.T. (1995). Long QT syndrome associated with syndactyly identified in females. *Am J Cardiol*. 76, 10, 744-745.
Markwardt, F. & Nilius, B. (1988). Modulation of calcium channel currents in guinea-pig single ventricular heart cells by the dihydropyridine Bay K 8644. *J Physiol*. 399, 559-575.
McDonald, T.F., Pelzer, S., Trautwein, W. & Pelzer, D.J. (1994). Regulation and modulation of calcium channels in cardiac, skeletal, and smooth muscle cells. *Physiol Rev*. 74, 365–507.
Mentrard, D., Vassort, G. & Fischmeister, R. (1984). Calcium-mediated inactivation of the calcium conductance in cesium-loaded frog heart cells. *J Gen Physiol*. 83, 1, 105-131.
Napolitano, C. & Antzelevitch, C. (2011). Phenotypical manifestations of mutations in the genes encoding subunits of the cardiac voltage-dependent L-type calcium channel. *Circ Res*. 108, 5, 607-618.
Napolitano, C., Bloise, R. & Priori, S.G. (2006). Gene-specific therapy for inherited arrhythmogenic diseases. *Pharmacol Ther*. 110, 1, 1-13.
Neef, S., Dybkova, N., Sossalla, S., Ort, K.R., Fluschnik, N., Neumann, K., Seipelt, R., Schöndube, F.A., Hasenfuss, G. & Maier, L.S. (2010). CaMKII-dependent diastolic

SR Ca2+ leak and elevated diastolic Ca2+ levels in right atrial myocardium of patients with atrial fibrillation. *Circ Res*. 106, 6, 1134-1144.

Ohrtman, J., Ritter, B., Polster, A., Beam, K.G. & Papadopoulos, S. (2008). Sequence differences in the IQ motifs of CaV1.1 and CaV1.2 strongly impact calmodulin binding and calcium-dependent inactivation. *J Biol Chem*. 283, 43, 29301-29311.

Opthof, T., Coronel, R., Vermeulen, J.T., Verberne, H.J., van Capelle, F.J. & Janse, M.J. (1993). Dispersion of refractoriness in normal and ischaemic canine ventricle: effects of sympathetic stimulation. *Cardiovasc Res*. 27, 11, 1954-1960.

Perrier, E., Kerfant, B.G., Lalevee, N., Bideaux, P., Rossier, M.F., Richard, S., Gomez, A.M. & Benitah, J.P. (2004). Mineralocorticoid receptor antagonism prevents the electrical remodeling that precedes cellular hypertrophy after myocardial infarction. *Circulation*. 110, 7, 776-783.

Peterson, B.Z., Lee, J.S., Mulle, J.G., Wang, Y., de Leon, M. & Yue, D.T. (2000). Critical determinants of Ca(2+)-dependent inactivation within an EF-hand motif of L-type Ca(2+) channels. *Biophys J*. 78, 4, 1906-1920.

Pietrobon, D. & Hess, P. (1990). Novel mechanism of voltage-dependent gating in L-type calcium channels. *Nature*. 346, 6285, 651-655.

Piot, C., Lemaire, S., Albat, B., Seguin, J., Nargeot, J. & Richard, S. (1996). High frequency-induced upregulation of human cardiac calcium currents. *Circulation*. 93, 1, 120-128.

Pitt, G.S., Zuhlke, R.D., Hudmon, A., Schulman, H., Reuter, H. & Tsien, R.W. (2001). Molecular basis of calmodulin tethering and Ca2+-dependent inactivation of L-type Ca2+ channels. *J Biol Chem*. 276, 33, 30794-30802.

Prystowsky, E.N., Camm, J., Lip, G.Y., Allessie, M., Bergmann, J.F., Breithardt, G., Brugada, J., Crijns, H., Ellinor, P.T., Mark, D., Naccarelli, G., Packer, D. & Tamargo, J. (2010). The impact of new and emerging clinical data on treatment strategies for atrial fibrillation. *J Cardiovasc Electrophysiol*. 21, 8, 946-958.

Qi, X., Yeh, Y.H., Chartier, D., Xiao, L., Tsuji, Y., Brundel, B.J., Kodama, I. & Nattel, S. (2009). The calcium/calmodulin/kinase system and arrhythmogenic afterdepolarizations in bradycardia-related acquired long-QT syndrome. *Circ Arrhythm Electrophysiol*. 2, 3, 295-304.

Qi, X.Y., Yeh, Y.H., Xiao, L., Burstein, B., Maguy, A., Chartier, D., Villeneuve, L.R., Brundel, B.J., Dobrev, D. & Nattel, S. (2008). Cellular signaling underlying atrial tachycardia remodeling of L-type calcium current. *Circ Res*. 103, 8, 845-854.

Qu, Y., Baroudi, G., Yue, Y. & Boutjdir, M. (2005). Novel molecular mechanism involving alpha1D (Cav1.3) L-type calcium channel in autoimmune-associated sinus bradycardia. *Circulation*. 111, 23, 3034-3041.

Richard, S., Charnet, P. & Nerbonne, J.M. (1993). Interconversion between distinct gating pathways of the high threshold calcium channel in rat ventricular myocytes. *J Physiol*. 462, 197-228.

Richard, S., Perrier, E., Fauconnier, J., Perrier, R., Pereira, L., Gomez, A.M. & Benitah, J.P. (2006). 'Ca(2+)-induced Ca(2+) entry' or how the L-type Ca(2+) channel remodels its own signalling pathway in cardiac cells. *Prog Biophys Mol Biol*. 90, 1-3, 118-135.

Rubart, M. & Zipes, D.P. (2005). Mechanisms of sudden cardiac death. *J Clin Invest*. 115, 9, 2305-2315.

Ryder, K.O., Bryant, S.M. & Hart, G. (1993). Membrane current changes in left ventricular myocytes isolated from guinea pigs after abdominal aortic coarctation. *Cardiovasc Res*. 27, 7, 1278-1287.

Samie, F.H., Mandapati, R., Gray, R.A., Watanabe, Y., Zuur, C., Beaumont, J. & Jalife, J. (2000). A mechanism of transition from ventricular fibrillation to tachycardia : effect of calcium channel blockade on the dynamics of rotating waves. *Circ Res*. 86, 6, 684-691.

Sather, W.A. & McCleskey, E.W. (2003). Permeation and selectivity in calcium channels. *Annu Rev Physiol*. 65, 133-159.

Schimpf, R., Wolpert, C., Gaita, F., Giustetto, C. & Borggrefe, M. (2005). Short QT syndrome. *Cardiovasc Res*. 67, 3, 357-366.

Schlotthauer, K. & Bers, D.M. (2000). Sarcoplasmic reticulum Ca(2+) release causes myocyte depolarization. Underlying mechanism and threshold for triggered action potentials. *Circ Res*. 87, 9, 774-780.

Schotten, U., Ausma, J., Stellbrink, C., Sabatschus, I., Vogel, M., Frechen, D., Schoendube, F., Hanrath, P. & Allessie, M.A. (2001). Cellular mechanisms of depressed atrial contractility in patients with chronic atrial fibrillation. *Circulation*. 103, 5, 691-698.

Schotten, U., de Haan, S., Neuberger, H.R., Eijsbouts, S., Blaauw, Y., Tieleman, R. & Allessie, M. (2004). Loss of atrial contractility is primary cause of atrial dilatation during first days of atrial fibrillation. *Am J Physiol Heart Circ Physiol*. 287, 5, H2324-2331.

Schotten, U., Haase, H., Frechen, D., Greiser, M., Stellbrink, C., Vazquez-Jimenez, J.F., Morano, I., Allessie, M.A. & Hanrath, P. (2003). The L-type Ca2+-channel subunits alpha1C and beta2 are not downregulated in atrial myocardium of patients with chronic atrial fibrillation. *J Mol Cell Cardiol*. 35, 5, 437-443.

Schouten, V.J. & Morad, M. (1989). Regulation of Ca2+ current in frog ventricular myocytes by the holding potential, c-AMP and frequency. *Pflugers Arch*. 415, 1, 1-11.

Schröder, F., Handrock, R., Beuckelmann, D.J., Hirt, S., Hullin, R., Priebe, L., Schwinger, R.H., Weil, J. & Herzig, S. (1998). Increased availability and open probability of single L-type calcium channels from failing compared with nonfailing human ventricle. *Circulation*. 98, 10, 969-976.

Schulze-Bahr, E., Wang, Q., Wedekind, H., Haverkamp, W., Chen, Q., Sun, Y., Rubie, C., Hordt, M., Towbin, J.A., Borggrefe, M., Assmann, G., Qu, X., Somberg, J.C., Breithardt, G., Oberti, C. & Funke, H. (1997). KCNE1 mutations cause jervell and Lange-Nielsen syndrome. *Nat Genet*. 17, 3, 267-268.

Shi, C. & Soldatov, N.M. (2002). Molecular determinants of voltage-dependent slow inactivation of the Ca2+ channel. *J Biol Chem*. 277, 9, 6813-6821.

Shimizu, W. (2005). Acquired forms of the Brugada syndrome. *J Electrocardiol*. 38, 4 Suppl, 22-25.

Shimizu, W., Aiba, T. & Antzelevitch, C. (2005). Specific therapy based on the genotype and cellular mechanism in inherited cardiac arrhythmias. Long QT syndrome and Brugada syndrome. *Curr Pharm Des*. 11, 12, 1561-1572.

Shimizu, W., Ohe, T., Kurita, T., Kawade, M., Arakaki, Y., Aihara, N., Kamakura, S., Kamiya, T. & Shimomura, K. (1995). Effects of verapamil and propranolol on early afterdepolarizations and ventricular arrhythmias induced by epinephrine in congenital long QT syndrome. *J Am Coll Cardiol*. 26, 5, 1299-1309.

Shinagawa, K., Shiroshita-Takeshita, A., Schram, G. & Nattel, S. (2003). Effects of antiarrhythmic drugs on fibrillation in the remodeled atrium: insights into the mechanism of the superior efficacy of amiodarone. *Circulation*. 107, 10, 1440-1446.

Shirokov, R. (1999). Interaction between permeant ions and voltage sensor during inactivation of N-type Ca2+ channels. *J Physiol*. 518 (Pt 3), 697-703.

Shorofsky, S.R. & January, C.T. (1992). L- and T-type Ca2+ channels in canine cardiac Purkinje cells. Single-channel demonstration of L-type Ca2+ window current. *Circ Res*. 70, 3, 456-464.

Sicouri, S., Timothy, K.W., Zygmunt, A.C., Glass, A., Goodrow, R.J., Belardinelli, L. & Antzelevitch, C. (2007). Cellular basis for the electrocardiographic and arrhythmic manifestations of Timothy syndrome: effects of ranolazine. *Heart Rhythm*. 4, 5, 638-647.

Sims, C., Reisenweber, S., Viswanathan, P.C., Choi, B.R., Walker, W.H. & Salama, G. (2008). Sex, age, and regional differences in L-type calcium current are important determinants of arrhythmia phenotype in rabbit hearts with drug-induced long QT type 2. *Circ Res*. 102, 9, e86-100.

Singh, B.N., Connolly, S.J., Crijns, H.J., Roy, D., Kowey, P.R., Capucci, A., Radzik, D., Aliot, E.M., Hohnloser, S.H. & Investigators, E.a.A. (2007). Dronedarone for maintenance of sinus rhythm in atrial fibrillation or flutter. *N Engl J Med*. 357, 10, 987-999.

Sipido, K.R., Volders, P.G., de Groot, S.H., Verdonck, F., Van de Werf, F., Wellens, H.J. & Vos, M.A. (2000). Enhanced Ca(2+) release and Na/Ca exchange activity in hypertrophied canine ventricular myocytes: potential link between contractile adaptation and arrhythmogenesis. *Circulation*. 102, 17, 2137-2144.

Slesinger, P.A. & Lansman, J.B. (1991). Reopening of Ca2+ channels in mouse cerebellar neurons at resting membrane potentials during recovery from inactivation. *Neuron*. 7, 5, 755-762.

Song, L.S., Pi, Y., Kim, S.J., Yatani, A., Guatimosim, S., Kudej, R.K., Zhang, Q., Cheng, H., Hittinger, L., Ghaleh, B., Vatner, D.E., Lederer, W.J. & Vatner, S.F. (2005). Paradoxical cellular Ca2+ signaling in severe but compensated canine left ventricular hypertrophy. *Circ Res*. 97, 5, 457-464.

Splawski, I., Timothy, K.W., Decher, N., Kumar, P., Sachse, F.B., Beggs, A.H., Sanguinetti, M.C. & Keating, M.T. (2005). Severe arrhythmia disorder caused by cardiac L-type calcium channel mutations. *Proc Natl Acad Sci U S A*. 102, 23, 8089-8096; discussion 8086-8088.

Splawski, I., Timothy, K.W., Sharpe, L.M., Decher, N., Kumar, P., Bloise, R., Napolitano, C., Schwartz, P.J., Joseph, R.M., Condouris, K., Tager-Flusberg, H., Priori, S.G., Sanguinetti, M.C. & Keating, M.T. (2004). Ca(V)1.2 calcium channel dysfunction causes a multisystem disorder including arrhythmia and autism. *Cell*. 119, 1, 19-31.

Starr, T.V., Prystay, W. & Snutch, T.P. (1991). Primary structure of a calcium channel that is highly expressed in the rat cerebellum. *Proc Natl Acad Sci U S A*. 88, 13, 5621-5625.

Takahashi, M. & Catterall, W.A. (1987). Dihydropyridine-sensitive calcium channels in cardiac and skeletal muscle membranes: studies with antibodies against the alpha subunits. *Biochemistry*. 26, 17, 5518-5526.

Tang, S., Mikala, G., Bahinski, A., Yatani, A., Varadi, G. & Schwartz, A. (1993). Molecular localization of ion selectivity sites within the pore of a human L-type cardiac calcium channel. *J Biol Chem*. 268, 18, 13026-13029.

Tanskanen, A.J., Greenstein, J.L., O'Rourke, B. & Winslow, R.L. (2005). The role of stochastic and modal gating of cardiac L-type Ca2+ channels on early after-depolarizations. *Biophys J*. 88, 1, 85-95.

Templin, C., Ghadri, J.R., Rougier, J.S., Baumer, A., Kaplan, V., Albesa, M., Sticht, H., Rauch, A., Puleo, C., Hu, D., Barajas-Martinez, H., Antzelevitch, C., Luscher, T.F., Abriel,

H. & Duru, F. (2011). Identification of a novel loss-of-function calcium channel gene mutation in short QT syndrome (SQTS6). *Eur Heart J.* 32, 9, 1077-1088.

Thiel, W.H., Chen, B., Hund, T.J., Koval, O.M., Purohit, A., Song, L.S., Mohler, P.J. & Anderson, M.E. (2008). Proarrhythmic defects in Timothy syndrome require calmodulin kinase II. *Circulation.* 118, 22, 2225-2234.

Thomas, G., Gurung, I.S., Killeen, M.J., Hakim, P., Goddard, C.A., Mahaut-Smith, M.P., Colledge, W.H., Grace, A.A. & Huang, C.L. (2007). Effects of L-type Ca2+ channel antagonism on ventricular arrhythmogenesis in murine hearts containing a modification in the Scn5a gene modelling human long QT syndrome 3. *J Physiol.* 578, Pt 1, 85-97.

Tiaho, F., Piot, C., Nargeot, J. & Richard, S. (1994). Regulation of the frequency-dependent facilitation of L-type Ca2+ currents in rat ventricular myocytes. *J Physiol.* 477 (Pt 2), 237-251.

Tomaselli, G.F. & Rose, J. (2000). Molecular aspects of arrhythmias associated with cardiomyopathies. *Curr Opin Cardiol.* 15, 3, 202-208.

Treinys, R. & Jurevicius, J. (2008). L-type Ca2+ channels in the heart: structure and regulation. *Medicina (Kaunas).* 44, 7, 491-499.

Tseng, G.N. (1988). Calcium current restitution in mammalian ventricular myocytes is modulated by intracellular calcium. *Circ Res.* 63, 2, 468-482.

Van Petegem, F., Clark, K.A., Chatelain, F.C. & Minor, D.L., Jr. (2004). Structure of a complex between a voltage-gated calcium channel beta-subunit and an alpha-subunit domain. *Nature.* 429, 6992, 671-675.

Van Wagoner, D.R., Pond, A.L., McCarthy, P.M., Trimmer, J.S. & Nerbonne, J.M. (1997). Outward K+ current densities and Kv1.5 expression are reduced in chronic human atrial fibrillation. *Circ Res.* 80, 6, 772-781.

Varró, A., Takács, J., Németh, M., Hála, O., Virág, L., Iost, N., Baláti, B., Agoston, M., Vereckei, A., Pastor, G., Delbruyère, M., Gautier, P., Nisato, D. & Papp, J.G. (2001). Electrophysiological effects of dronedarone (SR 33589), a noniodinated amiodarone derivative in the canine heart: comparison with amiodarone. *Br J Pharmacol.* 133, 5, 625-634.

Verduyn, S.C., Vos, M.A., Leunissen, H.D., van Opstal, J.M. & Wellens, H.J. (1999). Evaluation of the acute electrophysiologic effects of intravenous dronedarone, an amiodarone-like agent, with special emphasis on ventricular repolarization and acquired torsade de pointes arrhythmias. *J Cardiovasc Pharmacol.* 33, 2, 212-222.

Vinogradova, T.M., Zhou, Y.Y., Bogdanov, K.Y., Yang, D., Kuschel, M., Cheng, H. & Xiao, R.P. (2000). Sinoatrial node pacemaker activity requires Ca(2+)/calmodulin-dependent protein kinase II activation. *Circ Res.* 87, 9, 760-767.

Wang, Y., Tandan, S., Cheng, J., Yang, C., Nguyen, L., Sugianto, J., Johnstone, J.L., Sun, Y. & Hill, J.A. (2008). Ca2+/calmodulin-dependent protein kinase II-dependent remodeling of Ca2+ current in pressure overload heart failure. *J Biol Chem.* 283, 37, 25524-25532.

Weidmann, S. (1951). Effect of current flow on the membrane potential of cardiac muscle. *J Physiol.* 115, 2, 227-236.

Wellens, H.J., Tan, S.L., Bar, F.W., Duren, D.R., Lie, K.I. & Dohmen, H.M. (1977). Effect of verapamil studied by programmed electrical stimulation of the heart in patients with paroxysmal re-entrant supraventricular tachycardia. *Br Heart J.* 39, 10, 1058-1066.

Wibo, M., Bravo, G. & Godfraind, T. (1991). Postnatal maturation of excitation-contraction coupling in rat ventricle in relation to the subcellular localization and surface density of 1,4-dihydropyridine and ryanodine receptors. *Circ Res*. 68, 3, 662-673.

Wu, Y., Temple, J., Zhang, R., Dzhura, I., Zhang, W., Trimble, R., Roden, D.M., Passier, R., Olson, E.N., Colbran, R.J. & Anderson, M.E. (2002). Calmodulin kinase II and arrhythmias in a mouse model of cardiac hypertrophy. *Circulation*. 106, 10, 1288-1293.

Xiao, R.P., Cheng, H., Lederer, W.J., Suzuki, T. & Lakatta, E.G. (1994). Dual regulation of Ca2+/calmodulin-dependent kinase II activity by membrane voltage and by calcium influx. *Proc Natl Acad Sci U S A*. 91, 20, 9659-9663.

Xiong, L., Kleerekoper, Q.K., He, R., Putkey, J.A. & Hamilton, S.L. (2005). Sites on calmodulin that interact with the C-terminal tail of Cav1.2 channel. *J Biol Chem*. 280, 8, 7070-7079.

Yang, J., Ellinor, P.T., Sather, W.A., Zhang, J.F. & Tsien, R.W. (1993). Molecular determinants of Ca2+ selectivity and ion permeation in L-type Ca2+ channels. *Nature*. 366, 6451, 158-161.

Yarotskyy, V., Gao, G., Peterson, B.Z. & Elmslie, K.S. (2009). The Timothy syndrome mutation of cardiac CaV1.2 (L-type) channels: multiple altered gating mechanisms and pharmacological restoration of inactivation. *J Physiol*. 587, Pt 3, 551-565.

Yazawa, M., Hsueh, B., Jia, X., Pasca, A.M., Bernstein, J.A., Hallmayer, J. & Dolmetsch, R.E. Using induced pluripotent stem cells to investigate cardiac phenotypes in Timothy syndrome. *Nature*. 471, 7337, 230-234.

Yuan, W. & Bers, D.M. (1994). Ca-dependent facilitation of cardiac Ca current is due to Ca-calmodulin-dependent protein kinase. *Am J Physiol*. 267, 3 Pt 2, H982-993.

Yue, L., Feng, J., Gaspo, R., Li, G.R., Wang, Z. & Nattel, S. (1997). Ionic remodeling underlying action potential changes in a canine model of atrial fibrillation. *Circ Res*. 81, 4, 512-525.

Zhang, R., Dzhura, I., Grueter, C.E., Thiel, W., Colbran, R.J. & Anderson, M.E. (2005). A dynamic alpha-beta inter-subunit agonist signaling complex is a novel feedback mechanism for regulating L-type Ca2+ channel opening. *Faseb J*. 19, 11, 1573-1575.

Zimetbaum, P.J. (2009). Dronedarone for atrial fibrillation--an odyssey. *N Engl J Med*. 360, 18, 1811-1813.

Zuhlke, R.D., Pitt, G.S., Deisseroth, K., Tsien, R.W. & Reuter, H. (1999). Calmodulin supports both inactivation and facilitation of L-type calcium channels. *Nature*. 399, 6732, 159-162.

Zygmunt, A.C. & Maylie, J. (1990). Stimulation-dependent facilitation of the high threshold calcium current in guinea-pig ventricular myocytes. *J Physiol*. 428, 653-671.

Part 3

Pathophysiology of Cardiac Arrhythmias

7

Natural Protection Against Cardiac Arrhythmias During Hibernation: Significance of Adenosine

Tulasi Ram Jinka
Institute of Arctic Biology, University of Alaska Fairbanks, Fairbanks, AK, USA

1. Introduction

Hibernation is a physiological adaptation to periods of seasonal resource limitation (Carey et al., 2003a; Drew et al., 2007). Hibernators undergo several bouts of torpor during a hibernation season. Torpor in hibernation is a period of profound bradycardia, tachycardia, metabolic suppression and decreased core body temperature (Drew et al. 2007). Hibernation is characterized by alternating phases of torpor and euthermy that begins in the fall and continues until the hibernation season ceases in spring (Lyman, 1958; Geiser and Ruf, 1995; Boyer and Barnes, 1999). Based on whole-body metabolic rate and core body temperature each torpor bout consists of an entrance, steady-state, and arousal phases (Boyer and Barnes, 1999; Carey et al., 2003a; Heldmaier et al., 2004; Drew et al., 2007) (Fig.1). Successive torpor bouts are interrupted by a brief period (12-24h) of interbout euthermy.

Cardiac arrhythmia is described as any deviation from the normal sequence of electrical impulses resulting in slow (bradycardia), fast (tachycardia) or erratic hearbeats such as atrial and ventricle fibrillations and conduction disorders (Keating and Sanguinetti, 2001).

Cardiac arrhythmias are observed during hibernation (Chatfield and Lyman, 1950; Eagles et al., 1988; Milsom et al., 1993; Milsom et al., 1999; Toien et al., 2011). In spite of that no untoward effects such as ventricular fibrillation or heart failure are noticed in hibernators and the hearts remain functional even at a body temperature of 0°C (Johansson, 1996). Moreover, hibernators can rewarm to euthermic body temperature of about 36°C in a span of few hours (Lyman, 1958)(Fig1&2) without any cardiac or nervous system complications (Drew et al., 2007). In contrast, similar conditions in non-hibernators including humans lead to fatal cardiac complications and death (Nardone, 1955; Johansson, 1996; Drew et al., 2007). Unresolved intrinsic mechanisms protect the hibernating species against lethal cardiac arrhythmias at reduced body temperatures. Understanding the intrinsic functional mechanisms existing in hibernators can lead to novel therapies in treating several conditions such as cardiac arrest and stroke (Drew et al., 2007).

Patients with cardiac arrest are subjected to hypothermia in a clinical setting (Polderman, 2004; Polderman and Herold, 2009). However, inducing hypothermia beyond a certain level is not without complications. Patients subjected to temperatures colder than 30°C suffer cardiac arrhythmias (Polderman and Herold, 2009). Cooling more slowly should mimic similar drop in body temperature seen during torpor in hibernators and may thus avoid arrhythmias. The question is how to achieve this state where the temperature can be dropped below 30°C without any cardiac complications.

Difference exists between hibernators and nonhibernators in resisting ventricular fibrillation induced by hypothermia. Several factors are responsible including heart size (Surawicz, 1971).Hibernating animals vary in size (Geiser, 2004). Large hearts tend to develop ventricular fibrillations (Surawicz, 1971). Although bears are regarded as hibernators their body temperature does not fall below 30°C which is above the critical body temperature where ventricular fibrillations are noticed (Johansson, 1984; Eagles et al., 1988; Toien et al., 2011). This chapter discusses about small hibernators in general focusing on the role of nervous system regulation of cardiac function in the light of recent research findings and the importance of adenosine (Miyazawa et al., 2008; Jinka et al., 2011). This chapter gives an overview of hibernation physiology, various mechanisms regulating hibernation, cardiac arrhythmias observed during hibernation, functional difference between hibernator and a non-hibernator, especially in regard to heart function, and finally discusses novel findings and hypothesis that may be translated to treat certain medical conditions such as cardiac arrest and stroke to improve the outcome in such patients.

2. Phases of hibernation and cardiac arrhythmias

2.1 The entrance phase

A decrease in heart rate and metabolism prior to decrease in core body temperature is a characteristic phenomenon observed during entrance into hibernation (Lyman, 1958). Heart rate, metabolism and core body temperature gradually decline during the entrance phase until the core body temperature drops down to the lowest limit where the core body temperature is just above the ambient temperature (Boyer and Barnes, 1999; Tamura et al., 2005). Heart rate declines to 2-7 beats per minute (Dawe and Morrison, 1955) , metabolism drops to 2% of resting metabolic rate (Geiser, 1988; Buck and Barnes, 2000) and core body temperature drops to as low as -2.9° C (Barnes, 1989)(Fig.1&2).

2.1.1 Cardiac arrhythmias during entrance into hibernation

Evidence supports the central nervous system regulation during entrance into hibernation. Administration of adenosine agonist into the brain induces torpor in arctic ground squirrels (Jinka et al., 2011). By lowering the set-point (T_{set}) threshold below the actual hypothalamic temperature (T_{hy}) during entrance into hibernation a smooth entrance is facilitated. An occasional burst of body temperature paralleled by an increase in metabolism is observed when T_{hy} below $T_{set.}$ (Heller et al., 1977; Heldmaier et al., 2004). The changes in heart rate parallel the change in metabolic rate suggesting that entrance into hibernation is a highly regulated, orchestrated event of several physiological processes rather than a consequence of a drop in body temperature (Milsom et al., 1999).

A comparison between heart rate and temperature in hedgehogs during entrance into hibernation indicates a shift towards parasympathetic influence (Dawe and Morrison, 1955). Atropine is a parasympatholytic and increases heart rate by slowing of parasympathetic output. Administration of atropine during entrance into hibernation increased heart rate in hamsters (Lyman and O'Brien, 1963). Cardiac arrhythmias during entrance into hibernation are abolished by administration of atropine in marmots (Lyman, 1982). All these studies suggest that a well coordinated activation of parasympathetic system, preparatory initial changes in the heart rate, skipped beats and asystoles altogether are necessary for decline in heart rate and for a smooth entrance into hibernation (Milsom et al., 1999; Zimmer et al., 2000).

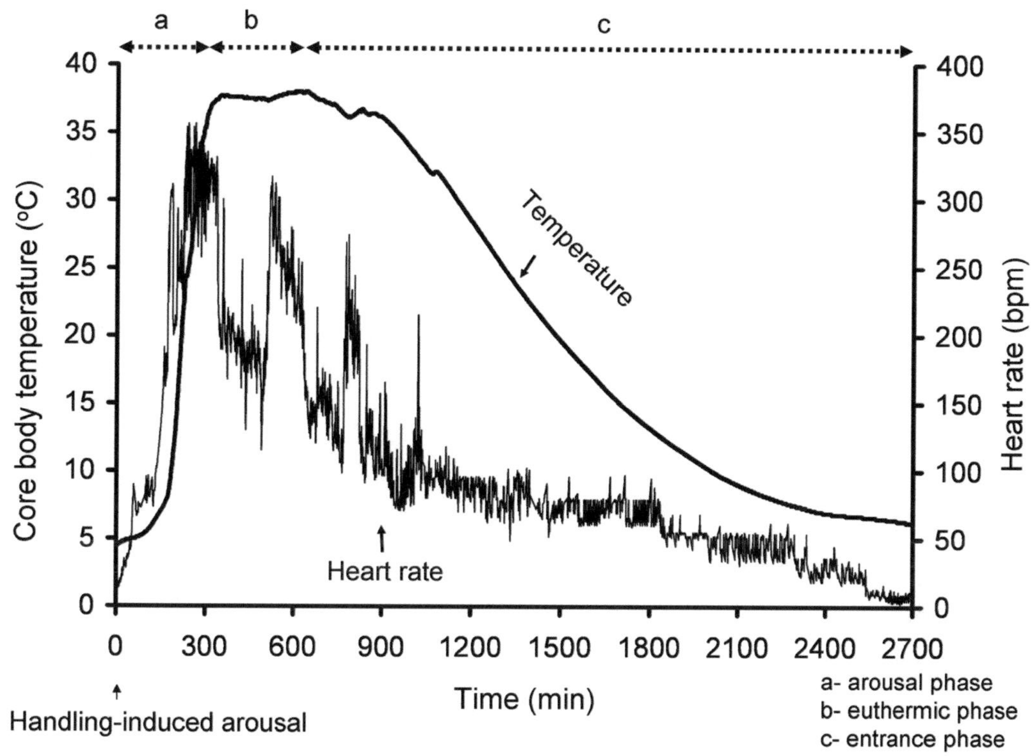

Fig. 1. Core body temperature was measured in an Arctic ground squirrel after arousal from torpor induced by gentle handling and until the animal entered another bout of torpor.
Core body temperature and heart rate were measured with an ip transmitter as described previously (Jinka et al., 2011). Torpor in hibernation is broadly divided into three phases- entrance, steady-state, and arousal (Boyer and Barnes, 1999; Carey et al., 2003a; Heldmaier et al., 2004; Drew et al., 2007). Entrance phase is followed by steady-state phase which lasts for 1-3 weeks before the arousal phase is initiated. Core body temperature in an Arctic ground squirrel can drop to as low as -2.9°C (Barnes, 1989) before it reaches steady-state phase. A fully aroused animal stays at euthermic body temperature of 35-37°C for about a day before another torpor bout ensues. Changes in heart rate reflect changes in core body temperature during a hibernation bout.

Several unique behavioral patterns of heart beats are noticed during entrance into hibernation. It is interesting to know how a hibernator can drastically reduce its heart rate during entrance into hibernation without any adverse effects. Heart rate drops prior to any changes in body temperature indicating that a decreased heart rate during entrance into hibernation is independent of body temperature. (Landau and Dawe, 1958; Lyman, 1958; Elvert and Heldmaier, 2005). Appearance of skipped beats is a characteristic feature exhibited by several species of hibernators during entrance into hibernation (Dawe and Morrison, 1955; Lyman, 1958; Twente and Twente, 1978; Lyman, 1982) (Fig.3). A drastic 50% fall in heart rate while a drop in body temperature by 0.6°C observed during initial stages of entrance into hibernation occurs around 33-34°C (Strumwasser, 1959).

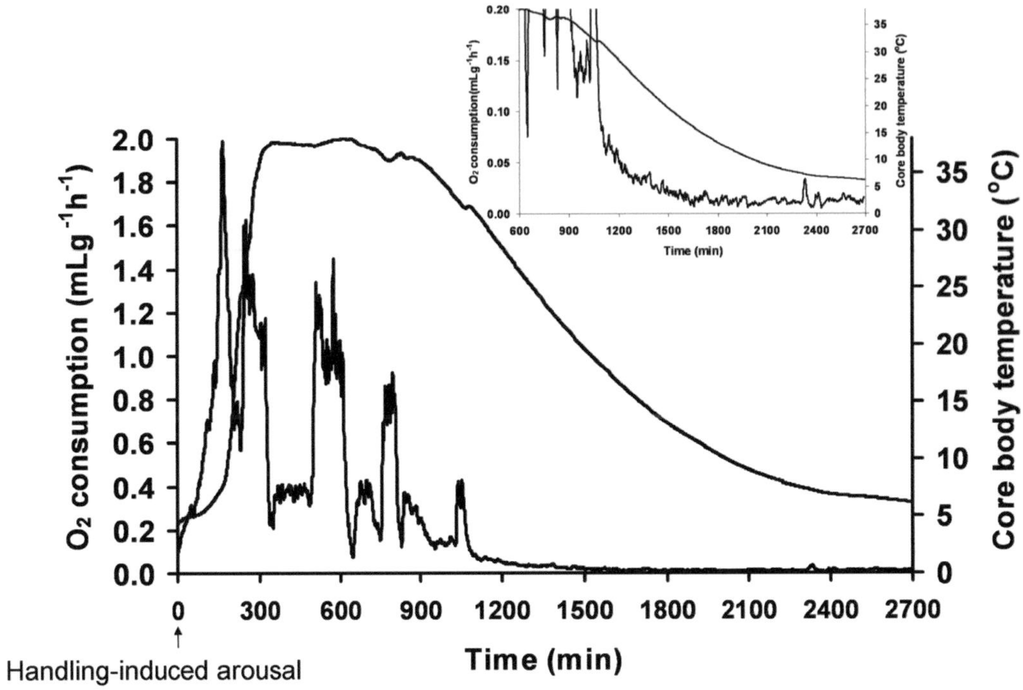

Fig. 2. Changes in core body temperature and whole animal oxygen consumption as measured in an Arctic ground squirrel after arousal from torpor was iniated by gentle handling and until the animal entered another bout of torpor.
Core body temperature was measured with an ip transmitter and oxygen consumption was measured using open flow respirometry as described previously (Jinka et al., 2011). The inset illustrates how oxygen consumption precedes a decline in core body temperature during entrance into torpor as shown on a smaller scale. Entrance into hibernation is characterized by a characteristic decline in whole animal oxygen consumption (metabolism) that precedes a decrease in core Tb (Lyman, 1958). [source: (Drew et al., 2009)]

2.2 The steady-state phase

Animal enters into a steady-state phase of hibernation after a few hours of initiation of torpor. Steady-state phase represents the nadir of mammalian heart rate, metabolism, and core body temperature (Drew et al., 2007) where the animal maintains its lowest heart rate, metabolism, and core body temperature for about 1-3 weeks (Boyer and Barnes, 1999; Buck and Barnes, 2000; Carey et al., 2003a). An occasional burst of activity paralleled with an increase in heart rate, metabolism and heat production is observed during this phase and is hypothesized as a measure to avoid decreases in body temperature beyond a certain point (Heldmaier et al., 2004).

2.2.1 Cardiac arrhythmias during steady state hibernation

Diastolic arrhythmias are noticed in deep hibernation (Twente and Twente, 1978; Milsom et al., 1999). Different opinions exist on the influence of sympathetic and parasympathetic systems on deep hibernation with no definitive conclusion (Milsom et al., 1999).

2.3 The arousal phase

Periodic arousals from hibernation are noticed in true hibernators (Lyman, 1958; Geiser and Ruf, 1995; Boyer and Barnes, 1999; Karpovich et al., 2009). A characteristic gradual increase in heart rate, metabolism and respiration followed by a gradual increase in core body temperature is observed during arousal from hibernation (Lyman, 1958). It is interesting to note that the rewarming from hibernation without any external source of heat suggests that hibernation is not a state of energy deficiency (Carey et al., 2003a). Animals attain a core body temperature of 35-37°C, then maintain euthermic body temperature for about a day before another hibernation bout starts (Boyer and Barnes, 1999; Carey et al., 2003b).

2.3.1 Cardiac arrhythmias during arousal from hibernation

Cardiac arrhythmias appear throughout arousal (Twente and Twente, 1978). Heart rate gradually increases in frequency as the body temperature increases (Lyman, 1958). The initial rapid increase in heart rate during arousal from hibernation is due to sympathetic activation (Milsom et al., 1993) and as such the increase in endogenous catecholamines are arrhythmogenic (Burn, 1961; Trautwein, 1963). Asystoles are followed by bradycardia during arousal from hibernation. Asystoles appear between 11-18°C during which period the heart rate falls below what it was before the appearance of asystolic episodes, and attains a regular rhythm and a higher rate as soon as the asystoles disappear at about 18°C (Eagles et al., 1988). This waxing and waning appearance of heart rate during arousal may be due to alternating sympathetic and parasympathetic dominance on the way to euthermia (Milsom et al., 1999). A ventricular bigeminy with a repetitive premature ventricular heart beats alternating with supraventricular beats is also demonstrated on ECG (Eagles et al., 1988). During mid to late arousal the heart rate, metabolism and respiratory frequency gradually reach a peak followed by body temperature under the influence of sympathetic tone until the animal reaches euthermia during which period the autonomic balance is restored (Lyman, 1958; Lyman and O'Brien, 1963; Twente and Twente, 1965; Lyman and O'Brien, 1969; Twente and Twente, 1978; Milsom et al., 1993).

3. Cardiac arrhythmias in hibernation vs hypothermia in hibernators

A study on ground squirrels revealed several differences in the ECG during hibernation and hypothermia (Dawe and Morrison, 1955; Nardone, 1955). A slow heart rate in hibernation is facilitated by a 40-70 fold increase in the duration of T-P segment suggesting a slowed SA node during hibernation. A 4-5 fold increase in duration of QRS complex is observed. About a 7 fold increase in the duration of P-R segment of an ECG indicates an increase in conduction time. On the other hand, a gradual decline in heart beats, appearance of right bundle branch block, and a notched QRS complex suggests a possibility of aberration in myocardial conduction. A reduced time span of QRS complex and a faster appearance of T wave soon after QRS complex were also noticed in hypothermia. Forced induction of hypothermia in Syrian hamsters induced J-waves and atrioventricular block while spontaneous hibernation had no adverse effect (Miyazawa et al., 2008). A study in ground squirrel has shown that decreased body temperature during spontaneous hibernation slows ventricular conduction velocity and increases excitation threshold thus avoiding arrhythmias at extreme low body temperatures (Fedorov et al., 2005).

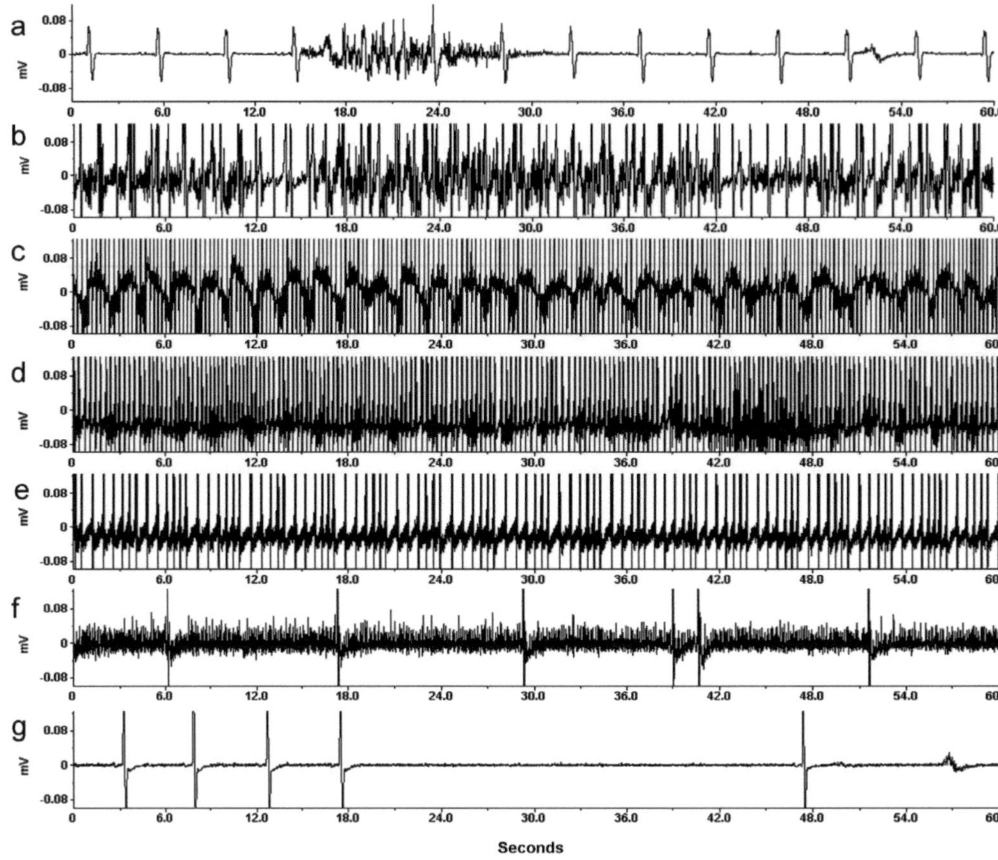

Fig. 3. Electrocardiogram of an arctic ground squirrel at different core body temperatures during different phases of hibernation.
Steady-state phase of hibernation is characterized by bradycardia with even beats as shown here at a body temperature of 4°C (a). An increase in heart rate occurs as soon as arousal is initiated as indicated in ECG at a body temperature of 5°C (b). A gradual progressive increase in heart rate is noticed through arousal phase at a body temperature of 20°C (c) until the animal reaches a euthermic body temperature of 37°C (d). Skipped beats and bradycardia follows as the animal prepares to enter into another torpor bout as represented by ECG at a body temperature of 36°C (e) and mid-entrance phase at 15°C (f). A brief pause in heart beats is a characteristic finding during the last stage of entrance phase (g) at a body temperature of 8°C.

4. Anatomical peculiarity of hibernator's heart

An insight into the anatomy of a hibernator's heart may provide clues as to how a hibernator can overcome heart failure under extreme hypothermia. The peculiar anatomy of the heart of a hibernator has been described by Walls in a hamster (Walls, 1942). Several interesting features of the conducting tissue have been identified in this study. Purkinje fibers are identified in the sino-atrial node, the pacemaker of the heart, and not in the atria suggesting that Purkinje fibers may have a function other than a simple conduction of the cardiac contraction impulse. The atrio-ventricular node has a compound nature of fibers which are similar to Purkinje type. Purkinje tissue is absent in the right ventricle and a limited amount of Purkinje tissue is present in the left ventricle whose wall is six times thicker than the right ventricle. In spite of limited Purkinje tissue distribution to the ventricles it is interesting to note that the heart is capable of about 450 beats per minute.

Gap junctions are specialized intercellular connections in the heart and are needed for conduction in the heart. Gap junctions ensure the propagation of action potentials between the myocytes and provide low resistance intercellular channels facilitating coordinated contraction of myocardium (Saitongdee et al., 2000). Connexins are gap junction proteins with four-membrane spanning domains. Among several types of connexins, connexin43 (Cx43) is the major connexin found in the mammalian heart (Beyer et al., 1987). Cx43 and Cx45 are upregulated in the hearts of hibernators (Gros and Jongsma, 1996; Fedorov et al., 2005; Van Der Heyden et al., 2007). Increased density of Cx43 has been identified in ventricular cardiomyocytes of hibernators during hibernation (Saitongdee et al., 2000). Cx43 density returned to normal control levels within 2 hours of arousal from torpor suggesting the importance of Cx43 and Cx45 in overcoming ventricular fibrillation during hibernation. (Saitongdee et al., 2000; Fedorov et al., 2005).

5. Adenosine in hibernation

A growing body of evidence supports the significance of adenosine in hibernation (Drew et al., 2007). Adenosine is a widely distributed inhibitory neuromodulator throughout the central nervous system including the brainstem, the principle cardiovascular control center (Mosqueda-Garcia et al., 1989; Barraco and Phillis, 1991). Adenosine decreases neuronal excitability and modulates the actions of other neurotransmitters (Dunwiddie and Masino, 2001). Adenosine acts through A1, A2a, A2b, and A3 receptors (Fredholm et al., 1994; Olah and Stiles, 1995; Dunwiddie and Masino, 2001). Endogenous adenosine is produced from multiple sources in the central nervous system, some sources associated to energy levels and functions as a homeostatic regulator in the CNS (White, 1977; Fredholm et al., 1994; Dunwiddie and Masino, 2001). Dephosphorylation of adenosine triphosphate (ATP) is one of the major sources of endogenous adenosine production where ATP released into synapse is metabolized to adenosine and mediates its effect through adenosine receptors (Fredholm et al., 1994; Dunwiddie and Masino, 2001).

5.1 Adenosine in induction of torpor during hibernation

Central nervous system regulation of hibernation is implicated by several studies (Drew et al., 2007; Jinka et al., 2011). Recent study has shown that administration of the adenosine A1 receptor agonist N^6-cyclohexyladenosine (CHA) into the lateral ventricle of arctic ground squirrel induces hibernation. CHA-induced hibernation is similar to natural spontaneous entrance into hibernation. Results indicate that onset of hibernation is regulated within the central nervous system through activation of A_1AR (Jinka et al., 2011). Studies focusing on specific sites in the brain including the hypothalamus and hippocampus indicate a prominent influence of CNS on hibernation (Heller and Colliver, 1974; Popov et al., 1992). Studies on central nervous system also direct towards involvement of adenosine, a neuromodulator in hibernation regulation (Shintani et al., 2005; Tamura et al., 2005; Jinka et al., 2011).

Successful translation of hibernation to non-hibernating species will open possibilities of applying the concept of metabolic suppression and low body temperature to humans in treating conditions such as stroke, hemorrhagic shock, cardiac arrest, cerebral ischemia, and multiorgan failure (Drew et al., 2007).

5.2 Significance of adenosine on dietary restriction induced hypothermia and cardiovascular regulation

Adenosine-induced hypothermia is mediated through A_1AR (Dunwiddie and Masino, 2001; Shintani et al., 2005). Adenosine modulates the cardiovascular system through numerous A_1AR in nucleus tractus solitarius (NTS) (Badman and Flier, 2005; Scislo et al., 2008) located in the brainstem which receives projections from hypothalamus, the thermoregulatory center in the brain (Scislo and O'Leary, 2006). Cardiovascular centers of the medulla are innervated by projections from the hypothalamus which alleviates cardiac arrhythmias by modulating the blood pressure (Willette et al., 1984; Lumb and Lovick, 1993; Kiely and Gordon, 1994; Hirasawa et al., 1996; Krukoff et al., 1997; Yang and Coote, 1998; Hardy, 2001). NTS influences cardiovascular system. Hypotensive responses in the cardiovascular system are mediated through A_1AR in NTS (White et al., 1996). Adenosine microinjections into the NTS result in a slow and regulated decrease in heart rate (Tseng et al., 1995; Phillis et al., 1997; Ho et al., 2008). Thus NTS and A_1AR contribute significantly towards induction of hypothermia and modulation of cardiovascular responses.

Dietary restriction is a dietary regimen defined by a decrease in food intake unassociated with malnutrition which lowers core body temperature, improves longevity, protects heart and attenuates progression of neurodegenerative diseases in animal models (Contestabile, 2009; Katare et al., 2009). These effects have been suggested to be through a reduction in metabolic demand (Ungvari et al., 2008) associated with a decrease in body temperature (Tb)(Conti et al., 2006). Mechanisms involved in induction of hypothermia are under investigation. Results from our studies have shown that DR-induced hypothermia is due to adenosine sensitization (Jinka et al., 2010). Our results have demonstrated that intraperitoneal administration of CHA (0.5mg/kg) in DR-sensitized rats induced a significant cooling undetected in ad libitum (AL) rats. However, it is not clear as to how the heart responds to this induced cooling in DR rats because hypothermia beyond a certain level is not without complications like cardiac arrhythmias (Polderman and Herold, 2009). It was shown that DR has certain beneficial effects on heart (Lee et al., 1999) including protection from arrhythmias (Johnson et al., 2006) although it is yet to be investigated whether these beneficial effects on heart are applicable under hypothermic conditions induced by the A_1AR agonists.

Central administration of A_1AR agonist-induced hypothermia in Syrian hamsters is free of cardiac arrhythmias while forced induction of hypothermia through intraperitoneal pentobarbital sodium causes J-waves and atrioventricular block (Miyazawa et al., 2008). Syrian hamsters undergo periods of food restriction, a process comparatively similar to dietary restriction, which prepares them to hibernate (Stamper et al., 1999). Dietary restriction influences NTS (Badman and Flier, 2005). Thus it can be hypothesized that centrally administered A_1AR agonist-induced hypothermia in dietary restricted rats may avoid cardiac arrhythmias.

5.3 Previous studies and results

In our previous studies we have shown that prolonged DR sensitizes A_1AR agonist-induced cooling. Sprague-Dawley rats were implanted with subcutaneous IPTT-300 transponders for monitoring body temperature. Rats were fed every other day for 27 days and then administered the A_1AR agonist, N^6-cyclohexyladenosine (CHA; 0.5mg/kg, ip). Respiratory rate (RR) and subcutaneous body temperature were monitored every day and after drug administration. A lower RR on day 20 and lower body temperature on day 22 were displayed by DR rats when compared to rats fed ad libitum and displayed a larger response to CHA. RR, a metabolic indicator, declined before body temperature in all cases suggesting that a decrease in oxidative metabolism associated with thermogenesis caused animals to cool. This is comparable to torpor because of prior changes in metabolism than body temperature as observed during hibernation (Lyman, 1958). An increased surface expression of A_1AR is demonstrated within the hypothalamus in DR rats. These results suggest that sensitization of thermoregulatory effects of endogenous adenosine through increased surface expression of A_1AR may play a role in enhanced hypothermia associated with DR. These results also suggest that a torpid like effect is seen with CHA-induced hypothermia in DR rats. However, it is not known from these studies as to how the heart responds to this CHA- induced hypothermia in DR rats (Jinka et al., 2010).

5.4 Hypothermia in hibernation vs hypothermia in A1AR stimulated DR rats

Hypothermia is seen in hibernators during torpor where their core body temperature (Tb) can reach to as low as -2.9°C (Barnes, 1989) without any complications. A sudden drop in metabolism followed by a decrease in core body temperature is the hallmark of hibernation (Lyman, 1958). CHA-induced hypothermia in DR rats resembled torpor in hibernators as there is a sudden decrease in respiration, an indicator of metabolism, followed by a slow decrease in body temperature (Jinka et al., 2010). Central administration of CHA in hibernators results in hypothermia without any untoward effects on heart while cardiac arrhythmias were seen with anesthetic-induced hypothermia (Miyazawa et al., 2008). Atrioventricular blocks and J-waves are observed in nonhibernators during induced hypothermia (Osborn, 1953; Brunson et al., 2005). Appearance of J-waves, also known as Osborne waves, indicates injury, delayed ventricular conduction, tissue anoxia or acidosis (Miyazawa et al., 2008). These studies suggest that an unidentified intrinsic mechanism in the heart of hibernators may be responsible for circumventing heart failure under extreme hypothermia.

5.5 Neuroprotection by induction of hypothermia and circumventing cardiac arrhythmias

Neuronal cell death is one of the major aftermaths of cardiopulmonary arrest and stroke. Under clinical setting, regulated hypothermia induced in the stroke patient in order to mitigate neuronal injury has proven to be helpful. Neuroprotection is evident in hibernators which experience extreme hypothermia. Thus inducing a hibernation-like state would be more beneficial in cardiac arrest patients. DR-induced cooling is well established in various rodents (Conti et al., 2006; Ungvari et al., 2008; Contestabile, 2009). What is novel in the recent research is that adenosine A1 receptor (A_1AR) agonist; CHA administration induces increased hypothermic response in DR rats (Jinka et al., 2010), although the response of the cardiovascular system is not measured. This CHA-induced hypothermia in DR rats is similar to the torpor seen in hibernation and this is achieved through sensitization of A_1AR in the brain's hypothalamus, the principle thermoregulatory center in the CNS. Recent study in hibernators also has shown that central administration of CHA induces cooling without cardiac arrhythmias (Miyazawa et al., 2008). Hence there is a possibility of circumventing cardiac arrhythmias in DR rats when hypothermia is achieved through central administration of CHA. Thus it can be hypothesized that A_1AR agonist-induced hypothermia in dietary restricted rats may avoid cardiac arrhythmias.

5.6 Hypothesized model

Sensitized adenosinergic system in DR rats acts through nucleus of the solitary tract (NTS), a primary integrative center for cardiovascular reflex. Adenosine in NTS modulates sympathetic, parasympathetic, and cardiovascular systems which in turn modulate arterial pressure, heart rate and vascular conductance by acting on and tuning the activity of the sympathetic and parasympathetic systems. The effect of adenosine may be one of the mechanisms behind cardioprotective effect (Fig.4) leading to generation of normal cardiac rhythms circumventing cardiac arrhythmias.

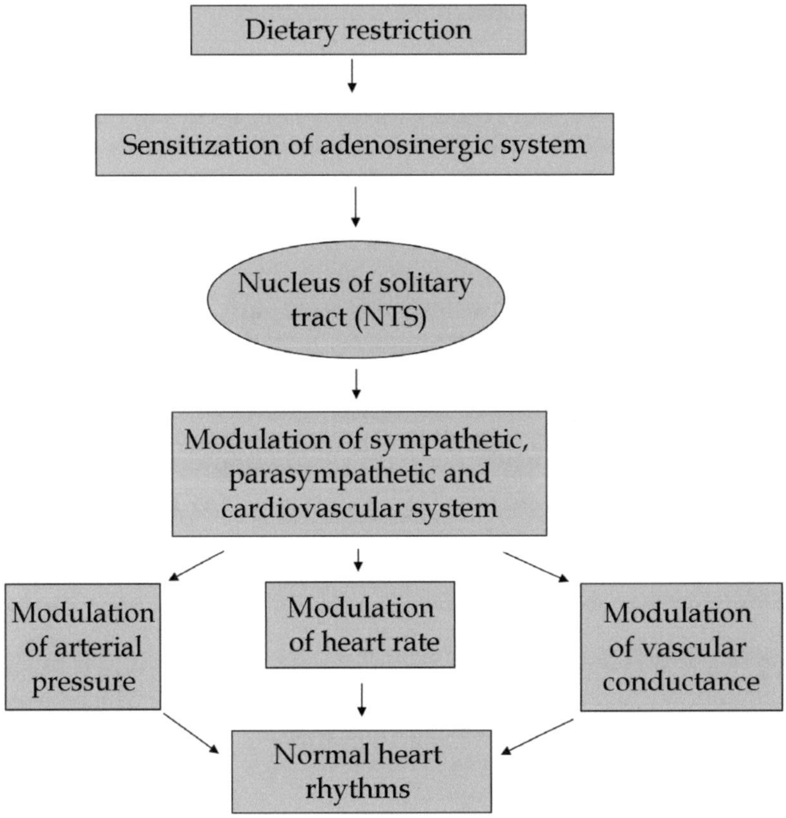

Fig. 4. Hypothesized model of dietary restriction induced cardioprotection.

6. Conclusion

Hibernators undergo a variety of complex morphological, behavioral, and physiological adaptive changes during hibernation period. Profound metabolic suppression, hypothermia, and bradycardia observed at the organismal level during the hibernation period have no harmful effects (Geiser, 1988; Barnes, 1989; Buck and Barnes, 2000; Drew et al., 2001; Zhou et al., 2001; Carey et al., 2003a; Heldmaier et al., 2004; Tamura et al., 2005; Ross et al., 2006; Drew et al., 2007). The hearts of hibernating mammals remain functional even at 0°C while the hearts of non-hibernating mammals becomes arrhythmic and stop functioning between 10°C and 15°C (Lyman, 1982; Caprette and Senturia, 1984; Burlington and Darvish, 1988). This implies that an intrinsic difference in functional mechanism may exist between the hearts of a hibernator and a non-hibernator enabling the hibernator to survive despite low body temperatures. Understanding the mechanisms regulating hibernation has the potential to develop therapies for conditions such as cardiac arrhythmias, hemorrhagic shock, stroke, cardiac arrest and cerebral ischemia (Drew et al., 2007).

7. Acknowledgements

Thanks to Kelly L. Drew, PhD; Barnes BM, PhD; Jeanette Moore, MS; Nichenametla SN,PhD; Dasari TR,DVM; Eega KR,DVM and Kampalli SB, DVM for their reviews. The author also thanks US Army Research Office W911NF-05-1-0280, Alaska Experimental Program to Stimulate Competitive Research (EPSCoR), and Institute of Arctic Biology at University of Alaska Fairbanks for research support.

8. References

Badman MK, Flier JS (2005) The gut and energy balance: visceral allies in the obesity wars. Science 307:1909-1914.

Barnes BM (1989) Freeze avoidance in a mammal: body temperatures below 0 degree C in an Arctic hibernator. Science 244:1593-1595.

Barraco RA, Phillis JW (1991) Subtypes of adenosine receptors in the brainstem mediate opposite blood pressure responses. Neuropharmacology 30:403-407.

Beyer EC, Paul DL, Goodenough DA (1987) Connexin43: a protein from rat heart homologous to a gap junction protein from liver. J Cell Biol 105:2621-2629.

Boyer BB, Barnes BM (1999) Molecular and metabolic aspects of hibernation. Bioscience 49:713-724.

Brunson CE, Abbud E, Osman K, Skelton TN, Markov AK (2005) Osborn (J) wave appearance on the electrocardiogram in relation to potassium transfer and myocardial metabolism during hypothermia. J Investig Med 53:434-437.

Buck CL, Barnes BM (2000) Effects of ambient temperature on metabolic rate, respiratory quotient, and torpor in an arctic hibernator. Am J Physiol Regul Integr Comp Physiol 279:R255-262.

Burlington RF, Darvish A (1988) Low-temperature performance of isolated working hearts from a hibernator and a non-hibernator. Physiol Zool 1988:387–395.

Burn JH (1961) The cause of fibrillation. Can Med Assoc J 84:625-627.

Caprette DR, Senturia JB (1984) Isovolumetric performance of isolated ground squirrel and rat hearts at low temperature. Am J Physiol 247:722–727.

Carey HV, Andrews MT, Martin SL (2003a) Mammalian hibernation: cellular and molecular responses to depressed metabolism and low temperature. Physiol Rev 83:1153-1181.

Carey HV, Rhoads CA, Aw TY (2003b) Hibernation induces glutathione redox imbalance in ground squirrel intestine. J Comp Physiol [B] 173:269-276.

Chatfield PO, Lyman CP (1950) Circulatory changes during process of arousal in the hibernating hamster. Am J Physiol 163:566-574.

Contestabile A (2009) Benefits of caloric restriction on brain aging and related pathological States: understanding mechanisms to devise novel therapies. Curr Med Chem 16:350-361.

Conti B, Sanchez-Alavez M, Winsky-Sommerer R, Morale MC, Lucero J, Brownell S, Fabre V, Huitron-Resendiz S, Henriksen S, Zorrilla EP, de Lecea L, Bartfai T (2006) Transgenic mice with a reduced core body temperature have an increased life span. Science 314:825-828.

Dawe AR, Morrison PR (1955) Characteristics of the hibernating heart. Am Heart J 49:367-384.

Drew KL, Rice ME, Kuhn TB, Smith MA (2001) Neuroprotective adaptations in hibernation: therapeutic implications for ischemia-reperfusion, traumatic brain injury and neurodegenerative diseases. Free Radic Biol Med 31:563-573.

Drew KL, Christian LS, Jinka TR, Hollen L, Dehn J (2009) "Natural" tolerance in hibernators: Can we learn from physiological and preconditioning against ischemic or hypoxic brain injury? In: Ischemic Tolerance of the Brain (Schaller BJ, ed), pp 1-44. Trivandrum: Research Signpost.

Drew KL, Buck CL, Barnes BM, Christian SL, Rasley BT, Harris MB (2007) Central nervous system regulation of mammalian hibernation: implications for metabolic suppression and ischemia tolerance. J Neurochem 102:1713-1726.

Dunwiddie TV, Masino SA (2001) The role and regulation of adenosine in the central nervous system. Annu Rev Neurosci 24:31-55.

Eagles DA, Jacques LB, Taboada J, Wagner CW, Diakun TA (1988) Cardiac arrhythmias during arousal from hibernation in three species of rodents. Am J Physiol 254:R102-108.

Elvert R, Heldmaier G (2005) Cardiorespiratory and metabolic reactions during entrance into torpor in dormice, Glis glis. J Exp Biol 208:1373-1383.

Fedorov VV, Li L, Glukhov A, Shishkina I, Aliev RR, Mikheeva T, Nikolski VP, Rosenshtraukh LV, Efimov IR (2005) Hibernator Citellus undulatus maintains safe cardiac conduction and is protected against tachyarrhythmias during extreme hypothermia: possible role of Cx43 and Cx45 up-regulation. Heart Rhythm 2:966-975.

Fredholm BB, Abbracchio MP, Burnstock G, Daly JW, Harden TK, Jacobson KA, Leff P, Williams M (1994) Nomenclature and classification of purinoceptors. Pharmacol Rev 46:143-156.

Geiser F (1988) Reduction of metabolism during hibernation and daily torpor in mammals and birds: Temperature effect or physiological inhibition? J Comp Physiol B 158:25-37.

Geiser F (2004) Metabolic rate and body temperature reduction during hibernation and daily torpor. Annu Rev Physiol 66:239-274.

Geiser F, Ruf T (1995) Hibernation versus daily torpor in mammals and birds : physiological variables and classification of torpor patterns Physiol Zool 68:935-966.

Gros DB, Jongsma HJ (1996) Connexins in mammalian heart function. Bioessays 18:719-730.
Hardy SG (2001) Hypothalamic projections to cardiovascular centers of the medulla. Brain Res 894:233-240.
Heldmaier G, Ortmann S, Elvert R (2004) Natural hypometabolism during hibernation and daily torpor in mammals. Respir Physiol Neurobiol 141:317-329.
Heller HC, Colliver GW (1974) CNS regulation of body temperature during hibernation. Am J Physiol 227:583-589.
Heller HC, Colliver GW, Beard J (1977) Thermoregulation during entrance into hibernation. Pflügers Arch 369:55-59.
Hirasawa M, Nishihara M, Takahashi M (1996) The rostral ventrolateral medulla mediates suppression of the circulatory system by the ventromedial nucleus of the hypothalamus. Brain Res 724:186-190.
Ho WY, Lu PJ, Hsiao M, Hwang HR, Tseng YC, Yen MH, Tseng CJ (2008) Adenosine modulates cardiovascular functions through activation of extracellular signal-regulated kinases 1 and 2 and endothelial nitric oxide synthase in the nucleus tractus solitarii of rats. Circulation 117:773-780.
Jinka TR, Toien O, Drew KL (2011) Season primes the brain in an arctic hibernator to facilitate entrance into torpor mediated by adenosine A1 receptors. J Neurosci 31:10752-10758.
Jinka TR, Carlson ZA, Moore JT, Drew KL (2010) Altered thermoregulation via sensitization of A1 adenosine receptors in dietary-restricted rats. Psychopharmacology (Berl) 209:217-224.
Johansson BW (1984) Cardiac responses in relation to heart size. Cryobiology 21:627-636.
Johansson BW (1996) The hibernator heart--nature's model of resistance to ventricular fibrillation. Cardiovasc Res 31:826-832.
Johnson JB, Laub DR, John S (2006) The effect on health of alternate day calorie restriction: eating less and more than needed on alternate days prolongs life. Med Hypotheses 67:209-211.
Karpovich SA, Toien O, Buck CL, Barnes BM (2009) Energetics of arousal episodes in hibernating arctic ground squirrels. J Comp Physiol [B].
Katare RG, Kakinuma Y, Arikawa M, Yamasaki F, Sato T (2009) Chronic intermittent fasting improves the survival following large myocardial ischemia by activation of BDNF/VEGF/PI3K signaling pathway. J Mol Cell Cardiol 46:405-412.
Keating MT, Sanguinetti MC (2001) Molecular and cellular mechanisms of cardiac arrhythmias. Cell 104:569-580.
Kiely JM, Gordon FJ (1994) Role of rostral ventrolateral medulla in centrally mediated pressor responses. Am J Physiol 267:H1549-1556.
Krukoff TL, Mactavish D, Jhamandas JH (1997) Activation by hypotension of neurons in the hypothalamic paraventricular nucleus that project to the brainstem. J Comp Neurol 385:285-296.
Landau BR, Dawe AR (1958) Respiration in the hibernation of the 13-lined ground squirrel. Am J Physiol 194:75-82.
Lee J, Yu BP, Herlihy JT (1999) Modulation of cardiac mitochondrial membrane fluidity by age and calorie intake. Free Radic Biol Med 26:260-265.

Lumb BM, Lovick TA (1993) The rostral hypothalamus: an area for the integration of autonomic and sensory responsiveness. J Neurophysiol 70:1570-1577.

Lyman CP (1958) Oxygen consumption, body temperature and heart rate of woodchucks entering hibernation. Am J Physiol 194:83-91.

Lyman CP, ed (1982) The hibernating state, Recent theories of hibernation. . New York: Academic Press.

Lyman CP, O'Brien RC (1963) Autonomic Control of Circulation during the Hibernating Cycle in Ground Squirrels. J Physiol 168:477-499.

Lyman CP, O'Brien RC (1969) Hyperresponsiveness in hibernation. Symp Soc Exp Biol 23:489-509.

Milsom WK, Burlington RF, Burleson ML (1993) Vagal Influence On Heart-Rate In Hibernating Ground-Squirrels. Journal Of Experimental Biology 185:25-32.

Milsom WK, Zimmer MB, Harris MB (1999) Regulation of cardiac rhythm in hibernating mammals. Comp Biochem Physiol A Mol Integr Physiol 124:383-391.

Miyazawa S, Shimizu Y, Shiina T, Hirayama H, Morita H, Takewaki T (2008) Central A1-receptor activation associated with onset of torpor protects the heart against low temperature in the Syrian hamster. Am J Physiol Regul Integr Comp Physiol 295:R991-996.

Mosqueda-Garcia R, Tseng CJ, Appalsamy M, Robertson D (1989) Modulatory effects of adenosine on baroreflex activation in the brainstem of normotensive rats. Eur J Pharmacol 174:119-122.

Nardone RM (1955) Electrocardiogram of the arctic ground squirrel during hibernation and hypothermia. Am J Physiol 182:364-368.

Olah ME, Stiles GL (1995) Adenosine receptor subtypes: characterization and therapeutic regulation. Annu Rev Pharmacol Toxicol 35:581-606.

Osborn JJ (1953) Experimental hypothermia; respiratory and blood pH changes in relation to cardiac function. Am J Physiol 175:389-398.

Phillis JW, Scislo TJ, O'Leary DS (1997) Purines and the nucleus tractus solitarius: effects on cardiovascular and respiratory function. Clin Exp Pharmacol Physiol 24:738-742.

Polderman KH (2004) Application of therapeutic hypothermia in the intensive care unit. Opportunities and pitfalls of a promising treatment modality--Part 2: Practical aspects and side effects. Intensive Care Med 30:757-769.

Polderman KH, Herold I (2009) Therapeutic hypothermia and controlled normothermia in the intensive care unit: practical considerations, side effects, and cooling methods. Crit Care Med 37:1101-1120.

Popov VI, Bocharova LS, Bragin AG (1992) Repeated changes of dendritic morphology in the hippocampus of ground squirrels in the course of hibernation. Neuroscience 48:45-51.

Ross AP, Christian SL, Zhao HW, Drew KL (2006) Persistent tolerance to oxygen and nutrient deprivation and N-methyl-D-aspartate in cultured hippocampal slices from hibernating Arctic ground squirrel. J Cereb Blood Flow Metab 26:1148-1156.

Saitongdee P, Milner P, Becker DL, Knight GE, Burnstock G (2000) Increased connexin43 gap junction protein in hamster cardiomyocytes during cold acclimatization and hibernation. Cardiovasc Res 47:108-115.

Scislo TJ, O'Leary DS (2006) Adenosine receptors located in the NTS contribute to renal sympathoinhibition during hypotensive phase of severe hemorrhage in anesthetized rats. Am J Physiol Heart Circ Physiol 291:H2453-2461.

Scislo TJ, Ichinose TK, O'Leary DS (2008) Stimulation of NTS A1 adenosine receptors differentially resets baroreflex control of regional sympathetic outputs. Am J Physiol Heart Circ Physiol 294:H172-182.

Shintani M, Tamura Y, Monden M, Shiomi H (2005) Characterization of N(6)-cyclohexyladenosine-induced hypothermia in Syrian hamsters. J Pharmacol Sci 97:451-454.

Stamper JL, Dark J, Zucker I (1999) Photoperiod modulates torpor and food intake in Siberian hamsters challenged with metabolic inhibitors. Physiol Behav 66:113-118.

Strumwasser F (1959) Thermoregulatory, brain and behavioral mechanisms during entrance into hibernation in the squirrel, Citellus beecheyi. Am J Physiol 196:15-22.

Surawicz B (1971) Ventricular fibrillation. Am J Cardiol 28:268-287.

Tamura Y, Shintani M, Nakamura A, Monden M, Shiomi H (2005) Phase-specific central regulatory systems of hibernation in Syrian hamsters. Brain Res 1045:88-96.

Toien O, Blake J, Edgar DM, Grahn DA, Heller HC, Barnes BM (2011) Hibernation in black bears: independence of metabolic suppression from body temperature. Science 331:906-909.

Trautwein W (1963) Generation and conduction of impulses in the heart as affected by drugs. Pharmacol Rev 15:277-332.

Tseng CJ, Ger LP, Lin HC, Tung CS (1995) Attenuated cardiovascular response to adenosine in the brain stem nuclei of spontaneously hypertensive rats. Hypertension 25:278-282.

Twente JW, Twente JA (1965) Effects of core temperature upon duration of hibernation Citellus lateralis. J Appl Physiol 20:411-416.

Twente JW, Twente J, eds (1978) Autonomic regulation of hibernation by Citellus and Eptesicus. New York: Academic Press.

Ungvari Z, Parrado-Fernandez C, Csiszar A, de Cabo R (2008) Mechanisms underlying caloric restriction and lifespan regulation: implications for vascular aging. Circ Res 102:519-528.

Van Der Heyden MA, Kok B, Kouwenhoven EN, Toien O, Barnes BM, Fedorov VG, Efimov IR, Opthof T (2007) Cloning, sequence analysis and phylogeny of connexin43 isolated from American black bear heart. DNA Seq 18:380-384.

Walls EW (1942) Specialized conducting tissue in the heart of the golden hamster (Cricetus auratus). J Anat 76:359-368 352.

White PJ, Rose'Meyer RB, Hope W (1996) Functional characterization of adenosine receptors in the nucleus tractus solitarius mediating hypotensive responses in the rat. Br J Pharmacol 117:305-308.

White TD (1977) Direct detection of depolarisation-induced release of ATP from a synaptosomal preparation. Nature 267:67-68.

Willette RN, Gatti PA, Sapru HN (1984) GABAergic mechanisms in the ventrolateral medulla alter vasopressor responses from the anterior hypothalamus. J Cardiovasc Pharmacol 6:476-482.

Yang Z, Coote JH (1998) Influence of the hypothalamic paraventricular nucleus on cardiovascular neurones in the rostral ventrolateral medulla of the rat. J Physiol 513 (Pt 2):521-530.

Zhou F, Zhu X, Castellani RJ, Stimmelmayr R, Perry G, Smith MA, Drew KL (2001) Hibernation, a model of neuroprotection. Am J Pathol 158:2145-2151.

Zimmer MB, Harris MB, Milsom WK (2000) Control of cardiac and ventilation frequencies during hibernation in ground squirrels. In: In Life in the Cold: Proceedings of the 11th International Hibernation Symposium (Klingenspor GHaM, ed), pp 159-167. Berlin, Heidelberg, New York: Springer-Verlag.

8

Neurohumoral Control of Heart Rate

Jones Bernardes Graceli, Diego França Pedrosa and Ágata Lages Gava
Federal University of Espirito Santo/UFES, Brazil

1. Introduction

It is well known that the heart generates and conducts electrical impulses, leading to a rhythmical contraction of the cardiac muscle. In normal situations, the atria contract about one sixth of a second ahead of ventricular contraction, allowing the filling of the ventricles before they pump the blood through the lungs and peripheral circulation. Additionally, all portions of the ventricles contract almost simultaneously, which is essential for a most effective pressure generation in the ventricular chambers. This rhythmical and conductive system is susceptible to damage by heart disease, especially by ischemia of the cardiac tissues. The result is often an abnormal heart rhythm and sequence of contraction of the heart chambers, leading to a reduction in pumping effectiveness, even to the extent of causing death (Hall, 2011).

Heart rate (HR) is not a static hemodynamic parameter but instead changes over time in response to physical and mental demands. HR is normally determined by spontaneous and periodic depolarizations of the sinoatrial node, the frequency of which is modulated by the sympathetic and parasympathetic divisions of the autonomic nervous system, the intrinsic cardiac nervous system, reflexes, and respiration. These neural systems also partially control cardiac contractility and conduction of electrical activity through the heart. As a result, HR (chronotropism), contractility (inotropism), and conduction (dromotropism) are adjusted to meet the changing needs of the body (Feldman et al, 2010).

2. Electrical activity of the heart

The properties of automaticity and rhythmicity are intrinsic to the cardiac tissue and considered a very complex phenomenon and, besides cellular mechanisms, integrative different factors are involved in cardiac pacemaking. The cardiac electrical events are initiated with changes in the permeability of the cell membrane, mainly to Na^+, K^+ and Ca^{2+} ions. Changes in cell membrane permeability alter the rate of ion passage across the membrane with the opening and closing of ion channels. Two main types of action potentials are observed in the heart: (A) fast action potentials, that occur in the normal myocardial fibers in the atria and ventricles and in the specialized conducting fibers (Purkinje´s fibers) and (B) slow action potentials, which are found in the sinoatrial (SA) node, the natural pacemaker of the heart, and in the atrioventricular (AV) node, the specialized tissue involved in conducting the cardiac impulse from atria to ventricles (Bouman and Jongsma, 1986).

In mammalian, the region of the heart that ordinarily generates impulses at the greatest frequency is the SA node. In humans, it lies in the groove where the superior vena cava joins the right atrium. It is a small, roughly rectangular region at the edge of the right atrium, bounded on two sides by the superior and inferior vena cava and on the other two by the interatrial septum and the crista terminalis, a part of the right atrial muscle over whose endocardial surface the pacemaking tissue of the SA node extends (Brown, 1982). The intact sinoatrial node is a heterogeneous structure and contains 2 principal types of cells: 1) small, round cells, which have few organelles and myofibrils; and 2) slender, elongated cells, which are intermediate in appearance between the round and the ordinary atrial myocardial cells. The round cells are probably the pacemaker cells, whereas the transitional cells probably conduct the impulses within the node and to the nodal margins (Verheijck et al., 2011; Verheijck et al., 2004; Tellez et al, 2006).

In the SA node cells, the upstroke of action potential is less steep, the plateau is not sustained and the depolarization is more gradual. However, the principal distinguish feature of a pacemaker resides in resting phase. In nonautonomic cells, the resting potential is constant, whereas in a pacemaker fiber there is as low depolarization that proceeds at steady rate until a threshold is attained, and then an action potential is triggered (Brown, 1982; Berne and Levy, 2009). In the pacemaker cells of the SA node the diastolic depolarization is attributed to at least 3 ionic currents: (1) an inward current (I_f), induced by hyperpolarization; (2) an inward Ca^{+2} current, (I_{Ca}); and (3) an outward K^+ current, I_K . The inward current (I_f) is carried mainly by Na^+ and the current is conducted through specific channels that differ from the fast Na^+ channels. This current becomes activated during the repolarization phase of the action potential, as the membrane potential becomes more negative than about -50mV. The more negative the membrane potential becomes at the end of repolarization, the greater is the activation of the I_f current. The second current responsible for diastolic depolarization is the slow inward current. This current is composed mainly of Ca^{+2} and therefore it is referred to as the Ca^{+2} current, (I_{Ca}). This Ca^{+2} current is carried mainly by T-type Ca^{+2} channels. Once the Ca^{+2} channels become activated, the influx of Ca^{+2} into the cell increases and accelerates the rate of diastolic depolarization, which then leads to upstroke of the action potential. The progressive diastolic depolarization mediated by the 2 inward currents, I_f and I_{Ca}, is opposed by a third current, an outward K^+ current, I_K . This efflux of K^+ tends to repolarize the cell after upstroke of the action potential. The outward K^+ current continues well beyond the time of maximum repolarization, but it diminishes throughout the end repolarization. Hence the opposition of I_K to the depolarizing effects of the 2 inward currents (I_{Ca} and I_f) gradually decreases (Brown, 1982; Berne and Levy, 2009).

From the SA node the cardiac impulse spreads radially throughout the right atrium along ordinary atrial myocardial fibers, at a conduction velocity of approximately 1m/sec. A special pathway, the anterior interatrial myocardial band, conducts the impulse from the SA node directly to the left atrium. Tree tracts, the anterior, middle, and posterior internodal pathways, constitute the principal routes to the conduction of the cardiac impulse from the SA to AV node. The AV node contains the same two cell types as the SA node, however the round cells are sparser and elongated cells preponderate. The AV node has been divided into three functional regions: 1) the AN region, the transitional zone between the atrium and the remnant node; 2) the N region, the midportion of the AV node; and 3) the NH region, the upper portion of the specialized conducting system for the ventricles. Usually, the AV node and the bundle of His constitute the only pathways to action potential conduction from atria to ventricles. The

conductive system passes subendocardially down the right side of the interventricular septum for about 1cm and divides into the right and left bundle branches. The right bundle branch is a direct continuation of the bundle of His and it proceeds down the right side of the interventricular septum. The left bundle branch, which is considerably thicker than the right, arises almost perpendicularly from the bundle of His and cross the interventricular septum. The right bundle branch and the two divisions of the left bundle branch ultimately subdivide into a complex network of conducting fibers called Purkinje´s fibers, which ramify over the subendocardial surfaces of both ventricles (Brown, 1982).
In the myocardium, the action potential generation includes 5 distinct phases: 1) Phase 0: the chemical and electrostatic forces both favor the entry of Na^+ into the cell through fast Na^+ voltage-gated channels to generate the upstroke; 2) Phase 1: the chemical and electrostatic forces both favor the efflux of K^+ through transient outward current (I_{to}) channels to generate early, partial repolarization; 3) Phase 2: during the plateau, the net influx de Ca^{2+} through L-type Ca^{2+} voltage-gated channels is balanced by the efflux of K^+ through rectifier (I_k), inwardly rectifying (I_{k1}) and I_{to} channels; 4) Phase 3: the chemical forces that favor the efflux of K^+ through I_k, I_{k1},I_{to} channels predominate over the electrostatic forces that favor the efflux of K^+ through these same channels; 5) Phase 4: the chemical forces that favor the efflux of K^+ through I_k and I_{k1} channels exceed very slightly the electrostatic forces that favor the influx of K^+ through these same channels (Berne and Levy, 2009).

3. Neural control of HR

The peripheral circulation distributes the cardiac output to the various organs and tissues according to their individual metabolic or functional needs while maintaining arterial blood pressure within a relatively narrow range. Regional blood flows can be efficiently regulated at the local level by the intrinsic ability of vessels to respond to various mechanical forces (e.g., wall tension and shear stress) as well as chemical stimuli (e.g., tissue metabolites and O_2). However, a perfect regulation of the peripheral circulation cannot be achieved only by the local vascular control mechanisms, but require the coordinating activity of central neural outflow to the heart and blood vessels (Thomas, 2011). In this field, the autonomic nervous system plays an important role to normal cardiovascular control and changes in autonomic balance has been related to several cardiovascular disorders, such as cardiac arrhythmias and hypertension (Workman, 2010; Pagani and Lucini, 2001).

3.1 The autonomic nervous system and cardiovascular control

The autonomic nervous system is responsible for the involuntary control of most visceral organs, including the heart and the interactions between the sympathetic and parasympathetic limbs play a critical role in cardiac electrical stability and arrhythmias generation. In general, sympathetic activation has a profound arrythmogenic potential (Schwartz et al., 1978, Schwartz 1984). Experimental stimulation of sympathetic nerves or stellate ganglia induces ECG repolarization changes and reduces the fibrillation threshold, facilitating ventricular fibrillation (Yanowitz et al, 1966; Podrid et al, 1990), while the use of β-adrenergic blocking agents can improve survival in patients following myocardial infarction (Gottlieb et al, 1998). On the other hand, vagal activation has a powerful antifibrillatory effect (Vanoli et al., 1991; De Ferrari et al., 1994). Therefore, autonomic imbalance could become either proarrythmic or anti-arrythmic based on which of the two components is going to prevail (Schwartz and De Ferrari, 2011).

Preganglionic fibers of autonomic nervous system are originated from central nervous system (CNS) at the level of the brainstem or sacral spinal cord (parasympathetic fibers) and the thoracic or lumbar spinal cord (sympathetic fibers). Both parasympathetic and sympathetic preganglionic fibers release acetylcholine which binds to nicotinic receptors located in the cell bodies of postganglionic neurons, leading to action potential generation. This synapse occurs in autonomic ganglia located outside of the CNS (Thomas, 2011).

The axons of postganglionic neurons innervate the effector tissues, including cardiovascular tissues. Parasympathetic neurons are distributed much more heterogeneously throughout the heart than sympathetic neurons. The density of parasympathetic innervation in the sinoatrial (SA) and AV nodes is considerably higher than in the surrounding atrial or ventricular tissue (Vaseghi and Shivkumar, 2008). Cardiac sympathetic innervation of the heart includes innervation of the SA node and myocardial cells. Based on norepinephrine content studies, a gradient exists in sympathetic innervation from atria to ventricles and from base to apex of the heart, indicating that the atria are most densely innervated, but the ventricles are also supplied with a sympathetic network, most densely at the base (Vaseghi and Shivkumar, 2008). Regarding the neurotransmitters, postganglionic parasympathetic fibers release acetylcholine, which binds to muscarinic receptors on the target tissue, while postganglionic sympathetic fibers release norepinephrine, which binds to either α or β adrenergic receptors (Thomas, 2011).

The effects of sympathetic and parasympathetic neurons on HR will be based on changes in the ion currents of SA node action potential generation. Norepinephrine release from post ganglionic sympathetic neurons will increase the slope of diastolic depolarization in SA node by the enhancement of the resting potential, while acetylcholine release from parasympathetic postganglionic neurons will decrease the slope of diastolic depolarization by hyperpolarization of the resting potential (Verrier and Tan, 2009). Additionally, sympathetic stimulation increases the rate of conduction as well as the level of excitability in all portions of the heart and augments greatly the force of contraction of all the cardiac musculature. Maximal stimulation can almost triple the frequency of heartbeat and can increase the strength of heart contraction as much as twofold. On the other hand, parasympathetic stimulation to the heart decreases the excitability of the A-V junctional fibers between the atrial musculature and the A-V node, thereby slowing the transmission of the cardiac impulse into the ventricles (Guyton and Hall, 2006).

Given the ability to modulate both HR and stroke volume, the autonomic nerves provide an important mechanism to rapidly adjust cardiac output to meet short-term changes in the body's needs (cardiovascular reflexes). In humans, there is a good deal of tonic vagal discharge and a moderate amount of tonic sympathetic discharge, showing a parasympathetic prevalence on the heart. Additional vagal discharge can further reduce HR, consequently cardiac output, whereas additional sympathetic discharge can increase HR and stroke volume and augment cardiac output. Conversely, withdrawal of tonic vagal or sympathetic discharge has opposing effects to increase or decrease cardiac output, respectively (Thomas, 2011).

4. Cardiovascular reflexes

It is well known that the maintenance of arterial pressure at adequate levels to perfuse the tissues is a basic requirement for survival. In cardiovascular system, among the mechanisms that act buffering arterial pressure fluctuations we can highlight the role of the neural reflexes. Such control is an important pathway to effect rapid changes in blood pressure and in the distribution of cardiac output that are essential to maintain a sufficient perfusion to vital organs, such as heart, brain and the kidney in face of physiological and environmental challenges. This rapid control of cardiovascular function is achieved through arterial and non-arterial reflexes that detect and correct changes in arterial blood pressure (baroreflex), blood volume (cardiopulmonary reflex) or chemical composition (chemoreflex) of the blood (Vasquez et al., 1997). It is important to notice that the effectiveness of these systems may be modulated by hormonal systems, such as angiotensin II and nitric oxide. The understanding of the key concepts about these reflexes under physiological conditions and the effects of hormonal substances on its functioning is an important step to clarify the development of arrhythmias.

4.1 Baroreflex

The baroreflex feedback loop is one of the most important mechanisms controlling arterial pressure. The main purpose of the baroreflex function is to provide a rapid and efficient stabilization of arterial blood pressure on a beat-to-beat basis by means of strategically located arterial sensors which are sensitive to high blood pressure and known as arterial baroreceptors. The baroreceptors endings are located in adventitia layer of carotid sinus and aortic arch with their soma located in the petrosal and nodose ganglia respectively. These receptors are mechano-sensitive and the distension of the vessels that occurs at each heart beat leads to action potential generation on these terminals which are transmitted to CNS, buffering arterial pressure fluctuations through changes in sympathetic and parasympathetic activity (Vasquez et al., 1997).

To achieve this precise control, the generated action potentials in each systole travel centrally to synapse onto neurons in the nucleus tractus solitarii (NTS) in the dorsal medulla. NTS neurons project to "higher" brain nuclei, as well as other nuclei in the brainstem that are critical for efferent sympathetic and parasympathetic activity (Loewy and Spyer, 1990). Projections from NTS are connected to the inhibitory neurons of caudal ventrolateral medulla (CVLM) that subsequently synapse to excitatory neurons in the rostral ventrolateral medulla (RVLM). RVLM exerts a tonic discharge upon the preganglionic sympathetic neurons, located in the intermediolateral column (IML) of the spinal cord (Kirkman and Sawdon, 2004). Therefore, activation of the baroreceptor afferents innervating the NTS causes excitation of neurons projecting to the CVLM, which in turn inhibits RVLM. These events lead to less activity from the RVLM to IML, reducing sympathetic efferent activity (Figure 1A). Several studies have demonstrated that disturbances in the normal functioning of these nuclei can be related to the development of arrhythmias. In example, Issa et al. (2005) showed that the central inhibition of the sympathetic drive using clonidine reduces the occurrence of ventricular tachycardia/ventricular fibrilation in a canine heart failure model.

In parallel, NTS neurons also synapse onto preganglionic vagal neurons localized within nucleus ambiguus (NA) and in the dorsal motor nucleus of the vagus (DMNX, Figure 1A). These neurons dominate the neural control of HR under normal conditions and also influence the prognosis of many cardiovascular disorders, such as sudden cardiac death, ventricular fibrillation, and myocardial ischemia (Wand et al, 2001). The axons from preganglionic cardiac vagal neurons travel down the vagus nerve and synapse onto postganglionic cardiac vagal neurons in cardiac ganglia. The synaptic innervation of cardiac vagal neurons is therefore critical for the tonic and reflex evoked changes in cardiac vagal activity that control HR.

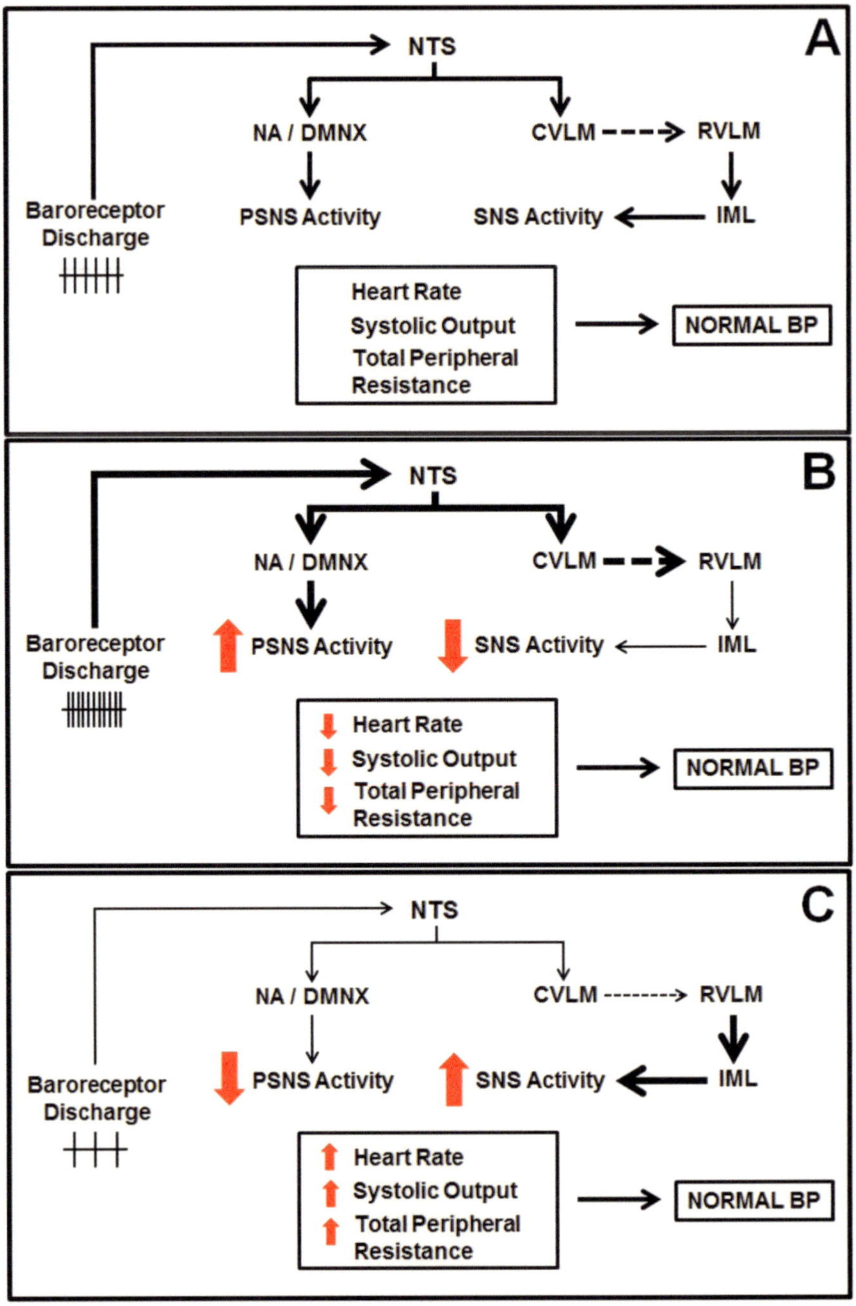

Fig. 1. Schematic diagram showing the baroreflex functioning during normal (A), increased (B) and decreased blood pressure (C). NTS: nucleus tractus solitarii, NA: nucleus ambiguus, DMNX: dorsal motor nucleus of the vagus, CVLM: caudal ventrolateral medulla, RVLM: rostral ventrolateral medulla, IML: intermediolateral column, PSNS: parasympathetic nervous system, SNS: sympathetic nervous system, BP: blood pressure. The continuous arrow and the dashed arrows indicate a stimulatory and an inhibitory synapse, respectively.

Therefore, when blood pressure rises, the baroreceptor afferent activity augments, leading to increased vagal activity and diminished sympathetic outflow. These effects will reduce HR and cardiac contractility, causing a decrease in cardiac output. Additionally, the fall the sympathetic activity to blood vessels also leads to vasodilation, diminishing the vascular resistance (Figure 1B). The reduced cardiac output and vascular resistance return blood pressure to its original level. On the other hand, a fall in blood pressure results in reduced baroreceptor afferent activity, causing a decrease in vagal activity and augmented sympathetic outflow (Figure 1C). These events increase cardiac output and vascular resistance, normalizing arterial blood pressure.

Experimentally, the baroreflex function can be evaluated through changes in arterial pressure. In bolus phenylephrine injections elicits increases in arterial pressure leading to reflex bradycardia and sodium nitroprusside injections reduces arterial pressure causing reflex tachycardia. Typical recordings of baroreflex evaluation are displayed in Figure 2.

4.2 Cardiopulmonary reflex

Despite the great importance of baroreflex in controlling arterial pressure, several investigations have demonstrated that the neural reflex of circulation also depends on cardiopulmonary reflex.

Cardiopulmonary receptors are found in low pressure portions of the circulation, such as walls of the atria and pulmonary arteries. These mechano-sensitive receptors are activated by the distension of the vessels walls, responding to changes in central blood volume (Thomas, 2011). The impulses arising from these receptors exert a tonic restraint on cardiac function and contribute to the physiological control of circulation. Cardiopulmonary reflexes are stimulated not only by changes in cardiac filling pressure but also by chemical agents, such as prostaglandins and serotonin (Vasquez et al., 1997). The cardiopulmonary fibers converge to the same pool of central neurons as the baroreceptors and act in a similar way (Spyer, 1990). Therefore, increased discharge of cardiopulmonary vagal afferent C fibers results in reflex enhancement of parasympathetic activity and decreased sympathetic outflow, leading to bradycardia, hypotension and apnea, also known as the Bezold-Jarisch reflex (BJR) (Kashihara, 2009). In addition, increased discharge of the cardiopulmonary receptors diminishes renal sympathetic outflow and pituitary release of vasopressin, thereby decreasing Na^+ and water reabsorption by the kidneys, increasing urine volume, and reducing blood volume. As changes in blood volume affect cardiac output and arterial pressure, this provides an additional mechanism by which the cardiopulmonary reflex contributes to blood pressure regulation (Thomas, 2011).

Interestingly, cardiopulmonary reflex may exert a tonic inhibitory influence in the arterial baroreflex sensitivity (Abboud and Thames, 1983). In pathological conditions, such as acute myocardial infarction, the reduction in baroreflex sensitivity could be explained by an increase in cardiopulmonary reflex sensitivity (Lacerda et al., 2007). Furthermore, the BJR activation might cause sudden cardiac death during ischemic injury (Robertson et al., 1985), since the overactivation of cardiopulmonary reflex together with baroreflex blunting might cause severe bradycardia and hypotension, placing the patient's life at risk due to the magnitude of sympathetic inhibition and vagal activation. These data demonstrate that the interplay between baroreflex and cardiopulmonary reflex may exert an important role in the progression of cardiovascular diseases and arrhythmias generation.

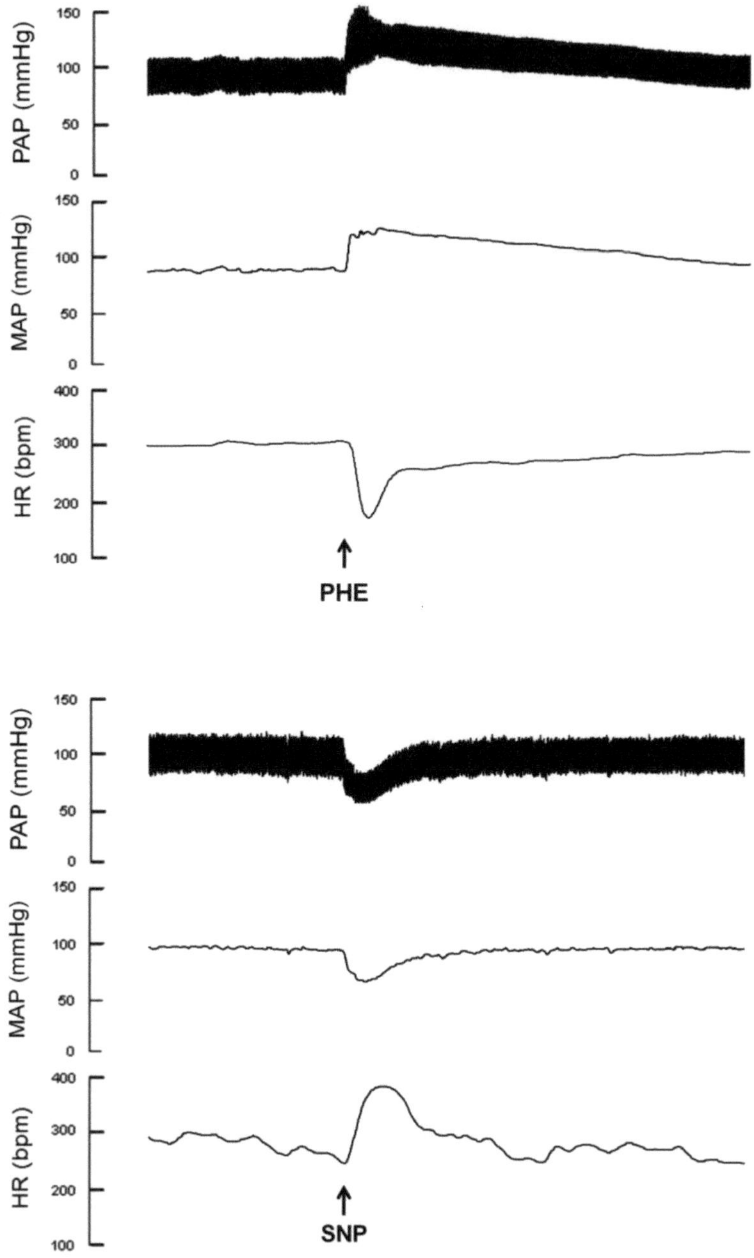

Fig. 2. Typical recordings of baroreflex evaluation in anesthetized rats. The phenylephrine-induced increase in arterial pressure leads to reflex bradycardia (upper panel) and the sodium nitroprusside-induced decrease in arterial pressure results in reflex tachycardia (lower panel). The images were generously provided by Professor Helder Mauad from Federal University of Espirito Santo, Brazil. Data from Pedrosa et al., 2009. PAP: pulsatile arterial pressure, MAP: mean arterial pressure, HR: heart rate, PHE: phenylephrine, SNP: sodium nitroprusside.

Experimentally, the cardiopulmonary reflex function can be evaluated through phenylbiguanide injections. Figure 3 shows typical recordings of changes in arterial pressure and HR during cardiopulmonary reflex test.

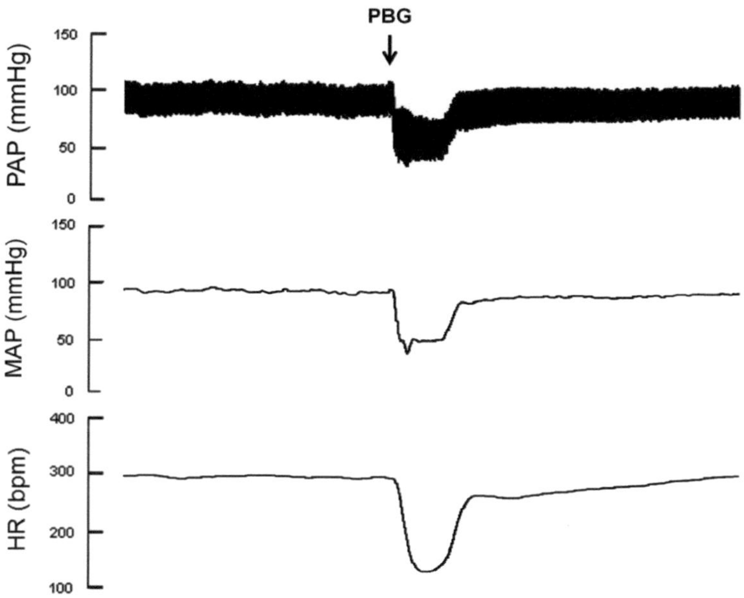

Fig. 3. Typical recordings of cardiopulmonary reflex evaluation in anesthetized rats. The activation of cardiopulmonary receptors is achieved by intravenous phenilbiguanide injections. The images were generously provided by Professor Helder Mauad from Federal University of Espirito Santo, Brazil. Data from Pedrosa et al., 2009. PAP: pulsatile arterial pressure, MAP: mean arterial pressure, HR: heart rate, PBG: phenybiguanide.

4.3 Arterial chemoreflex

The peripheral chemoreflex is considered one of the main mechanisms of control of the ventilatory responses to the changes in arterial O_2 and CO_2 concentrations. The peripheral chemoreceptors located in the carotid and aortic bodies, with afferents to the respiratory center in the medulla oblongata and the NTS, respond primarily to hypoxia (Guimarães et al., 2009). These chemo-sensitive receptors constantly receive information of arterial pO_2, pCO_2 e pH through a thin artery originated in the middle of the bifurcation of the common carotid artery that maintains these cells in close contact with blood gases (Vasquez et al., 1997). Increases in the firing rate of these neurons lead to a simultaneously activation of sympathetic outflow to blood vessels and increased vagal activity to the heart (Kara et al., 2003). Therefore, the excitation of the peripheral chemoreceptors produces an increased minute ventilation, systemic vasoconstriction and hypertension. The primary HR response to chemoreceptor stimulation is a parasympathetic mediated-bradycardia, but this mechanism is usually apparent only in the absence of ventilation. In the presence of the normal ventilatory response to hypoxia, tachycardia is generated by a lung inflation reflex that inhibits vagal outflow to the heart (Marshall, 1994). It is interesting to notice that, if blood pressure is within its normal range, the chemoreflex does not evoke a powerful cardiovascular response because of the predominant effect of the arterial baroreflex.

However, if blood pressure is low, generally below 80 mmHg, activation of the chemoreflex potentiates the vasoconstriction evoked by the baroreflex and helps to restore blood pressure to normal (Thomas et al., 2011).
The role of chemoreflex in cardiac arrhythmias have been already demonstrated. Patients with survived ventricular arrhythmias show significantly decreased chemoreflex sensitivity (Hennersdorf et al., 1997). The chemoreflex sensitivity is also considered as a marker of increased risk for ventricular tachyarrhythmias, since it shows a high positive predictive power in patients with prior myocardial infarction and who previously survived ventricular tachyarrhythmias (Hennersdorf et al., 2002). Central sleep apnea, which is associated with absent respiratory effort and results from instability in the chemoreflex control of breathing, is thought to predispose to cardiac arrhythmias generation (Leung et al., 2009).
Experimentally, the chemoreflex function can be evaluated through potassium cyanide injections. Figure 4 shows typical recordings of changes in arterial pressure and HR during chemoreflex test.

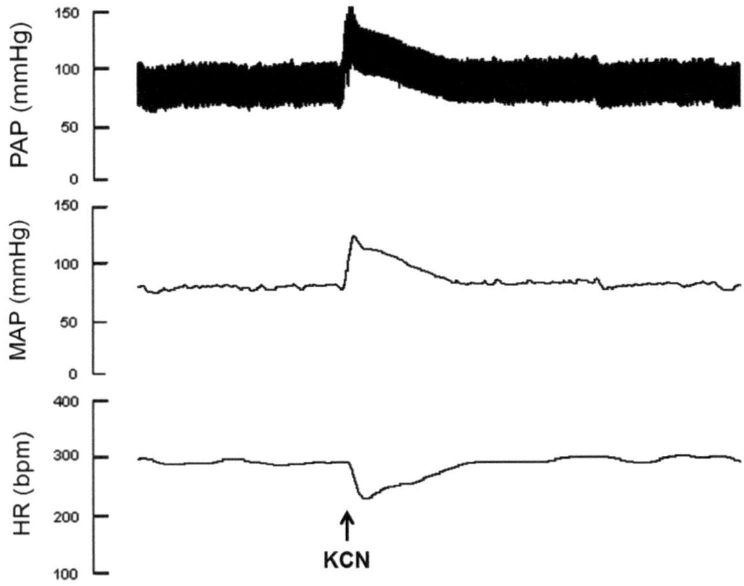

Fig. 4. Typical recordings of chemoreflex evaluation. The activation of chemoreflex is achieved by intravenous potassium cyanide injections. The images were generously provided by Professor Helder Mauad from Federal University of Espirito Santo, Brazil. Data from Pedrosa et al., 2009. PAP: pulsatile arterial pressure, MAP: mean arterial pressure, HR: heart rate, KCN: potassium cyanide.

5. Humoral control of HR

Several investigations have demonstrated that humoral systems can play a pivotal role in maintaining cardiac electric activity homeostasis and changes in their production and/or action pathways may contribute to various disorders in cardiac excitability. Additionally, the humoral systems can also modulate the autonomic nervous system and cardiovascular reflexes, demonstrating the importance of these substances in cardiovascular functioning.

5.1 Estrogen

The sexual hormones are related mainly with the control of reproductive function, however they can also modulate the cardiovascular function. Estrogen is the main female sex hormone in both humans and animal models. It is produced in the granulosa cells of the ovarian cortex through the conversion of androgen precursors by the aromatase enzyme, which in turn is modulated by the hormonal hypothalamic-pituitary axis (Filicori, 1986). The protective effects of estrogen on cardiovascular function have been already demonstrated by several investigations. Indeed, estrogen replacement therapy reduces the incidence of coronary artery disease (Rowland & Fregly, 1992; Farhat et al., 1996). Corroborating these data, Moyses et al. (2001) showed that estrogen treatment in ovariectomized female rats restored coronary vasodilation produced by serotonin in isolated hearts, and a bolus injection of 17ß-estradiol elicited a transient vasodilatory response in male and female normotensive (Santos et al., 2004) and spontaneously hypertensive rats (Santos et al., 2010).

It has been already demonstrated that estrogen levels are also related with the development of cardiac arrhythmias. During the menstrual cycle, estrogen levels rise and fall in women and these fluctuations are related with more frequent episodes with a longer duration of supraventricular tachycardia (Rosano et al., 1996). During perimenopause there is a marked decrease in ovarian estrogen production that is associated with an increase in HR (sinus tachycardia) and an enhancement in the frequency of palpitations and non-threatening arrhythmias, such as premature ventricular contractions (Rosano et al., 1996; Asplund and Aberg, 2003). During menopause a further decline in estrogen occurs and this event is associated with irregular heartbeats, palpitations, spasmodic chest pain and nightmares in women from 40 to 64 years old (Asplund and Aberg, 2003). Corroborating this data, hormonal replacement therapy (HRT) may decrease palpitations and other symptoms such as hot flashes, insomnia, and sweating (Grady et al., 2002). On the other hand, the Heart and Estrogen/Progestin Replacement Study (HERS) found no benefit to reduce cardiovascular events in women on HRT, which may even increase risk of thromboembolism during the first year (Grady et al., 2002). HRT has also being associated with lengthening the QT interval, although the relevance of this finding is not known (Gokce et al., 2005). Therefore, more investigations are necessary to better elucidate the benefits of HRT in preventing cardiac arrhythmias generations.

The mechanisms by which estrogen may affect the development of cardiac arrhythmias include changes ion channels expression and/or activity. Most of the studies demonstrate that estrogen exerts antiarrhythmic effects, possibly by acting the L-type Ca2+ channels, contributing to its cardioprotective actions (Nakajima et al., 1999). Ulrich et al (2007) demonstrated that estrogen inhibits ICaL through direct interactions of the steroid with the channel protein in a rate dependent way, leading to a decreased contraction. However, estrogen can also upregulates the sodium-calcium exchanger (NCX1) through a genomic mechanism mediated by estrogen receptors (ER), contributing to the enhanced propensity to early after depolarizations in female hearts (Cheng et al 2011).

It is well established that estrogen can cross the blood brain barrier and be accumulated in regions of the brain to bring about changes in neural activity, including in autonomic functions (Lee and McEwen, 2001). This modulation may occur via activation of ERs, since ER mRNAs expression have been identified in central areas controlling cardiovascular function such as, NTS, CVLM, RVLM and IML (Spary et al, 2009).

Several studies have demonstrated the effects of estrogen on cardiovascular reflexes. In ovariectomized female rats, intravenous estrogen supplementation significantly reduced sympathetic tone within 30 minutes and significantly increased parasympathetic tone within 5 minutes of administration (Saleh and Connel, 2000). Corroborating these findings, Flues et al (2010) demonstrated that ovariectomized rats supplemented with 17β estradiol presented an exacerbated vagal tonus when compared to ovariectomized rats. This study also showed that ovarian hormones deprivation induced a higher sympathetic activity to the heart. Additionally, Minson et al (2000) reported an increase of baroreflex sensitivity (BRS) in phases of menstrual cycle with estrogen preponderance. An enhanced BRS is associated with an increase in parasympathetic and/or a decrease in sympathetic tone (Rovere et al, 2000), and the degree of BRS depression is significantly correlated to an increased likelihood of cardiac arrhythmogenesis (Saleh et al, 2003). Taken together, those data indicate a beneficial effect of estrogen in autonomic balance and in arrhythmias prevention.

5.2 Testosterone

Testosterone, the major androgenic hormone is synthetized and released by the Leydig cells in the testis. It also gives rise to two other potent androgens: dihydrotestosterone and 5-alfa-androstenediol. Epidemiological and clinical studies indicate that testosterone status influence cardiovascular physiology and pathophysiology (Golden et al., 2002; Er et al., 2007).

The effects of testosterone on cardiac electric activity have been poorly investigated. Sanchez et al. (2009) showed that the acute administration of 5-alpha-dihydrotestosterone elicited a negative chronotropism effect and increased SA node recovery time, which could improve cardiac performance. The authors also suggested that this effect might be due to an interaction with the underlying mechanisms involved in the pacemaker activity (Mangoni and Nargeot, 2008) such as T-type Ca^{2+} channel and inward rectifier currents and a functional interaction with ionic pumps of plasma membranes. On the other hand, the acute treatment with testosterone enhanced the spontaneous beating frequency of cultured neonatal cardiomyocytes, which was associated with an increase in the level of expression of T-type Ca^{2+} channels (Michels et al., 2006). It has also been reported that androgens produce changes in the male heart phenotype and on electrophysiological properties, such as shortening of the QT interval in males after puberty (Rautaharju, 1992; Lehmann, 1997; Locati et al., 1998). These contradictory data may be related to different basal HR values among various mammalian species, and more studies are necessary to better elucidate the role of testosterone on cardiac electric activity.

Most of the research concerning the effects of gonadal hormones on the cardiovascular reflexes has focused on 17β-estradiol. However, other studies have provided evidence that androgens (including testosterone) play an important role in the control of cardiovascular function by modulation of cardiovascular reflexes (Caminiti et al., 2009). Steroids can cross the blood-brain barrier and act on the central nervous system, where androgen receptors in the central cardiovascular regulatory regions, such as NA and DMNX (Peuler et al., 1990; Pouliot et al., 1996) have been demonstrated. Therefore it is possible that androgens may act on brainstem vagal preganglionic neurons to modulate cardiomotor vagal activity. In accordance with this data, El-Mass et al. (2001) have shown that in male rats, castration caused a significant attenuation of baroreceptor control of reflex bradycardia versus no effect on reflex tachycardia. Testosterone replacement increased BRS to phenylephrine in castrated rats and restored reflex bradycardic responses to levels similar to those of sham-operated rats. The muscarinic blockade by atropine in sham-operated rats caused a substantial reduction in BRS to phenylephrine, an effect that was significantly attenuated by castration and restored to sham-operated levels after testosterone replacement, suggesting that testosterone facilitates baroreceptor control of reflex bradycardia. Moreover, the modulatory role of testosterone on baroreflex responsiveness appears to involve, at least partly, enhancement of cardiac vagal efferent activity. Corroborating these data, a long-term testosterone therapy (6 weeks) improves the baroreflex sensitivity in men with chronic heart failure (Caminiti et al., 2009). The blockade of androgen receptor with flutamide attenuates the enhancement of baroreflex bradycardia in sexually mature male rats, indicating that the effects of testosterone on BRS depend on the involvement of the androgen receptor (Ward and Abdel-Rahman, 2006).

Besides the testosterone-induced effects on baroreflex, this sexual hormone may also modulate the cardiopulmonary reflex and the chemoreflex. Bissoli et al (2009) demonstrated that long-term treatment (8 weeks) with supraphysiological doses of nandrolone decanoate reduces the sensitivity of BJR control of HR in male rats. The effects of testosterone on BJR seem to be time-dependent, since the same treatment for 4 weeks had no effects on BJR nor the basal HR (Andrade et al., 2008). Pereira-Junior et al. (2006) showed that 10 weeks of high-dose nandrolone decanoate treatment leads to dysfunction in tonic cardiac autonomic regulation, with marked impairment of parasympathetic cardiac modulation and sympathetic hyperactivity. Regarding the chemoreflex, data from castrated male cats suggest that testosterone increases the hypoxic and hypercapnic ventilatory responses and augmented carotid body sensitivity to hypoxia (Behan et al., 2003). In adult rats, however, castration had no effect on the ventilatory response measured at the end of hypoxia (Joseph et al., 2002). On the other hand, Bairam et al. (2009) demonstrated that gonadectomy increased the acute breathing frequency response to hypoxia in neonatal rats. Because the rapid increase in breathing frequency is attributed to peripheral chemoreceptor activation, these data suggest that testosterone attenuates carotid body function. Although several studies demonstrated contradictory results about the benefic or malefic effects of testosterone on the modulation of cardiovascular reflexes, the characterization of the mechanisms could lead to a better understanding of the effects of testosterone in cardiovascular system and to the development of new therapies.

5.3 Nitric oxide (NO)

Since the discovery of the signaling properties of nitric oxide (NO) (Ignarro et al. 1987), it has been suggested that this important molecule may be involved in many physiological processes, such as the control of cardiovascular function. NO is a free radical synthesized from L-arginine by three isoforms of nitric oxide synthase (NOS): NOS1 (neural), NOS2 (inducible), and NOS3 (endothelial) and all three isoforms have been shown to influence autonomic neural function in some manner (Schultz, 2009). NO generated at nerve synapses diffuses in an autocrine and paracrine way to influence both presynaptic and postsynaptic events on excitatory and inhibitory synapses. NO exerts its cellular actions by binding to guanylyl cyclase to activate cGMP production, which remains the only fully recognized physiological signal transduction mechanism for NO. In central neurons, cGMP then can have diverse effects on neuronal excitability. Cyclic GMP can directly bind to and modulate cyclic nucleotide-gated ion channels, bind to phosphodiesterases to impair cAMP hydrolysis, or most prominently, activate cGMP-dependent protein kinase which can directly or indirectly leads to phosphorylation of effector proteins or ion channels (Schultz, 2009).

The effects of NO on baroreflex have been already demonstrated by several investigations. Meyrelles et al (2003) have shown that adenovirus-mediated eNOS delivery to carotid sinus adventitia leads to a diminished baroreceptor activity. NO seems to have an inhibitory effect on sodium currents in baroceptor neurons (Li et al., 1999) and activates calcium dependent potassium channels, leading to membrane hyperpolarization (Bolotina et al., 1994).

Besides NO effects on baroreceptor afferents, NO also exerts effects on central nuclei regulating baroreflex function.

Intracerebroventricular injections of L-NAME (an inhibitor of NO synthases) caused an enhancement in baroreflex sensitivity, indicating that NO may exert an inhibitory effect upon baroreflex (Matsumura et al, 1998). This inhibition appears to occur in both sympathetic and parasympathetic component of baroreflex. Liu et al (1996) demonstrated that NO synthase blockade with L-NNA causes an increase in the baroreflex gain, which is prevented by L-arginine injections. This augmented sensitivity is blocked by the use of atropine, indicating an inhibitory effect of NO on the parasympathetic component of the reflex. NO also seems to exert sympatoinhibitory effects, as demonstrated by Zanzinger et al (1995) who show that L-NNA administration leads to an increased basal sympathetic tonus. On the other hand, Dias et al. (2005) demonstrated a stimulatory effect of NO in the central nuclei controlling cardiovascular function. In this study, the renal sympathoinhibition induced by activation of baroreceptors and cardiopulmonary receptors is attenuated by the microinjection of L-NAME in the NTS. The same investigators also demonstrated that NO increases the number of discharges evoked by excitatory amino acids in NTS neurons that receive vagal afferent inputs, and action potentials induced by iontophoretic application of AMPA in the NTS was reduced by L-NAME, indicating a excitatory effect of NO in this nucleus (Dias et al., 2003). Some studies also showed no effects of NO on baroreflex function. eNOS gene therapy did not alter baroreflex sensitivity and autonomic balance in C57 mice and was not able to prevent the increase in sympathetic tonus and the decrease parasympathetic activity to the heart in hypertensive mice (Gava et al., 2008).

In addition to the brain, emerging evidence suggests that NO can also influence sympathovagal function at the site of the end-organ itself, acting in sympathetic ganglia or vagal neurons. Neuronal nitric oxide synthase is localized in both intrinsic cardiac vagal neurons and stellate sympathetic ganglia innervating the SA node, indicating an important role NO in modulating of peripheral neuronal function (Herring and Paterson, 2009). In cholinergic neurons, NO seems to act increasing acetylcholine release through stimulation of soluble guanylate cyclase. The resultant generation of cGMP causes phosphodiesterase-3 inhibition, increasing cAMP-PKA dependent phosphorylation of N-type calcium channel and calcium-induced exocytotic release of acethycholine (Herring & Paterson, 2001). However, in the AV nodal cells, NO regulates AV excitabilility by muscarinic cholinergic attenuation of ICa-L (L-type calcium current), the mechanism likely involves the cGMP-stimulated phosphodiesterase (Han et al., 1997). In sympathetic ganglia, NO reduces the release of noradrenaline through a soluble guanylate cyclase–cGMP dependent pathway that reduces calcium influx (Schwartz et al. 1995; Wang et al. 2007), probably via stimulation of PDE2 and/or protein kinase G (Herring and Paterson, 2009). Despite some contradictory results, the role of NO in the modulating HR it is well established and the implication of changes in the NO production and/or activity for cardiovascular disease development remains an intriguing possibility of new targets for treating arrhythmias.

5.4 Renin-angiotensin-aldosterone system (RAAS)

The RAAS is a peptidergic cascade with endocrine characteristics and is considered one of the most important systems that participate of cardiovascular control. In the classical view of RAAS, angiotensinogen, an alfa-glycoprotein, is released from the liver and is cleaved in the circulation by the enzyme renin that is secreted from the juxtaglomerular apparatus of the kidney to form the decapeptide angiotensin I (Ang I). Ang I is then transformed into to the octapeptide angiotensin II (Ang II) by angiotensin converting enzyme (ACE), a membrane-bound metalloproteinase, which is predominantly expressed in high concentrations on the surface of endothelial cells in the pulmonary circulation. Ang II, considered the main effector peptide of the RAAS, acts on specific receptors (AT_1 and AT_2), for example, to induce vasoconstriction on vascular smooth muscle cells or to stimulate the release of aldosterone from the adrenal cortex (Paul et al., 2006).

Several lines of evidence suggest that Ang II may exert a direct modulation on cardiac ionic channels. Experiments have shown that stimulation of AT_1 receptor result in the inhibition of transient outward potassium channel in myocytes from rat or canine ventricle (Shimoni and Liu, 2003; Yu et al., 2000). Ang II also increases cardiac L-type Ca^{2+} current (ICaL) in isolated cat myocytes (Aiello and Cingolani, 2001). In this view, the RAAS activation may therefore significantly contribute to the pathogenesis of cardiac arrhythmias. On the other hand, Ang II decreased the current density of L-type Ca^{2+} current in SA node cells and reduces the auto rhythm of SA node cells via enhancing slowly activated delayed rectifier K^+ currents and reducing ICaL. Therefore, the elevated levels of Ang II may be involved in the occurrence of SA node dysfunction in cardiac pathophysiology (Sheng et al., 2011).

Numerous studies already demonstrated that Ang II plays a pivotal role in the neural regulation of cardiovascular system. High concentrations of AT_1 receptor and fibers with Ang II immunoreactivity have been described in the dorsomedial and ventrolateral areas of the medulla (Allen et al., 1998; Averill and Diz, 2000). It is well known that Ang II causes an increased sympathetic drive, particularly by means of central mechanisms. In dogs, acute (21 h) and chronic (5 days) infusion of Ang II caused a two- to threefold increase in Fos-Li immunoreactivity in the NTS and CVLM, leading to a baroreceptor suppression of sympathoexcitatory cells in the RVLM (Lohmeier et al, 2002). Lesions at either the area postrema or the subfornical organ attenuate angiotensin II-based hypertension, indicating a direct central sympathoexcitatory action of Ang II (Collister and Hendel, 2003; Collister and Hendel, 2005). Corroborating these data, experimental models of angiotensin II-dependent hypertension present an augmented sympathetic drive (Peotta et al., 2007) and patients with chronic angiotensin-dependent renovascular hypertension have generally demonstrated higher sympathetic levels, correlated with circulating angiotensin II concentrations (Grassi e Esler, 2002). Besides Ang II effects on sympathetic drive, this peptide also exerts effects on the parasympathetic component of the reflexes. Borges et al. (2008) demonstrated that mice with renovascular hypertension presented diminished cardiac vagal activity, and together with an enhanced cardiac sympathetic activity, contributed to a reduced baroreflex sensitivity in this animal model of hypertension. Moyses et al. (1994) also demonstrated a reduced cardiac vagal activity in renovascular hypertensive rats.

Although Ang II is considered the major effector of RAAS system, growing evidence have demonstrated an important role of angiotensin-(1-7) in cardiovascular regulation. This molecule can be formed from Ang I and Ang II fragments through an angiotensin-converting enzyme (ACE) independent pathway (Santos et al., 2007). It has been demonstrated that Ang-(1-7) actions are often contrary to those described for Ang II (Benter et al., 1993). In fact, regarding the neural control of circulation, several studies have provided evidence that endogenous Ang-(1-7) enhances the baroreceptor reflex bradycardia, while Ang II attenuates it (Campagnole-Santos, 1992; Sakima et al., 2007). The beneficial effect of Ang-(1-7) on cardiovascular reflexes was also demonstrated by Oliveira et al (1996) who showed that the central infusion of a selective Ang-(1-7) antagonist attenuates baroreflex and blocks the improvement in the reflex bradycardia produced by Ang-(1-7). The specific binding of Ang-(1-7) to its receptor (Mas receptor) seems to be a basic requirement for the maintenance of normal arterial blood pressure and cardiovascular reflex control, since Mas-knockout mice presented hypertension and altered cardiovascular reflexes (Moura et al., 2010).

5.5 Natriuretic peptides (NPs)

The NPs play an important role in the regulation of cardiovascular homeostasis maintaining blood pressure and extracellular fluid volume. There are four major natriuretic peptides (NPs) that have been isolated: atrial natriuretic peptide (ANP), brain natriuretic peptide (BNP), C-type natriuretic peptide (CNP), and Dendroaspis-type natriuretic peptide (DNP). NPs exert their biological effects by binding to three distinct cell surface receptors denoted NP receptors A, B and C (NPR-A, NPR-B and NPR-C) (Rose and Giles, 2008).

Several studies demonstrated that NPs affect the electrophysiology of the heart (Rose et al., 2004) and central nervous system (Trachte et al., 2003; Rose et al., 2005). Voltage-clamp studies demonstrated that CNP can inhibit L-type Ca^{2+} current (ICa-L) through NPR-C binding. This inhibition involves a decrease in adenylyl cyclase activity, which leads to reduced intracellular levels of cAMP (Rose et al., 2003). These results were also demonstrated in isolated myocytes from mouse SA node, that express several cAMP-sensitive currents, including ICa-L (DiFrancesco, 1993). Corroborating these data, inhibition of adenylyl cyclase decreases HR and increases the P–R interval, suggesting that the atrioventricular conduction system is slowed following the activation of NPR-C. These data are consistent with other studies demonstrating a key role for L-type Ca^{2+} channels in the intrinsic regulation of SA node function and the determination of HR (Zhang et al., 2002; Mangoni et al., 2003). The molecular mechanism(s) by which CNP–NPR-C effects are compartmentalized in animal models SA node myocytes is not clear and will require further investigation.

In addition to their effects on cardiac electric activity, NPs also exert effects on cardiovascular reflexes. Thomas et al. (2001) showed that ANP, BNP and CNP enhance bradycardic responses to cardiopulmonary chemoreceptor activation in conscious sheep. On the other hand, Tallarida et al. (1991) demonstrated that intravenous infusion of ANP did not substantially change the baroreflex cardiocirculatory responses to loading and unloading carotid and aortic baroreceptors. Some of the reported discrepancies may be attributed to the dose of ANP, preparation (e.g., synthetic peptide vs. atrial extract) or to experimental conditions (e.g., anaesthetized vs. conscious). The target site(s) for the NPs action on cardio-cardiac vagal reflexes is not clear and more studies are necessary to better elucidate the mechanisms involved in NP-induced changes in cardiovascular reflexes.

5.6 Thyroid hormones (TH)

Variations from euthyroid status affect virtually all physiological systems and the effects on the cardiovascular system are particularly pronounced (Levey and Klein, 1990). Hyperthyroidism causes tachycardia and cardiac arrhythmias whereas bradycardia, reduced cardiac output, and slowed relaxation result from hypothyroidism (Klein and Ojamaa, 2001). The actions of TH are mediated by two nuclear TH receptors (TRs)- α and- β, encoded by two separate genes (Yen, 2001). TR-α1 isoform represents 70% of the TRs and serves an important role in cardiac development (Mai et al., 2004) and the regulation of heart rate and contractility (Dilmann, 2010; Macchia et al., 2001). Corroborating these data, Wikström et al. (1998) demonstrated that TR-α1 knockout mice presented a 20% reduction in HR and a prolonged relaxation time. The molecular explanation for these results includes a diminished expression of the hyperpolarization activated cyclic nucleotide-gated potassium channel 2, which plays a pivotal role for pacemaking (Macchia et al., 2001).

Changes in thyroid status are associated with changes not only in cardiac and vascular function but also in autonomic regulation of the cardiovascular system (Levey and Klein, 1990). In example, Foley et al. (2001) evaluated the effect of thyroid status on arterial baroreflex control of lumbar sympathetic nerve activity (LSNA) and HR in conscious rats. The authors report that rats with hypothyroidism exhibit blunted baroreflex mediated increases in LSNA and HR and a downward shift in baroreflex control of HR compared with euthyroid rats. On the other hand, rats with hyperthyroidism presented normal baroreflex function and sympathetic tone to the vasculature. Although hypothyroidism has been associated with sympathovagal imbalance, current literature shows conflicting results with either increased sympathetic activity (Cacciatori et al., 2000), decreased sympathetic modulation (Gallet et al., 2008) or an increased vagal tone (Xing et al., 2001).

As observed, there is a complex relationship between humoral factors, neural systems (CNS and autonomic nervous system) and cardiac electric activity (Figure 5) and disturbances in these interactions may be related with the development of arrhythmias.

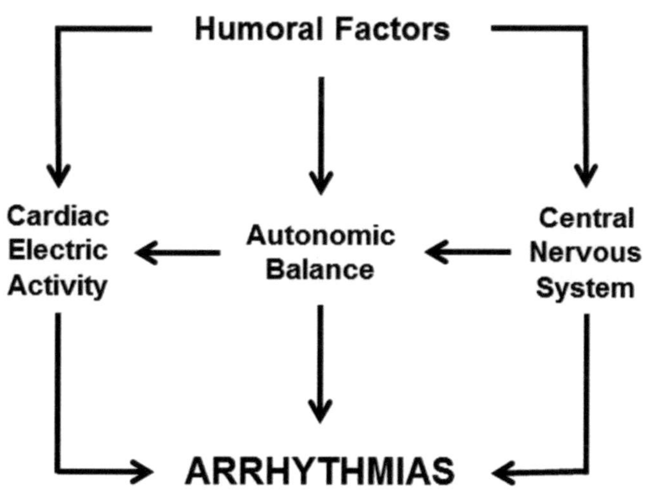

Fig. 5. Schematic diagram showing the interactions between humoral factors, cardiac electric activity, autonomic balance and central nervous system and their role in arrhythmias generation.

6. Perspectives

As observed, the normal control of HR depends on a complex interaction between neural and humoral factors and disturbances on these systems are strongly related with arrhythmias generation. The formation of an action potential in the SA node and its propagation throughout the heart involves several ion channels, mainly Na^+, K^+ and Ca^{+2}, and can be modulated by sympathetic and parasympathetic activation. The central outflow of autonomic nervous system is generated mainly in the brainstem and it involves the participation of diverse nuclei, such as NTS, CVLM and RVLM. The neuronal activity of these structures can be modulated by several hormones, including estrogen, testosterone, nitric oxide, angiotensin II, angiotensin (1-7), natriuretic peptides and thyroid hormones. Besides its effects on CNS, hormones can also regulate the release of neurotransmitters, the expression of ion channels and the activity of membrane transporters. Taken together, these data demonstrate the importance of neural and humoral systems in controlling cardiovascular function and brings out the possibility of new drug targets to treat arrhythmias.

7. Acknowledgments

We would like to acknowledge Professor Helder Mauad from Federal University of Espirito Santo - Brazil, who generously provided the typical recordings of baroreflex, cardiopulmonary reflex and chemoreflex evaluation displayed in Figure 2, 3 and 4.

8. References

Aiello, E.A. & Cingolani, H.E. (2001). Angiotensin II stimulates cardiac L-type Ca(2+) current by a Ca(2+)- and protein kinase C-dependent mechanism. *Am J Physiol Heart Circ Physiol,* Vol.280, No.4; pp.1528-1536, ISSN 0363-6135

Allen, A.M.; Moeller, I.; Jenkins, T.A.; Zhuo, J.; Aldred, G.P.; Chai, S.Y. & Mendelsohn, F.A.O. (1998). Angiotensin receptors in the nervous system. *Brain Res Bull,* Vol.47, pp. 17-28, ISSN 0361-9230

Andrade, T.U.; Santos, M.C.; Busato, V.C.; Medeiros, A.R.S.; Abreu, G.R. & Moyses, M.R. (2008). Higher physiological doses of nandrolone decanoate do not influence the Bezold-Jarisch reflex control of bradycardia. *Arch Med Res,* Vol.39, pp. 27-32, ISSN 0188-4409

Asplund, R. & Aberg, H.E. (2003). Nightmares, cardiac symptoms and the menopause. *Climacteric,* Vol.6, No.4, pp. 314-320, ISSN 1369-7137

Averill, D.B. & Diz, D. (2000). Angiotensin peptides and baroreflex control of sympathetic outflow: pathways and mechanisms of the medulla oblongata. Brain Res Bull, Vol.51, pp. 119-128, ISSN 0361-9230

Bairam, A.; Montandon, G.; Joseph, V.; Lajeunesse, Y. & Kinkead, R. (2009). Enhancement of the breathing frequency response to hypoxia by neonatal caffeine treatment in adult male rats: The role of testosterone. *Respiratory Physiology & Neurobiology,* Vol.165, pp. 261-265, ISSN 1569-9048

Behan, M.; Zabka, A.G.; Thomas, C.F. & Mitchell, G.S. (2003). Sex steroid hormones and the neural control of breathing. *Respir Physiol Neurobiol,* Vol.136, pp. 249-263, ISSN 1569-9048

Benter, I.F.; Diz, D.I & Ferrario, C.M. (2007). Cardiovascular actions of angiotensin(1-7). *Peptides,* Vol. 14, No.4, pp.679-684, ISSN 0196-9781

Berne, R.M.; Levy, M.N.; Koeppen, B.M. & Stanton, B.A. Berne & Levy physiology. ISBN 0721632564, Philadelphia, PA, Mosby:Elsevier, 2008.

Bissoli, N.S.; Medeiros, A.R.S.; Santosa, M.C.S.; Busatoa, V.C.W.; Jarskec, R.D.; Abreu, G.R.; Moysés, M.R.; Andrade, T.U. (2009). Long-term treatment with supraphysiological doses of nandrolone decanoate reduces the sensitivity of Bezold-Jarisch reflex control of heart rate and blood pressure. *Pharmacological Research,* Vol.59, pp. 379-384, ISSN 1043-6618

Bolotina, V.M.; Najibi, S.; Palaccino, J.J.; Pagano, J.P. & Cohen, R.A. (1994). Nitric oxide directly activates calcium-dependent potassium channels in vascular smooth muscle. *Nature,* Vol.368, pp. 850-853, ISSN 0028-0836

Borges, G.R. Salgado, H.C.; Silva, C.A.; Rossi, M.A.; Prado, C.M. & Fazan, R. Jr.(2008). Changes in hemodynamic and neurohumoral control cause cardiac damage in one-kidney, one-clip hypertensive mice. *Am J Physiol Regul Integr Comp Physiol,* Vol. 295, No.6, p.1904-1913, ISSN 0363-6119

Bouman, L.N. & Jongsma, H.J. (1986). Structure and function of the sino-atrial node: a review. *Eur Heart J,* Vol.7, No.2, pp. 94-104, ISSN 0195-668X

Brown HF. (1982). Electrophysiology of the sinoatrial node. *Physiol Rev,* Vol.62, No.2, pp. 505-530, ISSN 0031-9333

Cacciatori, V.; Gemma, M.L.; Bellavere,F.; Castello, R.; De Gregori, M.E.; Zoppini, G.; Thomaseth, K.; Mogheti, P. & Muggeo, M. (2000). Powerspectral analysis of heart rate in hypothyroidism. *European Journal of Endocrinology,* Vol.143, pp.327–333, ISSN 0804-4643

Caminiti, G.; Volterrani, M.; Iellamo, F.; Marazzi, G.; Massaro, R.; Miceli, M.; Mammi, C.; Piepoli, M.; Fini, M. & Rosano, G.M. (2009). Effect of long-acting testosterone treatment on functional exercise capacity, skeletal muscle performance, insulin resistance, and baroreflex sensitivity in elderly patients with chronic heart failure a double-blind, placebo-controlled, randomized study. *J Am Coll Cardiol,* Vol.54, No.10, pp. 919-27, ISSN 0735-1097

Campagnole-Santos, M.J.; Heringer, S.B.; Batista, E.N.; Khosla, M.C. & Santos, R.A. (1992). Differential baroreceptor reflex modulation by centrally infused angiotensin peptides. *Am J Physiol,* Vol.263, pp.89-94, ISSN 0002-9513

Collister, J.P. & Hendel, M.D. (2003). Role of the subfornical organ in the chronic hypotensive response to losartan in normal rats. *Hypertension,* Vol.41, pp. 576–582, ISSN 0194-911X

Collister, J.P. & Hendel, M.D. (2005). Chronic effects of angiotensin II and AT receptor antagonists in subfornical organ-lesioned rats. *Clin Exp Pharmacol Physiol,* Vol.32, pp. 462–466, ISSN 0305-1870

De Ferrari, G.M.; Vanoli, E. & Schwartz, P.J. (1994). Vagal activity and ventricular fibrillation. In: *Vagal control of the heart: experimental basis and clinical implications,* Levy, M.N. & Schwartz, P.J.. *Futura,* Armonk, NY, pp. 613–636, ISBN 0879935618

de Moura, M.M.; dos Santos, R.A.; Campagnole-Santos, M.J.; Todiras, M.; Bader, M.; Alenina, N. & Haibara, A.S. (2010). Altered cardiovascular reflexes responses in conscious Angiotensin-(1-7) receptor Mas-knockout mice. *Peptides,* Vol. 31, No.10, pp.1934-1939, ISSN 0196-9781

Dias, A.C.; Colombari, E. & Mifflin, S.W. (2003). Effect of nitric oxide on excitatory amino acid-evoked discharge of neurons in NTS. *Am J Physiol Heart Circ Physiol,* Vol.284, No.1, pp. 234-240, ISSN 0363-6135

Dias, A.C.; Vitela, M.; Colombari, E. & Mifflin, S.W. (2005). Nitric oxide modulation of glutamatergic, baroreflex, and cardiopulmonary transmission in the nucleus of the solitary tract. *Am J Physiol Heart Circ Physiol,* Vol.288, No.1, pp. 256-262, ISSN 0363-6135

DiFrancesco, D. (1993). Pacemaker mechanisms in cardiac tissue. *Annu Rev Physiol,* Vol. 55, pp.455–472, ISSN 0066-4278

Dillmann, W. (2010). Cardiac hypertrophy and thyroid hormone signaling. *Heart Fail Rev,* Vo.15, pp. 125-132, ISSN 1382-4147

El-Mas, M.M.; Afify, E.A.; Mohy El-Din, M.M.; Omar, A.G. & Sharabi, F.M. (2001). Testosterone facilitates the baroreceptor control of reflex bradycardia: role of cardiac sympathetic and parasympathetic components. *J Cardiovasc Pharmacol,* Vol.38, pp. 754-763, ISSN 0160-2446

Er, F.; Michels, G.; Brandt, M.C.; Khan, I.; Haase, H.; Eicks, M.; Lindner, M. & Hoppe, U.C. (2007). Impact of testosterone on cardiac L-type calcium channels and Ca2+ sparks: Acute actions antagonize chronic effects. *Cell Calcium,* Vol.41, pp. 467-477, ISSN 0143-4160

Farhat, M.Y.; Lavigne, M.C. & Ramwell, P.W. (1996). The vascular protective effects of estrogen. *FASEB. J,* Vol.10, pp. 615-624, ISSN 0892-6638

Feldman, D.; Elton, T.S.; Menachemi, D.M. & Wexler, R.K. (2010). Heart rate control with adrenergic blockade: Clinical outcomes in cardiovascular medicine. *Vasc Health Risk Manag,* Vol.6, pp. 387-397, ISSN 1176-6344

Filicori, M.; Santoro, N.; Merriam, G.R. & Crowley Jr, W.F. (1986). Characterization of the physiological pattern of episodic gonadotropin secretion throughout the human menstrual cycle. *J Clin Endocrinol Metab,* Vol.62, pp. 1136-1144, ISSN 0021-972X

Flues, K.; Paulini, J.; Brito, S.; Sanches, I.C.; Consolim-Colombo, F.; Irigoyen, M.C. & De Angelis, K. (2010). Exercise training associated with estrogen therapy induced cardiovascular benefits after ovarian hormones deprivation. *Maturitas,* Vol.65, pp. 267–271, ISSN 0378-5122

Foley, C.M.; McAllister, R.M. &, Hasser, E.M. (2001). Thyroid status influences baroreflex function and autonomic contributions to arterial pressure and heart rate. *Am J Physiol Heart Circ Physiol,* Vol.280, pp. 2061-2068, ISSN 0363-6135

Galetta, F.; Franzoni, F. Fallahi, P.; Tocchini, L.; Barccini, L.; Santoro, G. & Antonelli, A. (2008). Changes in heart rate variability and QT dispersion in patients with overt hypothyroidism. *European Journal of Endocrinology,* Vol.158, pp.85–90, ISSN 0804-4643

Gava, A.L.; Peotta, V.A.; Cabral, A.M.; Vasquez, E.C.; Meyrelles, S.S. (2008). Overexpression of eNOS prevents the development of renovascular hypertension in mice. *Can J Physiol Pharmacol,* Vol. 86, No.7, pp. 458-464, ISSN 0008-4212

Gökçe, M.; Karahan, B.; Yilmaz, R.; Orem, C.; Erdöl, C. & Ozdemir, S. (2005). Long term effects of hormone replacement therapy on heart rate variability, QT interval, QT dispersion and frequencies of arrhythmia. *Int J Cardiol,* Vol.99, No.3, pp. 373-379, ISSN 0167-5273

Golden, K.L.; Marsh, J.D.; Jiang, Y. (2002). Castration reduces mRNA levels for calcium regulatory proteins in rat heart. *Endocrine,* Vol.19, pp. 339-344, ISSN 1355-008X

Gottlieb, S.S.; McCarter, R.J. & Vogel, R.A. (1998). Effect of beta blockade on mortality among high-risk and low-risk patients after myocardial infarction. *N Engl J Med,* Vol.339, pp. 489-497, ISSN 0028-4793

Grady, D.; Herrington, D.; Bittner, V.; Blumenthal, R.; Davidson, M.; Hlatky, M.; Hsia, J.; Hulley, S.; Herd, A.; Khan, S.; Newby, L.K.; Waters, D.; Vittinghoff, E.; Wenger, N. & HERS Research Group. (2002). Cardiovascular disease outcomes during 6.8 years of hormone therapy: Heart and Estrogen/progestin Replacement Study follow-up (HERS II). *JAMA,* Vol.288, No.1, pp. 49-57, ISSN 0098-748

Grassi, G. & Esler, M. (2002). The sympathetic nervous system in renovascular hypertension: lead actor or "bit" player? *J Hypertens,* Vol.20, pp. 1071-1073, ISSN 0263-6352

Guimarães, G.V.; Belli, J.F.; Bacal, F. & Bocchi, E.A. (2011) Behavior of central and peripheral chemoreflexes in heart failure. *Arq Bras Cardiol,* Vol.96, No.2, pp. 161-167, ISSN 0066-782X

Guyton A.C. & Hall, J.E. *Textbook of Medical Physiology* (11th ed.): Elsevier Saunders, Philadelphia, PA, ISBN 072168307X, November, 2005

Han, X.; Kobzik, L.; Zhao, Y.Y.; Opel, D.J.; Liu, W.D.; Kelly, R.A. & Smith, T.W. (1997). Nitric oxide regulation of atrioventricular node excitability. *Can J Cardiol,* Vol.13, No.12, pp. 1191-201, ISSN 0828-282X

Hennersdorf, M.G.; Niebch, V.; Perings, C. & Strauer, B.E. (2002). Chemoreflex sensitivity as a predictor of arrhythmia relapse in ICD recipients. *International Journal of Cardiology, Vol.*86, pp. 169-175, ISSN 0167-5273

Hennersdorf, M.G.; Perings, C.; Kristovic, M. et al. (1997). Chemoreflex and baroreflex sensitivity among patients with survived sudden cardiac death. *Z Kardiol,* Vol.86, pp. 196-203, ISSN 0300-5860

Herring, N. & Paterson, D.J. (2001). Nitric oxide-cGMP pathway facilitates acetylcholine release and bradycardia during vagal nerve stimulation in the guinea-pig in vitro. *J Physiol,* Vol.535, No.Pt 2, pp. 507-518, ISSN 0022-3751

Herring, N. & Paterson, D.J. (2009). Neuromodulators of peripheral cardiac sympatho-vagal balance. *Exp Physiol,* Vol.94, No.1, pp. 46-53, ISSN 0144-8757

Ignarro, L.J.; Byrns, R.E.; Buga, G.M. & Wood, K.S. (1987). Endothelium-derived relaxing factor from pulmonary artery and vein possesses pharmacologic and chemical properties identical to those of nitric oxide radical. *Circ Res,* Vol.61, No.6, pp. 866-879, ISSN 0009-7330

Issa, Z.F; Ujhelyi, M.R. & Hildebrand, K.R. (2005). Intrathecal clonidine reduces the incidence of ischaemia-provoked ventricular arrhythmias in a canine post infarction heart failure model. *Heart Rhythm,* Vol.2, pp. 1122-1127, ISSN 1547-5271

Joseph, V.; Soliz, J.; Soria, R.; Pequignot, J.; Favier, R.; Spielvogel, H. & Pequignot, J.M. (2002). Dopaminergic metabolism in carotid bodies and high-altitude acclimatization in female rats. Am J Physiol Regul Integr Comput Physiol, Vol.282, pp. 765-7, ISSN 0363-6119

Kara, T.; Narkiewicz, K. & Somers, V.K. (2003). Chemoreflexes - physiology and clinical implications. *Acta Physiol Scand,* Vol.177, pp. 377-384, ISSN 0001-6772

Kashihara, K.M. (2009). Roles of arterial baroreceptor reflex during Bezold-Jarisch reflex. *Current Cardiology Reviews,* Vol.5, pp. 263-267, ISSN 1573-403X

Kirkman, E. & Sawdon, M. (2004). Neurological and humoral control of blood pressure. Anaesthesia and Intensive Care Medicine, Vol.11, pp. 159-165, ISSN 1472-0299

Klein, I. & Ojamaa, K. (2001). Thyroid hormone-targeting the heart. *Endocrinology,* Vol.142, pp. 11-12, ISSN 0013-7227

Koike, H.; Mark, A.L.; Heistad, D.D. & Schmid, P.G. (1975). Influence of cardiopulmonary vagal afferent activity on carotid chemoreceptor and baroreceptor reflexes in the dog. *Circ Res,* Vol.37, No.4, pp. 422-429, ISSN 0009-7330

Lacerda, J.E.C.; Consolim-Colombo, F.M.; Moreira, E.D.; Ida, F.; Silva, G.J.J.; Irigoyen, M.C. & Krieger, E.M. (2007). Influence of cardiopulmonary reflex on the sympathetic activity during myocardial infarction. *Autonomic Neuroscience: Basic and Clinical,* Vol. 133, pp. 128-135, ISSN 1566-0702

Lee, S.J., McEwen, B.S., 2001. Neurotrophic and neuroprotective actions of estrogens and their therapeutic implications. *Annu. Rev. Pharmacol. Toxicol.,* Vol.41, pp. 569-591, ISSN 0362-1642

Lehmann, M.H. (1997). QT prolongation in end-stage liver disease: a result of altered sex hormone metabolism? *Hepatology,* Vol.26, pp. 244, ISSN 0270-9139

Leung, R.S.T. (2009). Sleep-Disordered Breathing: Autonomic Mechanisms and Arrhythmias. *Progress in Cardiovascular Diseases,* Vol. 51, pp.324-338, ISSN 0033-0620

Levey, G.S. & Klein, I. (1990). Catecholamine-thyroid hormone interactions and the cardiovascular manifestations of hyperthyroidism. *Am J Med,* Vol.88, pp. 642-646, ISSN 0002-9343

Li, Z.; Chapleau, M.W.; Bates, J.N.; Bielefeldt, K.; Lee, H.C. & Abboud, F.M. (1998). Nitric oxide as an autocrine regulator of sodium currents in baroreceptor neurons. *Neuron,* Vol.20, pp. 1039-1049, ISSN 0896-6273

Liu, J.L.; Murakami, H. & Zucker, I.H. (1996). Effects of NO on baroreflex control of heart rate and renal nerve activity in conscious rabbits. *Am J Physiol,* Vol.270, No.6 Pt 2, pp. 1361-1370, ISSN 0363-6119

Locati, E.H.; Zareba, W.; Moss, A.J.; Schwartz, P.J.; Vincent, G.M.; Lehmann, M.H.; Towbin, J.A.; Priori, S.G.; Napolitano, C.; Robinson, J.L.; Andrews, M.; Timothy, K. & Hall, W.J. (1998). Age- and sex-related differences in clinical manifestations in patients with congenital long-QT syndrome: findings from the International LQTS Registry. *Circulation,* Vol.97, pp. 2237-2244, ISSN 0009-7322

Loewy, A.D. & K.M. Spyer. (1990). The central organization of reflex circulatory control. *Central Regulation of Autonomic functions,* Lowey, D. & Spyer, K.M. pp. 168-188, ISBN 0195051068, New York: Oxford University London/New York.

Lohmeier, T.E.; Lohmeier, J.R.; Warren, S.; May, P.J. & Cunningham, J.T. (2002). Sustained activation of the central baroreceptor pathway in angiotensin hypertension. *Hypertension,* Vol.39, pp. 550-556, ISSN 0194-911X

Macchia, P.E.; Takeuchi, Y.; Kawai, T.; Cua, K.; Gauthier, K.; Chassande, O.; Seo, H.; Hayashi, Y.; Samarut, J.; Murata, Y.; Weiss, R.E. & Refetoff, S. (2001). Increased sensitivity to thyroid hormone in mice with complete deficiency of thyroid hormone receptor α. *Proc Natl Acad Sci,* Vol.98, pp. 349-354, ISSN 0027-8724

Mai, W.; Janier, M.F.; Allioli, N.; Quignodon, L.; Chuzel, T.; Flamant, F. & Samarut, J. (2004). Thyroid hormone receptor α is a molecular switch of cardiac function between fetal and post natal life. *Proc Natl Acad Sci,* Vol.101, pp. 10332-10337, ISSN 0027-8424

Mangoni, M.E. & Nargeot, J. (2008). Genesis and regulation of the heart automaticity. *Physiol Rev,* Vol.88, pp. 919-982, ISSN 0031-9333

Mangoni, M.E.; Couette, B.; Bourinet, E.; Platzer, J.; Reimer, D.; Striessnig, J. & Nargeot, J. (2003). Functional role of L-type Cav1.3 Ca2+ channels in cardiac pacemaker activity. *Proc Natl Acad Sci USA,* Vol.100, pp.5543–5548, ISSN 1091-6490

Marshall, J.M. (1994). Peripheral chemoreceptors and cardiovascular regulation. *Physiological Reviews,* Vol.74, pp. 543-593, ISSN 0031-9333

Matsumura, K.; Abe, I.; Tsuchihashi, T. & Fujishima, M. (1998). Central nitric oxide attenuates the baroreceptor reflex in conscious rabbits. *Am J Physiol*, Vol.274, No.4 Pt 2, pp. 1142-1149, ISSN 0363-6119

Meyrelles, S.S.; Sharma, R.V.; Mao, H.Z.; Abboud, F.M. & Chapleau, M.W. (2003). Modulation of baroreceptor activity by gene transfer of nitric oxide to carotid sinus adventitia. *American Journal of Physiology*, Vol.284, pp. 1190-1198, ISSN 0363-6119

Michels, G.; Er, F.; Eicks, M.; Herzig, S. & Hoppe, U.C. (2006). Long-term and immediate effect of testosterone on single T-type calcium channel in neonatal rat cardiomyocytes. *Endocrinology*, Vol.147, pp. 5160-5169, ISSN 0013-7227

Minson, C.T.; Halliwill, J.R.; Young, T.M. & Joyner, M.J. (2000). Influence of the menstrual cycle on sympathetic activity, baroreflex sensitivity, and vascular transduction in young women. *Circulation*, Vol.101, pp.862-868, ISSN 0009-7322

Moysés, M.R.; Barker, L.A. & Cabral, A.M. (2001). Sex hormone modulation of serotonin-induced coronary vasodilation in isolated heart. *Braz J Med Biol Res*, Vol.34, pp. 949-958, ISSN 1678-4510

Moyses, M.R.; Cabral, A.M.; Marçal, D. & Vasquez, E.C. (1994). Sigmoidal curve-fitting of baroreceptor sensitivity in renovascular 2K1C hypertensive rats. *Braz J Med Biol Res*, Vol.27, No.6, pp.1419-1424, ISSN 0100-879X

Nakajima, T.; Iwasawa, K.; Oonuma, H.; Morita, T.; Goto, A.; Wang, Y. & Hazama, H. (1999). Antiarrhythmic effect and its underlying ionic mechanism of 17beta-estradiol in cardiac myocytes. *Br J Pharmacol*, Vol.127, No.2, pp. 429-440, ISSN 0007-1188

Pagani, M. & Lucini, D. (2001). Autonomic dysregulation in essential hypertension: insight from heart rate and arterial pressure variability. *Auton Neurosci*, Vol.90, No.1-2, pp. 76-82, ISSN 1566-070

Paul, M.; Poyan Mehr, A. & Kreutz, R. (2006). Physiology of local renin-angiotensin systems. *Physiol Rev*, Vol.86, No.3, pp.747-803, ISSN 0031-9333

Pedrosa, D.F.; Gava, P.L.; Benevides, M.C.A.; Mauad, H. (2009). Respostas das Microinjeções de Nicotina no Núcleo Ambíguo de Ratos Anestesiados. *Proceedings of XXVI Reunião Anual da FeSBE*, São Paulo, August 2009

Peotta, V.A.; Gava, A.L.; Vasquez, E.C.; Meyrelles, S.S. (2007). Evaluation of baroreflex control of heart rate in renovascular hypertensive mice. *Can J Physiol Pharmacol*, Vol. 85, No.8, pp. 761-766, ISSN 0008-4212

Pereira-Junior, P.P.; Chaves, E.A.; Costa-e-Sousa, R.H.; Masuda, M.O.; Carvalho, A.C.C. &, Nascimento, J.H.M. (2006). Cardiac autonomic dysfunction in rats chronically treated with anabolic steroid. *Eur J Appl Physiol*, Vol.96, pp. 487-494, ISSN 1439-6319

Petrashevskaya, N.N.; Koch, S.E.; Bodi, I. & Schwartz, A. (2002). Calcium cycling, historic overview and perspectives. Role for autonomic nervous system regulation. *J Mol Cell Cardiol*, Vol.34, No.8, pp.885-896, ISSN 0022-2828

Peuler, J.D.; Edwards, G.L.; Schmid, P.G. & Johnson, A.K. (1990). Area postrema and differential reflex effects of vasopressin and phenylephrine in rats. *Am J Physiol*, Vol.258, pp. 1255-1259, ISSN 0363-6135

Podrid, P.J.; Fuchs, T. & Cardinas, R. (1990). Role of the sympathetic nervous system in genesis of ventricular arrhythmia. *Circulation*, Vol.82, No.1, pp. 1103-1113, ISSN 0009-7322

Pouliot, W.A.; Handa, R.J. & Beck, S.G. (1996). Androgen modulates N-methyld-aspartate-mediated depolarization in CA1 hippocampal pyramidal cells. Synapse, Vol.23, pp. 10-19, ISSN 0887-4476

Rautaharju, P.M.; Zhou, S.H.; Wong, S., Calhoun, H.P.; Berenson, G.S.; Prineas, R. & Davignon, A. (1992). Sex differences in the evolution of the electrocardiographic QT interval with age. *Can J Cardiol,* Vol.8, pp. 690-695, ISSN 0828-282X

Robertson, D.; Hollister, A.S.; Forman, M.B. & Robertson, R.M. (1985). Reflexes unique to myocardial ischemia and infarction. *J Am Coll Cardiol,* Vol.5, pp. 99B-104B, ISSN 0735-1097

Rosano, G.M.; Leonardo, F.; Sarrel, P.M.; Beale, C.M.; De Luca, F. & Collins, P. (1996). Cyclical variation in paroxysmal supraventricular tachycardia in women. *Lancet,* Vol.347, No.9004, pp. 786-788, ISSN 0140-6736

Rose, R.A. & Giles, W.R. (2008). Natriuretic peptide C receptor signalling in the heart and vasculature. *J Physiol,* Vol.586, No.2, pp.353-66, ISSN 0022-3751

Rose, R.A.; Anand-Srivastava, M.B.; Giles, W.R. & Bains, J.S. (2005). C-type natriuretic peptide inhibits L-type Ca2+ current in rat magnocellular neurosecretory cells by activating the NPR-C receptor. *J Neurophysiol,* Vol.94, pp.612–621, ISSN 0022-3077

Rose, R.A.; Lomax, A.E. & Giles, W.R. (2003). Inhibition of L-type Ca2+ current by C-type natriuretic peptide in bullfrog atrial myocytes: an NPR-C-mediated effect. *Am J Physiol Heart Circ Physiol,* Vol.285, pp.2454–2462, ISSN 0363-6135

Rose, R.A.; Lomax, A.E.; Kondo, C.S.; Anand-Srivastava, M.B. & Giles, W.R. (2004). Effects of C-type natriuretic peptide on ionic currents in mouse sinoatrial node: a role for the NPR-C receptor. *Am J Physiol Heart Circ Physiol,* Vol. 286, pp.1970–1977, ISSN 0363-6135

Rowland, N.E.; & Fregly, M.J. (1992). Role of gonadal hormones in hypertension in the Dahl salt-sensitive rat. *Clin. Exp. Hypertens,* Vol.14, pp. 367-375, ISSN 1064-1963

Sakima, A.; Averill, D.B.; Kasper, S.O.; Jackson, L.; Ganten, D.; Ferrario, C.M.; Gallagher, P.E. & Diz, D.I. (2007). Baroreceptor reflex regulation in anesthetized transgenic rats with low glia-derived angiotensinogen. *Am J Physiol Heart Circ Physiol,* Vol.292, No.3, pp.1412-1419, ISSN 0363-6135

Saleh, T.M. (2003). The role of neuropeptides and neurohormones in neurogenic cardiac arrhythmias. *Curr Drug Targets Cardiovasc Haematol Disord,* Vol.3, No.3, pp. 240-253, ISSN 1568-0061

Saleh, T.M.; Connell, B.J. & Saleh, M.C. (2000). Acute injection of 17beta-estradiol enhances cardiovascular reflexes and autonomic tone in ovariectomized female rats. *Auton Neurosci,* Vol.84, No.1-2, pp. 78-88, ISSN 1566-0702

Sánchez, M.; Secades, L.; Bordallo, C.; Meana, C.; Rubín, J.M.; Cantabrana, B. & Bordallo, J. (2009). Role of Polyamines and cAMP-dependent Mechanisms on 5a-dihydrotestosterone-elicited Functional Effects in Isolated Right Atria of Rat. *J Cardiovasc Pharmacol,* Vol.54, pp. 310-318, ISSN 0160-2446

Santos, R.A. & Ferreira, A.J. (1994). Angiotensin-(1-7) and the renin-angiotensin system. *Curr Opin Nephrol Hypertens,* Vol.6, No.2, pp.122-128, ISSN 1062-4821

Santos, R.L.; Abreu, G.R.; Bissoli, N.S. & Moysés, M.R. (2004). Endothelial mediators of 17 beta estradiol-induced coronary vasodilation in the isolated rat heart. *Braz J Med Biol Res,* Vol.37, pp. 569-575, ISSN 1678-4510

Santos, R.L.; Marin, E.B.; Gonçalves, W.L.S.; Bissoli, N.S.; Abreu, G.R., & Moysés, M.R.(2010). Sex differences in the coronary vasodilation induced by 17 β-oestradiol in the isolated perfused heart from spontaneously hypertensive rats. *Acta Physiol,* Vol.200, pp. 203-210, ISSN 1748-1708

Schultz, H.D. (2009). Nitric oxide regulation of autonomic function in heart failure. *Curr Heart Fail Rep,* Vol.6, No.2, pp. 71-80, ISSN 1546-9530

Schwartz, P.J. & De Ferrari, G.M. (2011). Sympathetic–parasympathetic interaction in health and disease: abnormalities and relevance in heart failure. *Heart Failure,* Vol.16, pp. 101-107, ISSN 1573-7322

Schwartz, P.J. (1984) Sympathetic imbalance and cardiac arrhythmias. In: Randall, W.C. Nervous control of cardiovascular function, pp. 225-251, ISBN 0195033906, Oxford University Press, New York

Schwartz, P.J.; Brown, A.M.; Malliani, A. & Zanchetti, A. (1978) Neural mechanisms in cardiac arrhythmias, pp. 442, ISNB 0890042098, Raven Press, New York

Sheng, J.W.; Wang, W.Y. & Xu, Y.F. (2011). Angiotensin II decreases spontaneous firing rate of guinea-pig sino-atrial node cells. *Eur J Pharmacol,* Vol.660, pp.387-393, ISSN 0014-2999

Shimoni, Y. & Liu, X.F. (2003). Role of PKC in autocrine regulation of rat ventricular K+ currents by angiotensin and endothelin. *Am J Physiol Heart Circ Physiol,* Vol.284, No.4, pp.1168-1181, ISSN 0363-6135

Spary, E.J.; Maqbool, A. & Batten, T.F.C. (2009). Oestrogen receptors in the central nervous system and evidence for their role in the control of cardiovascular function. *Journal of Chemical Neuroanatomy,* Vol.38, pp. 185-196, ISSN 0891-0618

Tallarida, G.; Iellamo, F.; Raimondi, G.; Legramante, J.M.; Cassarino, S.; Marazza, D.; Di Nardo, P. & Peruzzi, G. (1991). On the role of neural mechanisms in the cardiocirculatory inhibitory action of alpha-human atrial natriuretic peptide in the anesthetized rabbit. *J Hypertens,* Vol.9,No.10, pp.935-45, ISSN 0263-6352

Thomas, C.J.; May, C.N.; Sharma, A.D. & Woods, R.L (2001). ANP, BNP and CNP enhance bradycardic responses to cardiopulmonary chemoreceptor activation in conscious sheep. *Am J Physiol Regul Integr Comp Physiol,* Vol.280, pp.282–288, ISSN 0363-6119

Thomas, G.D. (2011). Neural control of the circulation. *Advan in Physiol Edu,* Vol.35, pp. 28-32, ISSN 1043-4046

Trachte, G.J. (2003). Natriuretic peptides suppress protein kinase C activity to reduce evoked dopamine efflux from pheochromocytoma (PC12) cells. *Endocrinology,* Vol.144, pp.94–100, ISSN 0013-7227

Vanoli, E.; De Ferrari, G.M.; Stramba-Badiale, M.; Hull, S.S.; Foreman, R.D. & Schwartz, P.J. (1991). Vagal stimulation and prevention of sudden death in conscious dogs with a healed myocardial infarction. *Circ Res,* Vol.68, pp. 1471-1481, ISSN 0009-7330

Vaseghi, M. & Shivkumar, K. (2008). The Role of the Autonomic Nervous System in Sudden Cardiac Death. *Progress in Cardiovascular Diseases,* Vol.50, No.6, pp. 404-419, ISSN 0033-0620

Vasquez, E.C.; Meyrelles, S.S.; Mauad, H. & Cabral, A.M. (1997). Neural reflex regulation of arterial pressure in pathophysiological conditions: interplay among the baroreflex, the cardiopulmonary reflexes and the chemoreflex. *Brazilian Journal of Medical and Biological Research,* Vol.30, pp. 521-532, ISSN 0100-879X

Verrier, R.L. & Tan, A. (2009). Heart rate, autonomic markers, and cardiac mortality. *Heart Rhythm,* Vol.6, No.11, pp. 68-75, ISSN 1547-5271

Wang, L.; Henrich, M.; Buckler, K.J.; McMenamin, M.; Mee, C.J.; Sattelle, D.B. & Paterson, D.J. (2007). Neuronal nitric oxide synthase gene transfer decreases [Ca2+]i in cardiac sympathetic neurons. *J Mol Cell Cardiol,* Vol.43, No.6, pp.717-725, ISSN 0022-2828

Ward, G.R. & Abdel-Rahman, A.A. (2006). Orchiectomy or androgen receptor blockade attenuates baroreflex-mediated bradycardia in conscious rats. *BMC Pharmacol,* Vol.23, pp. 6-2, ISSN 1471-2210

Wikström, L.; Johansson, C.; Salto, C.; Barlow, C.; Campos Barros, A.; Baas, F.; Forrest, D.; Thorén, P. & Vennström, B. (1998). Abnormal heart rate and body temperature in mice lacking thyroid hormone receptor α1. *EMBO J,* Vol.17, pp. 455-461, ISSN 0261-4189

Workman, A.J. (2010). Cardiac adrenergic control and atrial fibrillation. *Naunyn Schmiedebergs Arch Pharmacol,* Vol.381, No.3, pp. 235-49, ISSN 0028-1298

Xing, H.; Shen, Y.; Chen, H.; Wang, Y. & Shen, W. (2001) Heart rate variability and its response to thyroxine replacement therapy in patients with hypothyroidism. *Chinese Medical Journal,* Vol.114, pp. 906-908, ISSN 0366-6999

Yanowitz, F.; Preston, J.B. & Abildskov, J.A. (1966). Functional distribution of right and left stellate innervation to the ventricles: production of neurogenic electrocardiographic changes by unilateral alteration of sympathetic tone. *Circ Res,* Vol. 28, pp. 416-428, ISSN 0009-7330

Yen, P.M. (2001). Physiological and molecular basis of thyroid hormone action. *Physiol Rev,* Vol.81, pp. 1097-1142, ISSN 0031-9333

Yu, H.; Gao, J.; Wang, H.; Wymore, R.; Steinberg, S.; McKinnon, D.; Rosen, M.R. & Cohen, I.S. (2000). Effects of the renin-angiotensin system on the current I(to) in epicardial and endocardial ventricular myocytes from the canine heart. *Circ Res,* Vol.86, No.10, pp.1062-1068, ISSN 0009-7330

Zanzinger, J.; Czachurski, J. & Seller, H. (1995). Inhibition of basal and reflex-mediated sympathetic activity in the RVLM by nitric oxide. *Am J Physiol,* Vol.268, No.4 Pt 2, pp. 958-962, ISSN 0363-6119

Zhang, Z.; Xu, Y.; Song, H.; Rodriguez, J.; Tuteja, D.; Namkung, Y.; Shin, H.S. & Chiamvimonvat, N. (2002). Functional roles of Cav1.3 (α1D) calcium channel in sinoatrial nodes: insight gained using gene-targeted null mutant mice. *Circ Res, Vol.* 90, pp.981–987, ISSN 0009-7330

9

Chronobiological Aspects of the Heart Rhythm Disorders at the Change of Pulmonary Ventilation in Rat Model

Pavol Svorc[1,2], Alexander Marossy[2], Pavol Svorc, Jr.[1], Sona Gresova[2], Marek Buzga[1] and Benjamin L. Fulton[2]
[1]Department of Physiology, Medical Faculty Ostrava University, Ostrava,
[2]Department of Physiology, Medical Faculty Safarik University, Kosice,
[1]Czech Republik
[2]Slovak Republic

1. Introduction

Presently is well established, that most physiological functions of living organisms fluctuate with a circadian dependence. Many experimental and clinical studies have demonstrated that cardiovascular functions show a marked circadian rhythmicity (Smith et al., 1987; Henry et al., 1990). Circadian fluctuations occur both in blood pressure and heart rate, but also in the ocurrence of ventricular dysrhythmias, the onset of cardiovascular symptoms, and the manifestations of cardiovascular diseases.

Ventricular fibrillation is the most dangerous type of arrhythmia in humans and belongs to the group of the most frequent causes of sudden death after myocardial infarction. The development of ventricular fibrillation is strengthened by the difference between the duration of the refractory period and irregular electrical activity in the various parts of the heart. The probability of the development of such irregular activity is increased by an increased resting excitability, a decreased conduction velocity, and an increase in automaticity (Fisch, 1973; Opie et al., 1979; Carmeliet, 1988). The resistance of the heart to these disorders is dependent on its electrical stability, which can be measured by several parameters such as the duration of the vulnerable period (Wegria et al., 1941; Axelrod et al., 1975), ventricular flutter threshold (Szekeres & Papp, 1967), excitability threshold (Jones & Klein, 1982), or ventricular fibrillation threshold (Wegria et al., 1941; Gerst et al., 1966).

Factors that contribute to the development of various cardiac disorders not only include local myocardial ischemia (Ferrier et al., 1985; Saint et al., 1992), but also hypoxia (Nishimura et al., 1989) and respiratory and metabolic acidosis (Gerst et al., 1966; Rogers et al., 1973; Kujanik et al., 1984; 1985). It is generally accepted that some disorders of pulmonary ventilation belong to the group of proarrhythmogenic factors. The effect of systemic hypoxia, hypercapnia and acidosis (consequences of hypoventilation or an apneic episode) were investigated not only in experimental studies (Kujaník et al., 1984; 1985, Tomori et al., 1997; 2000) but also in clinical ones (Guilleminault et al., 1983; Peter, 1990; Kujanik et al., 2000a; 2000b).

Surprisingly, only a few studies have described the time of day that experiments were conducted or the synchronization of animals to external environmental periodicity such as the light-dark (LD) cycle. This can be a problem because the LD cycle represents one of the strongest circadian synchronizers of endogenous animal rhythms. For this reason, circadian variability should be considered an important factor especially in cardiovascular studies.

2. Circadian rhythms of the electrical stability of the heart at the changes of the pulmonary ventilation

2.1 Circadian rhythm of the electrical stability of the heart during normal ventilation

In the cardiovascular system, most physiological phenomena (such as heart rate, blood pressure, atrioventricular conduction, etc), pathological events (cardiac ischemia, infarction, sudden cardiac death, etc.) as well as non-invasive cardiac electrophysiological phenomena (heart rate variability, T-wave alternans, QT dispersion, etc.) have circadian rhythms (Guo & Stein, 2002). Data regarding circadian patterns in arrhythmias reported in the medical literature are unclear because the data derived from almost all of the studies were confounded by a variety of factors extraneous to intrinsic arrhythmogenic activity (Portaluppi & Hermida, 2007).

Knowledge regarding circadian variations in the electrophysiological properties of the heart is needed for more precise estimation of the risk of occurrence of ventricular arrhythmia. QT dispersion is considered to be an index of spatial inhomogenity of repolarization duration; increased dispersion of ventricular repolarization is believed to increase the risk of ventricular arrhythmia. Circadian variation of QT dispersion was detected in healthy subjects and in patients with uncomplicated coronary artery disease, with a peak value in the morning hours shortly after awakening (Bissinger et al., 2008; Hansen et al., 2008). In patients with heart failure or previous myocardial infarction (Hansen et al., 2008), or in patients with diabetes mellitus and coronary artery disease (Bissinger et al., 2008), circadian variation of QT dispersion was not detected. Gunez et al. (2008) found that P-wave dispersion (a new parameter for assessing the risk of atrial fibrillation) and QT dispersion do not show diurnal variation in patients with either ischemic or nonischemic heart failure treated with optimal drug therapy.

The dependence of the electrophysiological parameters of ECG on the changing of LD cycles was also confirmed in experimental studies. The circadian fluctuation of the electrical stability of the heart, measured by ventricular arrhythmia threshold (VAT), was followed during normal ventilation, hypoventilation and hyperventilation in pentobarbital-anesthetized rats after adaptation to a daily LD cycle of 12h:12h, with the dark period from 18:00h to 6:00h for 4 weeks. The VAT was estimated as the minimal amount of electrical current (in mA) needed for elicitation of ventricular arrhythmias and was measured directly by electrical stimulation of the heart (in open-chest experiments). The stimulating electrodes (diameter 1 mm and 5 mm inter-electrode distance) were fixed at the base of the right ventricle of rats positioned supine. Cardiac stimulation (rectangular pulses with a frequency of 30 Hz, impulse lenght of 10 ms, stimulation duration of 400 ms) was triggered by the initial pulse of the R wave. Current intensity was increased progressively by steps of 0,2 mA until ventricular arrhythmias were obtained. The parameters of stimulation were chosen to apply at least one of the impulses during the vulnerable period provided that the duration of the stimulation covered a minimum of 2 to 3 heart cycles. The ventricular arrhythmias were of a mixed type with spontaneous mutual transitions between ventricular fibrillation, ventricular tachycardia and flutter which were comparable among the groups.

The 24h course of the VAT showed the highest susceptibility of the rat ventricular myocardium to arrhythmias between 12:00h and 15:00h and highest resistance between 24:00h and 03:00h under normoxic conditions (Svorc et al., 1994). Acrophase with confidence intervals were on -338⁰ (-288⁰; -7⁰), in time at 22:53h (19:20; 00:28h) with mesor 2,59 ± 0,53 mA and amplitude 0,33 ± 0,11 mA (Figure 1).

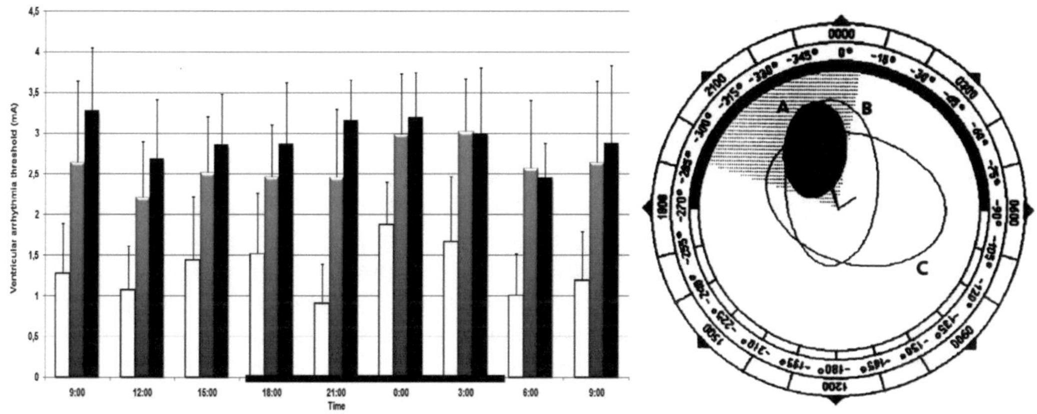

Fig. 1. Circadian rhythms of ventricular arrhythmia threshold during normal ventilation (gray columns), hypoventilation (empty columns) and hyperventilation (black columns); cosinor presentation of these rhythms during normoventilation (A), hypoventilation (B) and hyperventilation (C). Data are presented as mean ± SD. The dark bar indicates the dark cycle of the rat regime day.

Mechanisms responsible for the circadian changes in the vulnerability of the heart are probably multifactorial and are associated mainly with changes in electrophysiological properties of the myocardium. These are recognized as essential for the triggering and maintenance of arrhythmias. Portaluppi & Hermida (2007) summarized circadian rhythms of arrhythmia occurrence in humans, with peaks between 06:00h and 12:00h (ie. during the active part of the day). Similarly, during the day, when sympathetic output is enhanced and heart rate increased, P wave duration and its area, P-R interval, QRS duration and Q-T interval have been found to decrease. Estimated trough values usually occurred between 10:00h and 14:00h. During the night, following sympathetic withdrawal and parasympathetic dominance, the values of these electrical parameters increase, reaching their peak values between 12:00h and 06:00h. These changes are regulated mainly by the autonomic nervous system, which enables the heart to adapt to circadian fluctuations in demand by adjusting both its electrical activities and mechanical function (Guo & Stein, 2002).

In rats, the opposite tendency was observed. The highest vulnerability of the rat ventricular myocardium to arrhythmias occurred between 12:00h and 15:00h (non-active part of the day) and the highest resistance between 24:00h and 03:00h (active part). The possible mechanisms controlling the circadian rhythm of the VAT under normoxic conditions in rats can mainly be seen in the circadian alternations of the electrophysiological properties of the myocardium, which are determined to a large extent by a K^+ gradient (Fisch, 1973). Dispersion of duration of the refractory period (QT interval) is the result of the action of more ion currents (Ca^{2+}, Na^{+}, Cl^{-} and inward rectifying K^{+} current) (Amitzur et al., 2000), which depends mainly on intracellular K^{+} concentration (Froldi et al., 1994). The incidence of ventricular arrhythmias directly correlates with serum K^{+} decreasing with a higher K^{+} concentration (Curtis et al., 1985; Winslow et al., 1989). In circadian dependence, the peak of minimal myocardial vulnerability to ventricular arrhythmias coincides with the peak of the maximal K^{+} serum concentration in rats (Stoynev et al., 1986; Poulis et al., 1989; Granda et al., 1996). The speed of impulse conduction from atria to ventricles (PQ interval duration) depends on action potential amplitude, reflecting the active role of Na^{+} channels (Carmeliet , 1988; Amitzur et al., 2000). Statistically significant sodium circadian rhythm occurs in the dark part of the rat regime day (Granda et al., 1996), which can increase vulnerability of the heart mainly to the arrhythmias originating from disorders of impulse production and conduction. Thus, the circadian pacemaker controlling the rhythm of serum K^{+} likely plays a key role in the circadian control of the VAT in rats under normal ventilatory conditions.

The next mechanism directly controlling the circadian rhythm of the electrical stability of the heart, involves the autonomic nervous system. Circadian rhythms in the autonomic nervous system activity are well known and constitute major triggers of cardiac arrhythmias. Increased sympathetic activity accelerates heart rate, favors spontaneous depolarization, shortens the effective ventricular refractory period, and decreases the threshold for ventricular fibrillation. In contrast, increased parasympathetic activity slows heart rate, decreases atrioventricular (AV) nodal conduction and in the presence of baseline sympathetic neural activity, increases both the ventricular refractory period and the ventricular fibrillation threshold (VFT) (reviewed in Portaluppi & Hermida, 2007). This direct and clear dependence, described in humans and in larger experimental animals, was not confirmed in rats (Svorc et al., 1994). The course and acrophase of the circadian rhythm of heart rate did not correspond either to the course or to the acrophase of the circadian rhythm of the VAT. Loss of heart rate dependence on the LD cycle refers to the fact that pentobarbital anesthesia probably minimizes or disturbs the effect of the LD cycle on heart rate under conditions of normal pulmonary ventilation. These results are consistent with results of Bruguerolle's group, who demonstrated the pertubations of daily rhythm of heart rate, locomotor activity and body temperature in rats but under ketamine anaesthesia. Total anaesthesia can probably modify the acrophase, mesor and amplitude of some rhythms but without the loss of the total rhythmicity (Prudian et al., 1997; Pelissier et al., 1998).

2.2 Circadian rhythm of the electrical stability of the heart during hypoventilation

Hypoxic states of the heart result from disproportionate amounts of oxygen supplied to cardiac cells and the amount actually required by the cell. The degree of hypoxic injury does not only depend on the intensity and duration of the hypoxic stimulus, but also on the level of cardiac tolerance to oxygen deprivation. Such oxygen deprivation can result from systemic hypoxia or local ischemia with consequences of two different mechanisms of action at the cellular level. Systemic hypoxia is usually a generalized phenomenon diffusely involving the whole myocardium, whereas ischemia is confined to the area supplied by the affected coronary artery. In ischemia, there is not only a drop in the supply of oxygen and other substrates, but also a significant reduction in the clearance of metabolites. In contrast, in ischemic hypoxia (often described as „cardiac hypoxia“) there is a combined action of both ischemia and hypoxia, while perfusion results in partial elimination of metabolites.

Ischemic hypoxia is clinically manifested primarily in ischemic heart disease (coronary artery disease) and its acute form, myocardial infarction, whereas systemic hypoxia is associated with chronic cor pulmonale of various origin, cyanosis due to a hypoxemic congenital heart disease, exposure to low barometric pressure (e.g. at high altitudes and ventilatory disorders) (Ostadal et al., 1999).

The effects of ventilatory disorders on the heart were broadly investigated in more experimental animal studies and under various experimental conditions. Failure of, or decrease in pulmonary ventilation is associated with systemic hypoxia, hypercapnia and acidosis resulting in various disorders of cardiovascular system activity.

There are some clinical trials describing the circadian rhythmicity of the cardiovascular events associated with changes in pulmonary ventilation. We cite the study by Kujanik et al. (2010) who referred to the incidence of the supraventricular and ventricular extrasystoles in healthy elderly men at low (200 m) and moderate altitude (1350 m) in the circadian dependence. The moderate altitude with the lower pO_2 shifted the highest occurrence of supraventricular and vetricular extrasystoles to the other times of day and increased the incidence of extrasystoles compared to low altitude by 2-fold. The authors concluded that the increase in extrasystole occurrence at high altitudes is probably caused by higher hypobaric hypoxia and resulting sympathetic drive. Healthy men at elevated altitudes show circadian and several ultradian rhythms of single ventricular extrasystoles dependent on the level of hypoxia.

Sleep, ventilatory disorders, especially obstructive or central sleep apnea (OSA or CSA), are associated with neurohormonal and electrophysiological abnormalities that may increase the risk of sudden death from cardiac causes, especially during sleep. Gami et al. (2005) followed this dependence in 112 subjects who died suddenly from cardiac causes. They found that from midnight to 06:00h, sudden death from cardiac causes occurred in 46% of patients with OSA compared with 21% of individuals without OSA. Patients who experienced sudden death from cardiac causes from midnight to 06:00h, had a significantly higher apnea-hypopnea index than those with sudden death from cardiac causes during other intervals, and the apnea-hyponea index correlated directly with the relative risk of sudden death from cardiac causes from midnight to 06:00h. Thus, individuals with OSA experience a peak in sudden death from cardiac causes during the hours of sleep, which contrasts strikingly with the nadir of sudden death from cardiac causes during this period in people without OSA. Variation in the onset of myocardial infarction was found in patients with and without OSA. Myocardial infarction occurred between midnight and 06:00h in 32% of OSA patients and 7% of non-OSA patients. Of all patients who experienced a myocardial infarction between midnight and 06:00h, 91% had OSA (Kuniyoshi et al., 2008). These findings suggest that OSA may be a trigger for myocardial infarction in patients who experience nocturnal onset of myocardial infarction should be evaluated for OSA. Future research should address the effects of OSA therapy for prevention of nocturnal cardiac events. These studies refer to the fact that circadian rhythmicity may have practical relevance in screening for patients with OSA and may have prognostic clinical value in predicting future cardiovascular events (Gami et al., 2005; Kuniyoshi et al., 2008).

In experimental animal models, the link between disorders of pulmonary ventilation and the incidence of ventricular arrhythmias was also demonstrated in the circadian dependence. Otsuka & Watanabe (1990) followed the circadian rhythms of three types of bradyarrhythmia incidence in rats. The 24h chronogram of bradyarrhythmia incidence showed 2 peaks: the higher peak between 05:00h and 09:00h (immediately after the start of the light cycle) and the second one between 11:00h and 18:00h. The hourly distribution of the apnea index coincided with the highest peak of the 24h chronogram of bradyarrhythmia incidence in rats. In ketamine/xylazine-anesthetized rats from experiments performed by Bacova et al. (2010), RR and PQ interval duration showed the significant LD differences, except in the QT and QTc interval in spontaneously breathing animals. The initial significant LD differences in PQ interval and loss of dependence on LD cycle in the QT interval were preserved during short-term asphyxia induced by apneic episode (30 s to 60 s). In contrast, long-term asphyxia (90 s to 120 s) eliminated LD dependence in the PQ interval; however, significant LD differences were shown in the QT interval. It was concluded that myocardial vulnerability was dependent not only on changes in pulmonary ventilation but also on the LD cycle.

In our hypoventilatory rat model, hypoventilation-induced systemic hypoxia, hypercapnia and acidosis decreased the VAT and heart rate values in all measured intervals during a 24h period. The mesor (1, 33 mA), amplitude (0,14 mA) was decreased, and the circadian rhythm of the VAT was changed to biphasic with a smaller peak between 15:00h and 18:00h and higher peak between 24:00h and 03:00h. The hypoventilatory circadian rhythm of the VAT was not significant as revealed by the population mean cosinor (Svorc et al., 1997, 2000a) (Figure 1).

The decreased electrical stability of the heart during the course of the entire 24h period confirmed results from other electrophysiological studies investigating the effect of hypoxia on myocardium. The duration of the action potential was significantly decreased at the start of hypoxia in isolated hearts of rats (Perchenet and Kreher, 1995), rabbits (Baker et al., 2001), cats (Vleugels et al., 1980), guinea pigs (Sanguinetti et al., 1988) and dogs (Ferrier et al. 1985). The phase plateau of action potential shortened, and ATP content decreased (Noma, 1983). In isolated rabbit AV preparations, hypoxia impaired AV nodal conduction and depressed automaticity (Nishimura et al., 1989). In *in vivo* rabbit models, the sinus interval was gradually increased with duration of hypoxia. Atrio-His interval and His-ventricular intervals were prolonged (Sawanobori et al., 1995). The membrane potential was decreased, excitability and impulse conduction between Purkinje fibres and muscle tissue were depressed in isolated Purkinje fibres of papillary muscle from dogs (Ferrier et al. 1985).

In experiments using cats, hypercapnic hypoxemia produced N_2 inhalation and evoked all types of conduction blockades, supraventricular extrasystoles, peaked T waves, elevated ST segments and decreases in R waves (Tomori et al., 1997; 2000). In experiments conducted by Gerst et al. (1966) using dogs, pH changes owing to respiratory acidosis and alkalosis did not affect the electrical stability of the heart, measured by VFT. Neither respiratory acidosis nor hypoxia alone significantly changed the VFT, but together they increased the followed parameter in the canine ventricle (Rogers et al., 1973). Kujanik et al. (1985) described dynamic changes of the VFT in rats with various types of ventilation, but not its circadian dependence. The VFT was decreased during mild hypoxia and acidosis and increased during serious hypoxia and acidosis. The vulnerable duration period was prolonged during hypoventilation.

These disorders can be explained by a sudden increase in extracellular K^+ concentration, which plays a crucial role in the changes in resting membrane potential, and can produce ectopic activity as well as inhibition of the rapid reaction (Opie et al., 1979). The rapid increase in extracellular K^+ concentration is the result of K_{ATP} channel activation. It is

inactivated in normoxic conditions, but it is activated in hypoxic or anoxic conditions (Noma & Shibasaki, 1985; Sanguinetti et al., 1988; Daut et al., 1990; Billman et al., 1993). During ischemia, activation of K_{ATP} channels limits Ca^{2+} input into metabolically stressed cells. In ischemic regions, it can lead to the dispersion of refractory periods between normal and ischemic myocardium; thus, the blockade of K_{ATP} channels acts as an antiarrhythmic (Wolleben et al., 1989). On the other hand, no correlation between total ATP concentration and the electrical activity of the heart was found during relative hypoxia or ischemia of the myocardium (Kreher & Wedetti, 1986). We can suppose that the mechanism of K^+ current activation by hypoxia can also be responsible for changes in the electrical stability of the heart in circadian dependence, although the biphasic course of VAT is not specifically explained by this mechanism.
The control mechanisms responsible for the biphasic circadian course in the electrical stability of the heart during hypoventilation are not known, they are probably multifactorial and are mainly associatedwith changes in the electrophysiological properties of myocardium in hypoxic conditions. The biphasic course can be partly explained by the effect of histamine on rat ventricular arrhythmias under hypoxic conditions. Dai (1989) demonstrated that hypoxia and histamine can increase susceptibility to arrhythmias. If hypoxia does not alter the circadian rhythm of blood histamine levels, then increased myocardial susceptibility to arrhythmias can be in the certain range influenced by histamine under the hypoxic conditions. Our results from a hypoventilatory rat model support this hypothesis. The very close relationship is between rhythm of the electrical stability of the heart and the rhythm of histamine concentration in the blood. In a rat model, Catini & Legnaioli (1992) showed (upon synchronization to a natural lighted regime) that circadian oscillations in histamine concentration in the blood and in the thyroid gland are biphasic, with peaks at 07:50h and at 19:50h, in time the lowest VAT.

2.3 Circadian rhythm of the electrical stability of the heart during hyperventilation

In our experiments, hyperventilation increased the VAT at each measurement interval, but did not change the characteristic of its circadian rhythm. The 24h hyperventilatory rhythm of the VAT was non-significant, acrophase was shifted to -40^0 (02:40h), mesor was increased (2,91 mA) and amplitude was decreased (0,13 mA) (Figure 1) (Svorc et al., 2002). Although the results are not unequivocal, these ventilatory changes probably have a causal relationship with disorders of ion kinetics and/or ion distributions inside and outside of myocardial cells, and also with circadian dependence. From what is currently known, if the electrical stability of the heart is dependent on ion concentration changes, it follows that circadian rhythm of the VAT most probably behaves similarly to the circadian rhythms of the single ions. The unanswered question is how does light and dark act on ion kinetics ventilatory disorders and on return to normal ventilatory conditions, after synchronization to a 12h:12h LD regime?

3. The electrical stability of the heart in a hypoventilation/reoxygenation model

The onset and development of ventricular arrhythmias depends on many factors to which some disorders of pulmonary ventilation also belong. However, not all consider the effect of the recovery of oxygen delivery (reoxygenation) after hypoxic episodes to be the onset or development of ventricular arrhythmias. Reoxygenation after hypoxic episodes does not automatically normalize myocardial properties (electrophysiological and mechanical), but can increase the risk of onset of reoxygenation arrhythmias (Winslow et al., 1983; Perchenet & Kreher, 1995; Bilinska et al., 1996; Bernauer, 1997; Mubagwa et al., 1997; Shinmura et al., 1997; Guo et al. 2005).

Tissue hypoxia, for example in patients with sleep apnea, is an important factor in heart disease (Yokoe et al., 2003). Hypoxia and reoxygenation expose the myocardium to extremes in redox stress, which can result in the initiation of a series of cellular pathways leading to tissue injury and death. Myocardial hypoxia reduces left ventricular contractile performance (Tanonaka et al., 1989; Draper & Shah, 1997; Jeroudi et al., 1994; Kang et al., 2000); however, recovery of the contractile force was less than 10% and recovery of the myocardial high-energy phosphates during reoxygenation was approximately 40% (Tanonaka et al., 1989).

The study by Pahor et al. (1989) demostrated the antiarrhythmic effect of verapamil on spontaneous ventricular arrhythmias during reoxygenation after 15 min of glucose-free hypoxia and on programmed electrical stimulation-induced ventricular fibrillation in isolated Langendorff-perfused guinea pig hearts. Verapamil added during reoxygenation reduced the incidence of reoxygenation arrhythmias and ventricular fibrillation, but it had no effect on programmed stimulation-induced ventricular fibrillation. It is likely that verapamil exerts its antiarrhythmic effect by preventing cellular calcium overload during hypoxia and reoxygenation.

Hypoxia and mild acidosis progressively diminished the amplitude and duration of these slow-response action potentials, whereas reperfusion/reoxygenation progressively increased their amplitude even more than that in the control (prehypoxic value). Action potential duration increased (at all levels) during reperfusion compared with that in hypoxia and mild acidosis; however, action potential duration remained shorter than the control (prehypoxic level). The effects of hypoxia (and mild acidosis) and subsequent reoxygenation seem similar to the effects of elevating extracellular kalcium levels (increased inward current). From these experiments, one cannot, however, distinguish the effects of hypoxia on the inward currents from those on the outward currents (Bhattacharyya & Acharya, 1988). The response of hypoxic and acidotic ventricular muscle tissue to subsequent reoxygenation was studied by Bhattacharyya et al. (1991). Ventricular muscle tissue exhibited the different response to reoxygenation after hypoxia and acidosis: (1) arrhythmias, without much depolarization of the membrane potential; (2) oscillatory afterpotentials during the late diastole, which lessened in amplitude as the time of reoxygenation increased, but no arrhythmias; or (3) a pronounced slowed phase of repolarization (hump), but no arrhythmias. These different effects of reoxygenation did not occur if the concentration of K^+ in hypoxic and acidotic ventricular muscle tissue was much higher than 4.6 mM. Common to these three different responses was the prolongation of the action potential duration during reoxygenation at the 50% and 90% levels of repolarization (APD_{50} and APD_{90}) and a slight increase in the resting tension after 30 to 40 min. of reoxygenation.

Membrane potential changes of atrial fibroblasts in response to mechanical stress have been considered to modulate the rhythmic electrical activity of healthy hearts. It is suggested that cardiac arrhythmia after infarction is related to enhanced susceptibility of fibroblasts to physical stretch. It indicates that transmembrane currents in atrial fibroblasts are sensitive to changes in tissue oxygenation and altered electro-mechanical function of the ischemic heart may involve changes in the membrane potential of cardiac fibroblasts (Kamkin et al., 2003).

The proarrhythmogenic effect of reoxygenation was confirmed by several studies using various agents. For example, in the papillary muscles of guinea pigs, Ca^{2+} entry through Ca^{2+} channels apparently synchronized Ca^{2+} release from the sarcoplasmic reticulum, and a high concentration of D-600 apparently decreased the incidence of arrhythmias. Tetrodoxin and nicorandil decreased arrhythmias, probably by decreasing the Na^+ current or by increasing the ATP-sensitive K^+ current, respectively (Hayashida et al., 1996). Thus nicorandil antagonizes the cellular mechanisms that underlie the reoxygenation arrhythmias and prevent reoxygenation-induced arrhythmias (Xu et al., 1993). The effects of a selective blocker of Ca^{2+} influx by Na^+/Ca^{2+} exchange, KB-R7943, on the reoxygenation-induced arrhythmias and the recovery of developed tension after reoxygenation, were investigated in guinea pig papillary muscles. This blocker selectively inhibited the reverse mode of Na^+/Ca^{2+} exchange, attenuated reoxygenation-induced arrhythmic activity and prevented contractile dysfunction in guinea pig papillary muscles. These results suggest that Ca^{2+} influx by Na^+/Ca^{2+} exchange may play a key role in reoxygenation injury (Mukai et al., 2000).

It is well established that hypoxia followed by reperfusion may be fatal and result in generation of reactive oxygen species (ROS) and subsequent tissue damage (Danielsson et al., 2007) and is associated with additional damage to the myocardium by oxidation of cellular components and activation of the inflammatory cascade (Cerniway et al., 2002). Some of isoflurane's cellular actions, such as interference with intracellular Ca^{2+} handling, inhibition of the respiratory chain, and the capability to produce oxygen radicals, could result in impaired cellular function during ischemia/reoxygenation. When isoflurane was applied during ischemia/reperfusion, intracellular Ca^{2+}, oxygen radical formation, arrhythmic events, and contractile function were increased in rat cardiomyocytes. Furthermore, increased oxygen radical generation was detected in isoflurane-treated myocytes during reoxygenation. Isoflurane given during ischemia/reperfusion in a study by Dworschak et al. (2004) induced intracellular Ca^{2+} accumulation and impaired cell function. These potentially harmful effects were associated with diminished Ca^{2+} clearance and accelerated oxygen radical production. In clinical practice, reperfusion of ischemic myocardium usually occurs under high arterial oxygen levels. However, this might aggravate cardiac ischemia/reperfusion injury caused by excessive oxidative stress. In an experimental *in vivo* study, the cardioprotective role of hypoxic reoxygenation during initial reperfusion was assessed. Hypoxic reoxygenation at the onset of reperfusion attenuated myocardial ischemia/reperfusion injury and helped to preserve cardiac performance after myocardial ischemia in a pig model (Abdel-Rahman et al., 2009).

The mitochondrial K_{ATP} channel (mitoK_{ATP}) opening which can be triggered by activation of the angiotensin II (Ang II) type 1 receptor on ischemia/reperfusion causes ROS-induced ROS release. The electrophysiological actions of Ang II linked with the genesis of reperfusion arrhythmias were elucidated by clarifying the roles of Ang II and mitoK_{ATP} on cardiac impulse propagation. MitoK_{ATP} blocker and AT1 receptor blocker abolished conduction block and conduction delay induced by Ang II. This result demonstrated that a mitoK_{ATP} channnel blocker protectively associated with arrhythmogenesis properties during reoxygenation (Wakatsuki et al., 2009). The inhibition of inducible nitric oxide (NO) synthese (NOS) raises the peroxidative and apoptotic level in the hypoxic heart indicating that this isoform may have a protective effect on this organ against hypoxia/reoxygenation injuries, and challenges the conventional wisdom that isoforms of NOS are deleterious under these conditions. These findings could help in the design of

new treatments based on NO pharmacology against hypoxia/reoxygenation dysfunctions (Rus et al., 2011).
In contrast to previous evidence about the harmful effect of reoxygenation on myocardium, Milano et al. (2010) refer to the protective effect of chronic hypoxia against ischemia/reperfusion damage. In rat experiments, exposure to chronic hypoxia results in impairment of myocardial tolerance to ischemia/reperfusion, greater injury and reduced recovery of performance. Daily reoxygenation markedly reduced hypoxia-induced derangements by accelerating intrinsic adaptive changes in the myocardium. These findings correlate with enhanced NO signalling via up-regulation of the endothelial isoform of NOS.
Studies investigating the effect of ischemia/reperfusion or hypoxia/reoxygenation on the onset and development of ventricular arrhythmias concentrate mainly on the temporally current mechanical and metabolic changes in myocardial cells, often without respect to circadian dependence. The question remains whether vulnerability of the ventricles to arrhythmias is primarily changed only by the factors resulting from altered ventilation, or are there also natural factors (eg, environmental periodicities) that can influence the parameter being studied?

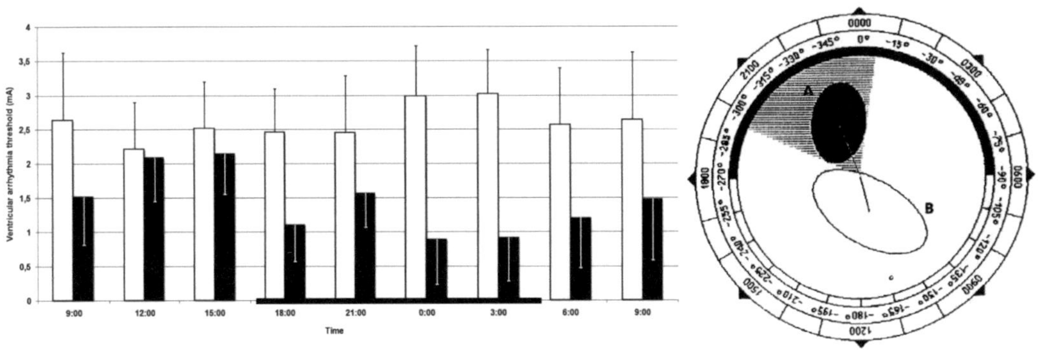

Fig. 2. Circadian rhythms of the ventricular arrhythmia threshold during normoventilation (empty columns) and reoxygenation after hypoventilation (black columns); cosinor presentation of these rhythms during normoventilation (A) and reoxygenation (B). Data presented as mean ± SD. The dark bar indicates the dark cycle of the rat regime day.

The analysis of VAT circadian rhythms was performed in a hypoventilation/reoxygenation group, in which pentobarbital anaesthetized animals were subjected to 20 min. of hypoventilation followed by 20 min. of reoxygenation. Reoxygenation expressively altered the VAT circadian rhythms inversely compared to the control group. Biphasic character was kept only after 5 min. of reoxygenation. 10, 15 and 20 min. of reoxygenation gradually changed the VAT circadian courses to inverse ones with the highest values between 12:00h and 15:00h and lowest values between 24:00h and 03:00h. The mesor was decreased (1,41 mA), amplitude was increased (0,57 mA) and acrophases was on -165^0 (Figure 2).
A more detailed analysis of the circadian VAT changes after 5., 10., 15. and 20. min. hypoventilation showed that the acrophases from 10., 15. and 20 min, of hypoventilation were nonsignificantly shifted compared to 5 min. of hypoventilation (Table 1). The characteristic biphasic course of the circadian rhythms of VAT was seen only after 10 min. of hypoventilation (Figure 3) (Svorc et al., 2000b, 2002).

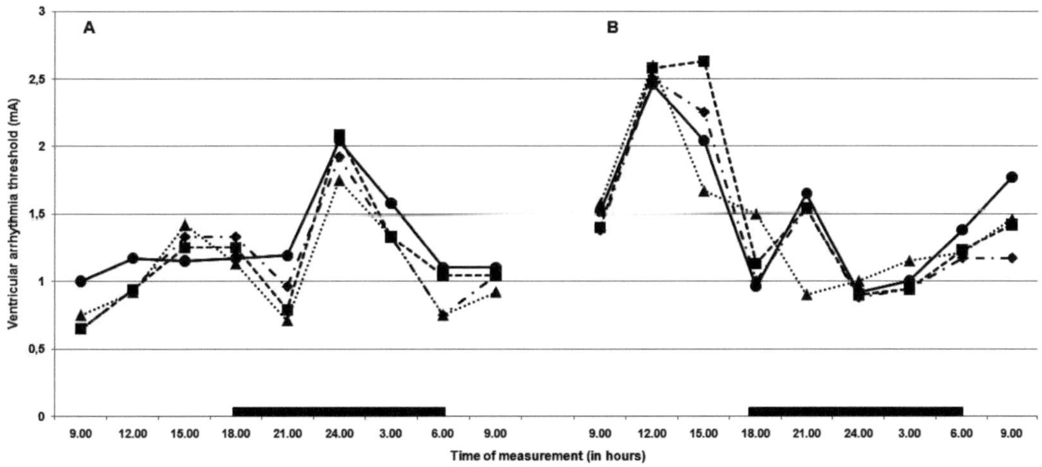

Fig. 3. Circadian rhythms of the ventricular arrhythmia threshold from hypoventilation/reoxygenation model after 5 min. (circles), 10 min. (squares), 15 min. (rhombus) and 20 min. (triangles) of the respective ventilation. A – initial hypoventilation, B – subsequent reoxygenation. The dark bar indicates the dark cycle.

	Initial hypoventilation				Subsequent reoxygenation			
	5 min.	10 min.	15 min.	20 min.	5 min.	10 min.	15 min.	20 min.
Mesor	1.32±0.1	1.17±0.2	0.15±0.2	0.12±0.1	1.41±0.1	1.41±0.1	1.29±0.1	1.42±0.1
Amplitude	0.33±0.2	0.33±0.2	0.35±0.2	0.20±0.2	0.41±0.2	0.48±0.1	0.37±0.2	0.53±0.1
Acrophase								
in degrees	-356±25	-11±37	-36±30	-30±58	-166±24	-165±17	-172±29	-156±10
in hours	23:50±1.40	00:44±2.28	02:24±2.00	02:50±2.32	11:04±1.36	11:00±1.08	11:28±1.56	10:24±0.4

Table 1. Parameters of the circadian rhythms of the ventricular arrythmia threshold (VAT) in a rat model of hypoventilation/reoxygenation.

Results from an experimental study involving ketamine/xylazine-anaesthetized rats (Svorc et al., 2005) indicated that although the electrical stability of the rat heart did not demostrate a dependence on LD cycle during normal pulmonary ventilation (probably an effect of ketamine/xylazine anaesthesia), hypoventilation/reoxygenation changed myocardial vulnerability by a manner dependent on LD cycle. It appears that rat myocardium is probably more sensitive to systemic asphyxia induced by hypoventilation and reoxygenation during the light (non-active) part of the day (Figure 4).

Hypoventilation and recovery of pulmonary ventilation produce different myocardial responses to electrical stimulation of the heart in individual animals. The reactions of animals to electrical stimulation under different ventilation conditions in both light parts of the day are shown in Table 2. A X^2-test was performed on the basis of these individual responses in the aspect of previous threshold values for evaluating the effect on the LD cycle. The significant effect of the LD cycle on the VAT changes was conformed for the period of hypoventilation ($p < 0{,}05$) as well as reoxygenation ($p < 0{,}01$), respectively.

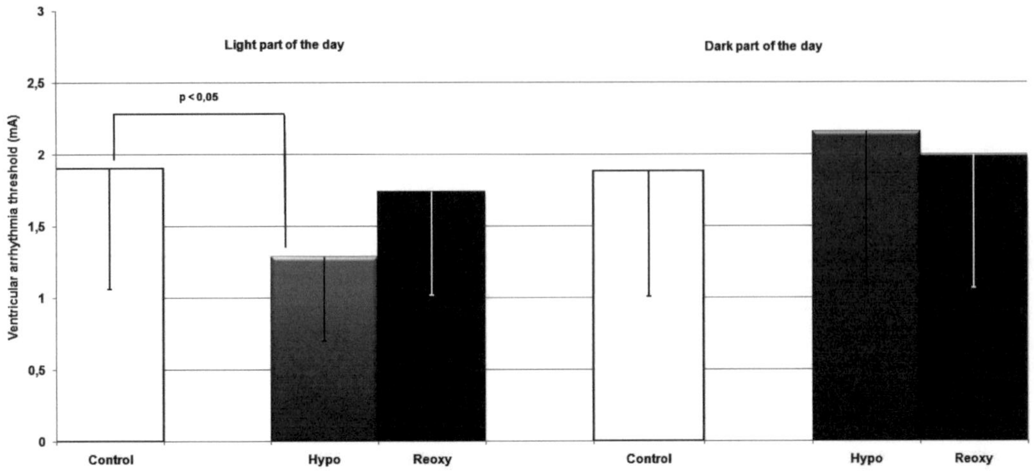

Fig. 4. The changes of the VAT in the hypoventilation (Hypo)/reoxygenation (Reoxy) rat model in the light and dark part of the regime day. Control - VAT value after the surgical interventions (tracheotomy, thoracotomy) and 5 min. stabilization at the parameters of normal artificial pulmonary ventilation (empty column - light and dark group). Hypo - the average VAT value from measurement after 5, 10, 15 and 20 min. of hypoventilation (gray columns). Reoxy - the average VAT value from measurement after 5, 10, 15 and 20 min. of reoxygenation (black columns).

	Hypoventilation vs. control		Reoxygenation vs. hypoventilation	
	Light	Dark	Light	Dark
VAT decrease	10/11 (90,9 %)	7/19 (36,8 %)	2/12 (18,2 %)	13/19 (68,4 %)
VAT increase	1/11 (9,1 %)	12/19 (63,2 %)	9/11 (81,8 %)	6/19 (31,6 %)

Table 2. Individual responses of animals to electrical stimulation of the heart. Numerator - number of animals with VAT changes against the previous VAT measurement, denominator - number of animals in experimental group.

As mentioned above, alterations in myocardial vulnerability depend mainly on changes in ion concentrations. LD differences in the electrical stability of the heart might reflect the LD differences in ion concentrations. In hypoxia/reoxygenation or ischemia/reperfusion models, more authors describe myocardial Ca^{2+} accumulation. Ca^{2+} overload in myocytes is one of the many causes of the reperfusion injury (Kamiyama et al., 1996; Mubagwa et al., 1997; Shinmura et al., 1997; Sharikabad et al., 2000). It was hypothetized that the delayed afterdepolarizations producing the substrate for arrhythmogenesis of the serious ventricular dysrhythmias (Ca-mediated, non re-entry arrhythmias) are the result of such Ca^{2+} overload (Whalley et al., 1995). Sharikabad et al. (2000) describe unchanged intracellular concentration of Ca^{2+} ions during hypoxia, but concentrations were 3 to 4 times higher during reoxygenation in isolated rat hearts. During reoxygenation of hypoxic rat cardiomyocytes there is a correlation between extracellular Ca^{2+} and ROS (the second factor involved in ischemia/reperfusion-induced cardiomyocyte damage), whereas the correlation between cell Ca^{2+} and ROS levels is less consistent. These results indicate that ROS levels during oxidative stress are at least partly dependent on extracellular Ca^{2+} concentration, but

ROS (H_2O_2) can increase or decrease cardiomyocyte Ca^{2+} accumulation during reoxygenation in a concentration-dependent manner (Sharikabad et al., 2004). Decrease of intracellular pH can also participate in the mechanism of myocardial reoxygenation damage. This decrease is mediated, at least in part, by anion exchange stimulation (Cl^-/HCO_3^- exchange) through protein kinase C activation. This exchange takes part in the reoxygenation-induced Ca^{2+} overload and in contractile dysfunction (Kawasaki et al., 2001). The decrease in electrical stability of the heart can also be the result of cellular K^+ loss during hypoxia (Shivkumar et al., 1997). Hypoxia (Perchenet & Kreher, 1995) significantly decreases action potential duration probably through the activation of the K_{ATP} channels and increased K^+ ion efflux. The inhibition of the outward K^+ currents showed the cardioprotective effect during reperfusion (Liu et al., 1993; Tosaki et al., 1996). The increase of intracellular concentration of Na^+ ions in myocardial cells, and Ca^{2+} overload, can contribute to the rise of reoxygenation arrhythmias (Takeo et al., 1995; Kamiyama et al., 1996; Shinmura et al., 1997).

Systemic hypoxia induced by hypoventilation changed the electrical stability of the rat heart in dependence on the LD cycle. Although the VAT decreased parallelly in both light parts of day during 20 min. hypoventilation, it was demonstrated that 1. The significant higher average VAT values were in the dark part of the day (active phase) versus the light part (non-active phase); 2. Rat hearts are more resistant to systemic hypoxia in the dark part of the day; and 3. The significant decrease of the VAT refer to the proarrhythmogenic effect of the systemic hypoxia only in the light part of day. These differences are probablya result of the changed myocardial reactivity to electrical stimulation dependent on the LD cycle.

Although reoxygenation returned VAT level to that of control values in both light (non-active) and dark (active) parts of the day, the problem remains that the VAT was significantly increased versus hypoventilatory value only in the light part of the day. The contrary tendency was found in the dark part of the day. The decrease in the dark part of the day probably signals the larger extent of the reoxygenation injury or increased sensitivity of the myocardium to the ventricular arrhythmias in the dark part of the day. This fact is supported by our previous results in rats under pentobarbital anaesthesia, where the nadir of the VAT circadian rhythm was found between 24:00h and 03:00h during reoxygenation (Svorc et al., 2000a).

The significant hypoventilatory LD differences in the thresholds show the different LD effects of hypoventilation–induced systemic asphyxia on the electrical stability of the rat heart. The higher values in the dark part of the day are probably the result of varying myocardial sensitivity to systemic asphyxia in the LD dependence, although there are more reports referring to the depressive effect of hypoxia on the circadian rhythms in rats (Bishop et al., 2000; 2001; Fenelon et al., 2000; Mortola & Seifert, 2000), in golden hamsters (Jarsky & Stephenson, 2000), and in humans (Bosco et al., 2003). An important and still unanswered question remains: whether the mechanisms responsible for altered myocardial vulnerability are mobilized mainly by hypoventilation-induced systemic asphyxia and reoxygenation with the additive effect of the LD cycle, or are they mobilized by the factors oscillating in the circadian dependence, with the additive effect of hypoventilation/reoxygenation?

4. Chronobiological aspects of preconditioning by systemic asphyxia

4.1 Ventricular arrhythmia threshold - A measure of the electrical stability of the heart

There is ample evidence that repeating brief periods of myocardial ischemia and reperfusion may provide protection against electrical instability of the heart evoked by subsequent ischemia/reperfusion injury. This mechanism, known as ischemic preconditioning (IPC), was first suggested by Reimer et al. (1981) and later elaborated on by Murry et al. (1986).

Similar cardioprotective effects, albeit of variable intensity, have been obtained after pre-treatment with repetitive episodes of hypoxia, which may provide clinical benefit over ischemia in that systemic blood flow into critical organs remains stable (Shizukuda et al., 1993). Most of the available information regarding hypoxic preconditioning (HPC) has come from *in vitro* studies on isolated perfused hearts using transient local hypoxia.

Therefore, it is important to know whether HPC with hypoventilation can also reduce experimentally induced ventricular arrhythmias or increase the electrical stability of the heart against the effect of a prolonged subsequent period of hypoventilation and reoxygenation. We hypothesized that 1. If hypoventilation, similar to ischemia, decreases the electrical stability of the heart, HPC with hypoventilation could have an effect comparable to IPC. Moreover, we focused on whether there were differences in the conditions and dynamics of the developing protective effects of myocardial PC applied during the light (nonactive) and dark (active) parts of the rat regime day and aimed to obtain an understanding of the chronophysiological aspects of this phenomenon in *in vivo* rat experiments; 2. If the autonomic nervous system participates in IPC-induced cardioprotection, it would also participate in the process of HPC. If the autonomic nervous system plays a role in HPC, the effect would depend on external periodicity because cardiovascular and autonomic nervous functions show dependence on 24h periodicity. Thus, the design was aimed to examine the effect of the LD cycle adaptation on the VAT, marker of the electrical stability of the heart, and on heart rate responses, as a marker of autonomic drive, during the post-anaesthetic state, hypoventilatory hypoxia and cardiac preconditioning induced by repeated asphyxias *in vivo* (Svorc & Bracokova, 2003; Svorc & Benacka, 2008; Svorc et al, 2011).

The main aim of these studies was to gain information about the chronophysiological aspect of cardioprotection by hypoventilation-induced asphyxia preconditioning in *in vivo* rat experiments. The experiments were performed in anaesthetized (ketamine/xylazine anaesthesia, ketamine 100 mg/kg [Narkamon, Prague] + xylazine 15 mg/kg [Rometar, Prague] i.m) rats (weight, 300 ± 15 g; 3 to 4 months of age). The rats were adaptated to a LD cycle of 12h:12h, with the dark part of day from 06:00h to 18:00h for 4 weeks and they were divided into 4 groups. During the experiments, all animals were subjected to 20 min of artificial hypoventilation-induced asphyxia, followed by a 20 min recovery period (reoxygenation). The first group of animals was not preconditioned (n = 19) and the other three experimental groups were preconditioned by one (1PC group; n = 9), two (2PC group; n = 15), and three (3PC group n = 11) 5 min cycles of hypoventilation (5 min), each separated by 5 min cycles of reoxygenation (Scheme 1).

The chest was opened by parasternal thoracotomy and after gentle mediastinal preparation, the heart was exposed. The VAT was estimated as the minimal amount of electrical current (mA) needed for elicitation of ventricular arrhythmias by direct electrical stimulation of the heart (400 ms series of rectangular pulses; frequency, 30 Hz; and 10 ms impulse lengths). Stimuli were triggered by the onset of the R wave in lead II of the ECG and the current intensity was increased progressively by steps of 0.2 mA until ventricular arrhythmias were obtained. Recovery of the sinus rhythm was spontaneous. Control recordings of VAT were performed after surgical interventions and a 5 min period of artificial ventilation with the parameters of the normal pulmonary ventilation. Values of VAT were measured in the 5th, 10th, 15th, and 20th min of hypoventilation and in the same intervals during ventilatory recovery.

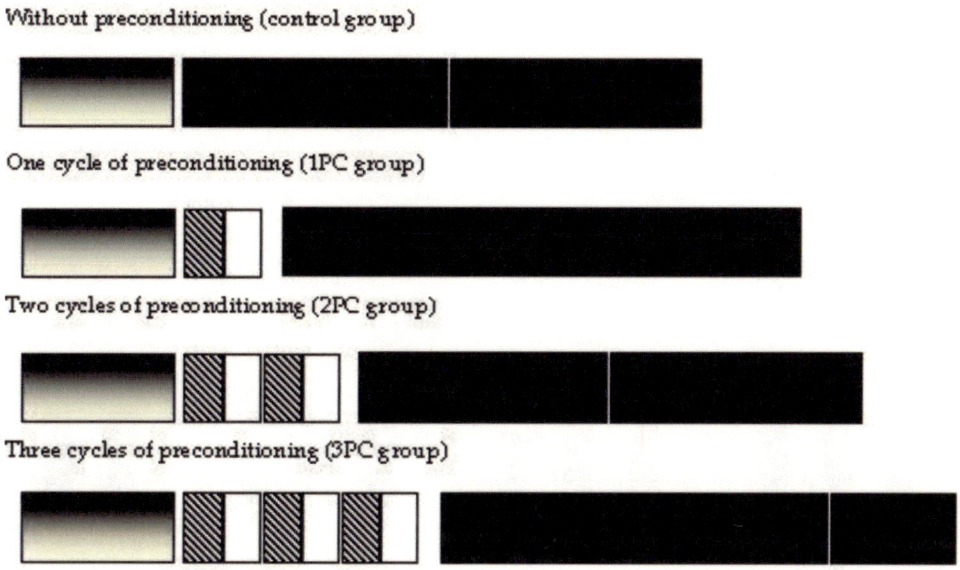

Scheme 1. Protocol of experiments using preconditioning (PC) by systemic asphyxia. The black-white columns refer to the initial phase of experiments with heating of the animals to the rectal temperature measured before the application of the anaesthetic agent, tracheotomy, thoracotomy, 5 min. period of stabilization (normal artificial ventilation at the parameters of the artificial ventilation V_T 1 ml/100 g of body weight and respiratory rate 50 breaths/min.). The hatched columns represent 5 min. cycles of PC by systemic asphyxia. The empty bars represent 5 min. cycles of reoxygenation, while the black columns represent 20 min. cycles of hypoventilation.

The measurement of heart rate (the mean value of the last 4 cycles) was performed in intact animals (before the surgical interventions in the supine position, spontaneous breathing), after tracheotomy and thoracotomy, after each minute of 5 min. stabilization (the parameters of the normal artificial ventilation), after each minute of PC cycles by systemic asphyxia and after each minute of 20 min. hypoventilation. Because the animals from each group passed through the same conditions from the start of the experiment, heart ratee were summed and one average value was calculated for intact animals (Ini), after the tracheotomy (Tr), thoracotomy (To), during the period of stabilization (Stabil) and during the single cycles of asphyxic PC.

Animals were artificially ventilated by humidified room air at the parameters of the initial ventilation and reoxygenation: respiratory rate 40 breaths/min. and tidal volume 1 ml/100g body weight. During experimental hypoventilatory asphyxia, the respiratory rate and tidal volume were reduced to 20 breaths/min and 0.5 ml/100g b.w., respectively. The respiratory effect of the ventilation was monitored by the analysis of the pH, pO_2, pCO_2, and O_2 saturation from blood samples taken from the femoral artery.

The control values of VATs in the experimental groups did not show any significant difference, although systematically higher values were found during the dark part of the day compared to the light part of the day (control light, 1,87 ± 0,80 mA vs. control dark, 2,12 ± 0,93 mA; 1PC light, 1,96 ± 0,73 mA vs. 1PC dark, 2,44 ± 0,68 mA; 2PC light, 2,19 ± 1,21 mA vs. 2PC dark, 2,48 ± 1,20 mA; and 3PC light, 2,32 ± 0,69 mA vs. 3PC dark, 1,85 ± 0,69 mA) (Figure 5).

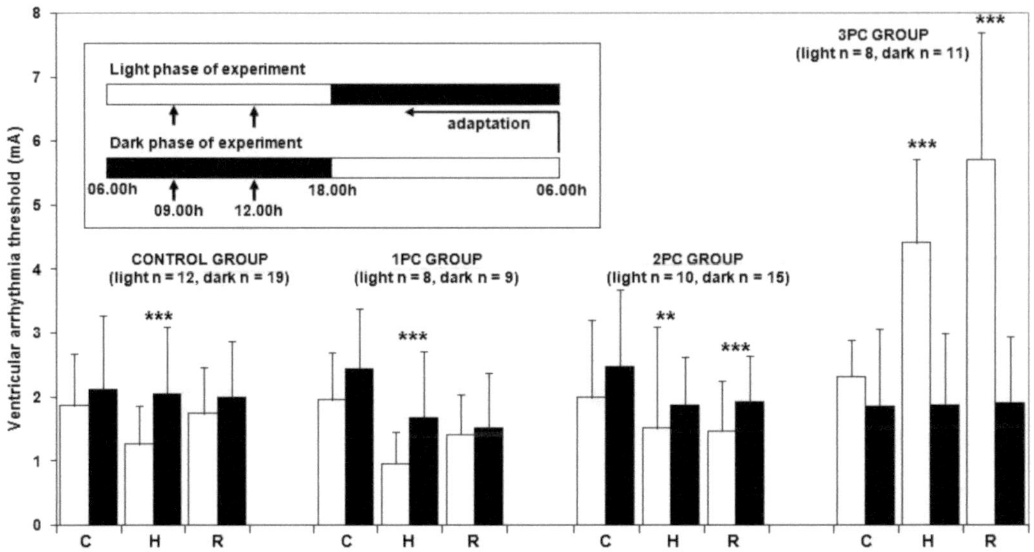

Fig. 5. Mean ± SD values of the ventricular arrhythmia threshold immediately before preconditioning (C), during 20 min. hypoventilatory asphyxia (H) following 20 min. reoxygenation (R) in the control animals (control group) and groups preconditioned by 1 (1PC group), 2 (2PC group) and 3 (3PC group) short cycles of hypoventilation-induced systemic hypoxia, hypercapnia and acidosis. Empty and black columns refer to light and dark parts of the day, respectively. Embedded scheme shows the timing of trials (arrows) in animals adapted to the light-dark cycle. *** $p < 0{,}001$, ** $p < 0{,}01$.

During the dark part of the day, hypoventilation non-significantly decreased the VAT in the group without PC (2,12 ± 0,93 mA [control] vs. 2,05 ± 0,85 mA [hypo]); in 1 PC (2,44 ± 0,68 mA [control] vs. 1,68 ± 0,87 mA [hypo]); and in 2 PC (2,48 ± 1,2 mA [control] vs. 1,87 ± 0,60 mA [hypo]). In the 3 PC group, the VAT was not changed and remained at the level of the pre-hypoventilatory value (1,85 ± 0,69 mA [control] vs. 1,87 ± 0,76 mA [hypo]). During the light part of the day, similar but significant VAT decreases were found in the group without PC and in the 1 PC group and non-significant decreases were found in the 2 PC group. In the 3 PC group, where the VAT was markedly increased ($p < 0{,}001$) above the control value. Significant LD differences were seen in all groups, with higher values in the dark part of the day, except the 3 PC group which had a higher VAT in the light part of the day. In the dark part of the day, reoxygenation after one and two cycles of HPC did not change and recovery of the VAT to control values and values from the period of hypoventilation (1 PC group, 2,44 ± 0,68 mA [control] vs. 1,68 ± 0,87 mA [hypo] vs. 1,53 ± 0,58 mA [reoxy]), (2 PC group, 2,48 ± 1,2 mA [control] vs. 1,87 ± 0,60 mA [hypo] vs. 1,93 ± 0,57 mA [reoxy]). In the group without preconditioning (2,12 ± 0,93 mA [control] vs. 2,05 ± 0,85 mA [hypo] vs. 2,00 ± 0,86 mA [reoxy]) and in the 3 PC group (1,85 ± 0,69 mA [control] vs. 1,87 ± 0,76 mA [hypo] vs. 1,91 ± 0,69 mA [reoxy]) the VAT was not changed and remained on the pre- and hypoventilatory levels. In the light part of the day, similar VAT changes were seen in all groups, except the 3 PC group, where the VAT was markedly ($p < 0{,}001$) increased versus control and hypoventilatory values. The higher VAT values were found in all groups, with higher values in the dark part of the day, except the 3 PC group, in which a higher VAT occurred in the light part of the day. A significant effect of the PC by the HPC was not confirmed by the χ^2 test nor for hypoventilation ($p < 0,09$) or for reoxygenation ($p < 0,64$) in the dark part of the day. In the light part, such significance was confirmed only for a prolonged period of hypoventilation ($p < 0,001$), but not during reoxygenation ($p < 0,39$).

A considerable intraindividual variability of results is a problem concerning mainly *in vivo* studies, which was also confirmed in our experimental groups. Such variability can be explained by production of spontaneous unpredictible alterations in the electrical stability of the heart induced by anaesthesia or hormonal and homeostatic reflexes operating only in intact animals (Lubbe et al., 1975).

LD differences in the VATs are probably a reflection of the changes in electrophysiological properties of the myocardium. These changes after HPC were also evident in the background of our observations. Possible mechanisms of protection might involve a faster shortening of the action potential (Tan et al., 1993; Ravingerova et al., 1998), also reflected as a shortening of refractoriness (Grover et al., 1994) during hypoxia after PC. Moreover, the duration of arrhythmic activity was significantly shorter in papillary muscles from the hearts of guinea pigs after HPD (Kamasaki et al., 1997), which refers to the fact that HPC can significantly attenuate arrhythmic activity. Unfortunately, these experiments were performed without LD dependence; therefore no information regarding the effect of HPC could be gained. Thus, the question remains whether the effects of these electrophysiological changes protecting the myocardium also depends on the LD cycle. Our results indirectly confirm the fact that the above described electrophysiological changes resulting from PC are probably more effective mainly during the light (nonactive) part of the rat regime day (Svorc et al., 2003).

The effect of PC also depends on the balance between the intensity of the first stimulus and the duration and severity of the prolonged stress. Following the changes in VAT during hypoventilation/reoxygenation, one cycle of HPC had an identical proarrhythmogenic effect in both light parts of the day, but with significantly higher values in the dark part of the day. However, the LD discrepancies in the VAT changes occurred during reoxygenation. In the light part of the day, reoxygenation partly recovered the VAT (antiarrhythmogenic effect), but in the dark part of the day, it was followed by a further decrease in VAT (proarrhythmogenic effect). In both light parts of the day, although hypoventilation/reoxygenation still decreased the VATs in the 2PC group, the decrease was not significant, values were higher than in the 1PC group, but with the preservation of LD differences. Reoxygenation was without effect. The three cycles of HPC stabilized the VAT in the dark part of the day, but a marked and significant cardioprotection against the hypoventilation/reoxygenation decrease of the electrical stability of the heart was detected in the light part, meaning that there are different reactions of the rat myocardium for the**HPC** in the dependence on the LD cycle.

Although the average hypoventilatory VAT value was lower in the 1PC group compared with the hypoventilatory VAT value from the control group (without HPC) in both light parts of the day, the VAT increased gradually in the dependence on the number of cycles of HPC. It appears that 1) one cycle of HPC is too weak of a stimulus for the production of cardioprotection in both light parts of the day; 2) the cardioprotection probably starts after two cycles of HPC in both light parts; and 3) the effect of HPC depends on the numbers of HPC cycles and the LD cycle - it is highlighted by three cycles of HPC.

The dependence of cardioprotection on the number of HPC cycles has been confirmed by others. In isolated rat hearts Testoni et al. (2000) and later Cerruti et al. (2002), showed that as long as the animals were exposed only to hypoxia (60 min.) and reoxygenation (60 min.), without HPC, the more severe atrial and right ventricle contractile disorders and less posthypoxic recovery (other endpoints of PC) were found. Whereas HPC by one 5 min.

cycle of hypoxia and subsequent 10 min. reoxygenation had a small effect, PC with two cycles of hypoxia exacerbated the contractile changes. O'Connor & Merrill (1995) referred to the fact that initial exposure to hypoxia can protect myocardium in *in vivo* conditions against arrhythmias during the second hypoxic period (significant percentage decrease of ectopy incidence). Blockade of cardiac β-adrenoceptors attenuated the incidence of arrhythmia in the second hypoxic period, demonstrating the possible role of catecholamines in the course of HPC. Myocardial ischemia, as well as non-ischemic hypoxia, stimulate efferent adrenergic nervous endings (Daly & Scott, 1963, 1964; Herrmann & Feigl, 1992), the assumption being that the ventricular arrhythmias induced by systemic hypoxia depend on intact adrenergic innervation (O'Connor & Merrill, 1993), which was also shown in our experiments. These interventions deliver possible protection by PC against electrogenic and mechanical effects of the prolonged ischemic period of the myocardium (Lasely et al., 1993). The differences in the number of cycles of hypoxia necessary for the mobilization of the cardioprotective mechanism in the prezent study and previous studies performed *in vitro* and *in vivo*, could be explained by different experimental procedures. Low-oxygen perfusion of isolated hearts *in vitro* (Testoni et al., 2000; Cerruti et al., 2002) may facilitate cardioprotection much sooner compared to an *in vivo* condition. The anaesthesia in *in vivo* experiments is an important variable, as is the animal species in use, e.g., ketamine anaesthesia inhibits PC with anoxia in rats (Ko et al., 1997), in rabbits (Han et al., 2002), and in our results, or α-chloralose in beagles (O'Connor & Merrill, 1993).

4.2 Heart rate – A measure of autonomic nervous system activity

Cyclic fluctuations based on subdiurnal, circadian or supradian cardiovascular responses are also influenced by the short- and long-term variability of the autonomic nervous system. Previous data showed that daily rhythmicity in sympathetic and parasympathetic nerve tone in healthy organisms is paralleled by corresponding changes in the electrophysiological properties of the myocardium (Cinca et al., 1986). Circadian variability in the autonomic nervous system might also represent a substantial influence on the electrical stability of the myocardium under pathological conditions including systemic hypoxia, pulmonary hypoventilation, asphyxia and acidosis (Meurling et al., 2001; Simantirakis et al., 2001; Watanabe et al., 2002).

It is known that both the hypoxic changes in the phasic and tonic drive od the autonomic nervous system and the alterations in the sensitivity of the myocardium to autonomic nervous drive, may also be involved in the effect of PC. It is now apparent that protection from IPC spreads from distant organs to the heart (Pell et al., 1998; Wolfrum et al., 2002) possibly via activation of the autonomic nervous system (Gho et al., 1996; Schoemaker & Van Heijningen, 2000; Liem et al., 2002; Wolfrum et al., 2002). It is possible that the release of local triggers of IPC activates the autonomic nervous system either directly (Schoemaker & Van Heijningen, 2000; Liem et al., 2002) or via sensory nerves (Tang et al., 1999; Xiao et al., 2001; Hu et al., 2002), and transfers the signal to the myocardium or other remote tissues.

Evidence exists that sympathovagal regulation might be related to the protective mechanism of IPC (Loukogeorgakis et al., 2005; Wu et al., 2005). IPC is mediated by sympathetic neurotransmitter release and α_1-adrenergic receptor stimulation (Banerjee et al., 1993; Cohen et al., 2001). Acetylcholine, the parasympathetic mediator, is also involved in the IPC triggering process (Cohen et al., 2001). The anti-arrhythmic protection afforded by IPC may be mediated by preservation of autonomic function (Miyazaki & Zipes, 1989). Other evidence implies that IPC may affect sympathovagal activity from the initial to the target effect (Airaksinen et al.,

1995; Pasceri et al., 1996). Brief coronary occlusion may result in severe autonomic reaction as measured by reduced heart-rate variability; however, the autonomic reaction after further coronary occlusion has been significantly smaller (Woo et al., 1994; Airaksinen al., 1995; Huikuri & Makikallio, 2001). These phenomena highlight the importance of cardiac autonomic regulation in the IPC protective process.

The above mentioned results clearly refer to probable autonomic nervous system participation in cardioprotection induced by IPC. Although HPC is less studied, it is known that pre-treatment with repetitive episodes of systemic hypoxia or hypoventilation-induced asphyxia under *in vivo* conditions evoked not only the similar cardioprotective effects (Shizukuda et al., 1993) but also showed marked LD dependence (Svorc et al., 2003). In the present, the date about the autonomic nervous system participation in HPC are absent and especially, in the dependence on the environment periodicities.

Results of a study with HPC show that the initial heart rate data measured in the intact spontaneously breathing ketamine/xylazine-anaesthetized animals (Ini) treated during the light part of the day (LP) were significantly lower compared to those from the dark part of the day (DP) (M ± SD, 231 ± 28 vs. 264 ± 31 beats/min. p < 0,001). Similar LD-dependent differences in the averaged heart rate values were maintained after tracheotomy, thoracotomy (To; LP 168 ± 39 vs. DP 218 ± 57 beats/min. p< 0.001) and after the onset of the artificial pulmonary ventilation (5 min after the onset, LP vs. DP, 202 ± 34 vs. 262 ± 44 beats/min p < 0,001). Interestingly, while the heart rate values in DP-treated animals usually returned to close to initial values within 1-5 min. of artificial ventilation (5 min, 262 ± 44 vs. Ini, 264 ± 31 beats/min,) similar recovery was not seen in LP-treated animals (5. min, 202 ± 34 vs. Ini 231 ± 28 beats/min. (Figure 6).

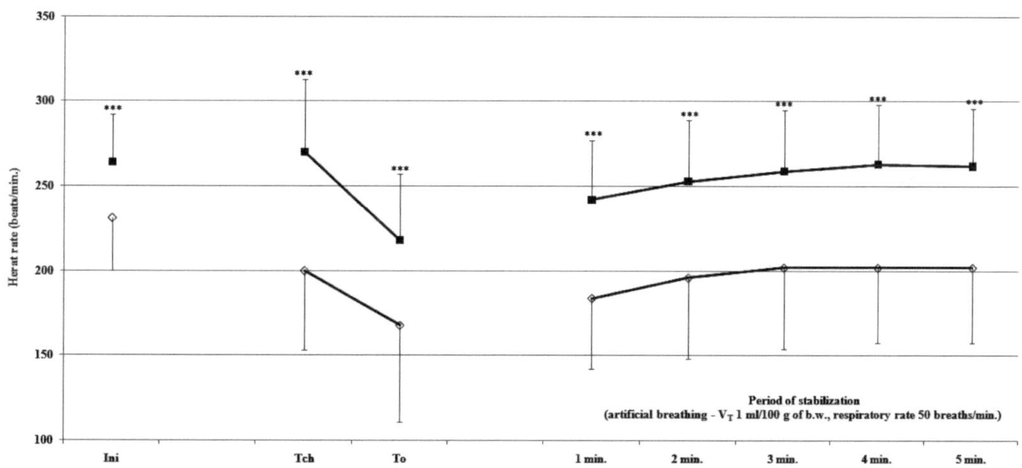

Fig. 6. The average heart rate (HR) values (mean ± SD) before, during and after the surgical interventions in the light (empty rhombus) and the dark (black square) part of the rat regime day. Ini – animals before the surgical interventions in ketamine/xylazine anaesthesia, spontaneous breathing), Tch – immediately after tracheotomy, To – immediately after thoracotomy and after 1., 2., 3., 4. and 5. min. of artificial ventilation (period of stabilization). *** p < 0,001 statistically significant differences between heart rates measured during the light and dark part of the rat regime day.

Statistically significant LD differences were found in each cycle of PC using hypoventilation-induced systemic asphyxia (Figure 7). HR changes in each cycle of asphyxic PC showed LD dependence. In the light period of the rat regime day, HR was significantly increased in the 5. min. vs. 1. min. in each cycle (1. cycle 203 ± 36 vs. 191 ± 35 beats/min., $p < 0,05$; 2. cycle 208 ± 36 vs. 190 ± 32 beats/min., $p < 0,01$; and 3. cycle 202 ± 34 vs. 189 ± 35 beats/min., $p < 0,01$). In the dark period, the significant differences between 1. min. and the 5. min. of each cycle were not detected (Figure 7).

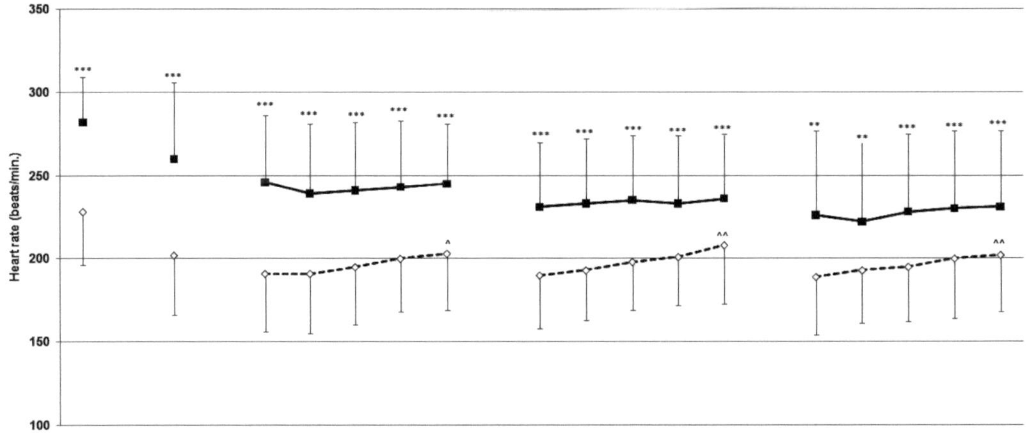

Fig. 7. Average values (mean ± SD) of heart rate during hypoventilation-induced asphyxia preconditioned cycles in the light (empty rhombus) and in the dark (black square) part of the rat regime day. Ini – average heart rate value from the anaesthetized rats before the surgical interventions and at the spontaneous breathing, Stabil – average heart rate value from the 5. min. of artificial ventilation. *** $p < 0,001$; ** $p < 0,01$ statistically significant differences between heart rates measured during the light and dark part of the rat regime day. ^ $p < 0,05$; ^^ $p < 0,01$ statistically significant heart rate difference between the 1. and 5. min. of the preconditioned hypoventilation-induced systemic asphyxia cycles.

In the light part of the day, the heart rate increased gradually with the duration of hypoventilation until the 10. to 11. min. mark in all experimental groups and with the followed stabilization in the control, 1PC and 2PC groups to the end of the asphyxic period. The next heart rate increase was seen only in the 3PC group with the significantly higher values in the 20. min. of hypoventilation against control, 1PC and 2PC groups (3PC vs. control, 235 ± 36 beats/min. vs. 215 ± 36 beats/min., $p < 0,05$; 3PC vs. 1PC, 235 ± 36 beats/min. vs. 196 ± 26 beats/min., $p < 0,01$ and 3PC vs. 2PC 235 ± 36 beats/min. vs. 209 ± 29 beats/min., $p < 0,002$). In the dark part of the day, the heart rate was stabilized in the course of the whole period of asphyxia in all experimental groups (Figure 8).

The spontaneously breathing rats under the ketamine/xylazine anaesthesia are in asphyxic conditions from the start of the experiment *in vivo*, independent of the LD cycle (Svorc et al., 2009). Thus, the disruptive effect of hypoxia on the LD-dependent differences in heart rate response curve was not demostrated, as suggested by the previously mentioned authors. One of the main conclusions from the present study was that heart rates were significantly and systematically higher in the dark part of the regime day than in the light part of the day, and also in asphyxic conditions even if the heart rate response curves in either condition practically paralleled one another.

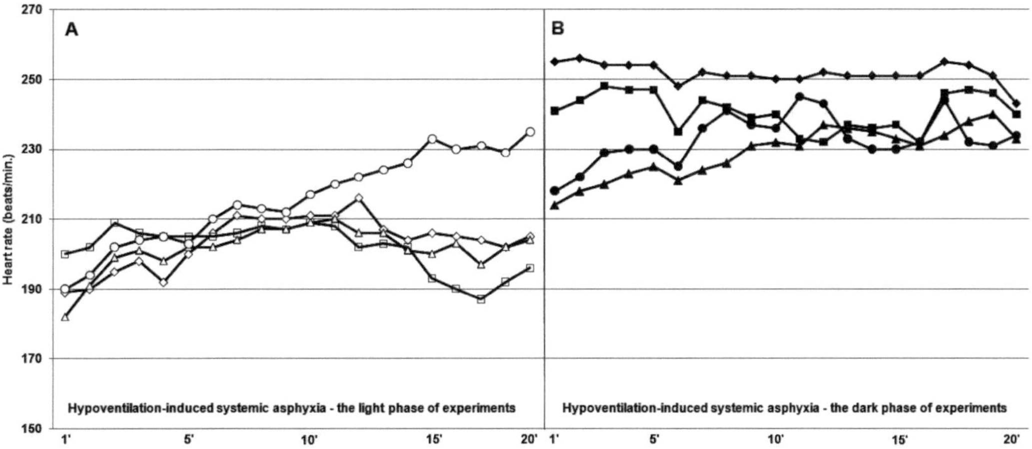

Fig. 8. Mean ± SD values of heart rate during hypoventilation-induced systemic asphyxia in the control group and in the groups pre-treated with a number of different preconditioning-cycles in the light (empty symbols) and the dark (filled symbols) parts of the rat regime day, respectively. Control group - rhombus, 1PC group - square, 2PC group - triangle and 3PC group - circle.

Interestingly, we found that this type of anaesthesia in rats expressively increases parasympathetic tone and decreases sympathetic drive, respectively. The results of heart-rate variability analysis show that in intact spontaneously breathing rats, power HF was significantly higher (light 19,387 ms^2; dark 3,129 ms^2) than power LF (light 0,974 ms^2; dark 0,432 ms^2) and there was also significant LD difference in both parameters ($p < 0.01$ for HF; $p < 0.02$ for LF) (Svorc, Jr. unpublished results). Although heart rates were on the level of bradycardia, the onset of asphyxia was regularly accompanied by a decrease in heart rate, which increased in intensity within a 5 min period in both light and dark parts of the day and persisted for the next 20 min. Atropine-resistant hypoxic bradycardia in rats was also reported by Kaplan et al. (2003) and in isolated ischemic rat hearts by Chanine et al. (1993) who explained that the response was due to a reduction of tissue noradrenaline in the ischemic rat myocardium. In contrast, in rats under moderate hypoxia, Ohkuwa et al. (2005) observed increased plasmatic noradrenaline levels as an indicator of increased sympathetic stimulation. The increase in heart rate was observed only after the first hour in the process of acclimatization the decrease was found with the amplitude reduction of the diurnal variation of heart rate (Kawaguchi et al., 2005). The relative contribution of afferent feedback, autonomic nervous drive and direct hypoxic effect on circulatory responses was examined by Hayashida et al. (1996) in conscious rats with or without chemoreceptor/baroreceptor input. In intact animals, they found that hypoxia facilitated sympathetic activity, while in chemodenervated animals hypoxia induced a decrease in blood pressure, heart rate and renal sympathetic activity. Nevertheless, their data from hypercapnic hypoxia suggest that CO_2–dependent chemical drive may contribute to larger parasympathetic influence to the heart, similar to asphyxia used in present work. In addition to differences in the hypoxic protocols, afferent inputs and behavioural state, sex-dependent differences may play an additional role. Hinojosa-Laborde & Mifflin (2005) reported increases in heart rate after exposure to intermittent hypoxia in males but not in females, in whom the response could even be opposite.

Adaptation in the light part of the day has an important effect on the efficiency of the PC mechanism *in vivo* as shown in our previous studies (Svorc et al., 2003). This later finding increases the practical value for pharmacological interventions, since the majority of the current data on the myocardial IPC or HPC come almost exclusively from in vitro studies. Significant LD cycle effects on heart rate responses, as a marker of autonomic nervous drive, were not reported previously during defined stages of open-surgery preparation.
In conclusion, the study showed that the effect of HPC depends on the LD cycle as well as on the number of PC cycles in *in vivo* conditions in rats. Cardioprotection against the hypoventilation/reoxygenation-induced decrease in the electrical stability of the heart likely begins to occur after two cycles of PC with asphyxia in both light parts of the rat regime day. If stabilization of the electrical stability of the heart is also considered to be a possible means of cardioprotection, then hypoventilation/reoxygenation myocardial injury is minimized only after 3 cycles of PC with asphyxia in the dark (active) part of the day, and the cardioprotection proved to be effective only after 3 cycles of PC by asphyxia in the light (nonactive) part.
This may suggest that while PC with 1-2 short asphyxias does not obviously alter LD-dependent differences in autonomic drive to the heart, several more cycles may eliminate the circadian effects. As to the variability and effects of PC by asphyxias, heart rate responses during the light part of the regime day obviously showed less pronounced dependence on the number of PC cycles and exhibited less interindividual variability than in the dark part of the day particularly during the first half of 20 min hypoventilatory challenge. In the group adapted to the light part of the regime day with 3 PC cycles, heart rate responses after 10 min of recovery lost obvious LD-dependence. Whether observed LD-dependent effects upon asphyxia merely reflect the variations in the autonomic nervous inputs, or represent more complex effects including remodelling of the PC mechanism, alterations in the sensitivity of cardiac conductive system, local effects of hypoxia and acidosis on myocardium remain unclear and require further study.

5. Conclusions

Cardiovascular responses show circadian fluctuations and significant dependence on the LD cycle in pentobarbital- and ketamine/xylazine-paralyzed rats, confirming that LD-related differences are not merely transient or procedure dependent. It is a systematic response assured by distinct neuro-humoral regulation during the light and dark parts of the day, and also under both types of anaesthesia.
This suggests that synchronization to local time may be an important factor in the evaluation of cardiovascular risks in patients also suffering from various respiratory disorders. Analyses of myocardial reactions to acute systemic asphyxia, and to reoxygenation are very important in cardiology because the myocardium reacts differently depending on synchronization to external environmental periodicity.

6. References

Abdel-Rahman, U.; Risteski, P.; Tizi, K.; Kerscher, S.; Bejati, S.; Zwicker, K.; Scholz, M.; U. Brandt, U. & Moritz, A. (2009). Hypoxic reoxygenation during initial reperfusion attenuates cardiac dysfunction and limits ischemia-reperfusion injury after cardioplegic arrest in a porcine model. *The Journal of Thoracic and Cardiovascular Surgery*, Vol. 137, No. 4, (Sep 2009), pp. 978-982, ISSN: 0022-5223.

Airaksinen, K.E.J.; Ylitalo, K.V.; Peuhkurinen, K.J.; Ikaheimo, M.J. & Huikuri H.V. (1995). Heart rate variability during repeated arterial occlusion in coronary angioplasty. *American Journal of Cardiology*, Vol. 75, No. 14, (May 1995), pp. 877–881, ISSN: 0002-9149.

Amitzur, G.; Schoels, W.; Visokovsky, A.; Levran, V.; Novikov, I.; Mueller, M.; Kraft, P.; Kaplinsky, E. & Eldar, M. (2000). Role of sodium channels in ventricular fibrillation: A study in nonischemic isolated hearts. *Journal of Cardiovascular Pharmacology*, Vol. 36, No. 6, (Dec 2000), pp. 785-793, ISSN: 0160-2446.

Axelrod, P.J.; Verrier, R.L. & Lown, B. (1975). Vulnerability to ventricular fibrillation during acute coronary arterial occlusion and release. *American Journal of Cardiology*, Vol. 36, No. 6, (Nov 1975), pp. 776-782, ISSN: 0002-9149.

Bacova, I.; Svorc, P.,Jr.; Kundrik, M. & Fulton, B.L. (2010). Light-dark dependence of electrocardiographic changes during asphyxia and reoxygenation in a rat model. *Central European Journal of Medicine*, Vol. 5, No. 5, (Oct 2010), pp. 611-619, ISSN: 1895-1058.

Baker, J.E.; Contney, S.J.; Singh, R.; Kalyanaraman, B.; Gross, G.J. & Bosnjak, Z.J. (2001). Nitric oxide activates the sarcolemmal K_{ATP} channel in normoxic and chronically hypoxic hearts by a cyclic GMP - dependent mechanism. *Journal of Molecular and Cellular Cardiology*, Vol. 33, No. 2, (Feb 2001), pp. 331–341, ISSN: 0022-2828.

Banerjee, A.; Locke-Winter, C.; Rogers, K.B.; Mitchell, M.B.; Brew, E.C.; Cairns, C.B.; Bensard, D.D. & AH Harken A.H.. (1993). Preconditioning against myocardial dysfunction after ischemia and reperfusion by an alpha 1-adrenergic mechanism. *Circulation Research*, Vol. 73, No. 4, (Oct 1993), pp. 656–670, ISSN: 1524-4571.

Bernauer, W. (1997). Concerning the effect of the K^+ channel blocking agent glibenclamide on ischaemic and reperfusion arrhythmias. *European Journal of Pharmacology*, Vol. 326, No. 2-3, (May 1997), pp. 147–156, ISSN: 0014-2999.

Bhattacharyya, M.L. & Acharya, S. (1988). Effects of hypoxia with mild acidosis and reoxygenation on slow response action potentials in canine myocardial tissues. *Jornal of Electrocardiology*, Vol. 21, No. 2, (Apr 1988), pp. 192-197, ISSN: 0022-0736.

Bhattacharyya, M.L.; Hughes, B. & Sarker, S. (1991). Different effects of reoxygenation on the electrical activity of ventricular muscle. *Journal of Electrocardiology*, Vol. 24, No. 4, (Oct 1991), pp. 363-369, ISSN: 0022-0736.

Bilinska, M.; Maczewski, M. & Beresewicz, M. (1996). Donors of nitric oxide mimic effects of ischaemic preconditioning on reperfusion induced arrhythmias in isolated rat heart. *Molecullar and Cellular Biochemistry*, Vol. 161, (Jul-Aug 1996), pp. 265–271, ISSN: 0300-8177.

Billman, G.E.; Avendano, C.E.; Halliwill, J.R. & Burroughs, J.M. (1993). The effects of the ATP-dependent potassium channel antagonist, glyburide, on coronary blood-flow and susceptibility to ventricular-fibrillation in unanesthetized dogs. *Journal of Cardiovascular Pharmacology*, Vol. 21, No. 2, (Feb 1993), pp. 197-204, ISSN: 0160-2446.

Bishop, B.; Silva, G.; Krasney, L.; Salloum, A.; Roberts, A.; Nakano, H.; Shucard, D.; Rifkin, D. & Farkas, G. (2000). Circadian rhythms of body temperature and activity levels during 63h of hypoxia in the rat. *American Journal of Physiology*, Vol. 279, No. 4, (Oct 2000), pp. R1378-R1385, ISSN: 0363-6119.

Bishop, B.; Silva, G.; Krasney, J.; Nakano, H.; Roberts, A.; Farkas, G.; Rifkin, D. & Shucard, D. (2001). Ambient temperature modulates hypoxic - induced changes in rat body temperature and activity differentially. *American Journal of Physiology,* Vol. 280, No. 4, (Apr 2001), pp. R1190-R1196, ISSN: 0363-6119.

Bissinger, A.; Markuszewski, L. & Rosiak, M. (2008). Value and circadian variations of QT dispersion in patients with diabetes mellitus and coronary artery disease. *Poland Merkury Lekarski*, Vol. 24, No. 140, (Feb 2008), pp. 90-94, ISSN: 14269686.

Bosco, G.; Ionadi, A.; Panico, S.; Faralli, F.; Gagliardi, R.; Data, P. & Mortola, J.P. (2003). Effects of hypoxia on the circadian patterns in men. *High Altitude Medicine and Biology*, Vol. 4, No. 3, (Fal 2003), pp. 305-318, ISSN: 1527-0297.

Carmeliet, E. (1988). Electrophysiology of cardiac arrhythmias. Recent developments. *Revista de Farmacologia Clinica y Experimental,* Vol. 5, No. 2, (1988), pp. 121-122, ISSN: 0213-0157.

Catini, C. & Legnaioli, M. (1992). Role of mast-cells in health - daily rhythmic variations in their number, exocytotic activity, histamine and serotonin content in the rat-thyroid gland. *European Journal of Histochemistry,* Vol. 36, No. 4, (1992), pp. 501-516, ISSN: 1121-760X.

Cerniway, R.J.; Morrison, R.R.; Byford, A.M.; Lankford, A.R.; Headrick, J.P.; Van Wylen, D.G.L. & Matherne, G.P. (2002). A_1 adenosine receptor overexpression decreases stunning from anoxia-reoxygenation: role of the mitochondrial K_{ATP} channel. *Basic Research in Cardiology*, Vol. 97, No. 3, (May 2002), pp: 232–238, ISSN: 0300-8428.

Cerruti, S.; Testoni, G.; Dalamon, V.; Kade, P.; Varela, A. & Savino, E.A. (2002). Effects of fasting and hypoxic preconditioning on the hypoxic-reoxygenated ventricular strips of the rat heart. *Journal of Physiology and Biochemistry*, Vol. 58, No. 2, (Jun 2002), pp. 95-101, ISSN: 1138-7548.

Cohen, M.V.; Yang, X.M.; Liu, G.S.; Heusch, G. & Downey, J.M. (2001). Acetylcholine, bradykinin, opioids, and phenylephrine, but not adenosine, trigger preconditioning by generating free radicals and opening mitochondrial K(ATP) channels. *Circulation Research*, Vol. 89, No. 3, (Aug 2001), pp. 273–278, ISSN: 0009-7330.

Chahine, R.; Adam, A.; Yamaguchi, N.; Gaspo, R.; Regoli, D. & Nadeau, R. (1993). Protective effects of bradykinin on the ischaemic heart: implication of the B1 receptor. *British Journal of Pharmacology*, Vol. 108, No 2, (Feb 1993), pp. 318–322, ISSN: 00071188.

Cinca, J.; Moya, A.; Figueras, J. Roma, F. & Rius, J. (1986) Circadian variations in the electrical properties of the human heart assessed by sequential bedside electrophysiologic testing. *American Heart Journal*, Vol. 112, No. 2, (Aug 1986), pp. 315-321, ISSN: 0002-8703.

Curtis, M.J.; Johnston, K.M. & Walker, M.J.A. (1985). Arrhythmias and serum potassium during myocardial ischaemia. *Medical Science*, Vol. 13, No. 8, (1985), pp. 688–689, IDS Number: APA98.

Dai S. (1989). Histamine enhances hypoxia-induced ventricular arrhythmias in isolated rat hearts. *Clinical and Experimental Pharmacology and Physiology,* Vol. 16, No. 12, (Dec 1989), pp. 925-931, ISSN: 0305-1870.

Daly, M.D.B. & Scott, M. (1963). The cardiovascular responses to stimulation of the carotic body chemoreceptors in the dog. *Journal of Physiology*, Vol. 165, No. 1, (Jan 1963), pp. 179-197, ISSN: 0022-3751.

Daly, M.D.B. & Scott, M. (1964). The cardiovascular effects of hypoxia in the dog with special reference to the contribution of the carotic body chemoreceptor. *Journal of Physiology*, Vol. 173, No. 2, (Aug 1964), pp. 201-214, ISSN: 0022-3751.

Danielsson, B.R.; Danielsson, C. & Nilsson, M.F. (2007). Embryonic cardiac arrhythmia and generation of reactive oxygen species: Common teratogenic mechanism for IKr blocking drugs. *Reproductive Toxicology*, Vol. 24, No. 1, (Jul 2007), pp. 42-56, ISNN: 0890-6238.

Daut, J.; Maierrudolph, W.; vonBeckerath, N.; Mehrke, G.; Gunther, K. & Goedel-Meinen, L. (1990). Hypoxic dilation of coronary-arteries is mediated by atp-sensitive potassium channels. *Science*, Vol. 247, No. 4948, (Mar 1990), pp. 1341-1344, ISSN: 0036-8075.

Draper, N.J. & Shah, A.M. (1997). Beneficial effects of a nitric oxide donor on recover of contractile function following brief anoxia in isolated rat heart. *Journal of Molecular and Cellular Cardiology*, Vol. 29, No. 4, (Apr 1997), pp.1195–1205, ISSN: 0022-2828.

Dworschak, M.; Breukelmann, D.& Hannon, J.D. (2004). The impact of isoflurane during simulated ischemia/reoxygenation on intracellular calcium, contractile function, and arrhythmia in ventricular myocytes. *Anesthesia and Analgesia*, Vol. 99, No. 5, (Nov 2004), pp. 1302-1307, ISSN: 0003-2999.

Fenelon, K.; Seifert, E.L. & Mortola, J.P. (2000). Hypoxic depression of circadian oscillations in sino-aortic denervated rats. *Respiration Physiology*, Vol. 122, No. 1, (Aug 2000), pp. 61-69, ISSN: 0034-5687.

Ferrier, G.R.; Moffat, M.P. & Lukas, A. (1985). Possible mechanisms of ventricular arrhythmias elicited by ischemia followed by reperfusion. *Circulation Research*, Vol. 56, No. 2, (1985), pp.184–194, ISSN: 0009-7330.

Fisch, Ch. (1973). Relation of electrolyte disturbances to cardiac arrhythmias. *Circulation*, Vol. 47, No. 2, (1985), pp. 408–419, ISSN: 00097322.

Froldi, G.; Pandolfo, L.: Chinellato, A; Ragazzi, E.; Caparrota, L. & Fassina, G. (1994). Protection of atrial function in hypoxia by high potassium concentration. *General Pharmacology*, Vol. 25, No. 3, (May 1994), pp. 401-407, ISSN: 0306-3623.

Gami, A.S.; Howard, D.E.; Olson, E.J. & Somers, V.K. (2005). Day-night pattern of sudden death in obstructive sleep apnea. *New England Journal of Medicine*, Vol. 352, No. 12, (Mar 2005), pp. 1206-1214, ISSN: 0028-4793.

Gerst, P.H.; Fleming, W.H. & Malm, J.R. (1966). A quantitative evaluation of the effects of acidosis and alkalosis upon the ventricular fibrillation threshold. *Surgery*, Vol. 59, No. 6, (Jun 1966), pp. 1050-1066, ISSN: 0039-6060.

Gho, B.C.; Schoemaker, R.G.; Van den Doel, M.A.; Duncker, D.J. & Verdouw, P.D. (1996). Myocardial protection by brief ischemia in noncardiac tissue. *Circulation*, Vol. 94, No. 9, (1996), pp. 2193–2200, ISSN: 0009-7322.

Granda, T.G.; Velasco, A. & Cachero, T.G. (1996). Circadian rhythms of plasma concentrations of Na^+ and K^+ and their urinary excretion in normal and diabetic rats. *Biological Rhythm Research*, Vol. 27, No. 1, (Feb 1996), pp. 31-42, ISSN: 0929-1016.

Grover, G.J.; D'Alonzo, A.J.; Sleph, P.G.; Dzwonczyk, S.; Hess, T. & Darbenzio, R.B. (1994). The cardioprotective and electrophysiological effects of cromakalim are attenuated by meclofenamate through a cyclooxygenase-independent mechanism. *Journal of*

Pharmacology and Experimental Therapeutics, Vol. 269, No. 2, (May 1994), pp. 536-540, ISSN: 0022-3565.

Guilleminault, C.; Conolly, S.J. & Winkle, R.A. (1983). Cardiac arrhythmia and conduction disturbances during sleep in 400 patients with sleep apnea syndrome. *American Journal of Cardiology*, Vol. 52, No. 5, (Sep 1983), pp. 490-494, ISSN: 0002-9149.

Gunez, Y.; Tuncer, M.; Guntekin, U.; Akdag, S. & Gumrukcuoglu, H.A. (2008). Lack of diurnal variation of P-wave and QT dispersions in patients with heart failure. *PACE – Pacing and Clinical Electrophysiology*, Vol. 31, No. 8, (Aug 2008), pp. 974-978, ISSN: 0147-8389.

Guo, Y.F. & Stein, P.K. (2002). Circadian rhythm in the cardiovascular system: Considerations in non/invasive electrophysiology. *Cardiac Electrophysiology Review*, Vol. 6, No. 3, (Sep 2002), pp. 267-272, ISSN: 1385-2264.

Guo, H.; Takahashi, S.; Cho, S.; Hara, T.; Tomiyasu, S. & Sumikawa, K. (2005). The effects of dexmedetomidine on left ventricular function during hypoxia and reoxygenation in isolated rat hearts. *Anesthesia and Analgesia, Vol.* 100, No. 3, (Mar 2005), pp. 629-635, ISSN: 0003-2999.

Han, J.; Kim, N.; Joo, H. & Kim, E. (2002). Ketamine abolishes ischemic preconditioning through inhibition of K_{ATP} channels in rabbit hearts. *American Journal of Physiology-Heart and Circulatory Physiology*, Vol. 283, No. 1, (Jul 2002), pp. H13-H21, ISSN: 0363-6135.

Hansen, S.; Rasmussen, V.; Torp-Pedersen, C. & Jemsen, G.B. (2008). QT intervals and QT dispersion determined from a 12-lead 24-hor Holter recording in patients with coronary artery disease and patients with heart failure. *Annals of Nonivasive Electrocardiology*, Vol. 13, No. 1, (Jan 2008), pp. 22-30, ISSN: 1082-720X.

Hayashida, Y.; Hirakawa, H.; Nakamura, T. & Maeda, M. (1996). Chemoreceptors in autonomic responses to hypoxia in conscious rats. In: *Frontiers in Arterial Chemoreception*, Zapata, P.; Eyzaguirre, C. & Torrance, R.W., pp. 439-442, Plenum Press, ISBN: 0-306-45490-4, New York.

Henry, R.; Casto, R. & Printz, M.P. (1990) Diurnal cardiovascular patterns in spontaneously hypertensive and Wistar-Kyoto rats. *Hypertension,* Vol. 16, No. 4, (Oct 1990), pp. 422-428, ISSN: 0194-911X.

Hinojosa-Laborde, C. & Mifflin, S.W. (2005). Sex differences in blood pressure response to intermittent hypoxia in rats. *Hypertension,* Vol. 46, No. 4, (Oct 2005), pp. 1016-1021, ISSN: 0194-911X.

Herrmann, S.C. & Feigl, E.O. (1992). Adrenergic blockade blunts adenosine concentration and coronary vasodilation during hypoxia. *Circulation Research*, Vol. 70, No. 6, (Jun 1992), pp. 1203-1216, ISSN: 0009-7330.

Hu, C.P.; Peng, J.; Xiao, L.; Ye, F.; Deng, H.W. & Li, Y.J. (2002). Effect of age on alpha-calcitonin gene-related peptide-mediated delayed cardioprotection induced by intestinal preconditioning in rats. *Regulatory Peptides*, Vol. 107, No. 1-3, (Jul 2002), pp. 137–143, ISSN: 0167-0115.

Huikuri, H.V. & Makikallio, T.H. (2001). Heart rate variability in ischemic heart disease. *Autonomic Neuroscience-Basic & Clinical*, Vol. 90, No. 1-2, Special Issue: Sp. Iss. SI, (Jul 2001), pp. 95–101, ISSN: 1566-0702.

Jarsky, T.M. & Stephenson, R. (2000). Effect of hypoxia and hypercapnia on circadian rhythms in the golden hamster (Mesocricetus aueatus). *Journal of Applied Physiology*, Vol. 89, No. 6, (Dec 2000), pp. 2130-2138, ISSN: 8750-7587.

Jeroudi, M.O.; Hartley, C.J. & Bolli, R. (1994) Myocardial reperfusion injury - role of oxygen radicals and potential therapy with antioxidants. *American Journal of Cardiology*, Vol. 73, No. 6, (Mar 1994), pp: B2–B7, ISSN: 0002-9149.

Jones, D.L. & Klein, G.J. (1982). Ventricular fibrillation threshold: Correlation with the repetitive ventricular response. *Circulation*, Vol. 66, pp. 11-74, ISSN: 1524-4539.

Kamasaki, Y.; Guo, A.C. & McDonald, T.F. (1997). Protection by hypoxic preconditioning against hypoxia-reoxygenation injury in guinea-pig papillary muscles. *Cardiovascular Research*, Vol. 34, No. 2, (Dec 1996), pp. 313-322, ISSN: 0008-6363.

Kamiyama, T.; Tanonaka, K.; Hayashi, J. & Takeo, S. (1996). Effects of aprindine on ischemia/reperfusion – induced cardiac contractile dysfunction of perfused rat heart. *Japanese Journal of Pharmacology*, Vol. 70, No. 3, (Mar 1996), pp. 227–234, ISSN: 0021-5198.

Kamkin, A.; Kiseleva, I.; Wagner, K.D.; Lozinsky, J.; Gunther, J. & Scholz, H. (2003). Mechanically induced potentials in atrial fibroblasts from rat hearts are sensitive to hypoxia/reoxygenation. *Pflugers Archiv-European Journal of Physiology*, Vol. 446, No. 2, (May 2003), pp. 169-174, ISSN: 0031-6768.

Kang, P.M.; Haunstetter, A.; Aoki, H.; Usheva, A. & Izumo, S. (2000). Morphological and molecular characterization of adult cardiomyocyte apoptosis during hypoxia and reoxygenation. *Circulation Research*, Vol. 87, No. 2, (Jul 2000), pp: 118–125, ISSN: 0009-7330.

Kaplan, J.L.; Gao, E.; deGaravilla, L.; Victain, M.; Minczak, B. & Dalsey, W.C. (2003). Adenosine A1 antagonism attenuates atropine-resistant hypoxic bradycardia in rats. *Academic Emergency Medicine*, Vol. 10, No. 9, (Sep 2003), pp. 923-930, ISSN: 1069-6563.

Kawaguchi, T.; Tsubone, H.; Hori, M.; Ozaki, H. & Kuwahara, M. (2005). Cardiovascular and autonomic nervous function during acclimatization to hypoxia in conscious rats. *Autonomic Neuroscience-Basic & Clinical*, Vol. 117, No. 2, (Feb 2005), pp. 97-104, ISSN: 1566-0702.

Kawasaki, H.; Otani, H.; Mishima, K.; Imamura, H. & Inagaki, C. (2001). Involvement of anion exchange in the hypoxia/reoxygenation-induced changes in pH_i and $[Ca^{2+}]_i$ in cardiac myocyte. *European Journal of Pharmacology*, Vol. 411, No. 1-2, (Jan 2001), pp. 35-43, ISSN: 0014-2999.

Ko, S.H.; Lee, S.K.; Han, Y.J.; Choe, H.; Kwak, Y.G.; Chae, S.W.; Cho, K.P. & Song, H.S. (1997). Blockade of myocardial ATP-sensitive potassium channels by ketamine. *Anesthesiology*, Vol. 87, No. 1, (Jul 1997), pp. 68-74, ISSN: 0003-3022.

Kreher, P. & Verdetti, J. (1986). Role of ATP in the maintenance of action-potential configuration of the isolated working rat-heart. *Cardiovascular Research*, Vol. 20, No. 2, (Feb 1986), pp. 89-99, ISSN: 0008-6363.

Kujanik, S.; Wilk, P. & Tomcova, D. (1984). Changes in the vulnerable period of the rat myocardium during hypoxia, hyperventilation and heart failure. *Physiological Bohemoslovaka*, Vol. 33, No. 5, (1984), pp. 470–480, ISSN: 0369-9463.

Kujanik, S.; Ivanco, I. & Svorc, P. (1985). Impairment of respiration and incidence of cardiac dysrhythmias. *Magazine Medical Faculty UPJŠ,* Vol. 28, (1985), pp. 3-20, ISSN: 67-356-87.

Kujanik, S.; Snincak, M.; Galajdová, K. & Rackova, K. (2000a). Cardiovascular changes during sudden ascent in a cable cabin to the moderate altitude. *Physiological Research,* Vol. 49, No. 6, (2000), pp. 729-731, ISSN: 0862-8408.

Kujanik, S.; Snincak, M.; Vokal, J.; Podracky, J. & Koval, J. (2000b). Periodicity of arrhythmias in healthy elderly men at the moderate altitude. *Physiological Research,* Vol. 49, No. 2, (2000), pp. 285–287, ISSN: 0862-8408. ***

Kujanik, S. & Mikulecky, M. (2010). Circadian and ultradian extrasystole thythms in healthy individuals at elevated versus lowland altitudes. *International Journal of Biometeorology,* Vol. 54, No. 5, (Sep 2010), pp. 531-538, ISSN: 0020-7128.

Kuniyoshi, F.H.S.; Garcia-Touchard, A.; Gami, A.S.; Romero-Corral, A.; van der Walt, C.; Pusalavidyasagar, S.; Kara, T.; Caples, S.M.; Pressman, G.S.; Vasquez, E.C.; Lopez-Jimenez, F. & Somers, V.K. (2008). Day-night variation of acute myocardial infarction in obstructive sleep apnea. *Journal of the American College Cardiolology,* Vol. 52, No. 5, (Jul 2008), pp. 343-346, ISSN: 0735-1097.

Lasely, R.D.; Anderson, G.M. & Mentzer, R.M. Jr. (1993). Ischemic and hypoxic preconditioning enhance postischemic recovery of function in the rat heart. *Cardiovascular Research,* Vol. 27, No. 4, (Dec 1992), pp. 565-570, ISSN 0008-6363.

Liem, D.A.; Verdouw, P.D.; Ploeg, H.; Kazim, S. & Duncker, D.J. (2002). Sites of action of adenosine in interorgan preconditioning of the heart. *American Journal of Physiology-Heart and Circulatory Physiology,* Vol. 283, No. 1, (Jul 2002), pp. H29–H37, ISSN: 0363-6135.

Liu, J.; Tanonaka, K.; Sanbe, A.; Yamamoto, K. & Takeo, S. (1993). Beneficial effects of quinidine on post - ischemic contractile failure of isolated rat hearts. *Journal of Molecular and Cellular Cardiology,* Vol. 25, No. 10, (Oct 1993), pp. 1249–1263, ISSN: 0022-2828.

Loukogeorgakis, S.P.; Panagiotidou, A.T., Broadhead, M.W.; Donald, A.; Deanfield, J.E. & MacAllister, R.J. (2005). Remote ischemic preconditioning provides early and late protection against endothelial ischemia-reperfusion injury in humans: Role of the autonomic nervous system. *Jornal of American College Cardiology,* Vol. 46, No. 3, (Aug 2005), pp. 450-456, ISSN: 0735-1097.

Lubbe, W.F.; Bricknell, O.L. & Marzagao, C. (1975). Ventricular fibrillation threshold and vulnerable period in the isolated perfused rat heart. *Cardiovascular Research,* Vol. 9, No. 5, (Sep 1975), pp. 613-620, ISSN: 0008-6363.

Meurling, C.J.; Waktare, J.E.P.; Holmqvist, F.; Hedman, A.; Camm, A.J.; Olsson, S.B. & Malik, M. (2001). Diurnal variations of the dominant cycle length of chronic atrial fibrillation. *American Journal of Physiology-Heart and Circulatory Physiology,* Vol. 280, No. 1, (Jan 2001), pp. H401-H406, ISSN: 0363-6135.

Milano, G.; Corno, A.F.; Samaja, M.; Morel S.; Vassalli G. & von Segesser L.K. (2010). Daily reoxygenation decreases myocardial injury and improves post-ischaemic recovery after chronic hypoxia. *European Journal of Cardio-thoracic Surgery,* Vol. 37, No. 4, (Apr 2010), pp. 942-949, ISSN: 1010-7940.

Miyazaki, T. & Zipes, D.P. (1989). Protection against autonomic denervation following acute myocardial infarction by preconditioning ischemia. *Circulation Research*, Vol. 64, No. 3, (Mar 1989), pp. 437–448, ISSN: 0009-7330.

Mortola, J.P. & Seifert, E.L. (2000). Hypoxic depression of circadian rhythms in adult rats. *Journal of Applied Physiology*. Vol. 88, No. 2, (Feb 2000), pp. 365-368, ISSN: 8750-7587.

Mubagwa, K.; Kaplan, P. & Flameng, W. (1997). The effects of ryanodine on calcium uptake by the sarcoplasmic reticulum of ischemic and reperfused rat myocardium. *Fundamental and Clinical Pharmacology*, Vol. 11, No. 4, (1997), pp. 315–321, ISSN: 0767-3981.

Mukai, M.; Terada, H.; Sugiyama, S.; Satoh, H. & Hayashi, H. (2000). Effects of a selective inhibitor of Na+/Ca2(+) exchange, KB-R7943, on reoxygenation-induced injuries in guinea pig papillary muscles. *Journal of Cardiovascular Pharmacology*, Vol. 3, No. 1, (Jan 2000), pp. 121-128, ISSN: 0160-2446.

Murry, C.E.; Jenning, R.B. & Reimer, K.A. (1986). Preconditioning with ischemia: a delay of lethal cell injury in ischemic myocardium. *Circulation*, Vol. 74, No. 5, (Nov 1986), pp. 1124-1136, ISSN: 0009-7322.

Nishimura, M.; Tanaka, H.; Homma, N.; Matsuzawa, T. & Watanabe, Y. (1989). Ionic mechanisms of the depression of automaticity and conduction in the rabbit atrioventricular node caused by hypoxia or metabolic inhibition and protective action of glucose and valine. *American Journal of Cardiology*, Vol. 64, No. 20, (Dec 1989), pp. J24–J28, ISSN: 0002-9149.

Noma, A. (1983). ATP-regulated K^+ channels in cardiac muscle. *Nature*, Vol. 305, No. 5930, (Sep 1983), pp. 147–148, ISSN: 0028-0836.

Noma, A. & Shibasaki, T. (1985). Membrane current through adenosine-triphosphate-regulated potassium channels in guinea-pig ventricular cells. *Journal of Physiology-London*, Vol. 363, No. Jun, (1985), pp. 463-480, ISSN: 0022-3751.

O'Connor, P.J. & Merrill, G.F. (1993). Sympathetic adrenergic nerves contribute to the ventricular arrhythmias of hypoxia in the dog. *Biomedical Letters*, Vol. 48, No. 190, (1993), pp. 163-170, ISSN: 0961-088X.

O'Connor, P.J. & Merrill, G.F. (1995). Ventricular arrhythmias caused by repeat exposure to hypoxia are dependent on duration of reoxygenation. *FASEB Journal*, Vol. 9, No. 5, (Mar 1995), pp. 387-391, ISSN: 0892-6638.

Ohkuwa, T.; Itoh, H.; Yamamoto, T.; Minami, C. & Yamazaki, Y. (2005). Effect of hypoxia on norepinephrine of various tissues in rats. *Wilderness and Environmental Medicine*, Vol. 16, No. 1, (Spr 2005), pp. 22-26, ISSN: 1080-6032.

Opie, L.H.; Nathar, D. & Lubbe, W.F. (1979). Biochemical aspects of arrhythmogenesis and ventricular fibrillation. *American Journal of Cardiology*, Vol. 43, No. 1, (Jan 1979), pp. 131–148, ISSN: 0002-9149.

Ostadal, B.; Ostadalova, I. & Dhalla, N.S. (1999). Development of cardiac sensitivity to oxygen deficiency: Comparative and ontogenetic aspects. *Physiol Res*, Vol. 79, No. 3, (Jul 1999), pp. 635-659, ISSN: 0031-9333.

Otsuka, K. & Watanabe, H. (1990). Experimental and clinical chronocardiology. *Chronobiologia*, Vol. 17, No. 2, (Apr-Jun 1990), pp. 135-163, ISSN: 0390-0037.

Pahor, M.; Bernabei, R. Gambassi, G. & Carbonin, P.U. (1989). Effects of verapamil on reoxygenation and programmed electrical stimulation-induced ventricular arrhythmias in the isolated heart. *International Journal of Cardiology,* Vol. 25, Suppl. 1, (1989), pp. S71-S79, ISSN: 0167-5273.

Pasceri, V.; Lanza, G.A.; Patti, G.; Pedrotti, P.; Crea, F. & Maseri, A. (1996). Preconditioning by transient myocardial ischemia confers protection against ischemia-induced ventricular arrhythmias in variant angina. *Circulation,* Vol. 94, No. 8, (Oct 1996), pp. 1850–1856, ISSN: 0009-7322.

Pelissier, A.L.; Gantenbein, M.; Prudian, F. & Bruguerolle, B. (1998). Influence of general anaethetics on circadian rhythms of heart rate, body temperature and locomotor activity in rats. *Sciences et Techniques de l Animal de Laboratoire,* Vol. 23, No. 2, (1998), pp. 91-98, ISSN: 0339-722X.

Pell, T.J.; Baxter, G.F.; Yellon, D.M. & Drew, G.M. (1998). Renal ischemia preconditions myocardium: role of adenosine receptors and ATP-sensitive potassium channels. *American Journal of Physiology - Heart and Circulatory Physiology,* Vol. 275, No. 5, (Nov 1998), pp. H1542–H1547, ISSN: 0363-6135.

Perchenet, L. & Kreher, P. (1995). Mechanical and electrophysiological effects of preconditioning in isolated ischemic/reperfused rat heart. *Journal of Cardiovascular Pharmacology,* Vol. 26, No. 5, (Nov 1995), pp. 831–840, ISSN: 0160-2446.

Peter, J.H. (1990). Sleep apnea and cardiovascular diseases. In: *Obstructive Sleep Apnea Syndrome: Clinical Research and Treatment,* Guilleminault, C. & Partinen, M., pp. 81-98, Raven Press, Ltd., New York, ISBN: 0-88167-585-7.

Portaluppi, F. & Hermida, R.C. (2007). Circadian thythms in cardiac arrhythmias and opportunities for their chronotherapy. *Advanced Drug Delivery Reviews,* Vol. 59, No. 9-10, (Aug 2007), pp. 940-951, ISSN: 0169-409X.

Poulis, J.A.; Roelfsema, F. & van der Heide, D. (1989). Circadian urinary electrolyte excretory rhythms in male and female rats. *Journal of Interdisciplinary Cycle Research,* Vol. 20, No. 1, (Feb 1989), pp. 35–47, ISSN: 0022-1945.

Prudian, F.; Gantenbein, M.; Pelissier A.L.; Attolini, L. & Bruguerolle, B. (1997). Daily rhythms of heart rate, temperature and locomotor activity are modified by anaesthetics in rats: A telemetric study. *Naunyn–Schmiedebergs Archives Pharmacology,* Vol. 355, No. 6, (Jun 1997), pp. 774-778, ISSN: 0028-1298.

Ravingerova, T.; Løkebø, J.E.; Munch-Ellingsen, J.; Sundset, R.; Tande, P. & Ytrehus, K. (1998). Mechanism of hypoxic preconditioning in guinea pig papillary muscles. *Molecular and Cellular Biochemistry,* Vol. 186, No. 1-2, (Sep 1998), pp. 53-60, ISSN: 0300-8177.

Reimer, K.A.; Hill, M.L. & Jennings, R.B. (1981). Prolonged depletion of ATP and the adenine nucleotide pool due to delayed resynthesis of adenine nucleotides following reversible myocardial ischemic injury in dogs. *Journal of Molecular and Cellular Cardiology,* Vol. 13, No. 2, (Feb 1981), pp. 229-39, ISSN: 0022-2828.

Rogers, R.M.; Spear, J.F.; Moore, E.N.; Horowitz, L.H. & Sonne, J.E. (1973). Vulnerability of canine ventricle to fibrillation hypoxia and respiratory acidosis. *Chest,* Vol. 63, No. 6, (Jun 1973), pp. 986–994, ISSN:0012-3692.

Rus, A.; del Moral, M.L.; Molina, F. & Peinado, M.A. (2011). Does inducible NOS have a protective role against hypoxia/reoxygenation injury in rat heart? *Cardiovascular Pathology,* Vol. 20, No. 1, (Jan-Feb 2011), pp. e17-e25, ISSN: 1879-1336.

Saint, K.M.; Abraham, S.; MacLeod, B.A.; McGough, J.; Yoshida, N. & Walker, M.J.A. (1992). Ischemic but not reperfusion arrhythmias depend upon serum potassium concentration. *Journal of Molecular and Cellular Cardiology,* Vol. 24, No. 7, (Jul 1992), pp. 701–710, ISSN: 0022-2828.

Sanguinetti, M.C.; Scott, A.L.; Zingaro, G.J.& Siegl P.K.S. (1988). BRL-34915 (Cromakalim) activates ATP-sensitive K^+ current in cardiac-muscle. *Proceedings of the National Academy of Sciences of the United States of America,* Vol. 85, No. 21, (Nov 1988), pp. 8360-8364, ISSN: 0027-8424.

Sawanobori, T.; Adaniya, H.; Yukisada, H. & Hiraoka, M. (1995). Role for ATP - sensitive K^+ channel in the development of A - V block during hypoxia. *Journal of Molecular and Cellular Cardiology,* Vol. 27, No. 1, (Jan 1995), pp. 647–657, ISSN: 0022-2828.

Schöemaker, R.G. & Van Heijningen, C.L. (2000). Bradykinin mediates cardiac preconditioning at a distance. *American Journal of Physiology - Heart and Circulatory Physiology,* Vol. 278, No. 5, (May 2000), pp. H1571–H1576, ISSN: 0363-6135.

Sharikabad, M.N.; Hagelin, E.M.; Halberg, I.A.; Lyberg, T. & Brørs, O. (2000). Effect of calcium on reactive oxygen species in isolated rat cardiomyocytes during hypoxia and reoxygenation. *Journal of Molecular and Cellular Cardiology,* Vol. 32, No. 3, (Mar 2000), pp. 441–452, ISSN: 0022-2828.

Sharikabad, M.N.; Østbye, K.M. & Brørs, O. (2004). Effect of hydrogen peroxide on reoxygenation-induced Ca^{2+} accumulation in rat cardiomyocytes. *Free Radical Biology and Medicine,* Vol. 37, No. 4, (Aug 2004), pp. 531-538, ISSN: 0891-5849.

Shinmura, K.; Tani, M.; Suganuma, Y.; Hasegawa, H.; Ebihara, Y.; Nakamura, Y. & Asakura, Y. (1997). Effects of alpha(1)-adrenoreceptor subtype blockade on ischemia - reperfusion injury. *Japanese Circulation Journal,* Vol. 61, No. 11, (Nov 1997), pp. 927–935, ISSN: 0047-1828.

Shivkumar, K.; Deutsch, N.A.; Lamp, S.T.; Khuu, K.; Goldhaber, J.J. & Weiss, J.N. (1997). Mechanism of hypoxic K loss in rabbit ventricle. *Journal of Clinical Investigation,* Vol. 100, No. 7, (Oct 1997), pp. 1782–1788, ISSN: 0021-9738.

Shizukuda, Y.; Iwamoto, T.; Mallet, R.T. & Downey, H.F. (1993). Hypoxic preconditioning attenuates stunning caused by repeated coronary artery occlusions in the dog heart. *Cardiovascular Research,* Vol. 27, No. 4, (Apr 1993), pp. 559-564, ISSN: 0008-6363.

Simantirakis, E.N.; Chrysostomakis, S.I.; Marketou, M.E.; Kochiadakis, G.E.; Vardakis, K.E.; Mavrakis, H.E. & Vardas, P. (2001). Atrial and ventricular refractoriness in paced patients - circadian variation and its relationship to autonomous nervous system activity. *European Heart Journal,* Vol. 22, No. 23, (Dec 2001), pp. 2192-2200, ISSN: 0195-668X.

Smith, T.L.; Coleman, T.G.; Stanek, K.A. & Murphy, W.R. (1987). Hemodynamic monitoring for 24 h in unanesthetized rats. *American Journal of Physiology,* Vol. 253, No. 6, (Dec 1987), pp. H1335-H1341, ISSN: 0002-9513.

Stoynev, A.G.; Ikonomov, O.C. & Vrabchev, N.C. (1986). Suprachiasmatic nuclei lesions do not eleminate the circadian rhythms of electrolyte excretion in the rat. *Physiology and Behavior,* Vol. 38, No. 5, (1986), pp. 657–662, ISSN: 0031-9384.

Svorc, P.; Wilk, P.; Murár, J. Podlubny I.; Kujanik S.; Bracokova I. & Murin M. (1994). Circadian rhythm of the ventricular fibrillation threshold in female Wistar rats. *Physiological Research,* Vol. 43, No. 6, (Sep 1994), pp. 355–358, ISSN: 0369-9463.

Svorc, P.; Podlubny, I.; Kujanik, S. & Bracokova, I. (1997). 24h rhythm of the vetricular fibrillation threshold during normal and hypoventilation in female Wistar rats. *Chronobiology International,* Vol. 14, No. 4, (Feb 1997), pp. 363–370, ISSN: 0742-0528.

Svorc, P.; Bracokova, I. & Podlubny, I. (2000a). Relation of ventricular fibrillation threshold to heart rate during normal ventilation and hypoventilation in female Wistar rats: A chronophysiological study. *Physiological Research,* Vol. 49, No. 6, (Mar 2000), pp. 711 -719, ISSN 0862-8408.

Svorc, P.; Bracokova, I.; Podlubny, I.; Kassayova, K.; Dorko, E. (2000b). Circadian rhythm of the ventricular fibrillation threshold in hypoventilation–reoxygenation model in female Wistar rats. *Bratislavske Lekarske Listy,* Vol. 101, No. 7, (Jun 2000), pp. 383–390, ISSN 0006-9248.

Svorc, P. & Podlubny, I. (2002). Modulatory influence of ventilator disorders on electrical stability of the rat heart. *Biomedicine and Pharmacotherapy,* Vol. 56 (suppl 2), (2002), pp. 327-332, ISSN 0753-3322.

Svorc, P. & Bracokova, I. (2003). Preconditioning by hypoventilation increases ventricular arrhythmia threshold in Wistar rats. *Physiological Research,* Vol. 52, No. 4, (Aug 2003), pp. 409-416, ISSN 0862-8408.

Svorc, P.; Benacka, R.; Petrasova, D; Bracokova, I. & Kujanik, S. (2005). Effect of systemic hypoxia and reoxygenation on electrical stability of the rat myocardium: Chronophysiological study. *Physiological Research,* Vol. 54, No. 3, (Dec 2005), pp. 319-325, ISSN 0862-8408.

Svorc, P. & Benacka, R. (2008). The effect of hypoxic myocardial preconditioning is highly dependent on the light-dark cycle in Wistar rats. *Experimental and Clinical Cardiology,* Vol. 13, No. 4, (Oct 2008), pp. 204-208, ISSN: 1205-6626.

Svorc, P.; Bracokova, I.; Bacova, I. & Svorcova, E. (2009). Acid-base balance and artificial controlled ventilation in Wistar rats: Chronobiological view. *Proceedings of The Third International Congress of Applied Chronobiology and Chronomedicine,* Akko, Israel, May 2009.

Svorc, P.; Bacova, I.; Benacka, R.; Svorc, P. Jr.; Galanova, R. & Fulton, B.L. (2011). Heart-rate changes in asphyxic preconditioning in rats depend on light-dark cycle. *Central European Journal of Medicine,* Vol. 6, No. 3, (Mar 2011), pp. 312-319, ISSN: 1895-1058.

Szekeres, L. & Papp, J.G. (1967). Effect of arterial hypoxia on the susceptibility to arrhythmias of the heart. *Acta Physiologica Academica Science Hungaria,* Vol. 32, (1967), pp. 143-162, ISSN: 0231-424X.

Takeo, S.; Liu, J.; Tanonaka, K.; Nasa, Y.; Yabe, K.; Tanahashi, H. & Sudo, H. (1995). Reperfusion at reduced flow rates enhances postischemic contractile recovery of perfused heart. *American Journal of Physiology-Heart and Circulatory Physiology,* Vol. 268, No. 6, (Jun 1995), pp. H2384–H2395, ISSN: 0363-6135.

Tan, H.L.; Mazon, P.; Verberne, H.J.; Sleeswijk, M.E.; Coronel, R.; Opthof, T. & Janse, M.J. (1993). Ischaemic preconditioning delays ischaemia induced cellular electrical uncoupling in rabbit myocardium by activation of ATP sensitive potassium channels. *Cardiovascular Research,* Vol. 27, No. 4, (Apr 1993), pp. 644-651, ISSN: 0008-6363.

Tang, Z.L.; Dai, W.Y.J.; Li, Y.J. & Deng, H.W. (1999). Involvement of capsaicin-sensitive sensory nerves in early and delayed cardioprotection induced by a brief ischaemia of the small intestine. *Naunyn-Schmiedebergs Archives of Pharmacology,* Vol. 359, No. 3, (Mar 1999), pp. 243-247, ISSN: 0028-1298.

Tanonaka, K.; Matsumoto, M.; Miyake, K.; Minematsu, R. & Takeo, S. (1989). Protective action of YM-12617, an α_1-adrenoceptor antagonist, on the hypoxic and reoxygenated myocardium. *European Journal of Pharmacology*, Vol. 165, No. 1, (Jun 1989), pp. 97-106, ISSN: 0014-2999.

Testoni, G.; Cerruti, S.; Kade, P.; Carregal, M.; Varela, A. & Savino, E.A. (2000). Effects of hypoxic preconditioning on the hypoxic-reoxygenated atria from fed and fasted rats. *Journal of Physiology and Biochemistry*, Vol. 56, No. 4, (Dec 2000), pp. 321-328, ISSN: 1138-7548.

Tomori, Z.; Benacka, R.; Tkacova, R. & Donic V. (1997). Dysrhythmias and ECG changes in experimentally induced apneic events. *Bratislavske Lekarske Listy*, Vol. 98, (Apr 1997), pp. 531–538, ISSN: 0006-9248.

Tomori, Z.; Benacka, R.; Donic, V. & Jakus, J. (2000). Contribution of upper airway reflexes to apnoea reversal, arousal, and resuscitation. *Monaldi Archive Chest Disease*, Vol. 55, No. 5, (Oct 2000), pp. 398–403, ISSN: 1122-0643.

Tosaki, A.; Engelman, D.T.; Engelman, R.M. & Das, D.K. (1996). The evolution of diabetic response to ischemia/reperfusion and preconditioning in isolated working rat hearts. *Cardiovascular Research*, Vol. 31, No. 4, (Apr 1996), pp. 526–536, ISSN: 0008-6363.

Vleugels, A.; Vereecke, J. & Carmeliet, E. (1980). Ionic currents during hypoxia in voltage-clamped cat ventricular muscle. *Circulation Research*, Vol. 47, No. 4, (May 1980), pp. 501–508, ISSN: 1524-4571.

Wakatsuki, D.; Shimojima, H.; Higashi, Y.; Suzuki, H. & Takeyama, Y. (2009). Inhibition of mitochondrial KATP channel can improve conduction delay induced by angiotensin II during early reoxygenation. *Journal of Molecular and Cellular Cardiology*, Vol. 46, No. 3, (Mar 2009), pp. 443, ISSN: 0022-2828.

Watanabe, M.; Nakagawa, M.; Nobe, S.; Ohie, T.; Takahashi, N.; Hara, M.; Yonemochi, H.; Ito, M. & Saikawa, T. (2002). Circadian variation of short-lasting asymptomatic paroxysmal supraventricular tachycardia. *Journal of Electrocardiology*, Vol. 35, No. 2, (Apr 2002), pp. 135-138, ISSN: 0022-0736.

Wegria, R.; Moe, G.K. & Wiggers, C.J. (1941). Comparison of the vulnerable periods and fibrillation threshold of normal and idioventricular beats. *American Journal of Physiology*, Vol. 133, (Jun 1941), pp. 651-657, ISSN: 1522-1539.

Winslow, E.; Marchall, R.J. & Hope, F.G. (1983). Comparative effects of fast - and slow - ion channel blocking agents on reperfusion – induced arrhythmias in the isolated perfused rat heart. *Journal of Cardiovascular Pharmacology*, Vol. 5: No. 6, (Nov-Dec 1983), pp. 928–936, ISSN: 0160-2446.

Winslow, E.; Walker, G. & Mason, R. (1989). Antiarrhythmic effects of selective β_1 – and β_2 – and nonselective β-adenoreceptor blockade in normokalaemic and dietary–induced hypokalaemic rats. *Journal of Cardiovascular Pharmacology*, Vol. 14, No. 5, (Nov 1989), pp. 673–680, ISSN: 0160-2446.

Whalley, D.W.; Wendt, D.J. & Grant A.O. (1995). Electrophysiologic effects of acute ischemia and reperfusion and their role in the genesis of cardiac arrhythmias. In: *Cardiac Arrhythmias: Mechanisms, Diagnosis and Management*, Podrid, P.J.; Kowey P.R., pp.109–130, Williams and Wilkins, Philadelphia. ISBN-13: 9780781724869.

Wolfrum, S.; Schneider, K.; Heidbreder, M.; Nienstedt, J.; Dominiak, P. & Dendorfer, A. (2002). Remote preconditioning protects the heart by activating myocardial PKC epsilon-isoform. *Cardiovascular Research*, Vol. 55, No. 3, (Aug 2002), pp. 583–589, ISSN: 0008-6363.

Wolleben, C.D.; Sanguinetti, M.C. & Siegl, P.K.S. (1989). Influence of ATP-sensitive potassium channel modulators on ischemia-induced fibrillation in isolated rat hearts. *Journal of Molecular and Cellular Cardiology*, Vol. 21, No. 8, (Aug 1989), pp. 783-788, ISSN: 0022-2828.

Woo, M.A.; Stevenson, W.G.; Moser, D.K. & Middlekauff, H.R. (1994). Complex heart rate variability and serum norepinephrine levels in patients with advanced heart failure. *Journal of the American College of Cardiology*, Vol. 23, No. 3, (Mar 1994), pp. 565–569, ISSN: 0735-1097.

Wu, Z.K.; Vikman, S.; Laurikka, J.; Pehkonen, E.; Iivainen, T.; Huikuri, H.V. & Tarkka, M.R. (2005). Nonlinear heart rate variability in CABG patients and the preconditioning effect. *European Journal of Cardio-Thoracic Surgery*, Vol. 28, No. 1, (Jul 2005), pp. 109-113, ISSN: 1010-7940.

Xiao, L.; Lu, R.; Hu, C.P.; Deng, H.W. & Li, Y.J. (2001). Delayed cardioprotection by intestinal preconditioning is mediated by calcitonin gene-related peptide. *European Journal of Pharmacology*, Vol. 427, No. 2, (Sep 2001), pp. 131–135, ISSN: 0014-2999.

Xu, Y.G.; Yang, X.Y.; Yao, R.M.; Yang, Y.Z. & Chen, H.Z. (1993). Protective effects of nicorandil on action-potentials in anoxia and reoxygenated ventricular myocardium of guinea-pig. *Acta Pharmacologica Sinica*, Vol. 14, No. 2, (Mar 1993), pp. 186-189, ISSN: 0253-9756.

Yokoe, T.; Minoguchi, K.; Matsuo, H.; Oda, N.; Minoguchi, H.; Yoshino, G.; Hirano, T. & Adachi, M. (2003). Elevated levels of C-reactive protein and interleukin-6 in patients with obstructive sleep apnea syndrome are decreased by nasal continuous positive airway pressure. *Circulation*, Vol. 107, No. 8, (Mar 2003), pp.1129–1134, ISSN: 0009-7322.

10

Late Ventricular Potentials in Cardiac and Extracardiac Diseases

Ioana Mozoş, Corina Şerban and Rodica Mihăescu
"Victor Babeş" University of Medicine and Pharmacy, Timisoara
Romania

1. Introduction

Late ventricular potentials (LVPs) are low amplitude, high frequency waveforms, appearing in the terminal part of the QRS complex of the electrocardiogram (Barbosa et al, 2002; Olinic & Zdrenghea, 1998), generated by diseased myocardium. They may extend in the ST segment (Zimmermann et al, 1983). Late ventricular potentials may be also defined as fragmented electrical activity, appearing in heterogeneous tissue areas, located at the border zone of a myocardial infarction (Fetsch, 1999). They are markers of an electrophysiological substrate for reentry ventricular tachycardia (VT) and sudden cardiac death (SCD) (Zipes et al, 2006).

Most of the clinical research in this field is focused on risk stratification of patients with a history of myocardial infarction (MI), but the role of LVPs in other cardiac and extracardiac diseases is also discussed. At present, there is considerable interest on improved tests for risk stratification of sudden cardiac death and appropriate selection of prophylactic implantable cardioverter defibrillator recipients.

2. History

Late ventricular potentials were first reported by Berberi and Simson in dogs (Engel et al, 2004). Berbari et al. (Berbari et al., 1978) first demonstrated that, using high-gain amplification, filtering and signal averaging, late potentials could be recorded. Initially, LVPs were obtained directly from the endocardium or epicardium, but they can be recorded from the body surface, as well. The amplitude of LVPs is too low to be detected on the standard surface ECG, requiring an amplified high-resolution ECG recording. Simson and Breithardt et al. first showed the clinical value of ventricular signal averaged electrocardiography (SAECG) for identification of patients with sustained VT (Breithardt et al., 1981; Simson, 1981).

By the end of the 1980s, LVPs were helpful for the diagnosis, risk stratification and therapy of patients with ventricular arrhythmias. The initial enthusiasm diminished over time due to variability in the sensitivity, but lately, its predictive value for VT and fibrillation (VF) has been re-evaluated (Frances, 2010).

SAECG was originally developed for use in patients with coronary artery disease and VT, but it has been subsequently applied to other groups of patients (Goldberger et al., 1994).

3. Recording of LVPs

The amplitude of LVPs is in the order of microvolts and can not be detected on the standard surface ECG, requiring an amplified high-resolution ECG recording for their identification (Santangeli et al, 2008). Thus, LVPs are recorded using SAECG (Olinic & Zdrenghea, 1998).
The leads are different from those used in standard 12-lead ECG. Most investigators use an XYZ lead system, made of three orthogonal bipolar electrode combinations (Engel et al, 2004) and high-pass filtering. The leads are combined into a vector magnitude, a measure that sums up the high frequency information contained in all these leads. This vector magnitude is called filtered QRS complex (Santangeli et al, 2008).
Considering the low intensity of LVPs, averaging of aproximately 300 ECG cycles is needed, in order to minimize the level of noise (Santangeli et al, 2008). The signal-to-noise ratio increases with the number of averaged beats (Gottfridsson et al, 2011).
Recording of LVPs using body surface mapping is, also, possible (Linnenbank et al, 2001).

3.1 Diagnosis criteria

LVPs are present, if, according to an international convention (Goldberger et al, 2008), 2 of the following criteria (variables of the filtered QRS) (Fig. 1) are positive:

- **SAECG-QRS** duration (**SA-QRS**)>120 ms. Other authors consider SA-QRS>114 ms (Breithardt et al, 1991; Lander et al, 1993)
- **LAS40**: low amplitude signal (duration of the terminal part of the QRS complex with an amplitude below 40 µV) >38 ms
- **RMS40**: root mean square signal amplitude of the last 40 ms of the signal < 20 µV.

Each laboratory should define its own normal values (Breithardt et al, 1991). Other authors (Askenazi et al, 1978) use two sets of criteria to classify SAECG results. SAECG-I criteria are positive if one or more variables are abnormal, and SAECG-II criteria are positive if two or more variables are abnormal.

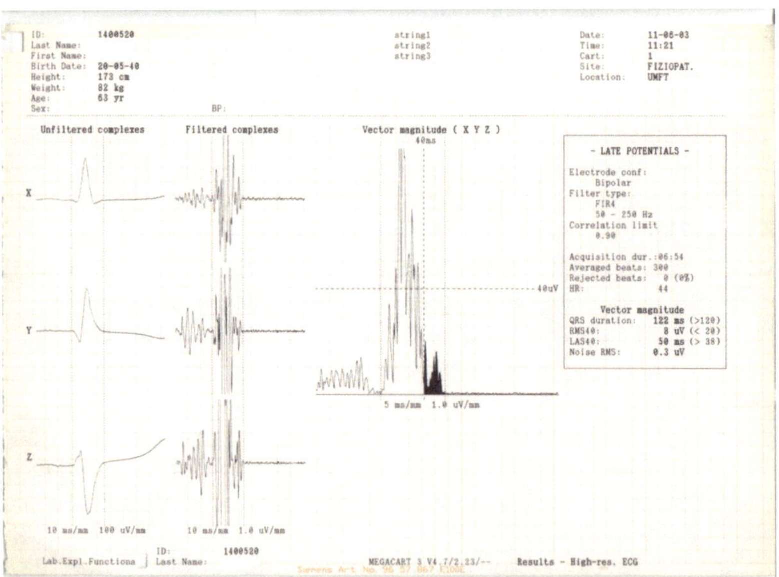

Fig. 1. Late ventricular potentials in a patient with an old inferior myocardial infarction.

Besides temporal domain analysis, frequency domain analysis allows identification of arrhythmia risk considering changes of ECG frequency components. Frequency domain analysis was not validated in clinical practice.

3.2 Limits

The amplitude of the signals is low, and averaging the electrocardiogram, amplifying it and filtering out the low frequencies is needed (Mehta & Camm, 1989; Santangeli et al, 2008). Several noise sources may appear in highly amplified recordings: artifacts from respiratory muscles, electronic noise arising from the electrodes, electrical power lines and other nearby electronic equipment (Engel et al, 2004). Despite technical improvement of the devices, electrical interferences and preexistent electrophysiological changes may cause false negative results. High-pass filters may attenuate or abolish LVPs (Santangeli et al, 2008).
Noise level was considered an important technical aspect influencing the results of the test. Steinberg and Bigger stated that the 0.3 μV level improves detection of late potentials (Steinberg & Bigger, 1989). The sensitivity of SAECG may be increased, by using a very low noise level (0.1 μV) (Frances, 2010). On the other hand, Engel et al. suggested that noise does not influence the SAECG variables and Christiansen et al. concluded that LVPs appear in healthy subjects at low noise levels (Christiansen et al, 1995; Engel et al, 1993).
The weakness of LVPs is the low positive predictive value. However, their negative predictive value for arrhythmic events is very high (Santangeli et al, 2008).
Difficulties may appear in detecting LVPs in patients with an anterior MI. Because of the early activation of the anterior regions during the normal sequence of electrical activation of the ventricles, delayed depolarization potentials of these regions after an anterior MI may not outlast the QRS complex, and therefore may be hidden within the QRS complex and not detected by SAECG (Santangeli et al, 2008).
Patients with a prolonged QRS complex duration, due to a bundle-branch block (BBB) or intraventricular conduction defect, have late-occurring depolarization potentials caused by these conduction disorders (Galinier et al, 1996). Separate LVPs criteria were used for patients with BBB: SA-QRS ≥145 ms, LAS40 ≥55 ms and RMS40≤17 μV (Galinier et al, 1996).
Assessment of LVPs using multiple channel electrocardiographs, allows the use of the method in patients with wide QRS complexes, identifying the origin of LVPs .

4. Predictive value of LVPs

LVPs characterize ventricular depolarisation and its signal is more stable and easy reproducible compared to the repolarisation process (Askenazi et al, 1978).
The positive predictive accuracy for malignant ventricular arrhythmias, in patients recovering from MI, of LVPs, ranges only from 8% to 29% (Santangeli et al, 2008). A high negative predictive value (90%) is mentioned for LVPs.

5. Pathophysiology of LVPs

LVPs represent delayed conduction through a diseased myocardium and indicate the presence of a potential **anatomical substrate** for **macroreentry** ventricular arrhythmias (Olinic & Zdrenghea 1998, Santangeli et al, 2008).
LVPs appear as a consequence of late ventricular depolarisation due to delayed impulse conduction in certain myocardial regions (Olinic & Zdrenghea 1998; Engel et al, 2004).

Decremental conduction appears in coronary heart disease due to decreased conduction speed in ischemic myocardium or due to a prolonged impulse propagation path (Breithardt et al, 1991).
Certain conditions must be met by the area that provides LVPs. First, **conduction must be slow** enough to enable reentry in the healthy tissue. Second, a 1/1 conduction should be mentained at **high frequencies**; otherwise a bidirectional block appears and reentry is imposible. Third, an uni**directional block** is needed, to allow depolarisation of the decremental zone in a single direction (Olinic & Zdrenghea, 1998).
If the lenght of the reentry circuit is not long enough, the amplitude of the potentials can not be detected on the surface ECG and LVPs are absent despite arrhythmia favorable conditions. This explains the reduced positive predictive value of LVPs for ventricular arrhythmia (Olinic & Zdrenghea, 1998).
In old MI, disorganised and asynchronous electrical activity arises from areas of surviving muscle at the border of a MI (Breithardt et. al, 1991; Savard et. al, 1997). Such areas are separated from each other by fibrous tissue, creating a disorganized, disconnected, heterogeneous network (Cain et al, 1996; Clayton, 2003). Considering other opinions, LVPs arise in the viable cells inside the necrotic and fibrotic mass, or in the injured myocardial fibers, with slow conduction (Cain et al, 1996; La Vecchia et al, 1998; Turrini et al, 1999).
An anatomical substrate, able to cause delayed conduction and produce LVPs, was reported in several other clinical conditions: dilated cardiomyopathy (Mancini et al, 1993), hypertrophic cardiomyopathy (Cripps et al, 1990), myocarditis, and infiltrative heart disease (Santangeli et al, 2008).
LVPs are favored by modified tissue architecture due to: necrosis, fibrosis or dystrophy, causing a delayed and fragmented depolarization. Fibrosis disturbs ventricular activity, separates myocardial bundles and prolongs conduction pathways (Cain et al, 1996). Anisotropic reentry is the result of fibrosis in addition to the density and distribution of gap junctions, which are responsible for variations in the conduction velocity (Kitamura et al, 2003; Peters et al, 1997). Some authors have demonstrated a close link between the distribution of the gap junctions, the specialized intercellular connections, and the development of reentrant arrhythmia in patients with healed MI and nonischemic dilated cardiomyopathy (Kitamura et al, 2003; Peters et al, 1997). The slow and discontinuous conduction caused by abnormalities in gap junction distribution and function form a **functional**, rather than anatomical, **substrate** for reentry (Santangeli et al, 2008).
To generate an arrhythmia needs a substrate (LVPs), but also a trigger and maintenance (Santangeli et al, 2008).
Arrhythmia triggers, such as acute ischemia, imbalance in autonomic tone, or the onset of clinical heart failure, may provide the link between the presence of LVPs and occurrence of spontaneous VT (Santangeli et al, 2008).
When sympathetic tone to the heart is augmented, vagal activation exerts a protective effect on ventricular vulnerability. Sympathetic stimulation unopposed by vagal activity induces ventricular electrical instability, increases susceptibility to ventricular fibrillation, resulting in a high risk of arrhythmia and SCD (Gussak & Antzelevitch, 2008). Myocardial infarction may damage nerve pathways, thereby limiting the potential of the vagus nerve to be activated (Gussak & Antzelevitch, 2008).
QRS prolongation may be explained by: intraventricular conduction disturbances and ventricular dilation, known to prolong ventricular conduction; and ventricular remodeling,

which increases tissue mass and slows conduction velocity. A correlation was found between QRS duration and end-diastolic volume after a few weeks after a MI. Some authors suggest that arrythmias are due to left ventricular dysfunction and do not depend on its etiology, considering that no differences were found in patients with myocardial ischemia or idiopathic cardiomyopathy (Kondo et al, 2001).
Reentry explains the appearance of LVPs mainly in old myocardial infarctions, due to scarring. An **abormal automatism** due to a recurrent acute MI can also cause LVPs. A significant proportion of deaths occuring after discharge are caused by an arrythmia focus due to acute ischemia, hence the lack of sensitivity of LVPs in predicting SCD (Savard et al, 1997). A prolonged QRS duration was suggested to be predictive for arrythmia SCD, regardless of arrythmia mechanism.
LVPs extend beyond the normal QRS complex due to the low velocity, and may be detected in the ST segment, as well (Barbosa et al, 2002; Cain et al, 1996). Abnormal intra-QRS potentials, as markers of reentry, may also appear (Lander et al, 1993).

6. Analysis of SAECG variables

Positivity criteria for LVPs (SA-QRS, LAS40 and RMS40) are significantly influenced by several factors: age, gender and myocardial infarction location (Barbosa et al, 2002; Savard et al, 1997). Criteria adjusted for sex, age and myocardial infarction location were developed only for SA-QRS, due to its higher predictive value for arrhythmic events (Lander et al, 1993).
SA-QRS measured by SAECG is higher in men than in women. This can be attributed to the greater myocardial mass. The significant increase of SA-QRS in aging MI patients was attributed to degenerative processes afecting conduction (Mozos, 2007).
All three SAECG variables showed significant predictive power for ventricular arryhthmic events. Several authors consider SA-QRS to have higher accuracy for arrhythmic events than any other combination of SAECG parameters (Ammann et al, 2004; Lander et al, 1993). Other authors concluded that RMS40 has the highest predictive value for ventricular arrhythmia (Nakai et al, 1988).
In patients with inferior myocardial infarction and documented episodes of sustained VT, all variables were significantly different (lower voltages, longer durations) compared to patients with anterior infarction (Barbosa et al, 2002). LVPs can be better identified at higher frequencies, confirming the high frequency of these signals.

7. The role of SAECG

The predictive value of SAECG for arrhythmic events after a MI (Savard et al, 1997) exceeds that of other tests such as left ventricular ejection fraction (LVEF) or ambulatory ECG. The existence of LVPs increases 6 to 8 times the risk of arrhythmic events after a MI and it is considered the best non-invasive method to identify postinfarction VT risk (Ho et al, 1993).
The widespread use of thrombolytic therapy, beta-blockers, antiplatelet therapy and revascularisation, lifetime changes and risk factor management, improved post-infarction survival. In this context and considering the proarrhythmic effects of antiarrhythmic drugs, it is important to identify patients with low risk. Due to its high negative predictive value, LVPs can play an important role in selecting patients for interventional studies. The role of SAECG as a screening test is limited due to the low positive predictive accuracy.

The behavior of LVPs on the body surface during programmed stimulation was evaluated by Ho et al (Ho et al, 1996), concluding that LVPs detected during sinus rhythm but lost after ventricular extrastimuli are often clinically irrelevant and may explain the false positive results and the reduced specificity of SAECG. LVPs revealed by ventricular extrastimuli but concealed during sinus rhythm may be clinically relevant and may explain some of the false negative results and the reduced sensitivity of SAECG.

8. Myocardial infarction (MI)

SAECG is still a very usefull method to identify MI patients at risk for lethal arrhythmic events (Huebner, 2010). In patients with **acute MI**, the electrophysiological substrate for LVPs gradually develop in the first 2 weeks of the acute event. LVPs were found in the first 3 hours after MI onset and their prevalence increased in the next 7-10 days. LVPs recorded in the first week were associated with subsequent ventricular dilation and may be due to cell slides (Zaman et al, 1993).

Once established, LVPs seem to remain indefinitely in most patients (Santangeli et al, 2008). LVPs can also disappear in the first year after an acute MI. Yang et al. consider that the prevalence of LVPs in the first week of a MI increases from 32% in the firs day to 52% in the days 7-10 (Yang et al, 1990).

Time-dependend changes have been also attributed to cell death in the border zone of the MI or resolution of myocardial ischemia (Goldberger et al, 1994).

In the second week and in **old myocardial infarction**, prevalence stabilizes at 25-35%. Savard et al. (Savard et al, 1997) consider that LVPs recorded after 5-15 days from an acute MI, are the best predictors of ventricular arrhythmia appearing in the first year. If LVPs are missing at hospital discharge, their subsequent appearance is unlikely (Kuchar et al, 1986). LVPs may disappear later due to reshuffle of the myocardial scar.

In the first year after a transmural infarction, the predictive value of LVPs is low for SCD, because factors like: unidirectional block, heart rate and autonomic imbalance are triggering repetitive arrythmias.

Patients with two MI (inferior and right ventricle) have a high prevalence of LVPs, independent of LVEF, and a high arrhythmia risk should be considered in those patients (Iltumur et al, 2001).

Prevalence of LVP is 7-10% in coronary heart disease without myocardial infarction.

Most studies on LVPs in MI patients were performed before the reperfusion era (Steinberg& Berbari, 1996). Studies investigating the effects of thrombolysis on LVPs reported controversial results. Bauer et al. (Bauer et al, 2005) suggested that LVP are of limited use for risk stratification in post infarction patients who received reperfusion/revascularization therapy. Zipes et al. considered that repermeabilisation of infarct related artery modifies the arrhythmogenic substrate and reduces the predictive power of LVPs (Zipes et al, 2006). The evidence for a benefit of thrombolysis on LVPs prevalence depended on the success of thrombolysis in achieving early and full coronary blood flow restoration (Hohnloser et al, 1994). LVPs were found in 25% to 65% of patients with an occluded infarct-related artery despite thrombolysis, but in only 6% to 34% of those with a patent infarct-related artery after thrombolytic therapy (Chew et al, 1990). Malik et al. showed that the usefulness of LVPs to predict subsequent arrhythmic events was significantly worse in patients who received thrombolytic therapy than in those who did not receive thrombolytic therapy (Malik et al, 1992). The controversial results may be due to the differences in therapy, lack of adequate randomization and controlled studies, different techniques of recording SA-ECG and criteria to define LVPs. Savard et al. demonstrated that the prevalence of arrhythmic events declined from 9.6% to 5.8% after trombolysis. Both the low positive predictive value (about 20%) and the high negative predictive value (97%) remained unchanged (Savard et al, 1997).

Percutaneous coronary interventions (PCIs) are associated with a significant reduction of the prevalence of LVPs (Santangeli et al, 2008). Bauer et al. showed that LVPs were significantly associated with SCD (Bauer et al, 2005). Ikeda et al. reported no significant prognostic role of LVPs for SCD/resuscitated cardiac arrest at a short-term follow-up of 3 to 6 months, but LVPs were independent predictors of sustained VT (Ikeda et al, 2002).

Reperfusion of severely ischemic myocardium may also lead to hemorrhages in the infarct core by extravasations of red blood cells through the damaged endothelium (Mather et al, 2010). The presence of hemorrhage was associated with a prolonged SA-QRS in patients with first ST-elevation acute MI, treated successfully with PCIs.

LVPs persist in patients not undergoing reperfusion, and may be caused by ventricular remodeling, involving fibrosis, redistribution of the fibers in the damaged region and one side left ventricular hypertrophy (LVH).

9. Cardiomyopathies

Cardiomyopathies are an important cause of SCD in young people.

Arrhythmogenic right ventricular cardiomyopathy/dysplasia (ARVC) is an inherited myocardial disease, characterized by fibro-fatty substitution of the right ventricle (Corrado & Thiene, 2006). The fibro-fatty areas can create reentry circuits, the substrate for repetitive ventricular arrhythmias and a delayed, fragmented activation font (Folino et al, 2006). The typical clinical manifestations are ventricular arrhythmias with left BBB pattern. LVPs were observed in more than 50% of patients with ARVC, and are minor diagnostic criteria in this setting (Santangeli et al, 2008). SAECG has shown particular reliability in ARVC, considering the classical location of the myocardial alterations in the right ventricle, which induce a delayed potential only in the terminal portion of QRS (Folino et al, 2006). Folino et al. (Folino et al, 2006) detected a progressive increase in delayed ventricular conduction, not associated with significant echocardiographic changes in patients with ARVC, and concluded that the baseline SAECG and echocardiographic parameters are useful in identifying patients with sustained VT. It was, also, hypothesized that the progression of the disease with an extension of fibro-fatty degeneration could completely isolate some infiltrated areas, with appearance of different preferential pathways of activation and reduction in late potentials (Folino et al, 2006).

A close correlation was found between SAECG and extent of disease (Nava et al, 2000). Turrini et al, found an increased percentage of fibrous tissue and a high risk for sustained ventricular arrhythmias in patients with LVPs and ARVC (Turrini et al, 1999). The sensitivity of SAECG for diagnosis of ARVC increased by using only 1 of 3 criteria (Kamath et al, 2011).

Santangeli et al (Santangeli et al, 2010) tested the association between noninvasive diagnostic criteria for ARVC and low voltage areas, detected at electroanatomic voltage mapping. SAECG abnormalities correlated with the presence of low voltage areas selectively in the right ventricular outflow tract, supporting the appropriateness of its inclusion among ARVC diagnostic criteria.

The prediction of sudden cardiac death is a major goal in the management of patients with **hypertrophic cardiomyopathy** (Cripps et al, 1990). Abnormal SAECGs were more prevalent in patients with hypertrophic cardiomyopathy compared to healthy controls, and were significantly associated with nonsustained VT on 48 h ECG Holter monitoring, but not with a family history of premature sudden cardiac death or a history of syncope (Cripps et al, 1990).

Fauchier et al. found a significantly higher incidence of severe ventricular premature beats in patients with **idiopathic dilated cardiomyopathy** (IDCM) and late ventricular potentials (Fauchier et al, 1991). Ohnishi et al. (Ohnishi et al, 1990) and Mancini et al. (Mancini et al, 1993) mentioned a high incidence of prospective arrhythmias and SCD in patients with a IDCM and abnormal SAECG. Kitamura et al (Kitamura et al, 2003) concluded that the heterogeneous expression of connexin 43 protein may contribute to impaired ventricular conduction and LVPs detected on SAECG in patients with IDCM. Patchy interstitial fibrosis adjacent to viable myocardium is commonly seen in dilated cardiomyopathy. Fibrosis decreases electrical coupling, slows the propagation of impulses between myocytes and can become the anatomical substrate for reentrant VT. Alterations of the gap junctions are accompanied by discontinuity of tissue structure, which includes the naturally occurring myocardial cell orientation and the collagen matrix formed by the fibrosis (Kitamura et al, 2003). The expression of connexin 43 was more decreased in patients with late ventricular potentials than in those without LVPs (Kitamura et al, 2003), but the degree of fibrosis seem not to influence the results.

10. Congenital heart defects

The predictive value of LVPs after repair of tetralogy of Fallot has been controversial. Al Balkhi et al. reported LVPs only 1 month after surgery in patients with tetralogy of Fallot, probably as a result of scarring (Al Balkhi et al, 2004). Zimmermann et al. found a correlation between inducibility of VT and LVPs (Zimmermann et al, 1991), but Giroud et al (Giroud et al, 1994) and Daliento et al. (Daliento et al, 1995) could not demonstrate a predictive value of LVPs alone in their studies. Janousek et al. found LVPs, and especially RMS40, to be predictive of spontaneous or induced VT in patients who underwent surgical correction of congenital cardiac disease (Janousek et al, 1995).

11. Heart failure (HF)

Patients with HF have a high SCD risk, despite therapeutic advances. Ventricular arrhythmias and SCD result from an interaction between a trigger and a substrate with neurohumoral factors (Bounhoure et al, 2010). The identification of the mechanisms of SCD in patients with HF is complicated by the different causes of HF. SCD risk correlates with the severity of congestive HF (Wilson et al, 1983). The high electrical instability in patients with post-infarction HF is due to structural inhomogeneities: patchy areas of fibrous tissue interdigitating with viable myocardium and scars. Interstitial fibrosis and hypertrophy are frequently seen on endomyocardial biopsies in patients with congestive HF. This can result in complex electrophysiological changes: abnormal impulse conduction with slow ventricular activation, changes in the refractory period responsible for ventricular arrhythmias (Bounhoure et al, 2010; Galinier et al, 1996).

There are conflicting results regarding the predictive value of LVPs for ventricular arrhythmias in HF patients. Small patient population studies (Meinertz et al, 1985; Middlekauff et al, 1990; Silverman et al, 1995) did not find SAECG to be predictive for SCD or ventricular arrhythmias in chronic HF. The studies by Mancini et al. and Galinier et al. found that the SAECG identified patients with congestive HF at high risk for death and/or ventricular tachycardia (Manicini et al, 1993; Galinier et al, 1996).

According to current guidelines, most patients with left ventricular dysfunction and symptomatic HF may benefit from implanted devices and resynchronization therapy. It is important but difficult to identify patients at risk, and LVPs , combined with other electrocardiographic stratification methods, etiologic and clinical information, may help to select the candidates (Bounhoure et al, 2010).

12. Brugada syndrome

Brugada syndrome is characterized by abnormal repolarization in the right ventricle, detected as ST elevation in the right precordial leads, and depolarization abnormality, detected as right bundle branch block and LVPs (Morita et al, 2008). Repolarization heterogeneity within the epicardium of the right ventricular outflow tract seems to be the origin of reentry arrhythmia (Morita et al, 2007). A reduced sodium current, due to mutations of the sodium channel gene SCN5A, slows the conduction velocity and causes conduction abnormalities. Conduction abnormalities provide a substrate for the degeneration of polymorphic VT into VF (Meregalli et al, 2005).

LVPs have been found in patients with the Brugada syndrome and might be helpful to identify patients at a higher risk of life-threatening arrhythmic events (Ikeda et al, 2001; Santangeli et al, 2008).

Kutsuzawa et al. (Kutsuzawa et al, 2011) reported two patients with Brugada syndrome and hypokalemia induced lethal events. Normalization of serum potassium concealed the typical ECG pattern, but LVPs persisted even at 18-month follow-up.

SAECG can detect not only LVPs, but also conduction abnormalities within the QRS complex: fragmented QRS (multiple spikes within the QRS complex) (Morita et al, 2008). It is considered that delayed activation within a small mass of ventricular tissue could produce LVPs and delayed activation in a larger ventricular mass can cause multiple spikes within the QRS complex. Fragmented QRS predicts syncope and VF in patients with Brugada syndrome (Morita et al, 2008).

13. Syncope

In patients with syncope of unknown cause, SAECG, combined with patient history and other diagnostic tests, can help identify or exclude a mechanism of VT as a cause of the syncope (Gang, et al, 1986; Santangeli et al, 2008).

14. Atrial fibrillation and flutter

It was hypothesized that the chaotic atrial activation in atrial fibrillation causes false-positive LVPs, making the analysis of SAECG very difficult (Buckingham et al, 1993; Halimi et al, 1994). But, atrial fibrillation rarely creates problems with time-domain analysis of the SAECG (Fitzgerald et al, 1996; Halimi et al, 1994). LVPs analysis provides similar results in atrial fibrillation and sinus rhythm, was concluded by Gottfridsson et al. (Gottfridsson et al, 2011) in a study including 82 patients with atrial fibrillation, undergoing electrical cardioversion, despite decrease of heart rate and prolongation of SA-QRS. Conflicting results were obtained by different authors, analyzing SAECG variables after cardioversion. Halimi et al (Halimi et al, 1994) mentioned significant changes of LAS40 and RMS40 after cardioversion. Buckingham et al (Buckingham et al, 1993) found no significant changes of SA-ECG parameters.

Atrial flutter waves occur during ventricular systole and mimic LVPs (Gatzoulis et al, 1993). In conclusion, atrial flutter can create significant errors in the automated time-domain analysis of the SAECG, and patients with atrial flutter should not undergo SAECG for postinfarction risk assessment (Fitzgerald et al, 1996).

15. Bundle branch block (BBB)

Increased QRS duration has been previously associated with increased mortality in patients with coronary heart disease and hypertensive patients (Brembilla-Perrot et al, 2001; Liew, 2011). Syncope and dizziness may be related either to atrio-ventricular conduction disturbances or to ventricular arrhythmias. On the other hand, the presence of intraventricular conduction defects interferes with the detection of LVPs (Brembilla-Perrot et al, 2001; Englund et al, 1995), and, thus, patients with BBB are often excluded from the SAECG studies. Therefore, the management of these patients needs special attention.

BBB decreased the specificity of the SAECG to predict VT risk in patients with dilated cardiomyopathy (Brembilla-Perrot et al, 1997). Among noninvasive parameters, only a prolonged SA-QRS (>165 ms) was a significant predictor of cardiac mortality (Brembilla-Perrot et al, 2001).

Delayed terminal conduction observed in incomplete right BBB may cause false positive LVPs (Manolis et al, 1997). In order to prevent false positive results, separate LVPs criteria were used for patients with BBB (Galinier et al, 1996).

16. Hypertension (HT)

A significant association has been demonstrated between hypertension and SCD (Yildirir et al, 2002). The risk of SCD due to ventricular arrhythmias was demonstrated by a prolonged QT interval or LVPs. The most important mechanisms by which HT predisposes to SCD are: the degree of left ventricular hypertrophy (LVH), interstitial fibrosis, myocardial or subendocardial scars, silent myocardial ischemia, diastolic dysfunction and disturbances in cardiac autonomic balance (Galinier et al, 1997; Kaftan AH & Kaftan O, 2000; Palatini et al, 1995; Yildirir et al, 2002). Coronary artery disease may interact with LVH in the genesis of ventricular arrhythmias and SCD (Galinier et al, 1997).

LVPs wer found by several authors in HT (Brune et al, 1991; Vester et al, 1992). Galinier et al. (Galinier et al, 1992) and Franchi et al. (Franchi et al, 1992) found a greater prevalence of LVPs in subjects with eccentric LVH than in those with concentric hypertrophy. Non-sustained VT has been found to have a prognostic value in HT patients (Galinier et al, 1997).

Vardas et al. (Vardas et al, 1994) and Palatini et al (Palatini et al, 1995) confirmed that a high prevalence of ventricular arrhythmias was associated with LVPs in HT patients. Only the E/A ratios were related to the presence of either LVPs or VT, and they were far lower in patients with LVPs (Palatini et al, 1995).

The initial reports of the Framingham Heart Study demonstrated the deleterious effect on survival of LVH (Kannel & Abbot, 1986; Levy et al, 1990). A downward trend in the prevalence of LVH was noticed in the last decades, which coincided with improved HT control (Priori et al, 2001). A lack of a relation between left ventricular mass and the occurrence of LVPs has been also reported by some authors (Panagides et al, 1990; Prisant et al, 1993; Rizzo et al, 2000).

Experimentally, LVH delays ventricular conduction and prolongs action potential duration. Electrocardiographic QRS duration and QT interval measures reflect these changes (Oikarinen et al, 2004). The increased QRS duration may be attributed to the increased thickness of the left ventricle wall and to intramural fibrosis, which distorts and prolongs transmural impulse propagation, or it could be a manifestation of intraventricular or interventricular conduction delay or block (Hancock et al, 2009). Alterations in ion channels due to hypertrophy were also mentioned as possible causes of QT interval prolongation in LVH (Hancock et al, 2009).

LVPs were present in both dippers and nondippers, and the values were significantly lower in dippers for SA-QRS and LAS40, and nondipper pattern was not linked to a worse arrhythmogenic substrate (Rizzo et al, 2000).

There is no study with power to show prognostic significance of LVPs in HT patients. All studies on LVPs in hypertensive patients have all been small scale, with short follow up.

17. Dyslipidemia and metabolic syndrome

The epidemiological association between elevated LDL cholesterol and risk of all manifestations of coronary artery disease including SCD is well established (Priori et al, 2001). A relation between **dyslipidemia** and electrical instability has been hypothesized. Gimaev et al. (Gimaev et al, 2009) evaluated the effect of disturbed lipid metabolism on SAECG characteristics and found LVPs in patients with high, moderately elevated, low and normal serum cholesterol. Hypercholesterolemia has been reported to induce proarrhythmic sympathetic neural sprouting and ventricular electrophysiologic remodeling, and an increased vulnerability to VF in a high-fat-fed animal model (Liu et al, 2003).

A significant correlation was found between serum cholesterol and SAQRS, LAS40 and RMS40 in patients with an old MI (Mozos & Hancu, 2010).

Clinical trials of lipid lowering in the primary prevention of coronary artery disease have not evaluated SCD risk, and have not sufficient statistical power to identify a significant reduction (Priori et al, 2001). Statins seem to have antiarrhythmic properties in addition to their lipid-lowering effects (Chu et al 2007; Abuissa et al, 2009).

Isolated **metabolic syndrome** is associated with an increase in left ventricular mass index and diastolic dysfunction, increasing the risk of cardiovascular disease (Aijaz et al, 2008). The prevalence of increased QT interval duration has been investigated with respect to single components of the metabolic syndrome (Strohmer et al, 2007).

18. Obesity

Patients with morbid obesity have high rates of sudden, unexpected cardiac death (Duflou et al, 1995). An increased prevalence of abnormal SAECG results has been found in obese patients without known clinical heart disease, and body mass index (BMI) can be considered as an independent predictor of abnormal SAECG results (Lalani et al, 2000). Mizia-Stec et al .

(Mizia-Stec et al, 2000) found an increased QT dispersion (QTd) in obese women, associated with LVH and significantly higher QTd in patients with late ventricular potentials.

The mechanism of death in these patients remains uncertain. Parasympathetic withdrawal, occuring with increasing obesity, conduction abnormalities, cardiomyopathy of obesity, the lipotoxicity of the myocardium induced by free fatty acids, released from hypertrophied adipocytes in obese persons with myocardial steatosis, structural heterogeneity due to fatty infiltration of the heart, myocyte hypertrophy, focal myocardial disarray, fibrosis and mononuclear cell infiltration could be involved (Alexander, 1985; Bharati & Lev, 1995; Duflou et al, 1995; Lalani et al, 2000). Particularly, with a concentric pattern of LVH, the prevalence of ventricular ectopic beats is substantially elevated in obese patients (Schunkert, 2002). The cardiomyopathy of morbid obesity, the most common cause of SCD in these patients, is characterized by cardiomegaly, left ventricular dilatation, and myocyte hypertrophy in the absence of interstitial fibrosis.

A BMI associated increase in chronic MI patients' SCD risk was mentioned by Mozos et al. and SAECG-QRS and LAS40 correlated with BMI in patients with an old MI (Mozos et al, 2007).

19. Diabetes mellitus and hyperglycemia

There is controversy in the literature as to whether glucose intolerance or diabetes mellitus are independent risk factors for SCD (Priori et al, 2001). Streptozocin experimentally induced diabetes impairs both depolarization and repolarization (Pacher et al, 1999). QT interval prolongation in diabetic patients has been attributed to autonomic neuropathy and insulin resistance, and in healthy non-diabetic subjects with high plasma glucose, to increased cytosolic calcium content, oxidative stress and enhanced sympathetic activity (Muntean et al, 2009).

Kowalewski et al. (Kowalewski et al, 2002) included 72 children with type 1 diabetes mellitus in his study and found an increased prevalence of abnormal SAECGs and LVPs. Diabetic children with LVPs had thicker left ventricular posterior wall and longer diabetes duration time than children without LVPs. Nonlinear regression model showed that duration of diabetes, cardiac autonomic neuropathy, and left ventricular posterior wall were the strongest independent parameters of LVPs occurrence.

An association between hyperglycemia on admission in patients with acute ST elevation MI and arrhythmias during hospitalization has been observed (Sanjuan et al, 2011). Stress hyperglycemia on admission was found to be a predictor of mortality and arrhythmias in patients with acute ST elevation MI and could be used in the stratification of risk in these patients (Pinto et al, 2008; Sanjuan et al, 2011).

20. End-stage renal failure and hemodialysis

Cardiac disease is the major cause of death in dialysis patients (Herzog et al, 2008). LVH with interstitial fibrosis, deposition of calcium and aluminum salts in the heart tissue often occur in patients with end-stage renal disease (ESRD) (Morales et al, 1998). Autonomic neuropathy and impairment of left ventricular functions have been frequently encountered in chronic renal failure and depend on the disease duration (Karayaylali et al, 2003). SCD risk due to ventricular arrhythmias is high in ESRD patients on hemodialysis (HD) (Dubrava et al, 2003; Sakhuja et al, 2009). SAECG parameters are abnormal in a significant proportion of patients with chronic renal failure (Girgis et al, 1999). The mentioned histological changes could represent a potential substrate for LVPs. LVH was already considered as SA-QRS prolonging factor in hypertensive patients (Vester et al, 1992) and associated with a high prevalence of LVPs in post-infarction HF patients (Mozos et al, 2009). This explanation appears unlikely in renal failure. Morales et al. did not detect significant differences in left ventricular mass between end-stage renal failure patients with and without late ventricular potentials before HD (Morales et al, 1998). Roithinger et al. did not find a significant association between mortality and LVPs or structural myocardial changes in HD patients, but a tendency towards an excess mortality of patients with coronary artery disease and compromised left ventricular function (Roithinger et al, 1992). On the other hand, Girgis et al. concluded that SAECG parameters improve with HD, and, decreased left ventricular dimensions, because of fluid removal during HD, (Girgis et al, 1999).

Volume, electrolyte, acid-base balance, heart rate and blood pressure changes appearing during HD, can trigger supraventricular and ventricular arrhythmias (Dubrava et al, 2003; Morales et al, 1998). Most of the studies performed in HD patients have focused on QRS amplitude and T wave (Morales et al, 1998). Abnormalities in SAECG were also mentioned in patients undergoing HD and peritoneal dialysis (Girgis et al, 1999; Ichikawa et al, 1997; Morales et al, 1998; Roithinger et al, 1992).

The prevalence of late ventricular potentials was 25% in the study of Morales et. al (Morales et al, 1998), including patients with a known history of myocardial infarction, and only 14% in another study including younger patients, with a lower prevalence of coronary heart disease (Roithinger et al, 1992). Ichikawa et al reported no LVPs before HD and abnormal SAECGs in only 2.4% of the patients (Ichikawa et al, 1997). Late ventricular potentials were attributed to underlying coronary heart disease with left ventricular dysfunction (Morales et al, 1998). Most of the studies reported improved SAECGs after HD.

Morales et al and Ichikawa et al reported a prolongation of SA-QRS duration after dialysis (Ichikawa et al, 1997; Morales et al, 1998), probably due to widening of the initial portion of the QRS, related to the acute reduction in serum potassium (Morales et al, 1998). Girgis et al. showed that only LAS40 and RMS40 change significantly after hemodialysis (Girgis et al, 1999). LAS40 was also significantly increased postdialysis in a study of Ichikawa et al, and the changes in LAS40 correlated with the changes in potassium in the high-K group (Ichikawa et al, 1997). Larger studies are needed to verify the effect of HD on time-domain SAECG parameters.

Animal studies demonstrated that hypokalemia-induced arrhythmogenicity is due to slowed conduction, prolonged ventricular repolarisation (caused by inhibition of outward potassium currents) and abnormal pacemaker activity (Osadchii, 2010). Hypokalemia effect on repolarisation is not uniform, causing amplified spatial repolarisation gradients and an unidirectional conduction block (Osadchii, 2010). Prolongation of action potential may be associated with shortening of the effective refractory period, facilitating reentry. Serum potassium between 4.6 and 5.3 mEq/l was associated with best survival in HD patients, and potassium <4 or ≥ 5.6 mEq/l was associated with increased mortality (Kovesdy et al, 2007). An insufficient decrease of serum potassium by hemodialysis was suggested to be an arrhythmogenic factor (Ichikawa et al, 1997).

21. Alcoholism

Acute alcoholic states, binge drinking, the "holiday heart syndrome" and liver cirrhosis are associated with prolonged QT intervals and an increased prevalence of cardiac arrhythmias and SCD (Day et al, 1993; Genovesi et al, 2008; Wever & Robles de Medina, 2004;). In contrast, case-control studies have demonstrated a protective effect of moderate alcohol consumption against sudden cardiac death (Priori et al, 2001; Vreede-Swagemakers et al, 1999). Alcohol inhibits the Na-K-ATPase, which alters the resting membrane potential, delays calcium binding and transport by the cardiac sarcoplasmic reticulum and impairs calcium channels (Lorsheyd & de Lange, 2005).

Life-threatening ventricular arrhythmias are found in alcoholics without heart disease (Moushmoush et al, 1991). Alcoholic cardiomyopathy is associated with localized delays in intraventricular conduction and nonuniform myocardial involvement (Luca, 1979).

Koskinen & Kupari did not find LVPs in chronic alcoholics without detectable heart disease (Koskinen & Kupari, 1993). The absence of LVPs does not exclude nonuniformity of alcohol induced myocardial changes.

Chronic heavy alcohol consumption increases left ventricular mass and may cause subclinical impairment in left ventricular function (Luca, 1979).

Pochmalicki et al. found LVPs in chronic alcoholics (Pochmalicki et al, 1997) and concluded that cronic alcohol intake, sufficient to cause histologically significant fatty liver, is ssociated with LVPs. LVPs could reveal early, preclinical myocardial lesions, and help to identify alcoholic patients at high risk of lethal arrhythmias.

22. Chronic obstructive pulmonary disease (COPD)

COPD is an independent risk factor for cardiovascular morbidity and mortality (Celli et al, 2010). Potential explanations for this association include: smoking, negative cardiac consequences of dynamic hyperinflation, exercise limitations and hypoxemia (Celli et al, 2010; Priori et al, 2001).

Carjea (Carjea, 2003) studied the prevalence and characteristics of late ventricular potentials in 90 patients with COPD compared to healthy subjects and found significant differences. The highest prevalence was noticed in moderate to severe cases.

23. Acromegaly

The heart is an end-organ of growth hormone action. A high prevalence of complex ventricular arrhythmias has been mentioned in patients with acromegaly, possible as a result of disordered left ventricular architecture and ventricular remodeling (Clayton, 2003).

The frequency of premature ventricular complexes increased with duration of acromegaly, and the severity of arrhythmia correlated with left ventricular mass but not with growth hormone levels (Kahaly et al, 1992). Structural heterogeneity in acromegalic heart is due to areas of hypertrophied myocytes, separated by fibrosis and cellular infiltrations (Clayton, 2003). Late ventricular potentials are frequently seen in active acromegaly, are associated with disease activity and may represent an early and sensitive parameter to detect myocardial injury (Herrmann et al, 2001). No association was found between presence of late ventricular potentials and left ventricular mass index. Longitudinal studies are needed to determine whether therapy changes the electrophysiological abnormalities.

Earlier studies showed that arrhythmias were as frequent before and after treatment of acromegaly, implying that fibrous tissue infiltration caused irreversible scarring (Hayward et al, 1987; Rodrigues et al, 1989).

24. Thalassemia

Beta–thalassemia, the impaired production of the beta hemoglobin chain, is associated with significant changes in heterogeneity of cardiac ventricular repolarization and SCD (Russo et al, 2011). In the late stages, frequent premature ventricular contractions and sustained ventricular tachycardia have been mentioned, related to cardiac death. Thalassemia patients require intensive blood transfusions due to severe anemia, and an increase in body iron burden occurs both in patients who are or are not receiving transfusions (Lekawanvijit & Chattipakorn, 2009).
The role of iron overload in causing conduction delays in the thalassemic heart is well documented and iron overload thalassemic cardiomyopathy may explain the occurrence of LVPs (Isma'eel et al, 2007), as well as changes in QRS duration and RMS40 voltage. The patchy nature of cardiac iron deposition may provide substrates for re-entry and risk of fatal arrhythmias (Lekawanvijit & Chattipakorn, 2009). Iron-overloaded cardiomyocytes have a smaller overshoot potential and shorter action potential duration than iron-free cardiomyocytes in the same heart and reduced Na^+ currents may be an underlying mechanism (Lekawanvijit & Chattipakorn, 2009). Further mechanisms related to tachyarrhythmias and SCD are changes in calcium homeostasis, elevated prostaglandin E2 to prostacyclin ratio, increased interleukin 1 level and lipid peroxidation.
Future large populations, long-term follow-up studies are needed to demonstrate further clinical consequences in iron overload cardiomyopathy.

25. Connective tissue and systemic diseases

Cardiovascular involvement is common in connective tissue diseases (Lazzerini et al, 2006), but myocardial involvement is seldom recognized clinically (Stanescu & Dan, 1992). Ventricular arrhythmias represent a major cause of SCD in autoimmune rheumatic diseases (Sefarovic et al, 2006). The mechanisms are probably multiple and myocardial fibrosis seems to play a pivotal role (Lazzerini et al, 2006). Lazzerini et al (Lazzerini et al, 2007) concluded that anti-Ro/SSA positive patients have a particularly high risk of developing ventricular arrhythmias.
The heart is one of the major organs involved in scleroderma. Ventricular arrhythmias are common among asymptomatic patients with **systemic sclerosis**, especially: premature ventricular contractions and non-sustained VT (Sefarovic et al, 2006). Patchy myocardial fibrosis represents an ideal substrate for reentry tachyarrhythmias. LVPs occurred in patients with diffuse progressive systemic sclerosis; a lower myocardial involvement was noticed in the CREST syndrome (Paradiso et al, 1996). Diffuse abnormalities of the cardiac tissue detected by SAECG may be present in patients with systemic sclerosis without cardiac symptoms and higher skin scores correlated with the presence of LVPs (Paradiso et al, 2002). Pignone et al (Pignone et al, 1994) found no correlation between LVPs and immunologic patterns, cutaneous and pulmonary involvement in 26 patients with systemic sclerosis.
Myocardial lesions in **systemic lupus erythematosus** are characterized by an increase in interstitial connective tissue and myocardial scarring (Paradiso et al, 2001). The most important cardiac manifestations of systemic lupus erythematosus are: pericarditis, lesions of valves, myocardium and coronary artery disease (Gomez-Leon Manduiano & Amezcua-Guerra, 2008). Sinus and atrial arrhythmias are more prevalent, but QT interval

prolongation, abnormalities in the autonomic tone and LVPs indicate high risk of developing life-threatening ventricular arrhythmias (Sefarovic et al, 2006). LVPs were recorded in patients with systemic lupus (Paradiso et al, 2001; Wranicz et al, 2001), and the depolarization abnormalities revealed by SAECG reflect a longer extent of myocardial fibrosis and echocardiography and SAECG alterations are markers of subclinical myocardial involvement. Increasing evidence suggest that anti-Ro/SSA antibodies may trigger rhythm disturbances due to an inhibiting cross-reaction with several cardiac calcium and potassium ionic channels (Lazzerini et al, 2010).

So far, the evidence related to electrocardiographic disturbances in this setting is restricted to studies with small number of patients (Teixeira, et al, 2010). The mechanisms of arrhythmias are related to the inflammatory process of pericarditis and myocarditis, atherosclerotic myocardial ischemia, increased sympathetic activity, vasculitis of small vessels with collagen deposits and anti-Ro/SSA antibodies (Lazzerini et al, 2010; Teixeira, et al, 2010).

Cardiac **sarcoidosis** affects the myocardium, pericardium and endocardium, and the disease may present with: atrioventricular and intraventricular conduction disturbances, ventricular arrhythmias and HF. Ventricular arrhythmias are among the main causes of SCD in cardiac sarcoidosis. LVPs on SAECG were mentioned and they were abolished after steroid therapy (Yodogawa et al, 2011).

26. Schizophrenia

Schizophrenia patients were also found to be positive for LVPs. Cardiac autonomic dysregulation in schizophrenia patients and use of psychiatric and/or non-psychiatric medications that affect conduction, may account for LVPs (Nashoni et al, 2010).

27. Influence of therapy on LVPs

LVPs are influenced by antiarrhythmic therapy, trombolytic drugs, anevrismectomy, percutaneous coronary interventions, coronary artery bypass surgery, statins, steroids.

The effect on the prevalence of LVPs of modern pharmacologic therapy in patients with acute MI has been assessed in several studies (Santangeli et al, 2008). Class I, II and III antiarrhythmics may reduce the prevalence of LVPs. Class IV antiarrhythmics (Verapamil) do not influence LVPs. Some class III antiarrhythmic drugs are able to prolong SA-QRS and LAS40, and may be associated with the occurence of LVPs.

Freedman and Steinberg showed that sodium channel blockers (quinidine, procainamide, imipramide) have preferential effects on slowly conducting tissue in patients with a history of VT, causing an important prolongation of LVPs (Freedman & Steinberg, 1991).

Santarelli et al, reported that LVPs were less frequent in acute MI patients treated with betablockers compared with those not treated with betablockers during hospitalization. This effect was found only in patients with a preserved LVEF (Santarelli et al, 1993).

No significant SAECG changes have been observed after Sotalol.

Adrenergic stimulation with adrenaline and isoprenaline, and parasympatholytic agents such as atropine, lead to significant changes in the signal averaged electrocardiogram in healthy subjects (Goldberger et al, 1994). Beta-adrenergic stimulation with isoproterenol led to a significant shortening of SA-QRS, and epinephrine prolonged the QRS duration. Increased alfa-adrenergic stimulation with phenylephrine and parasympathetic stimulation did not affect the SAECG. Parasympathetic blockade caused a mild decrease in the QRS duration. Changes in the RMS40 and LAS40 paralleled those of the QRS duration (Goldberger et al, 1994).

Junker et al, found in a substudy of the CONSENSUS II trial, a reduced prevalence of LVPs after the angiotensin converting enzyme inhibitor enalapril (Junker et al, 1995).

Lipid-lowering interventions reduce coronary events, VT/VF episodes, SCD and all-cause mortality (Liu et al, 2009). Recent studies have demonstrated that statins have antiarrhythmic properties in addition to their lipid-lowering effects (Abuissa et al, 2009; Chu et al 2007; Liu et al, 2009). Kayikcioglu et al. found a significant decrease of the prevalence of LVPs and ventricular arrhythmias in acute MI patients receiving pravastatin, irrespective of lipid level (Kayikcioglu et al, 2003). Pre-treatment with statin could reduce the reperfusion arrhythmias after acute myocardial infarction (Zhao et al, 2008). Most of the antiarrhythmic benefits after statin therapy observed in high cardiovascular risk patients might be explained by statins' pleiotropic effects: anti-ischemia, anti-inflammation, antihypertrophy, angiogenic and sympathetic effects (Chu et al, 2007). Statins achieve their antiarrhythmic drug action in part by preventing or reversing electrophysiologic remodeling induced by hypercholesterolemia, but they also have an independent antiarrhythmic effect (Liu et al, 2009).

The ratio between QTc and QRS changes caused by several antiarrhythmic drugs identifies patients with sustained VT risk, which appear despite therapy (Cain et al, 1996).

LVPs may disappear after coronary artery bypass surgery in acute MI patients (Bigger et al, 1997). Anevrisectomy is also known to reduce the prevalence of LVPs.

Corticosteroid therapy may be effective for ventricular arrhythmias in the early stage of cardiac sarcoidosis (Yodogawa et al, 2011).

28. Correlation and combination with other ECG methods

Several studies have mentioned correlations between surface standard 12-lead ECG and SAECG parameters. The relation between LVP and **QT dispersion** (QTd) (Ducceschi et al, 1996; Mozos, 2006), suggested that the existence of some slow conducting myocardial areas, related to positive LVPs, is associated with a higher inhomogeneity of ventricular repolarisation, expressed as a higher QTd. LAS40 and SA-QRS correlated with QT dispersion (Ducceschi et al, 1998).

QT intervals and Tpeak-Tend intervals were prolonged in post-infarction HF patients with LVPs. LVPs and SAECG parameters can be predicted using 12-lead ECG: QT intervals, QRS duration, T wave variables (Mozos et al, 2011). The significant association between SA-QRS and Tpeak-Tend interval and T wave amplitude was attributed to the extension of LVP into the ST segment.

Breithardt et al. (Breithardt et al, 1990) showed that the presence of LVPs was positively correlated with an **ECG score** based on R and Q wave duration and R/S ratio in MI patients with or without a history of sustained VT.

LVPs were not related to the frequency of **ventricular ectopic activity** and malignant premature ventricular contractions because each test assesses different components of arrhythmia susceptibility. The combination of the two abnormalities may identify a high-risk group for SCD (Middelkauff et al, 1990; Fauchier et al, 1991).

The combination of **T wave alternans** and SAECG, increases sensitivity, specificity, positive and negative predictive value for VT risk (Kondo et al, 2001).

SAECG and **body surface mapping** (BSM) provide complementary information in patients with an old MI, and an important, significant correlation was found between isointegral QRST maximum and LAS40 and RMS40 (Mozos et al, 2008). SAECG may be assessed using BSM, increasing its sensitivity in anterior and inferior MI (Ho, 1993). BSM may detect LVPs, undetected by SAECG, even if the underlying substrate is relative small or the electrodes are placed outside that area (Linnenbank et al, 2001). Analysis of isopotential maps of the terminal part of the QRS complex may provide additional information regarding LVPs distribution, slow conducting areas and VT origin (Faugere et al, 1986).

29. LVPs and other ventricular arrhythmia predictors

Despite the significant predictive value for arrhythmic events, LVPs show a low positive predictive accuracy, thus resulting in limited usefulness as a single variable to identify patients at high risk (Santangeli et al, 2008). Significantly impaired LVEF is an established predictor of SCD and is included in the current guidelines for primary prevention of SCD. But patients with a preserved LVEF are not included in the current guidelines (Liew, 2011).

Combination of LVPs with LVEF (Jain & Avasthi, 1992; Konta et al, Kudaiberdieva et al, 2003), ventricular volumes (Pollak et al, 1985), heart rate variability (Gomes et al, 2001), ventricular diskinezia (Olinic & Zdrenghea, 1998), programmed ventricular stimulation (Ho et al, 1996), atrial pacing (Steinbigler et al, 1999), a high Killip class (3 or 4) in a patient with a history of a MI, may improve the predictive value of LVPs for ventricular arrhythmias.

Kudaiberdieva et al (Kudaiberdieva et al, 2003) investigated incidence of ventricular tachycardia/ventricular fibrillation in relation with noninvasive arrhythmia risk markers in 54 patients with an old myocardial infarction. Logistic regression analysis revealed that the highest association with ventricular tachyarrhythmia had combination of LVPs and increased QT variability index, followed by combination of LVPs and left ventricular ejection fraction.

Standard methods fail to reveal late potentials in 20 to 30% of patients with ventricular arrhythmias after myocardial infarction (Steinbigler et al, 1999). Increase in heart rate may unmask late potentials in patients prone to malignant ventricular arrhythmias, because conduction in the arrhythmogenic area is critically slowed by an increased heart rate. Functional late potential analysis, with non-invasive clinical stress tests, should be performed in order to identify patients at risk of malignant ventricular arrhythmias, not identified with conventional late potential analysis (Steinbigler et al, 1999).

Epicardial mapping has demonstrated that during sinus rhythm, activation of the tissue critical to ventricular tachycardia is completed before the end of the QRS complex and is not detectable within the ST segment (Steinbigler et al, 1999). A shift of septal mid-QRS potentials toward the terminal QRS complex by critical slowing of conduction during increased heart rate, could explain the appearance of new late ventricular potentials. Different findings may be due to myocardial infarction location: an increase of QRS duration in patients with anterior infarction and an increase of magnitude and LAS40 in patients after inferior infarctions (Steinbigler et al, 1999).

Combining electrocardiography methods with other methods may help to select the candidates for pharmacological therapy, defibrillator implantation and resynchronization, in order to reduce overall mortality and SCD.

30. Conclusions

Sudden cardiac death, caused mainly by fatal ventricular arrhythmias, can be predicted using a practical and low-cost tool: SAECG. LVPs represent slowed conduction through a diseased myocardium and may form the substrate for life-threatening ventricular arrhythmias in patients with cardiac and extracardiac pathology. SAECG is altered due to a variety of physiological and pharmacologic conditions. Antiarrhythmic therapy, trombolytic drugs, anevrismectomy, percutaneous coronary interventions, coronary artery bypass surgery, statins and steroid therapy are able to influence LVPs. Late ventricular potentials have a high negative predictive value. When positive, LVPs help better stratify the arrhythmic risk of patients, alone or in combination with other methods, in several clinical settings.

31. References

Abuissa H, O'Keefe JH, Bybee KA. (2009). Statins as anti-arrhythmics: a systematic review part II: effects on risk of ventricular arrhythmias. *Clin Cardiol,* 23(10), pp. 542-52

Aijaz B, Ammar KA, Lopez-Jimenez F, et al. (2008). Abnormal cardiac structure and function in the metabolic syndrome: a population-based study. *Mayo Clin Proc,* 83(12), pp. 1350-7

Al Balkhi R, Beghetti M, Friedly B. (2004). Time course of appearance of markers of arrhythmia in patients with tetralogy of Fallot before and after surgery. *Cardiol Young,* 14, pp. 360–366

Alexander JK. (1985). The cardiomyopathy of obesity. *Prog Cardiovasc Dis,* 28, pp. 325-34

Ammann P, Bluzaite I, Roelli H, et al. (2004). Correlation of QT dispersion after Exercise Stress-Test with Coronary Artery Disease. *Elektronika ir Elektrotechnika,* 2(51), pp. 78-81

Askenazi J, Parisi AF, Cohn PF, et al. (1978). Value of the QRS complex in assessing left ventricular ejection fraction. *Am J Cardiol,* 41(3), pp. 494-499

Barbosa Benchimol PR, de Sousa MO, Correa Barbosa E, et al. (2002). Analysis of the Prevalence of Ventricular Late Potentials in the Late Phase of Myocardial Infarction Based on the Site of Infarction. *Arq Bras Cardiol,* 78, pp. 358-63

Bauer A, Guzik P, Barthel P, et al. (2005). Reduced prognostic power of ventricular late potentials in post-infarction patients of the reperfusion era. *Eur Heart J,* 26, pp. 755–761

Berbari EJ, Scherlag BJ, Hope RR, et al. (1978). Recording from the body surface of arrhythmogenic ventricular activity during the S-T segment. *Am J Cardiol,* 41, pp 697- 702

Bigger Jr JT. (1997). Prophylactic use of implanted cardiac defibrillators in patients at high risk for ventricular arrhythmias after coronary-artery bypass graft surgery. Coronary Artery Bypass Graft (CABG) Patch Trial Investigators. *N Engl J Med,* 337, pp. 1569

Bharati S & Lev M. (1995). Cardiac conduction system involvement in sudden death of obese young people. *Am Heart J,* 129, pp. 273-81

Bounhoure JP, Galinier M, Boveda S, et al. (2010). Ventricular arrhythmias, sudden death and heart failure. *Bull Acad Nat Med,* 194(6), pp. 997-1007

Breithardt G, Cain ME, El-Sherif N, et al. (1991). Standards for Analysis of Ventricular Late Potentials Using High - Resolution or Signal - Averaged Electrocardiography. *J Am Coll Cardiol*, 17(5), pp. 999-1006

Breithardt G, Hackstein N, Borggreffe M, et al. (1990). Diagnostiv value of electrocardiographic variables to predict the presence of ventricular late potentials. *J Am Coll Card*, 15, pp. 152-8

Breithardt G, Becker R, Seipel L, et al. (1981). Non-invasive detection of late potentials in man - a new marker for ventricular tachycardia. *Eur Heart J*, 2, pp. 1–11

Brembilla-Perrot B, Suty-Selton C, Houriez P, et al. (2001). Value of non-invasive and invasive studies in patients with bundle branch block, syncope and history of myocardial infarction. *Europace*, 3, pp. 187-194

Brembilla-Perrot B, Terrier de la Chaise A, Jacquemin L, et al. (1997). The signal-averaged electrocardiogram is of limited value in patients with bundle branch block and dilated cardiomyopathy in predicting inducible ventricular tachycardia or death. *Am J Cardiol*, 79(2), pp. 154-9

Brune S, Gonska BD, Fleischmann C, et al. (1991). Prevalence of late ventricular potentials in hypertensive patients. *J Cardiovasc Pharmacol*, 17(Suppl 2), pp. S46-7

Buckingham TA, Radin MM, Volgman AS, et al. (1993). Does atrial fibrillation cause false-positive late potentials? *Pacing Clin Electrophysiol*, 16(12), pp. 2222-6

Cain ME, Anderson JL, Arnsdorf MF, et al. (1996). Signal-Averaged Electrocardiography. ACC Expert Consensus Document. *J Am Coll Card*, 27(1), pp. 238-249

Carjea MI. (2003). Prevalence of late ventricular potentials in patients with chronic obstructive lung disease. *Pneumologia*, 52(3-4), pp. 181-3

Celli B, Decramer M, Leimer I, et al. (2010). Cardiovascular safety of tiotropium in patients with COPD. *Chest*, 137 (1), pp. 20-30

Chew EW, Morton P, Murtagh JG, et al. (1990). Intravenous streptokinase for acute myocardial infarction reduces the occurrence of ventricular late potentials. *BHJ*, 64, pp. 5

Christiansen EH, Frost L, Mlgaard H, et al. (1995). The signal-averaged ECG becomes late potential-positive at low noise levels in healthy subjects. *Eur Heart J*, 16, pp. 1731-5

Chu CS, Lee KT, Lee ST, et al. (2007). Effects of atorvastatin on ventricular late potentials and ventricular late potentials and repolarization dispersion in patients with hypercholesterolemia. *Kaohsiung J Med Sci*, 23, pp.217–24

Clayton RN. (2003). Cardiovascular function in acromegaly. *Endocrien Reviews*, 24, pp. 272-277

Corrado D & Thiene G. (2006). Arrhythmogenic right ventricular cardiomyopathy/dysplasia: clinical impact of molecular genetic studies. *Circulation*, 113, pp. 1634-37

Cripps TR, Counihan PJ, Frenneaux MP, et al. (1990). Signal-averaged electrocardiography in hypertrophic cardiomyopathy. *J Am Coll Cardiol*,15, pp. 956

Fauchier JP, Cosnay P, Babuty D, et al. (1991). Etude du potential arrythmogene des myocardiopathies. Les myocardiopathies dilatees. *Arch Mai Coeur*, 84, pp. 95-103

Daliento L, Caneve F, Turrini P, et al. (1995). Clinical significance of high-frequency, low amplitude electrocardiographic signals and QT dispersion in patients operated on for tetralogy of Fallot. *Am J Cardiol.*, 76, pp. 408–411

Day CP , James OF, Butler TJ, et al. (1993). QT prolongation and sudden cardiac death in patients with alcoholic liver disease. *Lancet*, 341, pp. 1423–8

Dubrava J, Fekete J, Lehotska A. (2003). Relation of ventricular late potentials and intradialytic changes in serum electrolytes, ultrafiltration, left ventricular ejection fraction and left ventricular mass index in haemodialysis patients. *Bratisl Lek Listy*, 104(12), pp. 388-392

Ducceschi V, Sarubbi B, Giasi A, et al.(1996). Correlation between late potentials duration and QTc dispersion: Is there a causal relationship? *Int J Cardiol*, 53(3), pp. 285-290

Ducceschi V, D'Andrea A, Sarubbi B, et al. (1998). Repolarization abnormalities in patients with idiopatic ventricular tachycardias. *Can J Cardiol.*, 14(12), pp. 1451-5

Duflou J, Virmani R, Rabin L, et al. (1995). Sudden death as a result of heart disease in morbid obesity. *Am Heart J*, 130, pp. 306-13

Engel G, Beckerman JG, Froelicher VF, et al. (2004). Electrocardiographic arrythmia risk testing. *Curr Probl Cardiol*, 29, pp. 357-432

Engel TR, Pierce DL, Murphy SP. (1993). Variation in late potentials and the reproducibility of their measurement. *Prog Cardiovasc Dis*, 35, pp. 247-62

Englund A, Rosenqvist M, Bergfeldt L. (1995). Use of signal-averaged electrocardiography for predicting inducible sustained monomorphic ventricular tachycardia in patients with bundle branch block with and without a history of syncope. *Am Heart J*, 130, pp. 481-8

Faugere G, Savard P, Nadeau RA, et al. (1986). Characterization of the spatial distribution of late ventricular potentials by body surface mapping in patients with ventricular tachycardia. *Circulation*, 74, pp. 1323-1333

Fetsch Th. (1999). Neue Methoden in der kardinalen Funktionsdiagnostik: Ventrikulare Spatpotentiale. *Deutsches Ärzteblatt*, 96(39), pp. A-2443/B-2105/C-1956

Fitzgerald DM, Hawthorne HR, Crossley GH, et al. (1996). Effects of atrial fibrillation and atrial flutter on the signal-averaged electrocardiogram. *Am J Cardiol*, 77(2), pp. 205-9

Folino AF, Bauce B, Frigo G, et al. (2006). Long-term follow-up of the signal-averaged ECG in arrhythmogenic right ventricular cardiomyopathy: correlation with arrhythmic events and echocardiographic findings. *Europace*, 8, pp. 423-29

Frances RJ. (2010). Low noise level unmasks late potentials on signal-averaged electrocardiography. *Exp Clin Cardiol*, 15(3), pp. e61-e64

Franchi F, Michelucci A, Padeletti L, et al. (1992). Arrhythmogenesis in left ventricular hypertrophy in mild to moderate essential hypertension. *G Ital Cardiol*, 23, pp. 905-18

Freedman RA & Steinberg JS. (1991). Selective prolongation of QRS late potentials by sodium channel blocking antiarrhythmic drugs: relation to slowing of ventricular tachycardia. *J Am Coll Cardiol*, 17, pp. 1017-25

Galinier M, Balanescu S, Fourcade J, et al. (1997). Prognostic value of arrhythmogenic markers in systemic hypertension. *Eur Heart J*, 18, pp. 1484-1491

Galinier M, Albenque JP, Afchar N, et al. (1996). Prognostic value of late potentials in patients with congestive heart failure. *Eur Heart J*, 17, pp. 264-271

Galinier M, Doazan JP, Albemque JP, et al. (1992). Cardiopathie hypertensive et potentiels tardifs ventriculaires. *Arch Mal Coeur Vaiss*, 85, pp. 1095-8

Gang ES, Peter T, Rosenthal ME, et al. (1986). Detection of late potentials on the surface electrocardiogram in unexplained syncope. *Am J Cardiol*, 58(10), pp. 1014-20

Gatzoulis KA, Biblo LA, Waldo AL, et al. (1993). Atrial flutter causes pseudo late potentials on signal-averaged electrocardiogram. *Am J Cardiol*, 71, pp. 251

Genovesi S, Dossi C, Vigano MR, et al. (2008). Electrolyte concentration during haemodialysis and QT interval prolongation in uraemic patients. *Europace*, 10, pp. 771–777

Gimaev RKh, Ruzov VI, Razin VA, et al. (2009). Effect of lipid metabolism disturbances on electrophysiologic heart remodeling in patients with hypertensive disease. *Klin Med*, 87(11), pp. 30-3

Giroud D, Zimmermann M, Adamec R, et al. (1994). Ventricular late potentials and spontaneous ventricular arrhythmias after surgical repair of tetralogy of Fallot. Do they have prognostic value? *Br Heart J*, 72, pp. 580–583

Girgis I, Contreras G, Chakko S Perez G, et al. (1999). Effect of hemodialysis on the signal-averaged electrocardiogram. *Am J Kidney Dis*, 34, pp. 1105-1113

Goldberger JJ, Cain ME, Hohnloser SH, et al. (2008). American Heart Association/American College of Cardiology Stratification Techniques for Identifying Patients at Risk for Sudden Cardiac Foundation/Heart Rhythm Society Scientific Statement on Noninvasive Risk and Council on Epidemiology and Prevention on Clinical Cardiology Committee on Electrocardiography and Arrhythmias. *J Am Coll Cardiol*, 52, pp. 1179-1199

Goldberger JJ, Ahmed MW, Parker MA et al. (1994). Assessment of effects of autonomic stimulation and blockade on the signal-averaged electrocardiogram. *Circulation*, 89, pp. 1656–64

Gomes JA, Cain ME, Buxton AE, et al. (2001). Prediction of long-term outcomes by signal-averaged electrocardiography in patients with unsustained ventricular tachycardia, coronary artery disease, and left ventricular dysfunction. *Circulation*, 104, pp. 436

Gomez-Leon Manduiano A & Amezcua-Guerra LM. (2008). Cardiovascular manifestations of systemic lupus erythematosus. *Arch Cardiol Mex*, 78(4), pp. 421-30

Gottfridsson C, Karlsson T, Edvardsson N. (2011). The signal-averaged electrocardiogram before and after electrical cardioversion of persistent atrial fibrillation – implications of the sudden change in rhythm. *J Electrocardiol*, 44, pp. 2420

Gussack I & Antzelevitch C. (2008). *Electrical Diseases of the Heart. Genetics, Mechanisms, Treatment, Prevention.* Springer, London

Halimi F, Le Heuzey JY, Lavergne T, et al. (1994). Limitations of ventricular late potentials in atrial fibrillation. *Arch Mal Coeur Vaiss*, 87(9), pp. 1201-6

Hancock EW, Deal BJ, Mirvis DM, et al. (2009). AHA/ACCF/HRS recommendations for the standardization and interpretation of the electrocardiogram: part V: electrocardiogram changes associated with cardiac chamber hypertrophy: a scientific statement from the American Heart Association Electrocardiography and Arrhythmias Committee, Council on Clinical Cardiology; the American College of Cardiology Foundation; and the Heart Rhythm Society. *J Am Coll Cardiol*, 53, pp. 992–1002

Hayward RP, Emanuel RW, Nabarro JDN. (1987). Acromegalic heart disease: influence of treatment of acromegaly on the heart. *QJ Med*, 62, pp. 41-58

Herrmann BL, Bruch C, Saller B, et al. (2001). Occurence of ventricular late potentials in patients with active acromegaly. *Clinical Endocrinology*, 55, pp. 201-207

Herzog CA, Mangrum JM, Passman R. (2008). Sudden cardiac death and dialysis patients. *Semin Dial*, 21(4), pp. 300-7

Ho DS, Daly M, Richards DA, et al. (1996). Behavior of late potentials on the body surface during programmed ventricular stimulation. *J Am Coll Cardiol*, 28(5), pp. 1283-91

Ho DS, Denniss RA, Uther JB, et al. (1993). Signal-averaged electrocardiogram. Improved identification of patients with ventricular tachycardia using a 28-lead optimal array. *Circulation*, 87(3), pp. 857-865

Hohnloser SH, Franck P, Klingenheben T, et al. (1994). Open infarct artery, late potentials, and other prognostic factors in patients after acute myocardial infarction in the thrombolytic era. *Circulation*, 90, pp. 1747

Huebner T, Goernig M, Schuepbach M, et al. (2010) Electrocardiologic and related methods of non-invasive detection and risk stratification in myocardial ischemia: state of the art and perspectives. *German Medical Science*, 8, Doc 27

Ichikawa H, Nagake Y, Makino H. (1997). Signal averaged electrocardiography in patients on hemodyalisis. *J Med*, 28, pp. 229-243

Ikeda T, Saito H, Tanno K, et al. (2002). T-wave alternans as a predictor for sudden cardiac death after myocardial infarction. *Am J Cardiol*, 89, pp. 79

Ikeda T, Sakurada H, Sakabe K, et al. (2001). Assessment of noninvasive markers in identifying patients at risk in the Brugada syndrome: insight into risk stratification. *J Am Coll Cardiol*, 37, pp. 1628

Iltumur K, Karabulut A, Temamogullari AV, et al. (2001). The relation between infarction localization and late potentials. *Anadolu Kardiyol Derg*, 1(2), pp. 76-79

Isma' eel H, Shamseddeen W, Taher A, et al. (2007).Ventricular late potentials among thalassemia patients. *Int J Cardiol*, 132(3), pp. 453-5

Jain P & Avasthi R. (2004). Corelation beteen dispersion of repolarization and ventricular ectopic beat frequency in patients with acute myocardial infarction: a marker for risk of arrhythmogenesis. *Int J Cardiol*, 93, pp. 69-73

Janousek J, Paul T, Bartakova H. (1995). Role of late potentials in identifying patients at risk for ventricular tachycardia after surgical correction of congenital heart disease. *Am J Cardiol*, 75, pp. 146–150

Junker A, Ahlquist P, Thayssen P, et al. (1995).Ventricular late potentials and left ventricular function after early enalapril treatment in acute myocardial infarction. *Am J Cardiol*, 76, pp. 1300

Kaftan AH & Kaftan O. (2000). QT intervals and heart rate variability in hypertensive patients. *Jpn Heart J*, 41(2), pp. 173-82

Kahaly G, Olshausen KV, Mohr-Kahaly S, et al. (1992). Arrhythmia profile in acromegaly. *Eur Heart J*, 13, pp. 51-56

Kamath GS, Zareba W, Delaney J, et al. (2011). Value of the signal-averaged electrocardiogram in arrhythmogenic right ventricular cardiomyopathy/dysplasia. *Heart Rhythm*, 8(2), pp. 256-62

Kannel WB & Abbot RD. (1986). A prognostic comparison of asymptomatic left ventricular hypertrophy and unrecognized myocardial infarction: the Framingham Study. *Am Heart J*, 111(2), pp. 391-7

Karayaylali I, San M, Kudaiberdieva G, et al. (2003). Heart rate variability, left ventricular functions, and cardiac autonomic neuropathy in patients undergoing chronic hemodialysis. *Ren Fail*, 25(5), pp. 845-53

Kayikcioglu M, Can L, Evrengul H, et al. (2003). The effect of statin therapy on ventricular late potentials in acute myocardial infarction. *Int J Cardiol*, 90, pp. 63

Kitamura H, Yoshida A, Ohnishi Y, et al. (2003). Correlation of connexin 43 expression and late ventricular potentials in nonischemic dilated cardiomyopathy. *Circ J*, 67, pp. 1017-1021

Kondo N, Ikeda T, Kawase A, et al. (2001). Clinical usefulnes of the combination of T-wave alternans and late potentials for identifying high-risk patients with moderately or severly impaired left ventricular function. *Jpn Circ J*, 65, pp. 649-653

Konta T, Ikeda K, Kubota I, et al. (1988). Relationship between late potentials and left ventricular function in patients with coronary artery disease. *Jpn Circ J*, 52(2), pp. 105-110

Koskinen P & Kupari M. (1993). Signal-Averaged Electrocardiography in Asymptomatic Alcoholics. *Am J Cardiol*, 17, pp. 254-255

Kovesdy CP, Regidor DL, Mehrotra R, et al. (2007). Serum and dialysate potassium concentrations and survival in hemodialysis patients. *Clin J Am Soc Nephrol*, 2, pp. 999-1007

Kowalewski MA, Urban M, Florys B, et al. (2002). Late potentials: Are they related to cardiovascular complications in children with type 1 diabetes? *Journal of Diabetes and its complications*, 16(4), pp. 263-270

Kuchar DL, Thorburn CW, Sammel NL. (1986). Late potentials detected after myocardial infarction: natural history and prognostic significance. *Circulation*, 74, pp. 1280

Kudaiberdieva G, Gorenek B, Goktekin O, et al. (2003). Combination of QT variability and signal-averaged electrocardiography in association with ventricular tachycardia in postinfarction patients. *J Electrocardiol*, 36(1), pp. 17-24

Kutsuzawa D, Arimoto T, Watanabe T, et al. (2011). Persistent abnormal value of late potential in Brugada syndrome associated with hypokalemia. *Ann Noninvasive Electrocardiol*, 16(1), pp. 104-6

Lalani AP, Kanna B, John J, et al. (2000). Abnormal Signal-Averaged Electrocardiogram (SAECG) in Obesity. *Obesity Research*, 8(1), pp. 20-28

Lander P, Berbari EJ, Rajagopalan CV, et al. (1993). Critical analysis of the Signal-averaged electrocardiogram. Improved identification of late potentials. *Circulation*, 87, pp. 105

La Vecchia L, Ometto R, Bedogni F, et al. (1998). Ventricular late potentials, interstitial fibrosis, and right ventricular function in patients with ventricular tachycardia and normal left ventricular function. *Am J Cardiol*, 15, pp. 790– 792

Lazzerini PE, Capecchi PL, Laghi-Pasini F. (2010). Anti-Ro/SSA antibodies and cardiac arrhythmias in the adult: facts and hypotheses. *Scand J Immunol*, 72(3), pp. 213-22

Lazzerini PE, Capecchi PL, Guideri F, et al. (2007). Comparison of frequency of complex ventricular arrhythmias in patients with positive versus negative anti-Ro/SSA and connective tissue diseases. *Am J Cardiol*, 100(6), pp. 1029-34

Lazzerini PE, Capecchi PL, Guideri F, et al. (2006). Connective tissue diseases and cardiac rhythm disorders: an overview. *Autoimmun Rev*, 5(5), pp. 306-13

Lekawanvijit S & Chattipakorn N. (2009). Iron overload thalassemic cardiomyopathy: Iron status assessment and mechanisms of mechanical and electrical disturbance due to iron toxicity. *Can J Cardiol*, 25(4), pp. 213-218

Levy D, Garrison RJ, Savage DD, et al. (1990). Prognostic implications of echocardiographically determined left ventricular mass in the Framingham Heart Study. *N Engl J Med*, 322, pp. 1561-6

Liew R. (2011). Electrocardiogram-based predictors of sudden cardiac death in patients with coronary artery disease. *Clin Cardiol*, 34 (8), pp. 466-473

Linnenbank AC, van Dessel PFHM, Potse M, et al. (2001). Localization of late potentials using body surface mapping. *Biomed Techn*, pp. 204-206

Liu YB, Wu CC, Lu LS, et al. (2003). Sympathetic Nerve Sprouting, electrical remodeling, and increased vulnerability to ventricular fibrillation in hypercholesterolemic rabbits. *Circ Res*, 92, pp. 1145-1152

Liu YB, Lee YT, Pak HN, et al. (2009). Effects of simvastatin on cardiac neural and electrophysiologic remodeling in rabbits with hypercholesterolemia. *Heart Rhythm*, 6(1), pp. 69–75

Lorsheyd A & de Lange DW. (2005). PR and QTc interval prolongation on the electrocardiogram after binge drinking in healthy individuals. *Neth J Med*, 2(63), pp. 59-63

Luca C. (1979). Electrophysiological properties of right heart and atrioventricular conducting system in patients with alcoholic cardiomyopathy. *Br Heart J*, 42, pp. 274-281

Malik M, Kulakowski P, Odemuyiwa O, et al. (1992). Effect of thrombolytic therapy on the predictive value of signal-averaged electrocardiography after acute myocardial infarction. *Am J Cardiol*, 70, pp. 21

Mancini DM, Wong KL, Simson MB. (1993). Prognostic value of an abnormal signal-averaged electrocardiogram in patients with nonischemic congestive cardiomyopathy. *Circulation*, 84, pp. 1083

Manolis AS, Chiladakis JA, Malakos JS, et al. (1997). Abnormal signal-averaged electrocardiograms in patients with incomplete right bundle-branch block. *Clin Cardiol*, 20(1), pp. 17-22

Mather AN, Fairbairn TA, Ball SG, et al. (2011). Reperfusion haemorrhage as determined by cardiovascular MRI is a predictor of adverse left ventricular remodelling and markers of late arrhythmic risk. *Heart*, 97, pp. 453-9

Meinertz T, Treese N, Kaspar W, et al. (1985). Determinant of prognosis in idiopathic dilated cardiomyopathy as determined by programmed electrical stimulation. *Am J Cardiol*, 56, pp. 337-41

Mehta D & Camm AJ. (1989). Signal-averaged electrocardiography and the significance of late potentials in patients with „idiopathic" ventricular tachycardia: a review. *Clicical Cardiology*, 12(6), pp. 307-12

Meregalli PG, Wilde AA, Tan HL. (2005). Pathophysiological mechanisms of Brugada syndrome: depolarization disorder, repolarization disorder, or more? *Cardiovasc Res*, 67, pp. 367-378

Middlekauff H, Stevenson W, Woo M, et al. (1990). Comparison of frequency of late potentials in idiopathic dilated cardiomyopathy and ischemic cardiomyopathy with advanced heart failure and their usefulness in predicting sudden death. *Am J Cardiol*, 66, pp. 1113-17

Mizia-Stec K, Mandecki T, Zahorska-Markiewicz B, et al. (2000). The QT interval dispersion and ventricular late potential in obese women. *Pol Merkur Lekarski*, 8(44), pp. 84-6

Morales MA, Gremigini C, Dattalo P, et al. (1998). Signal-averaged ECG abnormalities in haemodyalisis patients. Role of dialysis. *Nephrol Dial Transplant*, 13, pp. 668-673

Morita H, Kusano KF, Miura D, et al. (2008). Fragmented QRS as a marker of conduction abnormality and a predictor of prognosis of Brugada syndrome. *Circulation*, 118, pp. 1697-1704

Morita H, Zipes DP, Morita ST. (2007). Differences in the arrhythmogenicity between the canine right ventricular outflow tract and anteroinferior right ventricle in a model of Brugada syndrome. *Heart Rhythm*, 4, pp. 66-74

Moushmoush B & Abi-Mansour P. (1991). Alcohol and the heart. The long-term effects of alcohol on the cardiovascular system. *Arch Intern Med*, 151, pp. 36-42

Mozos I, Hancu M, Serban C, et al. (2011). Late ventricular potentials can be predicted from twelve-lead ECG in post-infarction heart failure. *International Journal of Collaborative Research on Internal Medicine & Public Health*, 3, pp. 53-63

Mozos I & Hancu M. (2010). High serum cholesterol and electrical instability in patients with an old myocardial infarction. *Atherosclerosis Supplements*, 11(2), pp. 109-222

Mozos I, Hancu M, Costea C, et al. (2009). Left ventricular hypertrophy and ventricular arrhythmia risk in post-infarction heart failure, In: *Proceedings of the IVth Congress of the Academy of Romanian Scientists „Quality of Life", October 15-17, 2009, Timisoara*, Candea V, Andea P, Popoviciu MO, Kilyeni St, pp. 335- 42, Orizonturi Universitare Publishing House, Timisoara, Romania

Mozos I, Hancu M, Cristescu A. (2008). The Relation between Late Ventricular Potentials and Isointegral QRST Body Surface Maps in Chronic Myocardial Infarction Patients, In: *XXVIII European Section Meeting of the International Society for Heart Research. Athens (Greece), May 28-31, 2008*, pp. 47-50, Medimond International Proceedings. Monduzzi Editore, Bologna, Italy

Mozos I. (2007). *Aspecte ale vulnerabilitatii la aritmii ventriculare in infarctul miocardic cronic*, Mirton Publishing House, Timisoara, Romania

Mozos I, Hancu M, Chiulan C, et al. (2007). Aspects of Electrical Instability in Obese Chronic Myocardial Infarction Patients, In: *Joint Meeting of the Slovak Physiological Society, the Physiological Society and the Federation of European Physiological Societies. Bratislava (Slovak Republic), September 11-14, 2007*, Strbak V, pp. 95-98, Medimond International Proceedings. Monduzzi Editore, Bologna, Italy

Mozos I. (2006). The relation between late ventricular potentials and electrocardiographic dispersion of ventricular activity in myocardial infarction patients. *Timisoara Medical Journal*, 2-3 (56), pp. 157-162

Muntean D, Varro A, Jost N, et al. (2009). *Translational research in cardiovascular disease: a cross-border approach.* Victor Babes Publishing House, Timisoara, Romania

Nakai K, Ito C, Koh E, et al. (1988). Relationship between the occurence of late potential on the body surface ECG and cardiac performance in myocardial infarction. *J Cardiol*, 18(1), pp. 207-215

Nashoni E, Strasberg B, Imbar S, et al. (2010). Late potentials in the signal-averaged electrocardiogram in schizophrenia patients maintained on antipsychotic agents. A preliminary naturalistic study. *European Neuropsychopharmacology*, 20, pp. 146-152

Nava A, Folino AF, Bauce B, et al. (2000). Signal-averaged electrocardiogram in patients with arrhythmogenic right ventricular cardiomyopathy and ventricular arrhythmias. *Eur Heart J*, 21, pp. 58-65

Ohnischi Y, Inoue T, Fukuzaki H. (1990).Value of the signal averaged electrocardiogram as a predictor of sudden death in myocardial infarction and dilated cardiomyopathy. *Jpn Circ J*, 54, pp. 127-36

Oikarinen L, Nieminen MS, Viitasalo M, et al. (2004). QRS Duration and QT Interval Predict Mortality in Hypertensive Patients with Left Ventricular Hypertrophy. The Losartan Intervention for Endpoint Reduction in Hypertension Study. *Hypertension*,43, pp. 1029-1034

Olinic N. & Zdrenghea D. (1998). *Cardiopatia ischemica.* Clusium Publishing House, Cluj-Napoca, Romania

Osadchii O. (2010). Mechanisms of hypokalemia-induced ventricular arrhythmogenicity. *Fundamental and Clinical Pharmacology*, 24(5), pp. 547-59

Pacher P, Ungvari Z, Nanasi PP, et al. (1999). Electrophysiological changes in rat ventricular and atrial myocardium at different stages of experimental diabetes. *Acta Physiol Scand*, 166(1), pp. 7-13

Palatini P, Maraglino G, Accurso V, et al. (1995). Impaired left ventricular filling in hypertensive left ventricular hypertrophy as a marker of the presence of an arrhythmogenic substrate. *Br Heart J*, 73, pp. 258-62

Panagides D, Amabile G, Deharo JC, et al. (1990). Etude des potentiels tardifs chez l'hypertendu. *Arch Mal Coeur Vaiss*, 83, pp. 1165-8

Paradiso M, Di Franco M, Musca A, et al. (2002). Ventricular late potentials in systemic sclerosis: relationship with skin involvement. *J Rheumatol*, 29(7), pp. 1388-92

Paradiso M, Gabrielli F, Masala C, et al. (2001). Evaluation of myocardial involvement in systemic lupus erythematosus by signal-averaged electrocardiography and echocardiography. *Acta Cardiol*, 56(6), pp. 381-6

Paradiso M, Gabrielli F, Coppotelli L, et al. (1996). Signal-averaged electrocardiography and echocardiography in the evaluation of myocardial involvement in progressive systemic sclerosis. *Int J Cardiol*, 53(2), pp. 171-7

Peters NS, Coromilas J, Severs NJ, et al. (1997). Disturbed connexin43 gap junction distribution correlates with the location of reentrant circuits in the epicardial border zone of healing canine infarcts that cause ventricular tachycardia. *Circulation,* 95, pp. 988 – 996

Pignone A, Matucci-Cerinic M, Becucci A, et al. (1994). Patterns of ventricular late potentials in systemic sclerosis: a noninvasive method in the study of cardiac involvement. *Ann Ital Med*, 9(3), pp. 141-5

Pochmalicki G, Genest M, Jibril H. (1997). Late ventricular potentials and heavy drinking. *Heart*, 78, pp. 163-165

Pollak SJ, Kertes PJ, Bredlau CE, et al. (1985). Influence of left ventricular function on signal averaged late potentials in patients with coronary artery disease with and without ventricular tachycardia. *Am Heart J*, 110(4), pp. 747-52

Priori SG, Aliot E, Blomstrom-Lundqvist C, et al. Task Force on Sudden Cardiac Death of the European Society of Cardiology. (2001). Task Force Report. *Eur Heart J*, 22(16), pp. 1374-1450

Prisant LM, Wylds AC, Carr AA, et al. (1993). Assessment of late potentials in patients with essential hypertension by the signal-averaged electrocardiogram with five year follow-up. *J Hypertens*, 7, pp. 497-503

Rizzo V, Di Maio F, Villatico Campbell S, et al. (2000). Left ventricular function, cardiac dysrhythmias, atrial activation, and volumes in nondipper hypertensive individuals with left ventricular hypertrophy. *Am Heart J*, 139, pp. 529-36

Rodrigues EA, Caruana MP, Lahiri A, et al. (1989). Subclinical cardiac dysfunction in acromegaly: evidence for a specific disease of heart muscle. *Br Heart J*, 62, pp. 185-194

Roithinger FX, Punzengruber C, Rossoll M, et al. (1992). Ventricularlate potentials in haemodyalisis patients and the risk of sudden death. *Nephrol Dial Transplant*, 7, pp. 1013-1018

Russo V, Rago A, Pannone B, et al. (2011). Dispersion of repolarization and beta-thalassemia major: the prognostic role of QT and JT dispersion for identifying the high-risk patients for sudden death. *Eur J Haematol*, 86(4), pp.324-31

Sakhuja R, Shah AJ, Hiremath S, et al. (2009). End-stage renal disease and sudden cardiac death. *Cardiac Electrophysiology Clinics*, 1(1), pp. 61-77

Santangeli P, Pieroni M, Dello Russo A, et al. (2010). Noninvasive diagnosis of electroanatomic abnormalities in arrhythmogenic right ventricular cardiomyopathy. *Circulation: Arrhythmia and Electrophysiology*, 3, pp. 632-8

Santangeli P, Infusino F, Sgueglia GA, et al. (2008). Ventricular late potentials: a critical overview and current applications. *J Electrocardiol*, 41, pp. 318-324

Santarelli P, Lanza GA, Biscione F, et al. (1993). Effects of thrombolysis and atenolol or metoprolol on the signal-averaged electrocardiogram after acute myocardial infarction. *Am J Cardiol*, 72, pp. 521

Savard P, Rouleau JL, Ferguson J, et al. (1997). Risk Stratification After Myocardial Infarction Using Signal-Averaged Electrocardiografic Criteria Adjusted for Sex, Age, and Myocardial Infarction Location. *Circulation*, 96, pp. 202-213

Schunkert H. (2002). Obesity and target organ damage: the heart. *International Journal of Obesity*, 26 (Suppl 4), pp. S15 – S20

Seferovic PM, Ristic AD, Maksimovic R, et al. (2006). Cardiac arrhythmias and conduction disturbances in autoimmune rheumatic diseases. *Rheumatology*, 45, pp. iv39-iv42

Silverman ME, Pressel MD, Bracken JC, et al. (1995). Prognostic value of the signal-averaged electrocardiogram and a prolonged QRS in ischemic and nonischemic cardiomyopathy. *Am J Cardiol*, 75, pp. 460-64

Simson MB. (1981). Use of signals in the terminal QRS complex to identify patients with ventricular tachycardia after myocardial infarction. *Circulation*, 64, pp. 235–42

Stanescu C & Dan GA. (1992). Myocardial involvement in systemic lupus erythematosus and systemic sclerosis - pulsed Doppler echocardiographic evaluation of left ventricular diastolic function. *Rom J Intern Med*, 30(4), pp. 243-8

Steinberg J & Berbari EJ. (1996). The signal-averaged electrocardiogram: update on clinical applications. *J Cardiovasc Electrophysiol*, 7, pp. 972

Steinberg JS & Bigger JT. (1989). Importance of the endpoint of noise reduction in analysis of the signal-averaged electrocardiogram. *Am J Cardiol*, 63, pp. 556-60

Steinbigler P, Haberl R, Jeleazcov C, et al. (1999). Functional changes of ventricular late potentials by provocation with increase of heart rate. *Europace*, 1, pp. 103-112

Strohmer B, Schernthaner C, Iglseder B, et al. (2007). Gender-specific effect of metabolic syndrome on rate adjusted QT interval in middle-aged participants of an atherosclerosis prevention program. *Wien Klin Wochenschr*, 119(17-18), pp. 544-52

Sanjuan R, Nunez J, Blasco ML, et al. (2011). Prognostic implications of stress hyperglycemia in acute ST elevation myocardial infarction. Prospective observational study. *Rev Esp Cardiol*, 64(3), pp. 201-7

Teixeira RA, Ferreira Borba E, Bonfa E, et al. (2010). Arrhythmias in systemic lupus erythematosus. *Bras J Rheumatol*, 50(1), 81-9

Turrini P, Angelini A, Thiene G, et al. (1999). Late potentials and ventricular arrhythmias in arrhythmogenic right ventricular cardiomyopathy. *Am J Cardiol*, 15, pp. 1214- 1219

Vardas PE, Simandirakis EN, Parthenakis FI, et al. (1994). Study of late potentials and ventricular arrhythmias in hypertensive patients with normal electrocardiograms. *Pacing Clin Electrophysiol*, 17, pp. 577-84

Vester EG, Kuhls S, Ochiulet-Vester J, et al. (1992). Electrophysiological and therapeutic implications of cardiac arrhythmias in hypertension. *Eur Heart J*, 13(Suppl D), pp. 70-81

Vreede-Swagemakers JJ, Gorgels AP, Weijenberg MP, et al. (1999). Risk indicators for out-of-hospital cardiac arrest in patients with coronary artery disease. *J Clin Epidemiol*, 52, pp. 601–7

Wever EFD & Robles de Medina EO. (2004). Sudden death in patients without structural heart disease. *J Am Coll Cardiol*, 43(7), pp. 1137-1144

Wilson JR, Schwartz JS, St John Sutton M, et al. (1983). Prognosis in severe heart failure: Relation to hemodynamic measurements and ventricular ectopic activity. *J Am Coll Cardiol*, 3, pp. 403-10

Wranicz JK, Cygankiewicz I, Zielinska M, et al. (2001). Non-invasive cardiac evaluation in patients with systemic lupus erythematosus. *J Med*, 32(3-4), pp. 195-206

Yang W, Horan LG, Flowers NC. (1990). An Analysis of Beat-By-Beat Recording of Late Potentials and His-Purkinje Signals in a Hospital Environment. *J Cardiovasc Electrophysiol*, 1, pp. 486-495

Yildirir A, Batur MK, Oto A. (2002). Hypertension and arrhythmia: blood pressure control and beyond. *Europace*, 4(2), pp. 175-82

Yodogawa K, Seino Y, Ohara T, et al. (2011). Effect of corticosteroid therapy on ventricular arrhythmias in patients with cardiac sarcoidosis. *Ann Noninvasive Electrocardiol*, 16(2), pp. 140-7

Zaman AG, Morris JL, Smyllie JH, et al. (1993). Late potentials and ventricular enlargement after myocardial infarction. A new role for high-resolution electrocardiography? *Circulation*, 88(3), pp. 905-914

Zhao J, Yang Y, Pei W, et al. (2008). Effect of statin therapy on reperfusion arrhythmia in patients who underwent successful primary angioplasty. *Clin Res Cardiol*, 97, pp. 147–151

Zimmermann M, Adamec R, de Lorgeril M, et al. (1983). Detection non invasve des potentiels tardifs de l'activation ventriculaire: identification et signification dans la maladie coronarienne. *Schwei Med Wschr*, 113, pp. 1678-1680

Zimmermann M, Friedli B, Adamec R, et al. (1991).Ventricular late potentials and induced ventricular arrhythmias after surgical repair of tetralogy of Fallot. *Am J Cardiol*, 67, pp. 873–878

Zipes DP, Camm AJ, Borggrefe M, et al. (2006). ACC/AHA/ESC 2006 Guidelines for Management of patients with Ventricular Arrhythmias and the Prevention of Sudden Cardiac Death. *J Am Coll Cardiol*, 48(5), pp. 247-346

11

Influence of Patern and Degree of Left Ventricular Hypertrophy on Cardiac Arrhythmias

Juraj Kunisek
Thalassotherapia Crikvenica, Special Hospital for Medical Rehabilitation, Crikvenica
Croatia

1. Introduction

1.1 Ventricular arrhythmias

A large number of clinical and epidemiological studies [1,2] have reported a correlation between the mass increase of the left ventricle (LV) and the risk of disease or death. The prevalence of left ventricular hypertrophy (LVH) in patients with essential hypertension may be as high as 40% (12%-70%) [3]. It has been suggested [4] that in patients with LVH sudden death may be associated with an increased number of ventricular extrasystoles (VPB), which is frequently observed in this population. In effect, a review by Lombardi et al. [5] indicated that nonsustained ventricular arrhythmias are an independent predictor of cardiac death in hypertensive patients.

Most frequently it concerns concentric hypertrophy with no enlargement of ventricular cavities, interpreted by multiplication of sarcomeras in a parallel arrangement. This type of hypertrophy is characterised by increased mass and increased relative wall thickness. In a smaller number of hypertensives LVH is initially eccentric, with a multiplication of sarcomeras in sequence in the process of which enlargement of the ventricular cavity is prevalent and thickening of the wall is only proportional or less marked. Although many hypertensive patients develop isolated septum hypertrophy, data on the structure and function of the myocardium and arrhythmias in hypertensive patients with this type of LVH are limited [6]. It would appear that concentric hypertrophy carries the greatest and eccentric hypertrophy a moderate risk of cardiovascular (CV) events [7]. Published data regarding arrhythmias are still conflicting and unconvincing [6,8]. It is unclear whether the greatest risk of CV events in the concentric type is due to arrhythmias or something else (ishaemia for inst.). According to some authors [9] the correlation between left ventricular mass (LVM) and ventricular arrhythmias is graded and permanent. Arrhythmias described in hypertensive patients with LVH are usually single premature ventricular contractions, frequently bigeminal or multiform, and more rarely ventricular tachycardia. [10].

1.2 Supraventricular arrhythmias

Risk of AF (and other supraventricular arrhythmias) is also increased in patients with left ventricular hypertrophy (LVH) [11]. Concentric hypertrophy appears to hold the highest risk [12]. Earlier investigations reported that LVH leads to diastolic dysfunction, decreased coronary blood flow reserve and the occurrence of ventricular and atrial arrhythmias. It appears that in the development of atrial arrhythmias, atrial volume overloading and the distension and dilatation of the myofibrils have a greater impact. This results from ventricular diastolic dysfunction (particularly of the left ventricle), due to hypertrophy and subsequent decreased compliance [13]. From the pathophysiological point of view, this is caused by the hypertrophy of cardiac myocytes, interstitial fibrosis and media hypertrophy of the arterioles. Microangiopathy can be diagnosed as the earliest sign of hypertensive heart disease, with diastolic dysfunction also being found as an early change. [14]. More recently, an increasing number of investigations conducted on supraventricular premature beats (SVPB) have documented enlarged atria in hypertrophic hypertensive hearts.

1.3 QT interval and QT dispersion

Marked left ventricular hypertrophy (LVH) is associated with potentially arrhythmogenic ventricular repolarization abnormalities and may generate conditions for QT interval (QTi) prolongation and increase QT dispersion (QTd)) [15,16]. Prolongation of QTc interval and QTd are risk markers for malignant ventricular arrhythmias (VA) and sudden cardiac death [17,18]. QT prolongation and dispersion are indicators for abnormalities in ventricular repolarization. This could suggest the presence of functional reentrant proarrhythmic circuits [19]. Defined as the difference between the longest and shortest QTi measured in any lead of the 12-lead electrocardiogram (ECG), QTd reflects the inhomogeneity in ventricular repolarisation. Both parameters include also depolarisation. Increased QTd has been shown to correlate positively to complex VA in many clinical conditions [17,20]. QTd and QTi correlate with the left ventricular mass index (LVMI) determined echocardiographically in a group of selected patients with essential hypertension [19,21,22]. Normal QTd values vary extensively from 10 to 71 ms. QTd is higher in cardiac patients in comparison to normal subjects. The probability is that only explicitly abnormal values (i.e., those >100 ms) outside error margins may potentially have a practical value, suggesting a markedly abnormal repolarisation [23]. Scarce data was published regarding QTc interval prolongation/QTd and complex ventricular arrhythmias in hypertensive patients with LVH [24,25], but which type of LVH has the greatest influence has been understudied (especially for the asymmetric type).

1.4 Discussion

Examined patients included in such studies should have essential hypertension and LVH confirmed by echocardiography. For that reason one must exclude congestive heart failure, known coronary disease (angina pectoris, previous myocardial infarction, percutaneous coronary interventions), heart surgery, valvular diseases, other cardiac diseases (previous myocarditis and hypertrophic obstructive cardiomyopathy in the absance of systemic hypertension), diabetes mellitus, alcoholics, mental disorders, overuse of non-antihypertensive drugs (psychiatric drugs: sedatives, psychopharmacs etc; antiparkinsonics, antirheumatics, analgesics and hormones), malignant or accelerated hypertension, stroke in the previous six months, patients with cancer, abnormal electrolytes, anemia, cardiopulmonary diseases, serum creatinine >140 μmol/L and abnormal thyroid function.

Study subjects usualy have long-term hypertension (average duration of 17 years in our sample) and excessive body weight. The majority subjects are physically inactive with elevated values of lipids and urea in serum [26].

Echocardiographic measurements confirme anthropological differences between genders [27]. Men have larger cardiac cavities and LVM. By indexing left ventricular mass according to the body surface (LVMI) this difference between genders is lost. Ejection fraction (EF) is most often very good (>60%). The values of mean LVMI, and in both genders are much higher than normal values (>170 g/m^2) Concentric LVH is the most frequent (63% in [26]), which is not in agreement with some earlier investigations [28]. Eccentric LVH, usually of a mild degree, is more frequently observed in male patients. This could be explained by the larger diameter of the cardiac cavity in men. Mild LVH, according to some authors [29], does not carry increased risk either of complex neither of simple ventricular arrhythmias.

Complex *ventricular arrhythmias* on ECG are usualy found in small number (4%) of patients. During Holter monitoring this percentage increased to over 40% of patients, and during the stress test it increased by additional 7,4% (in proportion to heart rate and blood pressure). Ventricular tachycardia can be found in 7-18% [26]. Some authors [24] found that concentric hypertrophy carries the greatest risk, and the eccentric a moderate risk of death and of CV complications. Nunez et al. [6] found equal prevalence and complexity of ventricular arrhythmias in hypertensive patients with concentric and asymmetric LVH. Some earlier investigations [8] reported an equal incidence of ventricular arrhythmias with regard to the morphological type of LVH and LVMI, similar to our results. Devereux et al. [30] also obtained a negative correlation. Only a small number of studies in the literature (not written in the English language) have monitored this correlation and obtained a statistical significance.

Atrial fibrillation associated with atrial dilatation is often observed in patients with hypertension [31]. About 40% of patients have paroxysmal atrial fibrillation or paroxysmal supraventricular tachycardia during Holter monitoring and additional 4% during the exercise test [32]. Until now it is unable to conclude whether any of the LVH types had a greater effect on the appearance of these arrhythmias.

The left atrial size significantly positively correlates with left ventricular hypertrophy degree, and it seems that a larger number of *supraventricular premature beats* for moderate and severe concentric LVH compared to mild concentric LVH, can bee found [32]. Schannwell et al. [13] also found greater prevalence of supraventricular arrhythmias proportional to the degree of LVH.

The largest left atrial diameters can bee found in patients with eccentric LVH and the higher prevalence of supraventricular premature beats in the concentric and eccentric type [32]. Some outhors [6,33] found significantly greater prevalence and complexity of supraventricular arrhythmias in patients with asymmetric LVH. The relationship between arrhythmias and concentric geometry appears more coherent if we consider that a recent study [34] reported an independent association of impaired left ventricular relaxation with concentric LV geometry. The abnormal diastolic function of LV and the stretch in LA may be less expressed in the asymmetric tipe of hypertrophy. In the context of epidemiology, this means that in patients with asymmetric left ventricular hypertrophy (about 9% of subjects) a lower incidence of arrhythmias should be expected. Concentric LVH is most frequently found in hypertensive patients, and it appears to cause the most severe diastolic left ventricular disfunction. Patients with eccentric LVH possibly have the largest LA dimension, and can have a slightly lower incidence of supraventricular premature beats then those with concentric LVH, meaning that the LA size is not the only factor that affecs the prevalence of supraventricular arrhythmias. Apart from mechanical remodeling, electrical remodeling that occures earlier should also be considered (change in the structure/function of ion channels and compounds, catecholamines, free oxygen radicals, angiotensin-converting enzyme, angiotensin II, cytokins and nitrogenous oxid), hypertrophy of media arteriola, dicrease in the coronary blood flow reserve and genetic factors (repeted expression of fetal genome isoforms, heme oxygenase-1[35]). These factors may differ in individual LVH forms.

Measurement of left atrial size from the parasternal long axis view using the 2-dimensional "M-mode" method is limited in accuracy for LA size quantification because of the irregular geometry of the LA and the angulations of the ultrasound beam [36]. Methods for measuring the LA volume are more appropriate for the assessment of the asymmetric remodelling of the LA chamber [37].

In patients with severe concentric and eccentric LVH higher values of the *QTc interval* can be find. Regarding the degree of LVH, a positive correlation with QTc length can be observed [38]. Not many articles investigating this correlation have been published in the literature [39,40]. In some [41] only 38 patients with essential hypertension and LVH were analyzed, and an attempt to classify them into groups with regard to LVH type was made. Their conclusion was that the QTc interval length correlates positively with LVMI and LVIDd. The longest QTc intervals were found in patients with LVH and complex arrhythmias. They also found that the incidence of complex ventricular arrhythmias was greater in patients with LVH, and that the prolonged QTc interval in these patients may be a good indicator for higher risk of arrhythmias. The mentioned authors also obtained the highest QTc interval values in patients with dilated (eccentric) LVH but the LVH type was not defined by calculating RWT, than by a simple addition of IVS and LVPW thickness. Patients with myocardial dilatation (with and without LVH) had the most severe arrhythmias. Measuring QTi only from the second lead represented a limitation to the study recognized by the authors. Other researchers also obtained the correlation between QTi and LVMI lengths [39,41]. QTc interval in patients with ventricular septal hypertrophy was significantly longer than in the normal group [42].

Higher values of the *QTdispersion* in severe concentric and eccentric LVH can also be find [38]. Manual assessment of the T-wave end is extremely unreliable. Regrettably, the existing automated methods have not proven to be advantageous. The main source of mistakes for readers and computers are the low amplitudes of T waves [43] and the border between the T and U wave or the P wave [44]. Increased QTc dispersion was associated with LVH, especially with its concentric variant in some studies [20,45]. In the LIFE study both concentric and eccentric LVH were associated with prolonged QTi and increased QTd [15]. In another study [46] QTd >60 ms and QTi >440 ms were associated with greater probability of LVH.

In our patients, the QTi length correlates with the VA incidence. QTc interval was also longer in patients having complex arrhythmias but the difference in relation to simple arrhythmias was not significant [38].

Several factors may influence the increased LV ectopic activity in patients with LVH. Increased stimulation of hypertrophic myocytes, fibrosis in hypertrophic myocardium that leads to electrophysiological inhomogeneity, distention of certain myocytes, increased oxygen requirement of the myocardium, damaged membrane porosity for various ions, and increased sympatic activity are possible pathophysiological factors for the increased incidence of ventricular arrhythmias [47,48].

In subjects without heart disease, during a 15-20 years follow-up period, prospective studies found significant correlation between prolonged QTc interval and increased risk for coronary events [49], cardiovascular (CV) mortality and all-cause mortality (mean follow-up of 4.9 years) [50], as well as for sudden cardiac death or CV death [51]. The Zutphen study [51] concluded that men with QTc interval >420 ms were at greater risk for CV death than men with shorter QTc interval. Increased QTd in patients with LVH and higher incidence of ventricular premature beats (VPB) or complex VA was also described by other authors [22,24,52]. Ichkhan et al. [22] found a significant correlation between QTd and LVM in hypertensive patients. They concluded that LVH and not hypertension *per se* leads to increased QTd, because hypertensive patients without LVH did not have an increased QTd. Ozdemir et al. [53] studing 80 patients with concentric LVH have found strong correlation between increased QTd and the incidence of VA. Other authors [33] obtained the highest influence of asymmetric LVH on QTd, but without correlation between VPB and QTd, neither between VPB and LVMI.

According to some investigations patients with increased QTd should be treated with angiotensin receptor blockers and nebivolol [54,55].

It is very important to *exclude the possible effect of* the extent of *antihypertensive therapy* and the types of antihypertensive drugs on the result. Discontinuation of all drugs seven days prior to ergometric examination and Holter monitoring is optimal. It is sometimes not possible to keep patients 7 days without antihypertensive and anti-arrhythmic drugs because a longer suspension of treatment could have threatened the patient or lead to reduced cooperation.. Shorter discontinuation can bee applied but the duration and the type of drugs should not differ between the examined groups.

2. Conclusion

In conclusion, The degree of LVH contributes more to the greater prevalence of VA then the LVH pattern. Given that this correlation (between the degree and VA) is most expressed in the concentric type (which is at the same time the most frequent pattern of LVH in hypertensive patients), the combination of severe degree and concentric type carries the greatest risk. Asymmetric LVH does not necessarily represent an increased risk. Concentric and eccentric types have a greater impact on the frequency of atrial arrhythmias. The prevalence of supraventricular premature beats correlates with the degree of left ventricular hypertrophy in the concentric type. QTc interval and QT dispersion tend to increase proportionally to the left ventricular mass probably only in the concentric and eccentric LVH type.

In clinical practice this means that patients with moderate and severe LVH (concentric in particular) should be tested by Holter monitoring and bicycle ergometry and treated with maximally tolerable doses of antihypertensives, particularly with angiotensin converting enzyme inhibitors/ angiotensin receptor blockers and also with outpatient training program.

3. References

[1] Hennersdorf MG, Strauer BE. Arterial hypertension and cardiac arrhythmias. J Hypertens 2001;19:167-77. Review.

[2] Yiu KH, Tse HF. Hypertension and cardiac arrhythmias: a review of the epidemiology, pathophysiology and clinical implications. J Hum Hypertens 2008; Mar 13; [Epub ahead of print]

[3] Coca A, Gabriel R, De la Figuera M, López-Sendón JL, Fernández R, Sagastagoitia JD, Garcia JJ, Barajas R. The impact of different echocardiographic diagnostic criteria on the prevalence of left ventricular hypertrophy in essential hypertension: the VITAE study. J Hypertens 1999;17:1471-80.

[4] Verdecchia P, Angeli F, Achilli P, Castellani C, Broccatelli A, Gattobigio R, Cavallini C. Echocardiographic left ventricular hypertrophy in hypertension: marker for future events or mediator of events? Curr Opin Cardiol 2007;22:329-34.

[5] Lombardi F, Terranova P. Hypertension and concurrent arrhythmias. Curr Pharm Des 2003;9:1703-13.

[6] Nunez BD, Lavie CJ, Messerli FH, Schmieder RE, Caravaglia GE, Nunez M. Comparison of diastolic left ventricular filling and cardiac dysrhythmias in hypertensive patients with and without isolated septal hypertrophy. Am J Cardiol 1994;74: 585-9.

[7] De Simone G, Palmieri V. Left ventricular hypertrophy in hypertension as a predictor of coronary events: relation to geometry [review]. Curr Opin Nephrol Hypertens 2002;11:215-20.

[8] Mammarella A, Paradiso M, Basili S, De Matteis A, Cardarello CM, Di Franco M, Donnarumma L, Labbadia G, Paoletti V. Morphologic left ventricular patterns and prevalence of high-grade ventricular arrhythmias in the normotensive and hypertensive elderly. Adv Ther 2000;17:222-9.

[9] Motz W. Arterial hypertension, left ventricular hypertrophy, and ventricular arrhythmias. Herzschrittmacherther Elektrophysiol. 2006;17:218-20.

[10] Galinier M, Pathak A, Fallouh V, Baixas C, Schmutz L, Roncalli J, Boveda S, Fauvel JM. Holter EKG for the hypertensive heart disease. [Article in French]. Ann Cardiol Angeiol 2002;51:336-40.

[11] Kannel WB, Wolf PA, Benjamin EJ, Levy D. Prevalence, incidence, prognosis, and predisposing conditions for atrial fibrillation: population-based estimates. Am J Cardiol 1998;82 (suppl):2-9N.

[12] Sierra C, de la Sierra A, Paré JC, Gómez-Angelats E, Coca A. Correlation between silent cerebral white matter lesions and left ventricular mass and geometry in essential hypertension. Am J Hypertens 2002;15:507-512.

[13] Schannwell CM, Steiner S, Hennersdorf MG, Strauer BE. Cardiovascular and organ impairment due to hypertension. Internist 2005;46:496-508. Review.

[14] Hennersdorf MG, Strauer BE. The heart in hypertension. Internist 2007;48: 236-45. Review.

[15] Oikarinen L, Nieminen MS, Viitasalo M, Toivonen L, Wachtell K, Papademetriou V, et al. Relation of QT interval and QT dispersion to echocardiographic left ventricular

hypertrophy and geometric pattern in hypertensive patients. The LIFE study. The Losartan Intervention For Endpoint Reduction. J Hypertens. 2001;19:1883-91.

[16] Galinier M, Balanescu S, Fourcade J, Dorobantu M, Albenque JP, Massabuau P, et al. Prognostic value of arrhythmogenic markers in systemic hypertension. Eur Heart J. 1997;18:1484-91.

[17] Haider AW, Larson MG, Benjamin EJ, Levy D. Increased left ventricular mass and hypertrophy are associated with increased risk for sudden death. J Am Coll Cardiol. 1998;32:1454–9.

[18] Kulan K, Ural D, Komsuoglu B, Agacdiken A, Goldeli O, Komsuoglu SS. Significance of QTc prolongation on ventricular arrhythmias in patients with left ventricular hypertrophy secondary to essential hypertension. Int J Cardiol. 1998;64:179–84.

[19] Facchini M, Malfatto G, Ciambellotti F, Riva B, Bragato R, Branzi G, et al. Markers of electrical instability in hypertensive patients with and without ventricular arrhythmias. Are they useful in identifying patients with different risk profiles? J Hypertens. 2000;18:763-8.

[20] Day CP, McComb JM, Campbell RW. QT dispersion in sinus beats and ventricular extrasystoles in normal hearts. Br Heart J. 1992;67:39-41.

[21] Chapman N, Mayet J, Ozkor M, Lampe FC, Thom SA, Poulter NR. QT intervals and QT dispersion as measures of left ventricular hypertrophy in a unselected hypertensive population. Am J Hypertens. 2001;14:455-62.

[22] Ichkhan K, Molnar J, Somberg J. Relation of left ventricular mass and QT dispersion in patients with systemic hypertension. Am J Cardiol. 1997;79:508-11.

[23] Malik M, Batchvarow VN. Measurement, interpretation and clinical potential of QT dispersion. J Am Coll Cardiol 2000;36:1749-66.

[24] Yildirir A, Batur MK, Oto A. Hypertension and arrhythmia: blood pressure control and beyond. Europace 2002;4:175-82.

[25] Saadeh A, Evans S, James M, Jones J. QTc dispersion and complex ventricular arrhythmiaas in untreated newly presenting hypertensive patients. J Hum Hypertens. 1999;13:665-9.

[26] Kunisek J, Zaputović L, Mavrić Z, Kunisek L, Bruketa-Markić I, Karlavaris R, Lukin-Eskinja K. Influence of the type and degree of left ventricular hypertrophy on the prevalence of ventricular arrhythmias in patients with hypertensive heart disease. Med Klin 2008;103:705-11.

[27] Verdecchia P, Schillaci G, Borgioni R, Gattobigio R, Ambrosio G, Porcellati C. Prevalent influence of systolic over pulse pressure on left ventricular mass in essential hypertension. Eur Heart J 2002;23:658-65.

[28] Wachtell K, Rokkedal J, Bella JN, Aalto T, Dahlof B, Smith G, Roman MJ, Ibsen H, Aurigemma GP, Devereux RB. Effect of electrocardiographic left ventricular hypertrophy on left ventricular systolic function in systemic hypertension. Am J Cardiol 2001; 87:54-60.

[29] Gatzoulis KA, Vyssoulis GP, Apostolopoulos T, Delaveris P, Theopistou A, Gialafos JH, Toutouzas PK. Mild left ventricular hypertrophy in essential hypertension: is it really arrhythmogenic? Am J Cardiol 2000;13:340-5.

[30] Devereux RB, Reichek N. Echocardiographic determination of left ventricular mass in men. Anatomic validation of the method. Circulation 1977;55:613-8.

[31] Lombardi F, Terranova P (2003) Hypertension and concurrent arrhythmias. Curr Pharm Des 9 (21):1703-13. Review.

[32] Kunišek J, Zaputović L, Žuvić Butorac M, Kunišek L, Lukin Eškinja K, Karlavaris R, Bruketa Markić I. The prevalence of supraventricular arrhythmias with regard to the type and degree of left ventricular hypertrophy in patients with hypertensive heart disease. Wien Klin Wochenschr 2008;120:171-7.

[33] Szymanski L, Mandecki T, Twardowski R, Mizia-Stec K, Szulc A, Jastrzebska-Maj E. QT dispersion and characteristics of left ventricular hypertrophy in primary hypertension. Pol Arch Med Wewn. 2002;107:19-27.

[34] de Simone G, Kitzman DW, Chinali M, Oberman A, Hopkins PN, Rao DC et al. (2005) Left ventricular concentric geometry is associated with impaired relaxation in hypertension: the HyperGEN study. Eur Heart J 26:1039-45.

[35] Bach FH. Heme oxygenase-1 as a protective gene. Wien Klin Wschr 2002;114 (suppl 4):1-3. Review.

[36] Wade MR, Chandraratna PA, Reid CL, Lin SL, Rahimtoola SH (1987) Accuracy of nondirected and directed M-mode echocardiography as an estimate of left atrial size. Am J Cardiol 60:1208-1211.

[37] Lang RM, Bierig M, Devereux RB, Flachskampf FA, Foster E, Pellikka PA et al. American Society of Echocardiography's Nomenclature and Standards Committee (2006) Task Force on Chamber Quantification. American College of Cardiology Echocardiography Committee. American Heart Association. European Association of Echocardiography, European Society of Cardiology. Recommendations for chamber quantification. Eur J Echocardiography 7:79-108.

[38] Kunišek J, Zaputović L, Čubranić Z, Kunišek L, Žuvić Butorac M, Lukin Eškinja K, Karlavaris R, Vučković Rapaić S. Do particular types of left ventricular hypertrophy influence the duration and dispersion of QT interval in hypertensive patients? EuroPRevent Congres Abstracts 2010;P353.

[39] Oikarinen L, Nieminen MS, Viitasalo M, Toivonen L, Wachtell K, Papademetriou V, et al. Relation of QT interval and QT dispersion to echocardiographic left ventricular hypertrophy and geometric pattern in hypertensive patients. The LIFE study. The Losartan Intervention For Endpoint Reduction. J Hypertens. 2001;19:1883-91.

[40] Porthan K, Virolainen J, Hiltuten TP, Viitasalo M, Väänänen H, Dabek J, et al. Relationship of electrocardiographic repolarization measures to echocardiographic left ventricular mass in men with hypertension. J Hypertens. 2007;25:1951-7.

[41] Kulan K, Ural D, Komsuoglu B, Agacdiken A, Goldeli O, Komsuoglu SS. Significance of QTc prolongation on ventricular arrhythmias in patients with left ventricular hypertrophy secondary to essential hypertension. Int J Cardiol. 1998;64:179–84.

[42] Kotajima N, Hirakata T, Kanda T, Yokoyama T, Hoshino Y, Tanaka T, et al. Prolongation of QT interval and ventricular septal hypertrophy. Jpn Heart J. 2000;41:463-9.
[43] McLaughlin NB, Campbell RWF, Murray A. Influence of T wave amplitude on automatic QT measurement. In: Computers in Cardiology. IEEE Computer Society Press. 1995;777-80.
[44] Macfarlane PW, Devine B, Latif S, McLaughlin NB, Shoat DB, Watts MP. Methodology of QRS interpretation in the Glasgow program. Methods Inf Med. 1990;29: 354-61.
[45] Pshenichnikov I, Shipilova T, Kaik J, Volozh O, Abina J, Lass J, et al. QT dispersion in relation to left ventricular geometry and hypertension in a population study. Scand Cardiovasc J. 2003;37:87-90.
[46] Salles G, Leocádio S, Bloch K, Nogueira AR, Muxfeldt E. Combined QT interval and voltage criteria improve left ventricular hypertrophy detection in resistant hypertension. Hypertension. 2005;46:1207-12.
[47] Tyoshima H, Park YD, Ishikawa Y, Nagata S, Hirata Y, Sakakibara H, et al. Effect of ventricular hypertrophy on conduction velocity of activation trend in the ventricular myocardium. Am J Cardiol. 1982;49:1938-45.
[48] Opherk D, Mall G, Zebe H, Schwarz F, Weihe E, Manthey J, et al. Reduction of coronary reserve, a mechanism for angina pectoris in patients with arterial hypertension and normal coronary arteries. Circulation. 1984;69:1-7.
[49] Schillaci G, Pirro M, Ronti T, Gemelli F, Pucci G, Innocente S, et al. Prognostic impact of prolonged ventricular repolarization in hypertension. Arch Intern Med. 2006;166:909-13.
[50] Oikarinen L, Nieminen MS, Viitasalo M, Toivonen L, Jern S, Dahlöf B, et al. LIFE Study Investigators. QRS duration and QT interval predict mortality in hypertensive patients with left ventricular hypertrophy: the Losartan Intervention for Endpoint Reduction in Hypertension Study. Hypertension. 2004;43:1029-34.
[51] Dekker JM, Schouten EG, Klootwijk P, Pool J, Kromhout D. Association between QT interval and coronary heart disease in middle-aged and elderly men. The Zutphen Study. Circulation. 1994;90:779-85.
[52] Mayet J, Shahi M, McGrath K, Poulter NR, Sever PS, Foale RA, et al. Left ventricular hypertrophy and QT dispersion in hypertension. Hypertension. 1996;28:791-6.
[53] Ozdemir A, Telli HH, Temizhan A, Altunkeser BB, Ozdemir K, Alpaslan M, et al. Left ventricular hypertrophy increases the frequency of ventricular arrhythmia in hypertensive patients. Anad Kardyol Derg. 2002;2:293-9.
[54] Miyajima K, Minatoguchi S, Ito Y, Hukunishi M, Matsuno Y, Kakami M, et al. Reduction of QTc dispersion by the angiotensin II receptor blocker valsartan may be ralated to its anti-oxidative stress effect in patients with essential hypertension. Hypertens Res. 2007;30:307-13.

[55] Galetta F, Franzoni F, Magagna A, Femia FR, Pentimone F, Santoro G, et al. Effect of nebivolol on QT dispersion in hypertensive patients with left ventricular hypertrophy. Biomed Pharmacother. 2005;59:15-9.

12

Sleep-Related Breathing Disorders and Cardiac Arrhythmia

Ahmad Salah Hersi
King Fahad Cardiac Center, College of Medicine, King Saud University, Riyadh, Saudi Arabia

1. Introduction

Sleep-disordered breathing (SDB) includes a range of conditions characterized by abnormalities in the frequency and/or depth of breathing during sleep. Cessations in breathing rhythm (apneas) are momentary and often cyclical, while reductions in breath amplitude (hypopneas) may be momentary or sustained (Dempsey et al., 2010). Obstructive sleep apnea (OSA)/hypopnea syndrome (HS), obesity hypoventilation syndrome, central sleep apnea (CSA), upper airway resistance syndrome, and Cheyne-Stokes respiration (CSR) are the primary sleep-related respiratory disorders.

Although CSA is accompanied by alterations in neural input, the obstruction characteristic of OSA, the most common form of SDB, is also neurally mediated (Veasey, 2009). Intermittent episodes of partial or complete obstruction of the upper airway during sleep characteristic of OSA result from collapse of the upper airway. The concomitant disruption of normal ventilation and sleep architecture is typically associated with snoring, repeated arousals from sleep, and daytime sleepiness (Bradley & Floras, 2003; Lattimore et al, 2003; Quan & Gersh, 2004; Shamsuzzaman et al; 2003;).

Prevalence studies indicate that SDB, and particularly OSA, are common problems worldwide, affecting millions of individuals. However, OSA is also considered to be largely undiagnosed (Young et al, 1993; Young et al, 2002; Lavie, 2007). In the United States, for example, the estimated proportions of adults with OSA who are not diagnosed range from 60% to 80%, with an even greater under diagnosis suspected for children (Carter III, 2008). The increasing prevalence can be intuitively associated with the global obesity epidemic; however, a reverse association has also been postulated based on emerging evidence that OSA promotes weight gain (Carter III, 2008).

The clinical relevance of OSA was thought for years to be limited to what was considered a benign but often annoying manifestation as snoring, ranging to the possibly serious consequences of daytime sleepiness affecting cognitive function and work performance, mental state, and driving ability. OSA is now known to be a risk factor for other serious conditions, and has been associated with increased cardiovascular morbidity and mortality (Bradley & Floras, 2009; Devulapally et al., 2009; Lattimore et al, 2003; Lopez-Jiminez et al., 2008). Cardiac arrhythmias are common in OSA, and the potential link between tachyarrhythmias and bradyarrhythmias and adverse outcomes in OSA patients continues to be an important area of research (Chan & Wilcox, 2010; Verrier & Josephson, 2009). However, the complex cascade of events triggered by OSA, the difficulty in determining cause and effect from the preponderance of observational studies addressing these issues, lack of standardization of variable definitions, and heterogeneous patient samples allowing the influence of a multitude of confounders have been a constraint to producing consistent and definitive explanatory. Study variations complicate comparisons among reports, and require that sufficient individual design details are considered when evaluating the results of each study. Despite these limitations, our rapidly expanding knowledge promises to provide guidance for the assessment and management of patients both with SDB and arrhythmias.

2. Epidemiology and diagnosis of SDB

The worldwide recognized prevalence of OSA accompanied by daytime sleepiness is estimated to be 3% to 7% for adult men and 2% to 5% for adult women in the general population, with higher risks reported for some subgroups (Punjabi, 2008). OSA with or without daytime sleepiness may reach 24% in men and 9% in women by middle age (Young et al., 1993).

The main risk factors for SDB include obesity, upper airway obstruction including abnormalities of craniofacial morphology, and male gender (Parati et al., 2007; Partinen, 1995; Young et al., 1993; Young et al., 2002). Age also plays a role; however, the effect of age on SDB prevalence is not linear. The Sleep Heart Health Study reported a plateau effect in age-related prevalence beginning at approximately 60 years of age (Young et al., 2002a). In addition, SDB in the elderly may be different from the typical SDB of middle age. In one study, increased age, obesity, and snoring were significantly associated with progression of apnea in subjects aged 30 to 60 years at baseline; however, other studies suggest little or no association among these and other common OSA correlates of middle age with OSA in the elderly (Young et al., 2002b).

2.1 REM and nonREM sleep

Sleep stages include rapid eye movement (REM) and nonREM sleep. NonREM sleep typically comprises 75% to 85% of the sleep time in adults, and is characterized by decreased metabolic demands, relative autonomic stability with dominant vagus nerve activity, high baroreceptor gain, and stable sympathetic nerve activity (Arias & Sanchez, 2007; Somers et al, 1993; Verrier & Josephson, 2009). During stage 4 of nonREM sleep, that is, during deep sleep, cardiovascular system input is reduced by more than half compared with that of wakefulness. Parasympathetic tone increases and sympathetic tone decreases durn nonREM sleep. The resultant increase in vagal nerve activity elicits bradycardia, and during the transition from nonREM to REM sleep bursts of vagal nerve activity can produce asystole or pauses in heart rhythm. REM sleep, occurring at approximately 90 minute intervals of increasing length during sleep, is characterized by surges in cardiac sympathetic nerve activity that can reach levels higher than those achieved during wakefulness, and is accompanied by suppression of efferent vagus nerve tone and reduced baroreceptor gain. During this time of increased brain excitability, breathing patterns are also irregular. The apneic events of SDB have been shown to occur in both REM and non-REM sleep; however, a recent study showed that when SDB occurred only during REM sleep, SDB was not associated with sleepiness, impaired quality of life, or difficulty maintaining sleep (Chami et al., 2010).

2.2 Diagnosing SDB

The polysomnogram is considered the "gold standard" for OSA diagnosis. Measuring multiple physiological signals during sleep, including electroencephalography, electro-oculography, electrocardiography, electromyography, nasal airflow, respiratory effort (thoracic and abdominal impedence), pulse oximetry, snoring (tracheal microphone), and leg and sleep position allows identification and classification of apneas and hypopneas.

Obstructive, central, and mixed apneas can be distinguished based on the presence of a ventilatory effort during the event. Decreased upper airway muscle activation can result in a collapsible pharyngeal airway and produce an obstructive event, which is not uncommon in the unstable ventilatory control experienced by patients with CSR and CSA, resulting in both central and obstructive events in these patients (Somers et al., 2008).

According to the American Academy of Sleep Medicine (AASM), an apnea is a complete cessation of airflow for ≥10 seconds (Iber et al., 2007). A hypoponea is a ≥30% decrease in airflow from baseline of ≥10 seconds associated with a 4% oxygen desaturation, or a ≥50% reduction in airflow from baseline for ≥10 seconds associated with either a 3% oxygen desaturation or electroencephalographic data supporting a cortical microarousal from sleep. The apnea-hypopnea index (AHI) quantifies the average number of apneas and hypopneas per hour of sleep. The AASM defines OSA categories based on AHI as well as the extent of daytime sleepiness, with mild OSA having an AHI of 5 to 15 (Table 1)(AASM, 2008). Some restrict using the term OSA to indicate an AHI ≥5, and reserve the term OSA syndrome (OSAS) for when symptoms are also present, especially excessive daytime sleepiness (EDS) (Lee et al., 2008; Young et al., 2002b).

Type	AHI	Attention Requirements of Activities Affected by Involuntary Sleepiness
Mild	5-15	Little (e.g., watching TV, reading)
Moderate	15-30	Some (e.g., meetings, presentations)
Severe	>30	More Active (e.g., talking, driving)

KEY: AHI - apnea/hypopnea index

Table 1. AASM Obstructive Sleep Apnea Classification

EDS is typically measured by a subjective rating using questionnaires that have 3 to 5 items (Lee et al., 2008). The Epworth Sleepiness Scale, comprising 8 questions, is also commonly used. Among the physiological disturbances produced by apneic events, oxygen desaturation indexes more reliably predict sleepiness relative to other polysomnographic parameters including sleep time, AHI, or arousal index (Engleman & Douglas, 2004; Kingshott et al., 2000; Tihonen et al., 1998).

Categorization of apnea is often arbitrary, and studies frequently use different definitions of OSA and its severity, which seriously complicates comparisons among reports. Although the AHI alone is often considered adequate to define the severity of OSA, polysomnography results are sometimes presented as the respiratory disturbance index (RDI), which includes respiratory event related arousals (RERAs) that do not technically meet the definition of apnea or hypopnea, in addition to hypopnic and apneic events.

3. Evidence linking SDB to arrhythymia

The multiple physiologic and anatomic events associated with sleep apneas are conducive to the development of cardiac arrhythmias. Several observational studies have shown an association between OSA and the spectrum of arrhythmias (Table 2). Some tachyarrhythmias, such as persistent supraventricular tachycardia, atrial fibrillation (AF) or flutter, and ventricular arrhythmias, in particular sustained or nonsustained ventricular tachycardia, have been shown in some studies to be more likely to occur in the setting of preexisting structural heart disease (Grimm et al., 1996).

3.1 Cardiac arrhythmias in community-based studies and in subjects referred for sleep testing

In the seminal study by Guilleminault et al. (1983), 48% of 400 patients with OSA were shown by 24-h Holter monitoring to have arrhythmias, which included 18% with bradycardia. There is some indication that longer monitoring may be warranted, as shown by the results in a small sample of 23 patients with moderate or severe OSA who underwent 2 months of monitoring with an insertable loop recorder (Simantirikas et al., 2004). Almost half (47%) were shown to have severe cardiac rhythm disturbances, of whom all but 2 had severe bradycardia.

In a study of 247 patients with OSAS who had been referred for polysomnography who were shown to have an AHI >=5 and daytime symptoms, 46 (18.6%) had rhythm disturbances during sleep (Olmetti et al., 2008). Tachyarrhythmias occurred in 35 (14.2%) and bradyarrhythmias in 11 (4.4%) patients. All bradyarrhythmias occurred during an episode of apnea or hypopnea, while 13 (37%) tachyarrhythmic events occurred either during the episode or during the subsequent phase of recovering ventilation. Premature ventricular complex events occurred throughout the recording interval without association with sleep or wakefulness. The OSA in bradyarrhythmia patients was significantly more severe than that in tachyarrhythmia patients. Although patients with bradyarrhythmia compared with those without arrhythmia had a significantly greater AHI (58.8 vs. 27.3; P=.02), mean desaturation amplitude (8.9 vs. 5.9; P=.03), and a lower oxygen saturation nadir (69% vs. 77%; P=.003), they were similar in BMI (34.5 vs. 36.1) and age (51.8 vs. 53.6). The prevalence of bradyarrhythmia was, however, significantly higher in patients with AHI >=30 (7.8%) compared with patients with AHI <30 (1.5%; OR 5.33; 95% CI: 1.13, 25.3; P=.03). Conversely, OSA patients with tachyarrhythmia were not different from those without arrhythmias with respect to AHI, mean desaturation amplitude, and oxygen saturation nadir, nor was the prevalence of tachyarrhythmia in patients with AHI >=30 (15.5%) different from that in patients with AHI <30 (13.0%). COPD was the only comorbidity associated with either arrhythmia, with tachyarrhythmia more common in patients who had both COPD and OSA than it was in patients who had OSA alone (OR 2.53; P=.03).

Study (N)	%	Arrhythmia
Tilkian et al., 1977 (15)	93	Marked sinus arrhythmia
	40	Extreme sinus bradycardia
	33	Asystole
	13	Second-degree AV block
	67	VA-complex premature ventricular beats
	13	VT
Guilleminault et al., 1983 (400)	18	Bradyarrhythmia
	2	Sustained VT
	11	Sinus arrest
	8	Second-degree AV block
	19	Frequent premature ventricular contractions
Flemons et al., 1993 (263)	1.3	Complex ventricular ectopy (including VT)
	2.6	Frequent premature ventricular beats
	1.3	Second-degree AV block
	5.2	Sinus arrest
Becker et al., 1995	7	Sinus arrest and AV block
Mooe et al., 1996 (121) Incident AF in CABG patients pre-discharge	32	AF with AHI >=5
	18	AF with AHI <5
Javaheri et al., 1998 (81)	22	AF (all patients with HF)
Simantirakis et al., 2004 (23)	48	Rhythm disturbances
Mehra et al., 2006 (566)	4.8	AF
	5.3	Nonsustained VT
	25	Complex ventricular ectopy
Mehra et al., 2009 (3135 men ≥65 years of age)	4.7	AF
	36	Complex ventricular ectopy

KEY: AF - atrial fibrillation, AHI - apnea/hypopnea index, AV - atrioventricular, CABG - coronary artery bypass graft, VA - ventricular arrhythmias, VT - ventricular tachycardia

Table 2. Prevalence of Cardiac Arrhythmias in Obstructive Sleep Apnea

The community-based Sleep Heart Health Study, which compared arrhythmia prevalence in 228 persons with (RDI ≥30) and 338 persons without (RDI <5) SDB, provided important data on the risk of complex arrhythmias in persons of both genders who were at least 46 years of age (Mehra et al., 2006). After adjusting for age, sex, BMI, and prevalent coronary artery disease (CAD), risk for arterial fibrillation (OR 4.02; 95% CI: 1.03, 15.74), nonsustained ventricular tachycardia (OR 3.40; 95% CI: 1.03, 11.20), and complex ventricular ectopy (OR 1.74; 95% CI: 1.11, 2.74) remained almost 2- to 4-fold greater in persons diagnosed with OSA.

Trigeminy, supraventricular tachycardia, and all conduction delay arrhythmias were not significantly different between subjects with and without SDB on univariate analysis.

Other community-based studies also failed to show an increase in conduction delays in persons with SDB compared with those without SDB. There was also no difference in conduction delay arrhythmias according to SDB severity in data from the elderly men in U.S. MrOS Sleep Study (Mehra et al., 2009), and conduction delay prevalences in subjects with and without OSA in the Norwegian Akershus Sleep Apnea Project (ASAP) were similar (Namtvedt et al., 2011).

The ASAP study, which included randomly recruited subjests from the general Norwegian population, showed similarities with other reports; for example, ventricular premature complexes occurred significantly more frequently both at night and during daytime in the presence of OSA, defined as AHI ≥5 (Namtvedt et al., 2011). Increases in AHI were significantly associated with an increased prevalence of ventricular premature complexes, which remained after adjusting for clinically relevant confounders. In addition to conduction delays, supraventricular arrhythmias, including atrial fibrillation, were not different between subjects with and without OSA in this study.

Diagnosis of 1456 Japanese patients suspected of having sleep apnea revealed 97.0% had at least mild (AHI ≥5) sleep apnea (Abe et al., 2010). CSA, defined as having more than 50% central apneas, was diagnosed in 62 patients. OSA in the remaining 1412 patients was classified according to mild, moderate, and severe OSA, using AASM levels. The occurrence of paroxysmal AF (P=.051), premature atrial complex (P=.005), premature ventricular complex (P=.004), sinus bradycardia (P=.036), and sinus pause (P<.001) were increased with increasing OSA severity. Nonsustained ventricular tachycardia and second- and third-degree atrioventricular block were not related to OSA severity; however, prevalence was very low, with no cases in subjects without OSA, and prevalence ranging from 1.0% to 1.3%, 0.3% to 1.3%, and 0% to 0.1% among OSA the 3 OSA severities for these 3 arrhythmias, respectively.

This was contrasted by data from the Sleep Heart Health Study where 5.3% of subjects with SDB had nonsustained ventricular tachycardia compared with 1.2% of subjects without SDB (P=.004)(Mehra et al., 2006). Complex ventricular ectopy (25.0% vs. 14.5%; P=.002) and atrial fibrillation (4.8% vs. 0.9%; P=.003) were also significantly more prevalent in subjects with SDB.

Other studies have failed to show a difference in atrial fibrillation prevalence between subjects with and without SDB, or in the prevalence of SDB in patients with and without atrial fibrillation (Roche et al., 2003). Requiring an AHI of at least 15 as diagnostic for OSA, a case control study failed to show a difference in OSA prevalence between 59 patients with lone atrial fibrillation (i.e., without chronic or acute risk factors) and controls who were age, gender, and co-morbidity matched controls (32% vs. 29%; P=0.67)(Porthan et al., 2004).

Another study (Leung et al., 2005) that excluded patients with a history of congestive heart failure (CHF), CAD, or stroke, enrolled 60 patients each without SBD, with CSA, and with OSA. The prevalence of atrial fibrillation was significantly higher in patients with CSA (27%) compared with OSA (1.7%) or no SBD (3.3%; P<.001). Patients with OSA had more hypertension and more extreme oxygen desaturation.

Nocturnal bradycardia was present in 17 of 239 (7%) patients with OSA who were diagnosed using a validated ambulatory recording device that measured heart rate, oxygen saturation, snoring, and body position (Becker et al., 1995; Koehler et al., 2000). Patients with bradycardia were then given polysomnograms. Two-thirds of 1575 bradyarrhythmic events recorded during 24-hour Holter ECG monitoring occurred during REM sleep, and all occurred concomitant with an apneic or hypopneic event. Oxygen saturation was similar in patients with and without bradyarrhythmia at the beginning of the apnea or hypopnea; however, end values were significantly lower in patients with bradyarrhythmia. RDI was significantly higher in patients with bradyarrhythmias, who had an RDI of at least 60. However, 80 patients with an RDI >=60 did not have bradyarrhythmia. BMI was also significantly higher in patients with bradyarrhythmias, and the authors concluded that the obesity and high RDI associated with the bradyarrhythmias may be interrelated in their development.

3.2 OSA in patients with cardiovascular disease

Javaheri et al. (1998) recruited 81 ambulatory men with stable heart failure for polysomnography and nocturnal Holter monitoring. In previous studies, these authors had used an AHI threshold of 20 to classify sleep apnea; however, for this study the threshold was set at AHI ≥15 to accommodate patients with a lower AHI but with significant arterial oxyhemoglobin desaturation. Forty-one (51%) patients had sleep apnea, with a mean AHI of 44 ± 19. Compared with patients without sleep apnea, patients with sleep apnea were more likely to have atrial fibrillation (22% vs. 5%; P=.026), with a non-significant higher prevalence of nocturnal ventricular tachycardia (51% vs. 37%; P=.23). The mean numbers of premature ventricular depolarizations (P=.0002) and couplets (P=.0001) were significantly higher in sleep apnea patients, with a non-significantly higher ventricular tachycardia rate (P=.07). When Sin et al. (1999) compared the prevalence and characteristics of CSA and OSA in 450 patients with CHF, the prevalence of CSA (33%) was similar to that of OSA (38%) using a threshold for SDB of AHI 10; however, atrial fibrillation was significantly greater in CSA patients (23.0%) compared with OSA patients (11.9%) and with patients without SBD (7.5%; P<.05).

Sleep apneas have been suggested to play a role in the recurrence of arrhythmias following successful therapy. In a study of 44 patients with sustained ventricular tachycardia without heart failure or other structural heart disease who underwent catheter ablation therapy, 17 (39%) were diagnosed with sleep apnea by polysomnography using a threshold of AHI ≥10 (Koshino et al., 2010). Arrhythmia recurrence in successfully ablated patients with apnea (5/11, 45%) was significantly greater than that in patients without sleep apnea (1/17, 6%; P=.02).

When sleep studies were performed in 45 patients with implantable cardioverter defibrillators (ICD), over half (57.87%) were diagnosed with SDB, using a threshold of AHI ≥10 (Zeidan-Shwiri et al., 2011). The mean number of ventricular arrhythmias was significantly higher in patients with SDB (P=.03). A significant increase in the number of ventricular arrhythmias occurred with increasing AHI quartiles (0–7, 8–11, 12–33, and 34–66 events/h; P=.003), as seen in other studies (e.g., ventricular premature complexes in the general population study of Namtvedt et al., 2011). Increases in ventricular arrhythmias in the ICD patients were predominantly related to increased ventricular arrhythmic events occurring from midnight to 6 a.m. SDB was a significant, independent predictor of nocturnal appropriate ICD therapy after adjusting for baseline variables including age, BMI, and serum creatinine (OR 3.8; 95% CI: 1.2, 12.1; P=.02). Similar results were reported by Serizawa et al. (2008), who enrolled 71 patients with heart failure and an ICD, of whom 47 (66%) were diagnosed with SDB, also using an AHI threshold of 10. Appropriate ICD therapies occurred more frequently in SDB patients (43%) compared with those without

SDB (17%; P=.029). In addition, ICD therapy from midnight to 6 a.m. was more frequent in patients with (34%) than in those without (13%) SDB (P=.046), and SDB was an independent predictor for appropriate ICD therapy in multivariate analysis (HR 4.05; 95% CI: 1.20 , 13.65; P=.015).

The recurrence rate of atrial fibrillation during 1-year of follow-up in 39 patients who underwent DC cardioversion for atrial fibrillation/atrial flutter was compared with that in 79 postcardioversion patients (controls) who did not have a previous sleep study (Kangala et al., 2003). Recurrence in 27 OSA patients who received no treatment for their OSA was 82%, compared with 42% for those with treated OSA (P=.013), and 53% in the control group (P=.009). Comparing nocturnal decrease in oxygen saturation in untreated OSA patients with recurrence of atrial fibrillation with that of untreated patients without a recurrence revealed a significantly greater decrease occurred in untreated OSA patients (18% vs. 8%; P=.034), who had a greater portion of sleep time with oxygen saturation <90% (23% vs. 4%; P=.063). The increased risk of recurrence of atrial fibrillation in untreated patients with OSA in this study prompted the authors to propose that patients with atrial fibrillation should be screened for OSA; and, similarly, OSA patients should be screened for atrial fibrillation.

Gami et al. (2004) compared the prevalence of OSA, diagnosed using the Berlin questionnaire, in 151 patients undergoing cardioversion for atrial fibrillation with the prevalence in 312 general cardiology practice patients.r Significantly more patients with atrial fibrillation had OSA compared with the general cardiology group (49% vs. 32%; P=.0004); with a multivariate adjusted OR for the association between atrial fibrillation and OSA of 2.19 (95% CI: 1.40, 3.42; P=.0006). To accommodate any misclassifications that might have occurred without using polysomnography for diagnosis, a separate analysis adjusted patient numbers per group using validation data acquired from 44 patients on whom polysomnography was performed. After decreasing OSA in the atrial fibrillation group by the false-positive rate and increasing it in the general cardiology group by the false negative rate, the difference in prevalence between the 2 groups remained statistically significant (48% vs. 37%, P=.022). These authors also concluded that the presence of OSA should be considered in all patients with atrial fibrillation, particularly those with obesity or hypertension. This should be considered particularly sage advice considering the current epidemic increase in atrial fibrillation and its associated morbidity and mortality (Steinberg, 2004).

The incidence of post surgical atrial fibrillation in 121 consecutive coronary artery bypass surgery patients was assessed by Mooe et al. (1996). All patients underwent preoperative diagnosis of disordered breathing, defined as AHI ≥5 or an oxygen desaturation index (ODI) ≥5. Atrial fibrillation was diagnosed in 25 of 78 (32%) patients with AHI ≥5 compared with 7 of 39 (18%) of patients with AHI <5 (P=.11), and in 19 of 49 (39%) patients with ODI ≥5 compared with 13 of 72 (18%) patients with an ODI <5 (P=.02). Using ODI ≥5, disordered breathing was an independent predictor of atrial fibrillation in a multiple-logistic regression model (RR 2.8, 95% CI: 1.2, 6.8).

In summary, these studies revealed some differences and similarities in the manifestation of arrhythmias associated with SDB. For example, bradyarrhythmias, premature ventricular complexes, and atrial fibrillation have been shown in some studies to be increased with increasing severity of SDB, while no effect of SDB severity was shown for tachyarrhythmias. Bradyarrhythmias occur with the apneic or hypopneic event, while tachycardias also occur during recovery. Finally, premature ventricular complexes have been shown to occur during waking hours as well as during sleep in patients with SDB. These results indicate the importance of identifying the mechanisms associating SDB with cardiac arrhythmias.

4. Pathophysiological mechanisms of arrhythmia in SDB

The exact mechanisms linking SDB and arrhythmia are not completely understood, as there are several complex and interrelated pathways by which arrhythmias may be produced or become more severe in the presence of SDB. Autonomic, hemodynamic, chemical, inflammatory, and metabolic mechanisms may be involved to varying degrees in relation to patient demographic and health characteristics (Figure 1). Research is ongoing, with the understanding that exploring the physiological effects of SDB should not be limited to sleep, as patients with sleep apnea exhibit elevated sympathetic nerve activity and blood pressure during wakefulness (Verrier & Josephson, 2009).

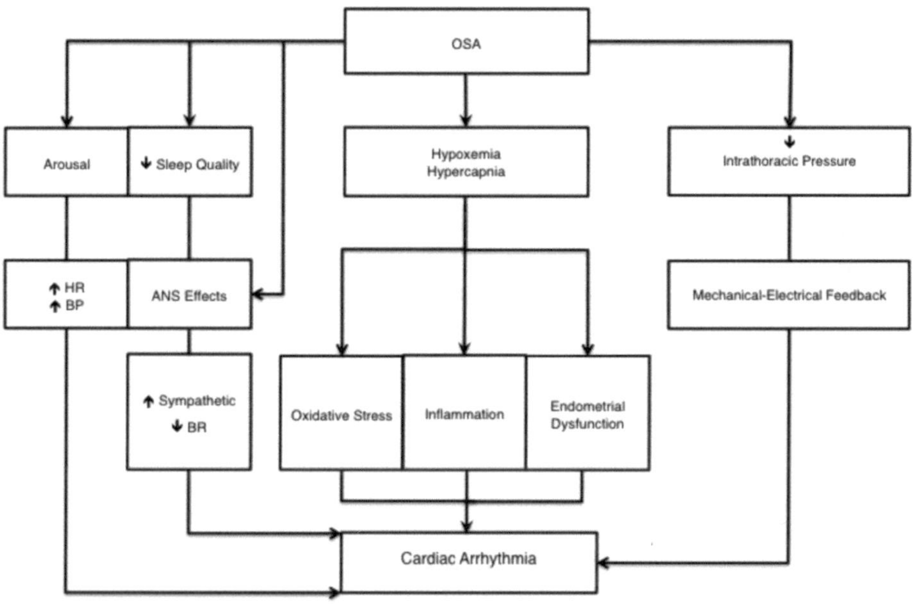

KEY: ANS – autonomic nervous system, BP – blood pressure, BR – barorecptor gain, OSA – obstructive sleep apnea

Fig. 1. Obstructive Sleep Apnea and Cardiac Arrhythmia – Possible Mechanisms

The increased risk of arrhythmias and sudden cardiac death in obesity is well known, and the common occurrence of SDB in obese subjects suggests overlapping mechanisms may contribute to arrhythmia development in these patients. Prolonged corrected QT (QTc) interval, increased vasomotor tone and ventricular instability, development of dilated cardiomyopathy, and impairment in autonomic nervous system cardiac modulation may be involved (Arias & Sanchez, 2007). Intermittent hypoxemia, sympathetic hyperactivity, and increased left-ventricular after load that occur secondary to each apneic event in OSA impose an additional burden.

The severity of OSA was shown to be independently associated with elevated inflammatory markers, including C-reactive protein (Shamsuzzaman et al., 2002), which is also elevated in atrial fibrillation (Chung et al., 2001). Decreases in some of these markers have been reported when OSA was treated with continuous positive air pressure (CPAP) therapy (Arias & Sanchez, 2007; Svatikova et al., 2003).

Some generalized mechanisms that may be involved with SDB and its effect on arrhymogenesis have been described, which are often linked to the specific type of arrhythmia evoked. For example, apneas are known to induce several arrythmogenic dysregulations including alterations in cardiac sympathetic and parasympathetic activity, myocardial hypoxemia (Schafer et al., 1997), and deformation of the cardiac chambers resulting from intrathoracic pressure fluctuations (Condos et al., 1987).

Mechanisms related to specific sleep stages may also impact the development of arrhythmias in SDB. REM-induced cardiac events may include both direct effects, such as alterations in electrophysiological stability, or indirect effects on heart rate and arterial blood pressure. Subsequent platelet aggregation or plaque disruption can be associated with the release of arrhythmogenic molecules. Metabolic imbalances can stimulate neural activity that results in myocardial ischemia or arrhythmias. Some studies have shown that arrhythmias were more common in SDB patients who had severe nocturnal hypoxemia during REM sleep (Findley et al., 1985; Shepard et al., 1985).

4.1 Ventricular arrhythmias

Surges in sympathetic nerve activity during REM sleep have been suggested to cause nocturnal ventricular arrhythmias and myocardial ischemia in patients with cardiovascular disease (Nowlin et al., 1965). The purported decrease in vagus nerve activity and unopposed cardiac sympathetic nerve activity in these patients may foster development of ventricular tachycardia and fibrillation (Verrier & Josephson, 2009).

The surge in arterial blood pressure and sympathetic nerve activity that occur with apneas may explain the temporal association between the apnea and the onset of nonsustained ventricular tachycardia (Monahan et al., 2009; Somers et al., 1995; Somers et al., 2008). In one sub-study from the Sleep Heart Health Study, polysomnograms from 57 patients with 62 episodes of paroxysmal atrial fibrillation or nonsustained vetricular tachycardia (NSVT) were reviewed (Monahan et al., 2009). Respiratory disturbances (apneas or hypopneas) occurring during hazard periods defined as the 90s intervals preceding an AF event were compared with those occurring during referent control periods in the same subject. Approximately three-fourths (n=47; 76%) of the events were NSVT, and two-thirds (68%) occurred in nonREM sleep (atrial fibrillation: 80%; NSVT: 64%). The overall risk of occurrence after a respiratory disturbance was 17.5-fold greater (95% CI: 5.3, 58.4) than the risk of an event during normal nocturnal breathing, and was similar for each arrhythmia type (atrial fibrillation OR: 17.9; NSVT OR: 17.4). When each variable was considered independently, there was no association between EEG-defined arousal or hypoxia and arrhythmia risk. Based on this data, the authors postulated that additional mechanisms may be involved in the link between sleep-related respiratory disturbances and arrhythmias, including large changes in intrathoracic pressure and stimulation of baroreflexes (Gami et al, 2008). However, they also suggested that the small number of respiratory disturbances in their study may have inhibited detection of an effect. In fact, others have suggested that the oxygen desaturation that occurs with apnea may be involved as an independent risk factor for ventricular arrhythmia (Bradley & Flores, 2003a; Bradley & Flores, 2003b).

4.1.1 The MrOS sleep study - A model for design and analysis of community-based studies

The MrOS Sleep Study, an ancillary cohort of the multicenter Osteoporotic Fractures in Men Study, enrolled 3135 men ≥65 years of age to explore the association of SDB with complex ventricular ectopy (CVE) and nocturnal atrial fibrillation in elderly men (Mehra et al., 2009). This elaborate study warrants detailed discussion. The design included clearly defined variables across SDB severities and types, supported by rigorous, standardized data collection from a large, community-based sample. The study investigated the occurrence of nocturnal CVE and atrial fibrillation as primary endpoints, and also evaluated the occurrence of any atrial arrhythmias, other ventricular arrhythmias, and conduction delay arrhythmias. Polysomnography data were used to produce RDI data, which provided an overall severity of SDB by including both obstructive and central apneas per hour, summarized into quartiles. The upper limit of the lowest quartile was only slightly above the commonly used threshold for SDB (<5.9 vs 5, respectively); therefore, the lowest quartile was approximately equivalent to no SDB. An obstructive AHI index (OAHI), limited to obstructive events, was also categorized by quartile. A Central Apnea Index (CAI) was created from categories made from the distribution of data for central apneas/hour of sleep. Categories were prepared from percent of total sleep time (TST) with arterial oxygen saturation <90% (defining hypoxia) that accommodated the right-skewed data distribution.

In the MrOS Sleep Study, 1048 (36%) subjects had CVE. There was a significant association between the fourth quartile of OAHI severity (RDI ≥23.9) and CVE (adjusted OR 1.37; 95% CI: 1.08, 1.75); however, the relationship between CSA and CVE was not significant after adjusting for confounders including cardiovascular disease. CVE was also associated with hypoxia, with both unadjusted and unadjusted ORs significant when at least 10% of TST was spent at <90% oxygen saturation (adjusted OR 1.62; 95% CI: 1.23, 2.14). The authors concluded that CVE is more likely to result in patients who experience intermittent hypoxia and collapse of the upper airway, which are triggers for intrathoracic pressure changes, blood pressure surges, and sympathetic nervous system activation. They compared their results to the study of Javaheri (2000), in which treatment of SDB resulted in reduced RDI and hypoxia.

4.2 Atrial fibrillation

Several studies in addition to those discussed in section 4.1 have explored potential mechanisms for atrial fibrillation to occur in the setting of SDB. Hypertension is an established risk factor for atrial fibrillation (Kannel et al. 1998; Chugh et al., 2001), and the relationship between OSA and both hypertension and left-ventricular hypertrophy has been documented (Arias & Sanchez, 2007; Nieto et al., 2000; Peppard et al., 2000). Data from OSA patients describe cardiac structural and functional changes, including right and left ventricular performance and left atrial enlargement (Otto et al., 2007; Romero-Corral et al., 2007). Shifts in transmural pressures and concomitant changes in cardiac chamber dimensions can occur in response to the futile ventilatory efforts during apnea (Condos et al., 1987; Hall et al., 1998), and may trigger stretch-activated ion channels in the atria (Franz & Bode, 2003) that can lead to atrial fibrillation. The mechanical effects of negative intrathoracic pressure can allow cardiac stretching, whereby a mechanical-electrical feedback mechanism could predispose to atrial fibrillation (Franz, 2000). These data support a mechanistic association of OSA with the development of atrial fibrillation; however, causation has not yet been proven.

Heart rate variability studies have shown that nocturnal atrial fibrillation is induced during periods of intense vagus nerve activity (Bettoni & Zimmerman, 2002). These vagally-mediated episodes of atrial fibrillation are usually preceded by bradycardia (Verrier & Yosephson, 2009). In addition, the apnea-induced hypoxemia, sympathetic nerve activity, and surges in blood pressure that can affect diastolic function by distending and remodeling atrial chambers may also contribute to atrial fibrillation development.

In a study of atrial fibrillation radiofrequency ablation in 424 patients, OSA was a significant risk factor for conduction recurrence after multivariable adjustment (RR 2.16; 95% CI: 1.32, 3.94; P=.01)(Sauer et al., 2006). This was postulated to be mechanistically related to left atrial electrical modeling, fibrosis, and chamber enlargement resulting from OSA (Gami et al., 2008).

In many studies of atrial fibrillation in association with OSA, oxygen saturation variables were independently predictive of atrial fibrillation, suggesting that hypoxemia is an important pathophysiological mechanism linking OSA and atrial fibrillation (Gami et al, 2008). In addition to decreased oxygen saturation, obesity, male gender, and coronary artery disease in persons 65 years of age, and heart failure in older subjects, have been shown to be associated with the development of atrial fibrillation in patients with apnea (Wang et al., 2004).

In the MrOS Sleep Study, atrial fibrillation had a stronger association with CSA than OSA (Mehra et al., 2009). Adjusted analysis revealed increasing severity of SDB was only significantly related to atrial fibrillation in patients with the most severe CSA (OR 2.69; 95% CI: 1.61, 4.47), which remained significant after excluding subjects without heart failure from the analysis. The effect of hypoxia on atrial fibrillation, however, was not significant. Although these results were based on self-reported heart failure, the authors suggested that their results agree with those of Leung et al. (2005), that atrial fibrillation is more strongly associated with CSA than OSA, even in the absence of heart failure. They concluded that it may be beneficial to screen patients with AF for CSA.

4.3 Bradyarrhythmias

While repeated hypoxemia and arousals enhance sympathetic nervous activity and may be involved with the tachyarrhymias seen in OSA, the simultaneous hypoxemia and apnea also induce the diving reflex, with cardiac parasympathetic vagal nerve activation and peripheral sympathetic activation that produces vasoconstriction in muscle, renal, and splanchnic, but not cerebral, vasculature (Daly et al., 1979; Madden et al., 1997; Somers et al., 1992). This may result in severe nocturnal bradyarrhythmia. In the study of 239 OSA patients by Becker et al. (1995), bradyarrhythmia occurred only during apnea and hypopnea. In some studies, these bradyarrhythmias occurred more frequently during REM sleep accompanied by at least a 4% decrease in oxygen saturation (Becker et al, 1995; Koehler et al., 1998; Koehler et al., 2000). Conversely, in the study by Guilleminault et al. (1983), in 3 patients extreme sinus bradycardia occurred during nonREM sleep, and sinus arrest was associated with apneas during REM sleep. These patients had both sinus arrest and extreme sinus bradycardia that were of similar duration.

The lack of a difference in conduction delay arrhythmias between subjects with and without SDB in both the MrOS Sleep Study (Mehra et al., 2009) and Sleep Heart Health Study (Mehra et al., 2006) was remarked by the authors to be at variance with the opinion that SDB is associated with increased vagal tone. They offered that there may be differences in the underlying comorbidities in these 2 studies compared with data from studies of clinic referral subjects that suggested an association of SDB with bradyarrhythmia and heart failure.

The clinical significance of these OSA-related arrhythmias is not completely understood, and their association with adverse outcomes warrants further investigation in studies designed to accommodate the numerous confounders influencing results. The possible relationship between nocturnal oxygen desaturation and arrhythmias and sudden death in heart failure patients was suggested 20 years ago (Davies et al., 1991). More recently, Gami et al. (2005) reported that sudden cardiac death in almost half of 78 heart failure patients with OSA occurred during sleeping hours from midnight to 6:00 a.m., significantly deviating from the typical time of death during early morning waking hours (6:00 a.m. to noon).

In summary, despite differences among studies and gaps in understanding the mechanisms by which SDB impacts arrhythmias, data suggest that patients with moderate to severe OSA are at increased risk for arrhythmias during sleep. the majority of data support the importance of identifying patients with SDB and treating them appropriately.

5. Treating OSA

Tracheostomy was the standard treatment for SDB until CPAP was introduced in 1981. Although CPAP is not as invasive as tracheostomy, it can present challenges. The equipment and devices can be cumbersome and annoying, with treatment compliance commonly less than 50% due to rhinitis, nose bleeds, facial abrasions, and improper fit (Gami et al., 2008; Veasey, 2009). Pressure must be titrated to a level high enough to prevent not only apneas and hyponeas, but also to prevent snoring that can cause arousal. However, pressure must also be kept at a level below what would cause sleep interference.

There have been no long-term, large, randomized controlled trials comparing OSA treatment with placebo on cardiovascular outcomes. Several studies, however, associated failing to treat OSA with increased mortality or morbidity (He et al., 1988). Data from 3 large observational studies that included a total of 2396 patients showed increased fatal and nonfatal cardiovascular outcomes in patients with severe OSA, compared with patients who were treated with CPAP (Buchner et al., 2007; Campos-Rodriguez et al., 2005; Marin et al., 2005).r One of the studies (Buchner et al., 2007) enrolled 449 patients, of whom 364 received OSA treatment, which provided a 64% cardiovascular risk reduction after adjusting for age, gender, cardiovascular risk factors, and baseline comorbidities.

In the Japanese study of the relationship between OSA and arrhythmias, 316 of 1047 patients with AHI ≥20 accepted treatment with CPAP therapy, and were re-evaluated an average of 3.9 weeks after polysomnography to determine the effectiveness of CPAP therapy and arrhythmia status (Abe et al., 2010). AHI and arousal index were among the OSA variables that were significantly improved with CPAP therapy ($P<.001$ for both). Premature atrial complex and nonsustained ventricular tachycardia were unchanged, as were the numbers of second- and third-degree AV block; however the latter were present in only 5 patients before treatment and 1 patient after treatment. The proportions of patients with premature ventricular complex, sinus bradycardia, pause, and paroxysmal atrial fibrillation were significantly decreased after treatment.

There is no clinical basis for treating nighttime atrial fibrillation differently from that occurring during the day. However, patients who have nocturnal onset of atrial fibrillation should be monitored for SDB and provided treatment with CPAP if warranted.

A recent study followed 47 OSA patients on CPAP for 12 months to assess changes in cardiac biomarkers from baseline (Colish et al., 2011). Systolic and diastolic abnormalities were reversed as early as 3 months after starting treatment, with additional improvements evident over 1-year as evidenced by transthoracic echocardiography and CMR. Levels of biomarkers, including CRP, did not change significantly during 12 months of follow-up, however.

Ventricular arrhythmias are assumed to be one of the major causes of sudden in heart failure. Screening for OSA in heart failure and treating patients may reduce the incidence of these fatal arrhythmias and improve survival.

Treating OSA has also been shown to resolve arrhythmias in many studies. Fifty OSA patients with arrhythmias in the study by Guilleminault et al. (1983) underwent tracheostomy, and after 3 to 6 months arrhythmias were no longer occurring in 46 patients. Arrhythmias in 4 patients with premature ventricular contractions decreased during sleep, and remained frequent during wakefulness.

Several other case series have shown that nocturnal cardiac rhythm disturbances were reduced following OSA treatment (Becker et al; 1995; Grimm et al., 2000; Harbison et al., 2000; Koehler et al, 1998; Tilkian et al., 1977). It was surprising, therefore, in a recent retrospective cohort study of 2626 patients with OSA, that CPAP use did not affect the incidence of atrial fibrillation (Gami et al., 2007). The authors commented that determining CPAP use in the retrospective study relied on subjective reporting with subsequent documentation in medical records. This precluded accurately determining frequency of use, compliance, and treatment outcome. In addition, in that study CPAP treatment was used by patients who had more severe OSA. These factors may have confounded the association between CPAP use and incident atrial fibrillation.

In the study of Beckers et al. (1995), only 1 of 17 patients with bradyarrhythmia did not achieve resolution of their arrhythmia after CPAP therapy. Similarly, OSA patients with severe cardiac rhythm disturbances reported by Simantirakis et al. (2004) experienced a significant reduction in bradycardias from a median of 5.5 per week in the 8-week pre-treatment period to 0.5 per week in the first 8 weeks of CPAP therapy (P=.028). No bradycardias or pauses were reported beginning 5 months after starting treatment through 14 months of follow-up.

In response to reports noting an association between OSA and bradyarrhythmias, several studies were performed in the last 10 years exploring the potential for pacemakers to resolve OSA. As reviewed by Simantirakis & Vardas (2006), positive results were reported from a small study of patients with CSA but not in several studies of OSA. These authors postulated that in patients with predominantly OSA, the functional changes elicited by atrial overdrive pacing have no effect on the anatomical obstructions that cause the apnea. In CSA, functional and autonomic nervous system changes were able to affect the pathophysiological causes of respiration disturbances during sleep. The recent ACC/AHA/HRS Guidelines for Device-Based Therapy of Cardiac Rhythm Abnormalities (Eptsein et al., 2008) conclude that results of randomized controlled trials (RCTs) failed to suggest a role for atrial overdrive pacing in OSA, and that CPAP has been shown to be highly effective. However,r the possible role of cardiac pacing in patients with OSA who continue to have persistent bradycardia episodes despite CPAP has not been confirmed. Data from a subsequent meta-analysis by Baranchuk et al. (2009) of 10 crossover RCTs in patients with AHI >=15 that enrolled 175 patients revealed that atrial overdrive pacing caused a significant 4.65 episode/h reduction in AHI (P=.01). However, this was substantially less than that achieved with CPAP treatment reported in the literature and the mean 42.5 episode/h reduction achieved in the 3 studies in the meta-analysis that included CPAP arms. The authors concluded that, although it was statistically significant, the reduction on atrial overdrive pacing was not clinically significant, and that patients with sleep apnea should not be treated with cardiac pacing unless there is a conventional indication. Conversely, studies suggest that increased parasympathetic input to the heart may be the main mechanism for nocturnal bradycardias (reviewed by Bradley & Flores, 2009). Therefore, treatment of OSA-induced nocturnal bradycardia may obviate the need for cardiac pacing; however, more studies are needed.

6. Future directions

Since the first suggestion was made of an association between OSA and cardiovascular morbidity and mortality, a rapidly expanding volume of observational data link OSA with the development of arrhythmias. Much research must be done, however, to answer the numerous questions that remain. In addition to larger epidemiological studies, randomized controlled trials must be performed that use robust designs similar to those used in cardiovascular intervention trials, with standardized definitions and adequate control of confounders.

A major issue with properly investigating OSA and arrhythmias in both research and clinical settings is the expense and limited availability of sleep laboratories for the diagnosis of OSA. Once OSA is suspected, although other forms of diagnosis have been used, polysomnography remains the gold standard for diagnosis. Ambulatory in home devices may become a reasonable alternative, particularly in developing countries that have availability, access, and cost constraints (Ng et al., 2009). Many other methods are being investigated, and reports suggest some of these may be appropriate for initial screening in suspected cases, followed by full polysomnography when warranted.

The Berlin questionnaire has been used as the diagnostic test in some studies, and has been validated as part of one study (Gami et al., 2004). It has also been shown to be comparable to other checklists and questionnaires that have been suggested as being valid screening tools (Chung et al., 2008a,b).

The high prevalence of SDB in patients on cardiac pacing prompted several investigations of the potential for diagnosing OSA in patients who have rate-responsive pacemakers with minute ventilation sensors (Simantirakis & Vardas, 2006). These devices could provide preliminary screening for SDB, subsequent monitoring of correlations between arrhythmias and apnea/hypopnea events, and evaluate therapeutic efficacy. Limitations include the inability to distinguish between central and obstructive apneas and to recognize specific sleep stages. However, its benefits can be acquired by interrogating extant devices without additional cost in patients with pacemakers; therefore, this may be useful in patients who are already on permanent pacemakers, but does not justify pacemaker placement without a clinical indication.

Data have shown that OSA in the setting of cardiac arrhythmias may confer a higher risk of stroke and cardiovascular events (Marin et al., 2005) on affected patients,r and early treatment of OSA in these patients may reduce cardiovascular morbidity (Kanagala et al., 2003; Barcena & Fang, 2007). Putting these understandings into practice is necessary. The importance of this is exemplified by considering the association between sleep apnea and heart failure, which has not resulted in increased vigilance or therapy. For example, despite the high prevalence (40% to 60%) of sleep apnea in heart failure, a recent study was reported summarizing data in U.S. Medicare files for over 30,000 incident heart failure patients, of whom only 4% were suspected to have sleep apnea (Javaheri et al., 2011). Less than half of these received testing and treatment, and were shown to have significantly greater 2-year

survivals compared with patients who were not tested (P<.0001) or were tested but not treated (P=.009). Policies for addressing issues relating to SDB and arrhythmia should be developed and implemented.
In summary, continuing research should focus on acquiring high quality, standardized data. As new data are acquired, policies should be developed and implement to assure screening for and treating SDB is available to high risk populations.

7. Conclusions

Many studies suggest that there is a significant association between SDB and increased prevalence and incidence of cardiac arrhythmias. The pathophysiological pathways between arrhythmias and SDB have not been clearly defined, but apnea-induced hypoxia, intrathoracic pressure changes, inflammation, and autonomic instability that can lead to adverse cardiovascular consequences are presumed to be involved. Larger epidemiological studies and RCTs are required to define the association and its mechanisms, which should control for confounding and apply standardized definitions. While studies are limited, initial results suggest that intervention with CPAP may be effective in reducing the arrhythmia burden in the OA population, however, additional RCTs are necessary.

8. References

AASM. Obstructive Sleep Apnea. American Academy of Sleep Medicine. 2008. Available from http://www.aasmnet.org/resources/factsheets/sleepapnea.pdf

Abe, H.; Takahashi, M.; Yaegashi, H., et al. (2010). Efficacy of Continuous Positive Airway Pressure on Arrhythmias in Obstructive Sleep Apnea Patients. *Heart Vessels*, Vol.25, No.1, (January 2010), pp. 63–9

Arias, M. & Sánchez, A. (2007). Obstructive Sleep Apnea and Its Relationship To Cardiac Arrhythmias. *J Cardiovasc Electrophysiol.* Vol.18, No.9, (September 2007), pp. 1006-14

Baranchuk, A.; Healey, J.; Simpson, C., et al. (2009). Atrial Overdrive Pacing in Sleep Apnoea: A Meta-Analysis. *Europace*, Vol.11, No.8, (August 2009), pp. 1037–40

Barcena, J. & Fang, J. (2007). Diagnosis And Treatment of Sleep Apnea in Heart Disease. *Curr Treat Options Cardiovasc Med,* Vol.9, No.6, (December 2007), pp. 501–9

Becker, H.; Brandenburg, U.; Peter, J., et al. (1995). Reversal of Sinus Arrest and Atrioventricular Conduction Block in Patients with Sleep Apnea During Nasal Continuous Positive Airway Pressure. *Am J Respir Crit Care Med,* Vol.151, No.1, (January 1995), pp. 215–8

Bettoni, M. & Zimmerman, M. (2002). Autonomic Tone Variations Before the Onset of Paroxysmal Atrial Fibrillation. *Circulation,* Vol.105, No.23, (June 2002), pp. 2753–9

Bradley, T. & Floras, J. (2003). Sleep Apnea and Heart Failure. I: Obstructive Sleep Apnea. *Circulation,* Vol.107, No.12, (April 2003), pp. 1671–8

Bradley, T. & Floras, J. (2003). Sleep Apnea and Heart Failure, II: Central Sleep Apnea. *Circulation*. Vol.107, No.13 (April 2003), pp. 1822–6

Buchner, N.; Sanner, B.; Borgel, J., et al. (2007). Continuous Positive Airway Pressure Treatment of Mild to Moderate Obstructive Sleep Apnea Reduces Cardiovascular Risk. *Am J Respir Crit Care Med,* Vol.176, No.12, (December 2007), pp. 1274–80

Carter III, R. & Watenpaugh, D. (2008). Obesity and Obstructive Sleep Apnea: Or is it OSA and Obesity? *Pathophysiology*, Vol.15, No.2, (August 2008), pp. 71–77

Chami, H.; Baldwin, C.; Silverman, A., et al. (2010). Sleepiness, Quality of Life, and Sleep Maintenance in REM versus non-REM Sleep-disordered Breathing. *Am J Respir Crit Care Med*. Vol.181, No. 9 (May 2010), pp. 997–1002

Campos-Rodriguez, F.; Pena-Grinan, N.; Reyes-Nunez, N., et al. (2005). Mortality in Obstructive Sleep Apnea- Hypopnea Patients Treated with Positive Airway Pressure. *Chest*, Vol.128, No.2, (August 2005), pp. 624–33

Chan, K. & Wilcox, I. (2010). Obstructive Sleep Apnea: Novel Trigger and Potential Therapeutic Target for Cardiac Arrhythmias. *Expert Rev Cardiovasc Ther*, Vol.8, No.7, (July 2010), pp. 981-94

Chugh, S.; Blackshear, J.; Shen, W., et al. (2001). Epidemiology and Natural History of Atrial Fibrillation: Clinical Implications. *J Am Coll Cardiol*, Vol.27, No.2, (February 2001), pp. 371-8

Chung, F.; Yegneswaran, B. & Liao, P. (2008). STOP Questionnaire: A Tool to Screen Patients for Obstructive Sleep Apnea. Anesthesiology, Vol.108, No.5, (May 2008), pp: 812–21

Chung, F.; Yegneswaran, B.; Liao, P., et al. (2008). Validation of the Berlin Questionnaire and American Society of Anesthesiologists Checklist as Screening Tools for Obstructive Sleep Apnea in Surgical Patients. *Anesthesiology*, Vol.108, No.5, (May 2008), pp. 822–30

Chung, M.; Martin, D.; Sprecher, D., et al. (2001). C-reactive Protein Elevation in Patients with Atrial Arrhythmias: Inflammatory Mechanisms and Persistence of Atrial Fibrillation. *Circulation*, Vol.104, No.24, (December 2001), pp. 2886–91

Colish, J.; Walker, J.; Elmayergi, H., et al. (2011). Obstructive Sleep Apnea: Effects Of Continuous Positive Airway Pressure On Cardiac Remodeling As Assessed By Cardiac Biomarkers, Echocardiography, And Cardiac Mri. *Chest*, Published online before print August 11, 2011, doi: 10.1378/chest.11-0615

Condos, W. Jr.; Latham, R.; Hoadley, S., et al. (1987). Hemodynamics of the Mueller Maneuver in Man: Right and Left Heart Micromanometry and Doppler Echocardiography. *Circulation*, Vol.76, No.5, (November 1987), pp. 1020-8

Daly, M.; Angell-James, J. & Elsner, R. (1979). Role of Carotid-Body Chemoreceptors and Their Reflex Interactions in Bradycardia and Cardiac Arrest. *Lancet*. Vol.1, No.8819, (April 1979), pp. 764 -7

Davies, S.; John, L.; Wedzicha, J., et al. (1991). Overnight Studies in Severe Chronic Left Heart Failure: Arrhythmias and Oxygen Desaturation. *Br Heart J*, Vol.65, No.2, (February 1991), pp. 77-83

Dempsey, J.; Veasey, S.; Morgan, B., et al. (2010). Pathophysiology of Sleep Apnea. *Physiol Rev*, Vol.90, No.1, (January 2010), pp. 47–112

Duvalapally, K; Pongonis Jr., R. & Khayat, R. (2009). OSA: The New Cardiovascular Disease: Part II: Overview of Cardiovascular Diseases Associated with Obstructive Sleep Apnea. *Heart Fail Rev*. Vol.14, No.3, (September 2009), pp. 155–164. doi:10.1007/s10741-008-9101-2.

Engleman, H. & Douglas, N. (2004). Sleep. 4: Sleepiness, cognitive function, and quality of life in obstructive sleep apnoea/hypopnoea syndrome. *Thorax*, Vol.59, No.7, (July 2004), pp. 618–22

Epstein, A.; DiMarco, J.; Ellenbogen, D., et al. (2008). ACC/AHA/HRS 2008 Guidelines for Device-Based Therapy of Cardiac Rhythm Abnormalities: A Report of the

American College of Cardiology/ American Heart Association Task Force on Practice Guidelines. J *Am Coll Cardiol*, Vol.51, No.21, (May 2008), pp. e1–62

Findley, L.; Wilhoit, S.; Suratt, P. (1985). Apnea Duration and Hypoxemia During REM Sleep in Patients with Obstructive Sleep Apnea. *Chest*, Vol.87, No.4, (April 1985), pp. 432-6

Franz, M. (2000). Mechano-electrical Feedback. *Cardiovascular Research*, Vol.45, No.2, (January 2000), pp: 263-6

Franz, M. & Bode, F. (2003). Mechano-electrical Feedback Underlying Arrhythmias: The Atrial Fibrillation Case. *Prog Biophys Mol Biol*, Vol.82, No.1-3, (May-July 2003), pp. 163–74

Gami, A.; Pressman, G.; Caples, S., et al. (2004). Association of Atrial Fibrillation and Obstructive Sleep Apnea. *Circulation*, Vol.110, No.4, (July 2004), pp. 364–7

Gami, A. & Somers, V. (2008). Implications of Obstructive Sleep Apnea for Atrial Fibrillation and Sudden Cardiac Death. *J Cardiovasc Electrophysiol*, Vol.19, No.9, (September 2008), pp. 997–1003

Gami, A.; Howard, D.; Olson, E., et al. (2005). Day-night Pattern of Sudden Death in Obstructive Sleep Apnea. *N Engl J Med*, Vol.352, No.12, (March 2005), pp. 1206–14

Grimm, W.; Hoffmann, J.; Menz, V., et al. (1996). Electrophysiologic Evaluation of Sinus Node Function and Atrioventricular Conduction in Patients with Prolonged Ventricular Asystole During Obstructive Sleep Apnea. *Am J Cardiol*, Vol.77, No.15, (June 1996), pp. 1310–14

Grimm, W.; Koehler, U.; Fus, E., et al. Outcome of patients with sleep apnea-associated severe bradyarrhythmias after continuous positive airway pressure therapy. *Am J Cardiol*, Vol.86, No.6, (September 2000), pp. 688–92

Guilleminault, C.; Connolly, S. & Winkle, R. (1983). Cardiac Arrhythmia and Conduction Disturbances During Sleep in 400 Patients with Sleep Apnea Syndrome. *Am J Cardiol*, Vol.52, No.5, (September 1983), pp. 490–4

Hall, M.; Ando, S.; Floras, J., et al. (1998). Magnitude and Time Course of Hemodynamic Responses to Mueller Maneuvers in Patients with Congestive Heart Failure. *J Appl Physiol*, Vol.85, No.4, (October 1998), pp. 1476–84

Harbison, J.; O'Reilly, P. & McNicholas, T. (2000). Cardiac Rhythm Disturbances in The Obstructive Sleep Apnea Syndrome: Effects of Nasal Continuous Positive Airway Pressure Therapy. *Chest*, Vol.118, No.3, (September 2000), pp. 591–5

He, J.; Kryger, M.; Zorick, F., et al. (1988). Mortality and Apnea Index in Obstructive Sleep Apnea. Experience in 385 Male Patients. *Chest*, Vol.94, No.1, (July 1988), pp. 9–14

Iber, C.; Ancoli-Israel, S.; Chesson, A., et al. (2007). The AASM Manual For The Scoring of Sleep and Associated Events: Rules, Terminology, and Technical Specifications. Vol. 1. Westchester, Illinois: American Academy of Sleep Medicine; 2007

Javaheri, S. (2000). Effects of Continuous Positive Airway Pressure on Sleep Apnea and Ventricular Irritability in Patients with Heart Failure. *Circulation*, Vol.101, No.4 (February 2000), pp. 392-7

Javaheri, S., Ben Caref, E.; Chen, E., et al. (2011). Sleep Apnea Testing and Outcomes in a Large Cohort of Medicare Beneficiaries with Newly Diagnosed Heart Failure. *Am J Respir Crit Care Med*, Vol.183, No.4, (February 2011), pp. 539-46

Javaheri, S.; Parker, T.; Liming, J., et al. (1998). Sleep Apnea in 81 Ambulatory Male Patients With Stable Heart Failure. Types and Their Prevalences, Consequences, and Presentations. *Circulation,* Vol.97, No.21, (June 1998), pp. 2154-9

Kanagala, R.; Murali, N.; Friedman, P., et al. (2003). Obstructive Sleep Apnea and the Recurrence of Atrial Fibrillation. *Circulation,* Vol.107, No.20, (May 2003), pp. 2589–94

Kingshott, R.; Vennelle, M.; Hoy, C., et al. (2000). Predictors of Improvements in Daytime Function Outcomes with CPAP Therapy. *Am J Respir Crit Care Med,* Vol.161, No.3 (March 2000), pp. 866–71

Kannel, W.; Wolf, P., & Benjamin, E. 1998). Prevalence, Incidence, Prognosis, and Predisposing Conditions for Atrial Fibrillation: Population-Based Estimates. *Am J Cardiol,* Vol.82, No.8A, (October 1998), pp. 2N-9N

Koehler, U.; Becker, H.; Grimm, W, et al. (2000). Relations Among Hypoxemia, Sleep Stage, and Bradyarrhythmia During Obstructive Sleep Apnea. *Am Heart J,* Vol.139, No.1, (January 2000), pp. 142-8

Koehler, U.; Fus, E.; Grimm, W., et al. (1998). Heart Block in Patients with Obstructive Sleep Apnoea: Pathogenetic Factors and Effects of Treatment. *Eur Respir J,* Vol.11, No.2, (February 1998), pp. 434–9

Koshino, Y.; Satoh, M.; Katayose, Y., et al.: (2010). Sleep Apnea and Ventricular Arrhythmias: Clinical Outcome, Electrophysiologic Characteristics, and Follow-Up After Catheter Ablation. *J Cardiol,* Vol.55, No.2, (March 2010), pp. 211–6

Lavie, P. (2007). Insomnia and Sleep-disordered Breathing. *Sleep Medicine,* Vol.8, No.Supp 4, (December 2007), pp. S21-S25

Lee, W.; Nagubadi, S.; Kryger, M., et al. (2008). Epidemiology of Obstructive Sleep Apnea: a Population-based Perspective. *Expert Rev Respir Med.* Vol.2, No.3, (June 2008), pp. 349–64, doi:10.1586/17476348.2.3.349.

Leung, R.; Huber, M.; Rogge, T., et al. (2005). Association Between Atrial Fibrillation and Central Sleep Apnea. *Sleep,* Vol.28, No.12, (December 2005), pp. 1543–6

Madden, B.; Shenoy, V.; Dalrymple-Hay, M., et al. (1997). Absence of Bradycardic Response to Apnea and Hypoxia in Heart Transplant Recipients with Obstructive Sleep Apnea. *J Heart Lung Transplant,* Vol.16, No.4, (April 1997), pp. 394–7

Marin JM, Carrizo SJ, Vicente E, Agusti AG. (2005). Long-term Cardiovascular Outcomes in Men With Obstructive Sleep Apnoea-Hypopnoea with or Without Treatment With Continuous Positive Airway Pressure: An Observational Study. *Lancet,* Vol.365, No.9464, (March 2005), pp. 1046–53

Mehra, R.; Stone, K.; Varosy, P., et al. (2009). Nocturnal Arrhythmias Across a Spectrum of Obstructive and Central Sleep-disordered Breathing in Older Men. *Arch Intern Med* Vol.169, No.12, (June 2009), pp. 1147-55

Mooe, T.; Gullsby, S.; Rabben, T., et al. (1996). Sleep-Disordered Breathing: A Novel Predictor of Atrial Fibrillation After Coronary Artery Bypass Surgery. *Coron Artery Dis,* Vol.7, No.6, (June 1996), pp. 475-8

Monahan, K.; Storfer-Isser, A.; Mehra. R., et al. (2009). Triggering of Nocturnal Arrhythmias by Sleep-Disordered Breathing Events. *J Am Coll Cardiol,* Vol.54, No.19, (November 2009), pp. 1797-804

Namtvedt, S.; Randby, A.; Einvik, G., et al. (2011). Cardiac Arrhythmias in Obstructive Sleep Apnea (From The Akershus Sleep Apnea Project). *Am J Cardiol,* 27 July 2011, ISSN 0002-9149, DOI: 10.1016/j.amjcard.2011.06.016

Ng, T.; Chan, T.; To, K., et al. (2009). Validation of a Portable Recording Device (Apnealink) for Identifying Patients with Suspected Obstructive Sleep Apnoea Syndrome. *Internal Medicine Journal,* Vol.39, No.11, (November 2009), pp. 757–62

Nieto, F.; Young, T.; Lind, B., et al. (2000). Association of Sleep-disordered Breathing, Sleep Apnea, and Hypertension in a Large Community-Based Study. *JAMA,* Vol.283, No.14, (April 2000), pp. 1829-36

Nowlin, J.; Troyer, W. Jr.; Collins, W., et al. (1965). The Association of Nocturnal Angina Pectoris with Dreaming. *Ann Intern Med,* Vol.63, No.6, (December 1965), pp. 1040–6

Olmetti, F.; La Rovere, M.; Robbi, E., et al. (2008). Nocturnal Cardiac Arrhythmia in Patients with Obstructive Sleep Apnea. *Sleep Med,* Vol.9, No.5 (July 2008), pp. 471–2

Parati, G.; Lombardi, C. & Narkiewicz, K. (2007). Sleep Apnea: Epidemiology, Pathophysiology, and Relation to Cardiovascular Risk. *Am J Physiol Regul Integr Comp Physiol,* Vol.293, No.4, (October 2007). Pp. R1671–83

Partinen, M. (1995). Epidemiology of Obstructive Sleep Apnea Syndrome. *Curr Opin Pulm Med,* Vol.1, No.6, (November 1995), pp. 482–7

Peppard, P.; Young, T.; Palta, M., et al. (2000). Prospective Study of the Association Between Sleep-Disordered Breathing and Hypertension. *N Engl J Med,* Vol.342, No.19, (May 2000), pp. 1378-84

Porthan, K.; Melin, J.; Kupila, J., et al. (2004). Prevalence of Sleep Apnea Syndrome in Lone Atrial Fibrillation: A Case-Control Study. *Chest,* Vol.125, No.3, (March 2004), pp. 879–85

Punjabi, N. (2008). The Epidemiology of Adult Obstructive Sleep Apnea. *Proc Am Thorac Soc,* Vol.5, No.2, (February 2008), pp. 136–143

Roche, F.; Xuong, A.; Court-Fortune, I., et al. (2003). Relationship Among the Severity of Sleep Apnea Syndrome, Cardiac Arrhythmias, and Autonomic Imbalance. *Pacing Clin Electrophysiol,* Vol.26, No.3, (March 2003), pp. 669–77

Sauer, W.; McKernan, M.; Lin, D., et al. (2006). Clinical Predictors and Outcomes Associated with Acute Return of Pulmonary Vein Conduction During Pulmonary Vein Isolation for Treatment of Atrial Fibrillation. *Heart Rhythm,* Vol.3, No.9, (September 2006), pp. 1024-8

Schafer, H.; Koehler, U.; Ploch, T., et al. (1997). Sleep-related Myocardial Ischemia and Sleep Structure in Patients with Obstructive Sleep Apnea and Coronary Heart Disease. *Chest,* Vol.111, No.2 (February 1997), pp. 387–93

Serizawa, N.; Yumino, D.; Kajimoto, K., et al. (2008). Impact of Sleep-disordered Breathing on Life-threatening Ventricular Arrhythmia in Heart Failure Patients with Implantable Cardioverter-defibrillator. *Am J Cardiol,* Vol.102, No.8, (October 2008), pp. 1064-8

Shepard, J.; Garrison, M.; Grither, D., et al. (1985). Relationship of Ventricular Ectopy to Oxyhemoglobin Desaturation in Patients with Obstructive Sleep Apnea. *Chest.* Vol.88, No.3 (September 1985), pp. 335–40

Simantirakis, E. & Vardas, P. (2006). Cardiac Pacing in Sleep Apnea: Diagnostic and Therapeutic Implications. *Europace,* Vol.8, No.11, (November 2006), pp. 984-7

Simantirakis, E.; Schiza, S.; Marketou, E., et al. (2004). Severe bradyarrhythmias in Patients with Sleep Apnoea: The Effect Of Continuous Positive Airway Pressure Treatment: A Long-Term Evaluation Using an Insertable Loop Recorder. *Eur Heart J*, Vol.25, No.12, (June 2004), pp. 1070–6

Sin, D.; Fitzgerald, F.; Parker, J., et al. (1999). Risk Factors for Central and Obstructive Sleep Apnea in 450 Men and Women with Congestive Heart Failure. *Am J Respir Crit Care Med,* Vol.160, No.4, (October 1999), 1101–6

Somers, V.; Dyken, M.; Clary, M., et al. (1995). Sympathetic Neural Mechanisms in Obstructive Sleep Apnea. *J Clin Invest,* Vol.96, No.4, (October 1995), pp. 1897–904

Somers, V.; Dyken, M.; Mark, A., et al. (1992). Parasympathetic Hyperresponsiveness and Bradyarrhythmias During Apnoea in Hypertension. *Clin Auton Res,* Vol.2, No.3, (June 1992), pp. 171–6

Somers, V.; Dyken, M.; Mark, A., et al. (1993). Sympathetic Nerve Activity During Sleep in Normal Subjects. *N Engl J Med.* Vol.328, No.9, (May 1993), pp. 303–7

Somers, V.; White, D.; Amin, R., et al. (2008). Sleep Apnea and Cardiovascular Disease. An American Heart Association/American College of Cardiology Foundation Scientific Statement From the American Heart Association Council for High Blood Pressure Research Professional Education Committee, Council on Clinical Cardiology, Stroke Council, and Council on Cardiovascular Nursing. *Circulation,* Vol.118, No.10, (September 2008), pp. 1080-111

Steinberg, J. (2004). Atrial Fibrillation: An Emerging Epidemic? *Heart.* Vol.90, No.3, (March 2004), pp. 239-40

Svatikova, A.; Wolk, R.; Shamsuzzaman, A., et al. (2003). Serum Amyloid A in Obstructive Sleep Apnea. *Circulation,* Vol.108, No.12, (September 2003), pp. 1451-4

Tiihonen, M. & Partinen, M. (1998). Polysomnography and Maintenance of Wakefulness Test as Predictors of CPAP Effectiveness in Obstructive Sleep Apnea. *Electroencephalogr Clin Neurophysiol,* Vol.107, No.6, (December 1998), pp. 383–6

Tilkian, A.; Guilleminault,; Schroeder, J., et al. (1977). Sleep-induced Apnea Syndrome. Prevalence of Cardiac Arrhythmias and Their Reversal After Tracheostomy. *Am J Med,* Vol.63, No.3, (September 1977), pp, 348–58

Veasey, S. (2009). Obstructive Sleep Apnea, In: *Encyclopedia of Neuroscience,* M.D. Binder, N. Hirokawa, U. Windhorst U, (Eds.), 975-981, Springer, 978-3-540-29678-2, Berlin, Germany

Verrier, R. & Josephson, M. (2009). Impact of Sleep on Arrhythmogenesis. *Circ Arrhythm Electrophysiol,* Vol.2, No.4, (August 2009), pp. 450-9

Young, T.; Palta, M., Dempsey, J., et al. (1993). The Occurrence of Sleep-Disordered Breathing Among Middle-aged Adults. *N Engl J Med,* Vol.328, No.17, (April 1993), pp. 1230-5

Young, T.; Peppard, T. & Gottlieb, D. (2002a). Epidemiology of Obstructive Sleep Apnea: a Population Health Perspective. *Am J Respir Crit Care Med,* Vol.165, No.9, (May 2002), pp. 1217-39

Young, T.; Shahar, E.; Nieto, F., et al. (2002b). Predictors of Sleep-disordered Breathing in Community-Dwelling Adults: The Sleep Heart Health Study. *Arch Intern Med,* Vol.162, No.8, (April 2002), pp. 893-900

Wang, T.; Parise, H.; Levy, D., et al. Obesity and the Risk of New-Onset Atrial Fibrillation. *JAMA,* Vol.292, No.20, (November 2004), pp. 2471–7

Zeidan-Shwiri, T.; Aronson, D.; Atalla, K., et al. (2011). Circadian Pattern of Life-Threatening Ventricular Arrhythmia in Patients With Sleep-Disordered Breathing and Implantable Cardioverter-defibrillators. *Heart Rhythm.* Vol.8, No.5, (May 2011), pp. 657–62

13

Approach to Ventricular Arrhythmias in the Pediatric Intensive Care Unit

Jong-Hau Hsu, Jiunn-Ren Wu*, Zen-Kong Dai and I-Chen Chen
Department of Pediatrics, Kaohsiung Medical University Hospital and College of Medicine, Kaohsiung Medical University, Kaohsiung, Taiwan

1. Introduction

Ventricular arrhythmia was once regarded uncommon in infants and children, since most cardiac arrests were thought to be hypoxia-induced bradycardia followed by asystole. Furthermore, ischemic heart disease, the basis for many of the ventricular arrhythmias in adults, is rare in pediatric patients. However, with the advent of pediatric critical care, improved techniques of extracorporeal life support, increasing awareness of genetic abnormalities, and a growing population of patients with congenital heart diseases, ventricular arrhythmia is being recognized more frequently in pediatric patients, and is becoming a larger management issue.

Pediatric critical care is a special field that rapid diagnosis and intervention are often essential. These interventions may be life-saving or sometimes debilitating, depending on their appropriateness and timeliness. The spectrum of cardiac arrhythmias in the pediatric intensive care unit (PICU) ranges from those that are immediately life threatening to those with little or no hemodynamic consequences. However, patients in the PICU often have hemodynamic instability, poor cardiac reserve or structural cardiac defects so that they are especially vulnerable to arrhythmia-induced cardiac dysfunction. Therefore, early recognition and prompt management of life-threatening ventricular arrhythmias are essential aspects of the care that must be provided to these patients. Indeed, given with the heterogeneity of diseases and complexity of structural heart defects in the pediatric critical care setting, treatment must frequently be provided in the PICU even before the specific cardiac diagnosis is made. To meet this challenge, the management of life-threatening ventricular arrhythmias in children will be the most effective if these arrhythmias are anticipated by the pediatric intensivist.

The aims of this chapter are to provide an update, from the standpoint of pediatric critical care, regarding comprehensive concepts of (1) non-cardiac clinical entities associated with ventricular arrhythmias, such as electrolyte imbalance, hypothermia, infection and drugs; (2) cardiac entities associated with ventricular arrhythmias, such as dilated cardiomyopathy, hypertrophic obstructive cardiomyopathy, and congenital heart diseases post cardiac surgery;

---

* Corresponding Author

(3) genetic abnormalities associated with ventricular arrhythmias, including conditions such as long QT syndrome, arrhythmogenic right ventricular cardiomyopathy, and Brugada syndrome; and (4) management of ventricular arrhythmias in the PICU.

2. Non-cardiac clinical entities associated with ventricular arrhythmias

In a multidisplinary PICU, although it is appropriate to consider ventricular arrhythmias as a problem of cardiac origin, other noncardiac etiologies should not be overlooked. Table 1 shows the systemic causes of ventricular arrhythmias.

Electrolyte imbalance	Hyperkalemia Hypokalemia Hypomagnesemia Hypocalcemia
Hypothermia	Cold stress Therapeutic hypothermia Extracorporeal life support
Infectious	Systemic viral infections causing myocarditis Systemic bacterial infections causing endocarditis Sepsis-induced cardiomyopathy
Drugs	Catecholamine Quinidine Procainamide Digitalis Psychotropic medications
Traumatic	Displacement of central venous catheters

Table 1. Systemic clinical entities associated with ventricular arrhythmia

2.1 Electrolyte imbalance

Serum electrolyte imbalance is very common in patients in the PICU for many non-cardiac reasons. Potassium is the one with the greatest chances to cause ventricular arrhythmias (Schaefer et al., 2005). For, example, we have previously demonstrated a case of life-threatening ventricular arrythmias and hyperkalemia induced by tumor lysis syndrome during the surgical biopsy (Lee et al., 2007). Hyperkalemia causes electrocardiographic changes before it reaches the serum potassium levels that cause arrhythmia. With modest hyperkalemia, the T wave will become narrow and peaked. Pediatric patients with faster resting heart rates tend to have narrower T waves, and peaked T waves may not be immediately evident. The QRS widens with higher levels of potassium. With extremely high serum potassium, ventricular tachycardia and fibrillation will ultimately occur. Hypokalemia causes prolonged QT-U interval and prominent U waves. Although less common than hyperkalemia, hypokalemia may also induce polymorphic ventricular tachycardia or ventricular fibrillation. Different from the devastating effect of potassium, imbalance of serum calcium and magnesium rarely cause significant arrhythmia.

2.2 Hypothermia

Hypothermia can slow the rate of sinus rhythm induce ventricular arrhythmia. Mild hypothermia results in the development of QT interval prolongation. Deep hypothermia results in AV block and subsequently ventricular arrhythmia and fibrillation (Pilichou et al., 2006). With the emergence of hypothermia as a critical management in the ICU, such as to improve the outcome especially in the survivors of out-of-hospital cardiac arrest and neonatal asphyxia, ventricular arrhythmia can be a growing issue to be concerned. Indeed, recent case reports have demonstrated occurrences of ventricular tachycardia, fibrillation, and Torsade de pointes during the procedure of hypothermia (Schaefer et al., 2005; Matsuhashi et al., 2010), suggesting that monitoring temperature levels is very important as the risk of life-threatening may induced by deep hypothermia less than 32°C.

2.3 Infection

Systemic infection may cause sinus tachycardia due to an increase in metabolic demand. Endocarditis near the normal conduction system may cause AV block by direct damaging conduction system. Myocarditis, one of the most common pediatric acquired heart diseases, is often associated with ventricular tachyarrhythmia. Myocarditis may not always be the primary source of infection but may complicate systemic infection, such as viremia or viral encephalitis For example, enteroviral infection is one of the most common causes of fulminant myocarditis secondary to systemic infection in the setting of pediatric critical care (Figure 1.). Rheumatic heart disease, a complication of group A streptococcal infection, may cause transient or permanent AV block and sinus node dysfunction. Lyme disease, transmitted by the bite of a tick infected with Borrelia burgdorferi, is also known to cause AV block and other cardiac conduction abnormalities (Lo et al., 2003).

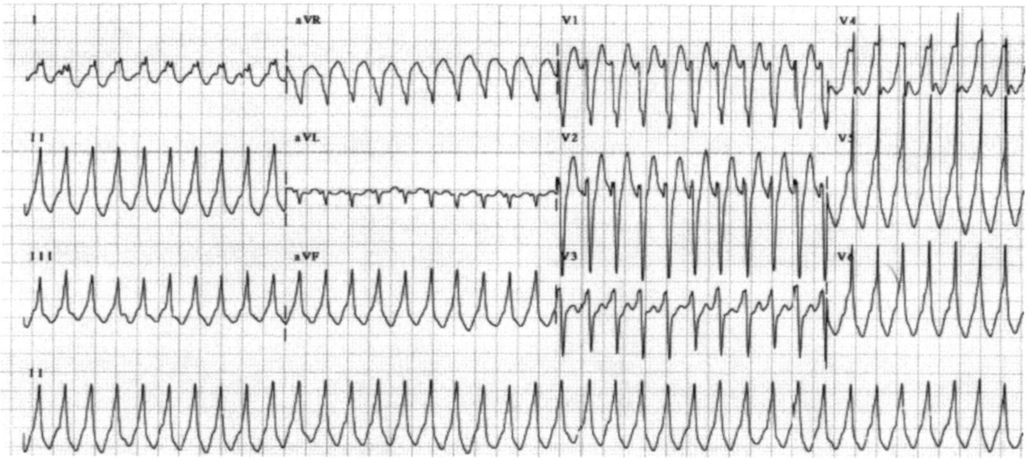

Fig. 1. EKG of ventricular tachycardia in a child with enteroviral encephalitis complicated with fulminant myocarditis.

2.4 Drugs

Drugs commonly administered in the PICU such as exogenous catecholamines, digoxin, and antiarrhythmic drugs may possess potential proarrhythmic effects. Although the arrhythmic effects of exogenous catecholamines are usually immediately recognized and treated, digoxin toxicity may be more difficult to be recognized due to its insidious effect. Renal function impairment in critically ill patients and administration of medications affecting digoxin metabolism are common in the PICU. Digitalis toxicity can result in many forms of arrhythmia. Treatment of digitalis toxicity has been simplified with the availability of digoxin-immune Fab antibody therapy. Toxicity with other antiarrhythmic drugs has become less frequent, such as the use of quinidine and procainamide.

3. Cardiac entities associated with ventricular arrhythmias

In the PICU, ventricular arrhythmias are often associated cardiac diseases. We herein discuss common cardiac diseases including dilated cardiomyopathy, hypertrophic cardiomyopathy and congenital heart diseases.

3.1 Dilated cardiomyopathy

Dilated cardiomyopathy (DCM) is the most common severe cardiomyopathy, accounting for more than 50% of pediatric cardiomyopathy (Jefferies et al., 2010). Etiology of DCM includes immunologic, familial, metabolic, infectious, toxic and neuromuscular causes. These patients are prone to ventricular arrhythmia. Treatment is targeted at symptoms, ventricular dysfunction and underlying rhythm disturbance. Prophylactic use of implantable cardiac defibrillator in the pediatric population is not well established as in adults with ischemic cardiomyopathies. In patients with muscular dystrophy, DCM is also common and may be a potential cause of mortality in these patients due to ventricular arrhythmia. Figure 3 shows non-sustained ventricular tachycardia and a premature ventricular contraction in a patient with Duchenne muscular dystrophy complicated with DCM.

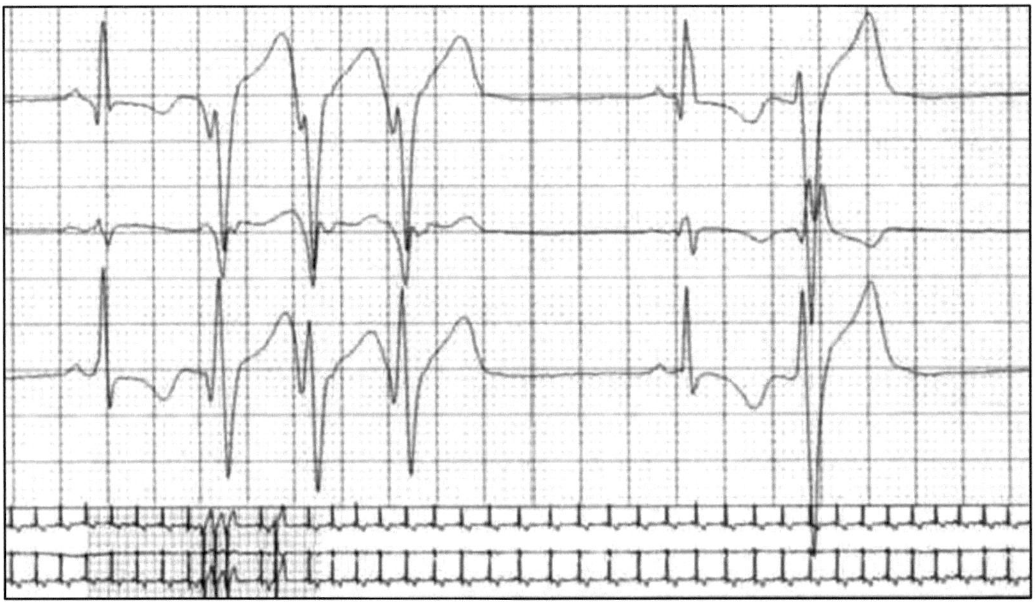

Fig. 2. A patient of Duchenne muscular dystrophy with dilated cardiomyopathy presented with chest pain. The Holter EKG record revealed non-sustained ventricular tachycardia and a premature ventricular beat.

3.2 Hypertrophic cardiomyopathy

Patients with hypertrophic cardiomyopathy comprise a subgroup with myocardial disease that is prone to ventricular arrhythmias. Left ventricular outflow tract obstruction may cause coronary artery insufficiency and myocardial ischemia, thus resulting in ventricular arrhythmias. Microscopically, hypertrophic cardiomyopathy shows disorganization of the cardiac muscle cells, a substrate for arrhythmia. Indeed, this microscopic finding seems to put these patients at risk regardless of the degree of outflow tract obstruction. Non-sustained ventricular tachycardia is common in children with hypertrophic cardiomyopathy. Clinical risk factors of sudden death include family history of cardiac arrest, increased QRS duration, myocardial bridging of the left coronary artery, increased QT dispersion, ventricular wall thickness, exercise-induced hypotension, and syncope.

3.3 Congenital heart disease post cardiac surgery

Ventricular arrhythmia has a reported incidence of 1–5% among pediatric patients and adults who have had palliative surgery for congenital heart disease (CHD) (Gatzoulis et al., 2000; Deanfield et al., 1980; Vetter et al., 1982; Kavey et al., 1982). With the advent of surgical technique and postoperative care, ventricular arrhythmia and sudden death have been reported as causes of early, intermediate and late morbidity and mortality (Garson et al., 1979). Congenital heart diseases are associated with various types of arrhythmia, depending on specific lesions, as shown in Table 3.

Congenital heart disease	arrhythmia
Tetralogy of Fallot	Atrial tachycardia
Double outlet right ventricl	Ventricular tachycardia Sinus node dysfunction
Transposition of the great arteries	Ventricular arrhythmias Atrioventricular block
Ebstein's anomaly	Supraventricular tachycardia
Ventricular septal defect repair	Heart block Ventricular arrhythmias
Atrial septal defect	Atrial tachycardia
Atrial septal defect repair	Sinus node dysfunction

Table 2. Congenital heart disease and associated arrhythmias

Occurrence of ventricular arrhythmia is particularly well known after the repair of tetralogy of Fallot (TOF). To relieve the obstruction of right ventricular outflow tract in TOF, it is always necessary for the surgeon to make a right ventricular outflow tract incision, to augment the outflow tract region, and repair the ventricular septal defect with a patch. Thus, the scar after surgical procedures may create a complex substrate for the development of arrhythmias.

Postoperative ventricular arrhythmias have been previously found in 5-10% of patients on the 12-lead ECG and in 40-60% on 24-hour Holter EKG in patients undergoing surgery (Garson et al., 1990). The advent of surgical techniques and repair at a younger age have led to a significant reduction in the incidence of arrhythmias. In fact, transatrial repair has been confirmed to have a beneficial effect on the incidence of ventricular arrhythmias. For example, a study comparing the incidence of arrhythmias in two groups of patients who underwent transventricular or transatrial repair showing that in the former group, 39.4% had significant ventricular arrhythmias, while in the latter group only 2.8% had significant arrhythmias (Dietl et al., 1994).

In addition to ventricular arrhythmias, sudden cardiac death is also an important issue and has been reported in 1.5-5% of patients after repair of TOF. In fact, ventricular arrhythmias have been regarded as a controversial etiological factor of sudden cardiac death (Garson et al., 1980; Katz et al., 1982; Quattlebaum et al., 1975). For example, it has been reported that previous ventricular arrhythmias were found in 100%of patients who died suddenly, compared to 12%of those who did not (Garson et al., 1985). On the other hand, another study followed patients with TOF post surgery for 12 years and found no correlation between the degree of ventricular arrhythmias and sudden death (Cullen et al., 1994). Therefore, some studies were aimed to elucidate the relationship between ECG indices and the risk of ventricular tachycardia and sudden death. A QRS duration >180 ms was found to be a very sensitive predictor for the development of VT and sudden death (Gatzoulis et al., 1995), so is the use of a transannular patch in combination with severe pulmonary valve insufficiency (Gatzoulis et al. , 2000). Furthermore, QT dispersion has also been suggested as risk factor of sustained ventricular tachycardia (Gatzoulis et al., 1997). Factors associated with the development of ventricular tachycardia in patients with TOF are summarized in Table 2.

Older age at repair
Earlier surgical era
Residual ventricular septal defect
Prior systemic-to-pulmonary artery shunt
Trans-annular right ventricular outflow tract patch
Right ventricular pressure overload
Right ventricular volume overload
Ventricular arrhythmias
Atrial arrhythmias
Complete heart block
QRS duration >180 mini-seconds

Table 3. Proposed risk factors for ventricular tachycardia and sudden death after repair of tetralogy of Fallot

Patients with other cardiac lesions may also be at risk for ventricular arrhythmias. Patients with aortic stenosis seem to be the highest risk group (Wolfe et al., 1993), with an increased mortality risk in patients with greater outflow tract gradients. Thus, all patients with repaired and unrepaired congenital heart disease should be considered at increased risk for ventricular arrhythmias and associated morbidity, including sudden death.

Notably, some atypical forms of supraventricular tachycardia can mimic ventricular tachycardia, such as supraventricular tachycardia with right bundle branch block after repair of TOF or double outlet of right ventricle (Figure 3). However, a wide QRS complex tachycardia in a patient who is hemodynamically unstable should be treated as ventricular tachycardia until proven otherwise.

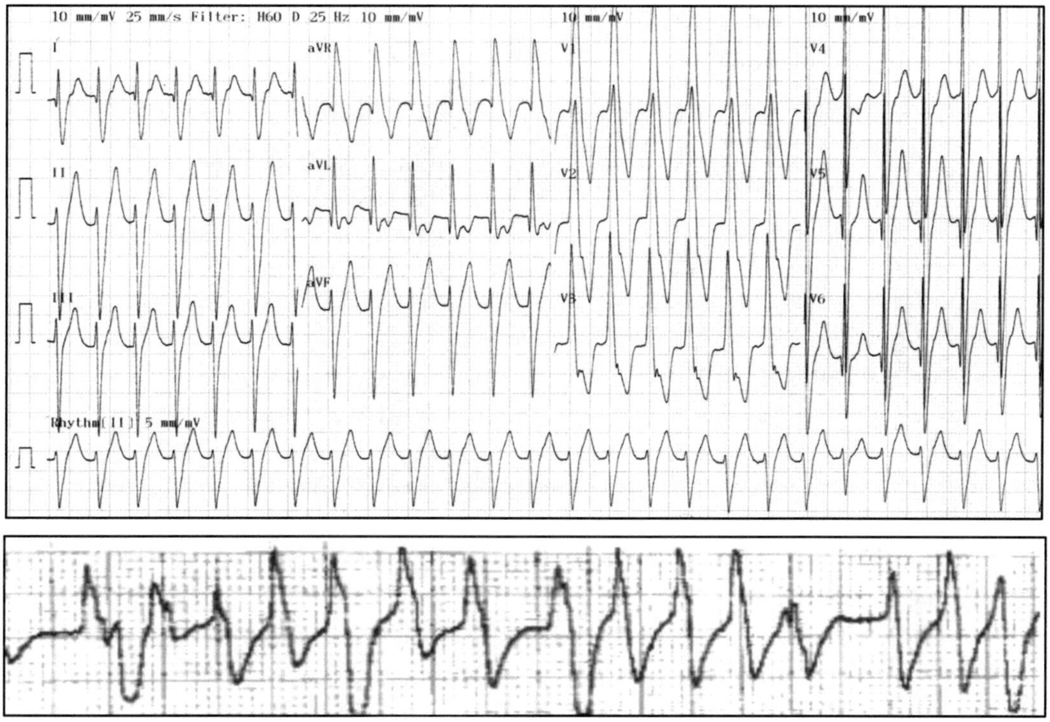

Fig. 3. Upper panel: The EKG of a patient with double outlet of right ventricle post palliative repair. Even with wide QRS, the inverted p wave following every QRS in aVL suggests supraventricular tachycardia instead of ventricular tachycardia. Lower panel: Another episode of ventricular tachycardia recorded in the lead II EKG strip in the same patient.

4. Genetic abnormalities associated with ventricular arrhythmias

Various forms of genetic abnormality-associated with ventricular arrhythmia may place a child at risk for sudden cardiac death. Although some diseases are clinically obvious, cardiovascular collapse may be the first symptom in others. Studies of sudden cardiac death and ventricular arrhythmia have therefore focused on identification of patients with the genetic abnormalities, including long QT syndrome, arrhythmogenic right ventricular dysplasia and Brugada syndrome.

4.1 Long QT syndrome

The congenital long QT syndrome (LQTS) is a rare but important clinical disorder, with the prevalence of 1 to 2500 live births. It includes two hereditary variants under the unifying name of "Long QT syndrome" (Schwartz et al., 1975). One is associated with deafness, Jervell and Lange-Nielsen syndrome (Jervell et al., 1957; Schwartz et al., 2006), and one is not, Romano-Ward syndrome (Romano et al., 1963; Ward et al., 1964). Long-QT syndrome has been subdivided into types based on the gene in which causative mutations occur. The most prevalent forms are LQT1 and LQT2 (mutations in potassium channels), and LQT3 (mutation in a sodium channel). The clinical manifestations of the disease may be life-threatening including syncope, cardiac arrest and sudden death. Electrocardiographic and genetic features of LQTS are discussed below.

4.1.1 Electrocardiographic features

4.1.1.1 QT interval duration

The Bazett's correction for heart rate remains a very useful clinical tool. Conventionally, QTc values in excess of 440 ms are considered prolonged; however, values up to 460 ms may still be normal among females (Merri et al., 1989). The longer QT values among women and becoming evident only after puberty suggest a role for hormonal changes (Stramba et al., 1995). Even though syncope occurs also in patients with modest QT prolongation or even with a normal QT interval., however, it is believed that the longer the QT, the greater is the risk for malignant arrhythmias. In fact, when QTc exceeds 500–550 ms, there is a definite increase in risk (Priori et al., 2003; Moss et al., 1991)

4.1.1.2 T wave morphology

In LQTS both the duration of repolarization and its morphology are altered. The T wave is often biphasic or notched because of regional differences in the time course of ventricular repolarization, especially prominent in the precordial leads. (Figure 4)

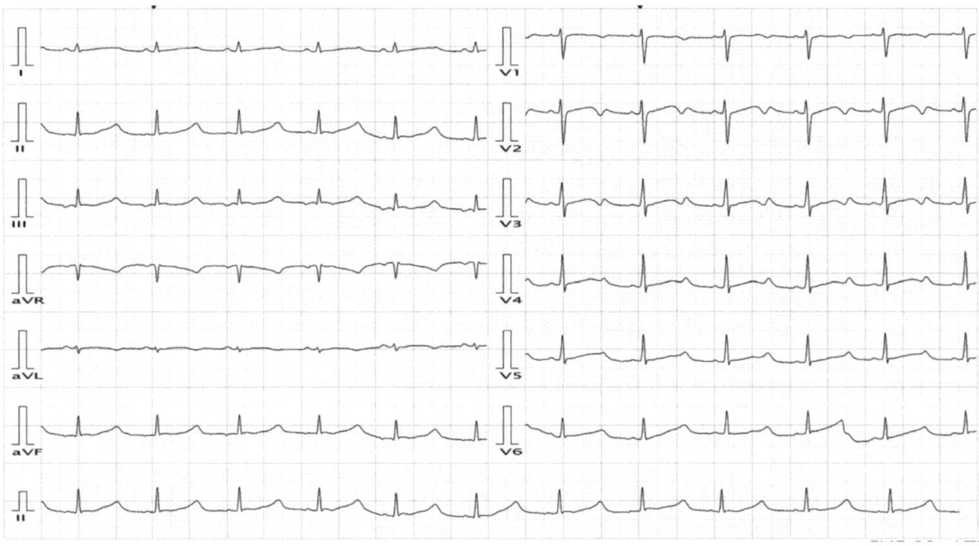

Fig. 4. The 12-lead EKG of a 13 year-old girl with long QT syndrome with the clinical presentation of recurrent syncopes. The QTc is 645 ms, with typical biphasic T waves in V2 and V3.

4.1.1.3 T wave alternans

Beat-to-beat alternation of the T wave is a marker of electrical instability suggesting the diagnosis of LQTS. It may be present at rest but most commonly appears during emotional or physical stresses and may sometimes precede torsades de pointes.

4.1.1.4 Sinus pauses

Sudden pauses in sinus rhythm longer than 1.2 seconds that are not related to sinus arrhythmia may be present in LQTS patients and may contribute to the initiation of ventricular arrhythmias. Their occurrence in LQT3 patients represents an important warning signal that warrants further life-saving management.

4.1.2 Genetic etiologies of LQTS

Since 1995, following the first identification of the first three LQTS genes associated with the most frequently encountered LQTS variants LQT1, LQT2, and LQT3, there has been growing identifications of genes associated with LQTS (Wang et al., 1995; Curran et al., 1995; Wang et al., 1996) including the genes for LQT4 through LQT10 (Table 3)

LQTS subtypes	Gene	Prevalence (%)
LQT1	*KCNQ1*	50
LQT1	*KCNQ1*	35
LQT2	*KCNH2*	10
LQT3	*SCN5A*	<5
LQT4	*ANK2*	<5
LQT5	*KCNE1*	<5
LQT6	*KCNE2*	<5
LQT7	*KCNJ2*	<5
LQT8	*CACNA1c*	<5
LQT9	*CAV3*	<5
LQT10	*SCN4B*	<5

Table 4. Long QT syndrome (LQTS) subtypes, disease-associated genes and prevalenc

4.1.3 Association between sudden infant death syndrome and LQTS

Sudden infant death syndrome (SIDS) is the leading cause of sudden death during the first year of life. The causes of SIDS remain a mystery, even with a lot of theories focused on dysfunctional control of respiratory or cardiac function (Schwartz et al., 1988). However, there are some evidence showing the association between SIDS and LQTS. For example, a large cohort study measuring the QT interval during the first week of life in more than 30,000 infants and following them for occurrence of SIDS demonstrated that infants who died of SIDS had a longer QTc than the survivors and the victims from other causes (Schwartz et al., 1998). In addition, in a study of Norway (Arnestad et al., 2007), based on 201 SIDS victims and 187 controls, mutations in LQTS genes were identified. These data justify the rationale of neonatal ECG screening and the guidelines proposed by the Task Force of the European Society of Cardiology (Schwartz et al., 2002) Therefore, future aim is the prevention of those sudden deaths due to unrecognized LQTS which may result in SIDS.

4.2 Arrhythmogenic right ventricular dysplasia

Arrhythmogenic right ventricular dysplasia (ARVD) is a predominantly genetically determined and heritable form of cardiomyopathy that may lead to right ventricular failure, ventricular arrhythmias, and sudden cardiac death. It is uniquely characterized by the replacement of myocytes by adipose and fibrous tissue in histology. The estimated prevalence of ARVD ranges from 1 in 2,000 to 1 in 5,000, with a predominance in men than women, with an approximate ratio of 3:1 (Corradoet al., 2006). Twelve genes have been identified to be associated with ARVD (Table 4). These genes are responsible for encoding several components of the cardiac desmosome. Dysfunctional desmosomes cause defective cell adhesion proteins, such as plakoglobin (JUP), desmoplakin (DSP), plakophilin-2 (PKP-2), and desmoglein-2 (DSG-2) consequently cause loss of electrical coupling between cardiomyocytes, leading to death of cardiomyocyte, fibrous replacement of myocardium and finally arrhythmias (Rampazzo et al., 2002 ; McKoy et al., 2000; Gerull et al., 2004; Pilichou et al., 2006). Diagnosis is based on the finding a combination of characteristic abnormalities in family history, electrocardiography, cardiac imaging especially MRI and biopsy.

ARVD type	Chromosome/locus	Gene codes	Mode of transmission
ARVD type 1	14q23 - q24	TGFβ-3	Autosomal dominant
ARVD type 2	1q42 - q43	RyR2	Autosomal dominant
ARVD type 3	14q12 - q22		Autosomal dominant
ARVD type 4	2q32		Autosomal dominant
ARVD type 5	3q23	Transmembrane protein 43	Autosomal dominant
ARVD type 6	10p12 - p14		Autosomal dominant
ARVD type 7	10q22		Autosomal dominant
ARVD type 8	6p24	Desmoplakin(DSP)	Autosomal dominant
ARVD type 9	12p11	Plakophilin-2(PKP2)	Autosomal dominant
ARVD type 10	18q12	Desmoglein-2(DSG2)	Autosomal dominant
ARVD type 11	18q12.1	Desmocollin-2(DSC2)	Autosomal dominant
ARVD type 12	17q21	Plakoglobin(JUP)	Autosomal dominant
Naxos Disease	17q21	Plakoglobin(JUP)	Autosomal recessive

Table 5. Genes mutations associated with arrhythmogenic right ventricular dysplasia

Therapeutic options are limited due to the progressive course of ARVD. Competitive athletics should be avoided. It is generally believed that patients who meet the Task Force criteria for ARVD are at high risk for sudden cardiac death and should undergo ICD placement (Marcus et al., 2010). The role of electrophysiologic study and catheter ablation in ARVD is not well established, and but it is frequently used as a palliative measure in the setting of refractory ventricular tachycardia. Even though sotalol may be effective in patients with ARVD and ventricular tachycardia, heart transplantation is the choice for patients with refractory ventricular arrhythmias and progressive heart failure.

4.3 Brugada syndrome

Brugada syndrome is a genetic disease characterized by the occurrence of cardiac arrhythmias and sudden cardiac death in young individuals without evidence of structural heart disease. In fact, Brugada syndrome is associated with structural and functional abnormalities in the sodium channel. Because of the absence of structural heart abnormalities, Brugada syndrome is classified as a cardiac "channelopathy".

Genetic studies have determined that more than one gene is capable of causing this syndrome. Initially, mutations in only one gene, SCN5A, encoding the cardiac sodium channel, have been identified. Recently, flourishing gene mutations have been identified, such as mutations in the CACNA1c and CACNB2b genes, coding the calcium channels, and mutations in the KCNE3 gene, coding a subunit of the potassium channel (Antzelevitch et al., 2007; Delpón et al., 2008). There is some evidence showing that the electrical disorders associated with Brugada syndrome are mainly located in the right ventricle, particularly in the outflow tract of right ventricle. These patients typically present an ECG pattern characterized by ST segment elevation in the right precordial leads and a RBBB (Brugada et al., 1992).

Brugada syndrome is thought to be responsible for 4% to 12% of all sudden cardiac death and for up to 20% of sudden cardiac death in subjects without structural heart disease (Brugada et al., 2002). Sudden cardiac death associated with Brugada syndrome is caused by polymorphic ventricular tachycardia or ventricular fibrillation (Antzelevitch et al., 2006). Unfortunately, because the ECG is often dynamic and concealed, it is difficult to estimate the real prevalence of this disease (Nademanee et al., 1997). However, it is believed that the prevalence is less frequent in western countries and higher in Southeast Asia. In fact, Brugada syndrome is considered to be the major cause of natural death in young individuals in Thailand and the Philippines (Miyasaka et al., 2001; Donohue et al., 2008).

5. Management of ventricular arrhythmias in the PICU

The major issue for a pediatric intensivist regarding management of ventricular arrhythmias in the PICU is to cope with postoperative arrhythmias in patients with congenital heart diseases (CHD). In these patients, ventricular arrhythmias may occur in the early postoperative stage, caused by surgical procedure, or in the late stage, caused by a residual structural defect or scar tissue. In addition to early and late postoperative management, catheter ablation and implantable cardioverter-defibrillators (ICD) will also be discussed in this section.

5.1 Early postoperative ventricular arrhythmias

Early postoperative arrhythmias are defined as occurrence within the first 10 days after surgery. Patients with CHD who have hemodynamically unstable early postoperative ventricular tachycardia or ventricular fibrillation require immediate treatment, as suggested by the AHA guidelines for cardiopulmonary resuscitation. After stabilizing the airway and breathing, cardiopulmonary resuscitation should be started immediately (Kleinman et al., 2010). If the ventricular tachycardia persists after cardiopulmonary resuscitation, synchronized electrical cardioversion (0.5–1.0 J/kg) should be administered. If a second shock (2.0 J/kg) is unsuccessful, amiodarone or procainamide should be considered before administering a third shock. If the ventricular arrhythmias are successfully converted to sinus rhythm, potential causes for the ventricular arrhythmias must be identified. In patients without identifiable causes, close observation and administration of intravenous antiarrhythmic medications are necessary.
Amiodarone is the antiarrhythmic treatment for pulseless ventricular tachycardia recommended by the AHA Committee on Resuscitation guidelines. Amiodarone dosing should adhere to the following regimen for pediatric patients: an intravenous bolus administered at 5–10 mg/kg and then maintenance infusion at 5–15 mg/kg/day. The safety and efficacy of amiodarone has been documented in studies performed in children with CHD (Drago F et al., 1998). For patients with stable ventricular tachycardia, the dosage and desired levels of antiarrhythmic medications are shown in Table 6.

Drug	Dosage	Desired level
Propranolol	0.05 - 0.1 mg/kg/dose q6h	20 - 150 ng/ml
Procainamide	Loading: 5 - 15 mg/kg in 30 min Infusion: 20 – 80 μg/kg/min	4 – 8 μg/ml
Lidocaine	Loading: 1 - 2 mg/kg in 30 min Infusion: 10 – 50 μg/kg/min	1-5 μg/ml
Mexiletine	3 - 5 mg/kg/dose q8h	0.5 - 2.0 μg/ml
Amiodarone	Loading: 5 - 10 mg/kg in 30 min Infusion: 5 - 15 mg/kg/day	1.5 - 2.5 μg/ml

Table 6. Pharmacologic management of ventricular tachycardia in pediatric patients.

5.2 Late postoperative ventricular arrhythmias

All patients with CHD who have undergone surgery are at risk of late postoperative ventricular arrhythmias. Therefore, they require follow-up for routine electrocardiography to evaluate the patient's conduction system for potential bundle branch block. Evaluation of sinus node function, abnormalities of ST and T wave, and premature ventricular contraction are important, since these abnormalities can trigger the occurrence of ventricular tachycardia or sudden death in these patients. In addition, Holter EKG can detect asymptomatic ventricular arrhythmias in patients with CHD, for example in up to 9% of postoperative TOF (Chandar et al., 1990). Furthermore, the electrophysiologic study with programmed ventricular stimulation may have a role in the risk stratification because some investigators found that the induction of polymorphic VT could predict VT and sudden cardiac death (Khairy et al., 2004). The most common types of CHD associated with postoperative ventricular arrhythmia are listed in Table 7.

Tetralogy of Fallot
Trasposition of great arteries
Aortic stenosis
Ventricular septal defect
Atrail septal defect, secundum type
Atrial septal defect, primum type
Aortic coarctation
Pulmonary stenosis

Table 7. Types of congenital heart defects commonly associated with postoperative ventricular arrhythmia.

5.3 Catheter ablation

There is some recent evidence addressing the role of catheter ablation in the treatment of ventricular tachycardia in CHD patients. For example, in a study of 10 patients with TOF who received noncontact mapping due to hemodynamically unstable ventricular tachycardia (Kriebelet al., 2007), ablation was achieved in eight patients and for all of them ventricular tachycardia was not inducible at the end of the procedure. Another study of electroanatomical contact mapping and catheter ablation in patients with ventricular tachycardia after repair of CHD demonstrated that isthmuses between patches and tricuspid annulus, right ventricular outflow tract, or pulmonary annulus were responsible for the reentrant tachycardias (Zeppenfeld et al., 2007). Ablation of these isthmuses abolished all ventricular tachycardias. Accordingly, there is a potential role for ventricular tachycardia ablation in patients after repair of CHD.

5.4 Implantable cardioverter-defibrillators

An implantable cardioverter-defibrillator (ICD) is recommended in CHD patients with a positive ventricular stimulation in the electrophysiology study. However, it is sometimes highly technical to implant a cardioverter-defibrillator transvenously in these patients due to their structural anomaly and small size of these patients. In addition, implanting a transvenous ICD system in patients with intracardiac shunting is not recommended, because the risk of thromboembolic events. The implantation of a transvenous ICD in patients younger than 8 years of age can be a high-risk procedure because of complications such as venous occlusion, infection or wound dehiscence because of limited prepectoral tissue.

Surgical implantation is required when an ICD cannot be implanted transvenously. As such, the generator or device is implanted in the abdomen with the leads sewn into the epicardium. This surgical method is associated with some complications including postpericardiotomy syndrome, constrictive pericarditis, lead-induced trauma and lead failure (Stefanelli et al., 2002; Ketteringet al., 2004). Recent reports have described less invasive ways to implant an epicardial ICD in patients who are either too small or have mixing lesions (Cannon et al., 2006; Snyder et al., 2007). An additional problem is that patients may receive inappropriate shocks for sinus tachycardia due to improper programming. Accordingly, before programming an ICD in a patient with repaired CHD, patients should undergo exercise testing to determine their peak heart rate. Notably, some patients require adjuvant therapy with either nadolol or amiodarone, even with an ICD, to limit their peak heart rate and decrease chances of inappropriate shocks.

6. Conclusions

Ventricular tachycardias in the setting of PICU are a diverse group of rhythm disorders different from those seen in the adults with ischemic heart disease. They are not only different in ventricular substrates and etiologies, but also in the electrophysiologic mechanisms. Furthermore, ventricular arrhythmia after surgery for CHD requires a comprehensive evaluation including the clinical state of the patient, the cardiac anatomy, previous surgical history, and the electrophysiologic patterns of the arrhythmia. Most importantly, ventricular arrhythmia is an important cause of sudden death in the infants and children, so pediatric intensivists should be familiar with risk factors and emergent management of these life-threatening scenarios to ensure a better outcome.

7. Acknowledgment

We appreciate the assistance by Miss Hung Jui Feng to edit this manuscript.

8. References

Antzelevitch, C. Brugada syndrome. *Pacing Clin Electrophysiol*, Vol.29, No.10, (October2006), pp. 1130-1159, ISSN 1703-814

Antzelevitch, C.; Pollevick, GD.; Cordeiro, JM. Casis, O.; Sanguinetti, MC.; Aizawa, Y.; Guerchicoff, A.; Pfeiffer, R.; Oliva, A.; Wollnik, B.; Gelber, P.; Bonaros, EP. Jr.; Burashnikov, E.; Wu, Y.; Sargent, JD.; Schickel, S.; Oberheiden, R.; Bhatia, A.; Hsu, LF.; Haïssaguerre, M.; Schimpf, R.; Borggrefe, M. & Wolpert, C, Loss-of-function mutations in the cardiac calcium channel underlie a new clinical entity characterized by ST-segment elevation, short QT intervals, and sudden cardiac death. *Circulation*, Vol.115, No.4, (Janurary2007), pp.442-9, ISSN 1722-4476

Arnestad, M.; Crotti, L.; Rognum, TO.; Insolia, R.; Pedrazzini, M.; Ferrandi, C.; Vege, A.; Wang, DW.; Rhodes, TE.; George, AL.; Jr. & Schwartz, PJ. Prevalence of long QT syndrome gene variants in sudden infant death syndrome. *Circulation*, Vol.115, No.3, (Janurary2007), pp. 361-367, ISSN 17210-839

Brugada, P.; Brugada, J. Right bundle branch block, persistent ST segment elevation and sudden cardiac death: a distinct clinical and electrocardiographic syndrome. *J Am Coll Cardiol*, Vol.20, No.6, (November1992), pp. 391-1396, ISSN 1309-182

Brugada, J.; Brugada, R.; Antzelevitch, C.; Towbin, J.; Nademanee, K. & Brugada, P. Long-term follow-up of individuals with the electrocardiographic pattern of right bundle-branch block and ST-segment elevation in precordial leads V1 to V3. *Circulation*, Vol.105, No.1, (Janurary2002), pp. 73-78, ISSN 1177-2879

Cannon, BC.; Friedman, RA.; Fenrich, AL.; Fraser, CD.; McKenzie, ED. & Kertesz, NJ. Innovative techniques for placement of implantable cardioverter-defibrillator leads in patients with limited venous access to the heart. *Pacing Clin lectrophysiol*, Vol.29, No.2, (February2006), pp. 181–187, ISSN 1649-2305

Chandar, JS.; Wolff, GS.; Garson, A.; Jr.; Bell, TJ.; Beder, SD.; Bink-Boelkens, M.; Byrum, CJ.; Campbell, RM.; Deal, BJ. & Dick, M 2nd. et al. Ventricular arrhythmias in postoperative tetralogy of Fallot. *Am J Cardiol*, Vol.65, No.9(March1990), pp. 655-661, ISSN 1689-93510

Corrado, D. & Thiene, GC. Arrhythmogenic right ventricular cardiomyopathy/dysplasia: clinical impact of molecular genetic studies. *Circulation*, Vol.113, No.13, (April2006) pp. 1634–1647, ISSN 1658-5401

Curran, ME.; Splawski, I.; Timothy, KW.; Vincent, GM.; Green, ED. & Keating, MT. A molecular basis for cardiac arrhythmia: HERG mutations cause long QT syndrome. *Cell*, Vol.80, No.5, (March1995), pp. 795-803, ISSN 7889-573

Cullen, S.; Celermajer, DS.; Franklin, RC.; Hallidie-Smith, KA. & Deanfield, JE. Prognostic significance of ventricular arrhythmia after repair of tetralogy of Fallot: a 12-year prospective study. *J Am Coll Cardiol*, Vol.23, No.5, (April1994), pp. 1151-1155, ISSN 8144-782

Deanfield, JE.; McKenna, WJ. & Hallidie-Smith, KA. Detection of late arrhythmia and conduction disturbances after correction of tetralogy of Fallot. *Br Heart J*, Vol.44, No.3, (September1980) , pp. 248–253, ISSN 742-6182

Delpón, E.; Cordeiro, JM.; Núñez, L.; Thomsen, PE.; Guerchicoff, A.; Pollevick, GD.; Wu, Y.; Kanters, JK.; Larsen, CT.; Hofman-Bang, J.; Burashnikov, E.; Christiansen, M. & Antzelevitch, C. Functional effect of KCNE3 mutation and its role in the development of Brugada syndrome. *Circ Arrhythm Electrophysiol*. Vol.1, No.3, (August2008), pp. 209-218, ISSN 1912-2847

Dietl, CA.; Cazzaniga, ME.; Dubner, SJ.; Perez-Balino, NA.; Torres, AR. & Favaloro, RG. Life-threatening arrhythmias and RV dysfunction after surgical repair of tetralogy of Fallot. Comparison between transventricular and transatrial approaches. *Circulation*, Vol.90, No.5, (November1994), pp. II7-12, ISSN 7955-286

Donohue, D.; Tehrani, F.; Jamehdor, R.; Lam, C. & Movahed, MR. The prevalence of Brugada ECG in adult patients in a large university hospital in the western United States. *Am Heart Hosp J*. Vol.6, No.1, (November2008), pp. 48-50, ISSN 1825- 9122

Drago, F.; Mazza, A.; Guccione, P.; Mafrici, A.; Di Liso, G. & Ragonese, P. Amiodarone used alone or in combination with propranolol: a very effective therapy for tachyarrhythmias in infants and children. *Pediatr Cardiol*, Vol.19, No.6, (November1998), pp. 445–449, ISSN 9770-567

Garson, A.; Jr.; Nihill, MR.; McNamara, DG. & Cooley, DA. Status of adult and adolescent after repair of tetralogy of Fallot. *Circulation*, Vol.59, No.6, (June1979), pp. 1232–1240, ISSN 436-215

Garson, A.; Jr. Gillette, PC.; Gutgesell, HP.& McNamara, DG. Stressinduced ventricular arrhythmia after repair of tetralogy of Fallot. *Am J Cardiol*, Vol.46, No.6, (December1980), pp. 1006-1012, ISSN 7446-414

Garson, A.; Jr.; Randall, DC.; Gillette, PC.; Smith, RT.; Moak, JP.; McVey, P. & McNamara, DG. Prevention of sudden death after repair of tetralogy of Fallot: Treatment of ventricular arrhythmias. *J Am Coll Cardiol* , Vol.6, No.1, (July1985), pp. 221-227, ISSN 4008-776

Gatzoulis, MA.; Till, JA.; Redington, AN. Depolarization-repolarization inhomogeneity after repair of tetralogy of Fallot. The substrate for malignant ventricular tachycardia? *Circulation*, Vol.95, No.2, (Janurary1997), pp. 401-404, ISSN 9008-456

Gatzoulis, MA.; Till, JA. Somerville, J. & Redington, AN. Mechanoelectrical interaction in tetralogy of Fallot. QRS prolongation relates to right ventricular size and predicts malignant ventricular arrhythmias and sudden death. *Circulation*, Vol.92, No.2, (July1995), pp. 231-237, ISSN 7600-655

Gatzoulis, MA.; Balaji, S.; Webber, SA. Siu, SC.; Hokanson, JS.; Poile, C.; Rosenthal, M.; Nakazawa, M.; Moller, JH.; Gillette, PC.; Webb, GD. & Redington, AN. Risk factors for arrhythmia and sudden cardiac death late after repair of tetralogy of Fallot: a multicentre study. *Lancet*, Vol.356, No.9234, (september2000), pp. 975-981, ISSN 11041-139825.

Gerull, B.; Heuser, A.; Wichter, T.; Paul, M.; Basson, CT.; McDermott, DA.; Lerman, BB.; Markowitz, SM.; Ellinor, PT.; MacRae, CA.; Peters, S.; Grossmann, KS.; Drenckhahn, J.; Michely, B.; Sasse-Klaassen, S.; Birchmeier, W.; Dietz, R.; Breithardt, G.; Schulze-Bahr, E. & Thierfelder L. Mutations in the desmosomal protein plakophilin- 2 are common in arrhythmogenic right ventricular cardiomyopathy. *Nat Genet*, Vol.36, No.11, (November2004), pp. 1162–1164, ISSN 1548-9853

Jefferies, JL.; Towbin, JA. Dilated cardiomyopathy. *Lancet*, Vol.375, No.9716, (February2010), pp. 752–7622, ISSN 2018-9027

Jervell, A.; Lange-Nielsen, F. Congenital deaf-mutism, functional heart disease with prolongation of the Q-T interval, and sudden death. *Am Heart J*, Vol.54, No.1, (July1957), pp. 59-68. ISSN 1343-5203

Katz, NM.; Blackstone, EH.; Kirklin, JW.; Pacifico, AD. & Bargeron, LM. Jr. Late survival and symptoms after repair of tetralogy of Fallot. *Circulation*, Vol.65, No.2, (February1982), pp. 403-410, .ISSN 7053-900

Kavey, RE.; Blackman, MS. & Sondheimer, HM. Incidence and severity of chronic ventricular dysrhythmias after repair of tetralogy of Fallot. *Am Heart J*, Vol.103, No.3, (March1982) pp. 342-350, ISSN 7064-767

Kettering, K.; Mewis, C.; Dörnberger, V.; Vonthein, R.; Bosch, RF.; Seipel, L. & Kühlkamp, V. Long-term experience with subcutaneous ICD leads: a comparison among three different types of subcutaneous leads. *Pacing Clin Electrophysiol*, Vol.27, No.10, (October 2004), pp. 1355-1361, ISSN 1551-1244

Khairy, P.; Landzberg, MJ.; Gatzoulis, MA.; Lucron, H.; Lambert, J.; Marçon, F.; Alexander, ME. & Walsh, EP. Value of programmed ventricular stimulation after tetralogy of Fallot repair: a multi center study. *Circulation* , Vol.109, No.16, (April2004), pp. 1994-2000, ISSN 1505-1640

Kleinman, ME.; Chameides, L.; Schexnayder, SM.; Samson, RA.; Hazinski, MF.; Atkins, DL.; Berg, MD.; de Caen, AR.; Fink, EL.; Freid, EB.; Hickey, RW.; Marino, BS.; Nadkarni, VM.; Proctor, LT.; Qureshi, FA.; Sartorelli, K.; Topjian, A.; van der Jagt, EW. & Zaritsky, AL. Part 14: pediatric advanced life support: 2010 American Heart Association Guidelines for Cardiopulmonary Resuscitation and Emergency Cardiovascular Care. *Circulation*, Vol.122, No.18, (November2010), pp. S876-908. ISSN 2095-6230

Kriebel, T.; Saul, JP. Schneider, H.; Sigler, M. & Paul, T. Noncontact mapping and radiofrequency catheter ablation of fast and hemodynamically unstable ventricular tachycardia after surgical repair of tetralogy of Fallot. *J Am Coll Cardiol*, Vol.50, No.22, (November2007), pp. 2162–2168, ISSN 1803-6455

Lee, MH.; Cheng, KI.; Jang, RC.; Hsu, JH.; Dai, ZK. & Wu, JR. Tumour lysis syndrome developing during an operation. *Anaesthesia*, Vol.62, No.1, (Janurary2007), pp. 85-87. ISSN 1715-6233

Lo, R.; Menzies, DJ.; Archer, H. & Cohen, TJ. Complete heart block due to Lyme carditis. *J Invasive Cardiol*, Vol.15, No.6, (June2003), pp. 367-369, ISSN 1277-7681

Marcus, FI.; McKenna, WJ.; Sherrill, D.; Basso, C.; Bauce, B.; Bluemk, DA.; Calkins, H.; Corrado, D.; Cox, MG.; Daubert, JP.; Fontaine, G.; Gear, K.; Hauer, R.; Nava, A.; Picard, MH.; Protonotarios, N.; Saffitz, JE.; Sanborn, DM.; Steinberg, JS.; Tandri, H.; Thiene, G.; Towbin, JA.; Tsatsopoulou, A.; Wichter, T. & Zareba, W. Diagnosis of arrhythmogenic right ventricular cardiomyopathy /dysplasia: proposed modification of the task force criteria. *Circulation*. Vol.121, No.13, (Arpil2010), pp. 1533–1541, ISSN 2017-2911

Matsuhashi, T.; Sato, T.; Aizawa, Y. & Takatsuki, S. Recurrent Torsade de Pointes during mild hypothermia therapy for a survivor of sudden cardiac arrest due to drug-induced long-QT syndrome. *J Cardiovasc lectrophysiol*, Vol.21, No.4, (April2010), pp. 462-463, ISSN: 1984-5813

McKoy, G.; Protonotarios, N. & Crosby, A. Tsatsopoulou A, Anastasakis A, Coonar A, Norman M, Baboonian C, Jeffery S, McKenna WJ, Identification of a deletion in plakoglobin in arrhythmogenic right ventricular cardiomyopathy with palmoplantar keratoderma and woolly hair (Naxos disease). *Lancet* , Vol.355, No.9221, (June2000), pp. 2119–2124, ISSN 1090-2626

Merri, M.; Benhorin, J.; Alberti, M.; Locati, E. & Moss, AJ. Electrocardiographic quantitation of ventricular repolarization. *Circulation,* Vol.80, No.5, (November1989), pp. 1301-1308, ISSN 2805-26

Miyasaka, Y.; Tsuji, H.; Yamada, K.; Tokunaga, S.; Saito, D.; Imuro, Y.; Matsumoto, N. & Iwasaka, T. Prevalence and mortality of the Brugada-type electrocardiogram in one city in Japan. *J Am Coll Cardiol*, Vol.38, No.3, (September2001), pp. 771-774, ISSN 1152-7631

Moss, AJ.; Schwartz, PJ.; Crampton, RS.; Tzivoni, D.; Locati, EH.; MacCluer, J.; Hall, WJ.; Weitkamp, L.; Vincent,GM. & Garson, A. Jr. The long QT syndrome. prospective longitudinal study of 328 families. *Circulation*, Vol.84, No.3, (September1991), pp. 1136-1144, ISSN 1884-444

Nademanee, K. Sudden unexplained death syndrome in Southeast Asia. *Am J Cardiol,* Vol.79, No.6A, (March1997), pp. 10-1, ISSN 9080-856

Pilichou, K.; Nava, A.; Basso, C.; Beffagna, G.; Bauce, B.; Lorenzon, A.; Frigo, G.; Vettori, A.; Valente, M.; Towbin, J.; Thiene, G.; Danieli, GA. & Rampazzo, A. Mutations in desmoglein-2 gene are associated to arrhythmogenic right ventricular cardiomyopathy. *Circulation*, Vol.113, No.9, (March2006), pp. 1171–1179, ISSN 1650-5173

Priori, SG.; Schwartz, PJ.; Napolitano, C.; Bloise, R.; Ronchetti, E.; Grillo, M.; Vicentini, A.; Spazzolini, C.; Nastoli, J.; Bottelli, G.; Folli, R.& Cappelletti, D. Risk stratification in the long-QT syndrome. *N Engl J Med*, Vol.348, No.19, (May2003), pp.1866-1874, ISSN 1273-6279

Quattlebaum, TG.; Varghese, J.; Neill, CA. & Donahoo, JS. Sudden death among postoperative patients with tetralogy of Fallot. A follow-up study of 243 patients for an average of 12 years. *Circulation*, Vol.54, No.2, (August1975), pp. 289-293, ISSN 9390-26

Romano, C.; Gemme, G. & Pongiglione, R.. Aritmie cardiache rare dell'eta pediatrica. *Clin Pediat*, Vol.45, (September1963), pp. 656-683, ISSN 1415-8288

Rampazzo, A.; Nava, A.; Malacrida, S.; Beffagna, G.; Bauce, B.; Rossi, V.; Zimbello, R.; Simionati, B.; Basso, C.; Thiene, G. Towbin, JA & Danieli, GA. Mutation in human desmoplakin domain binding to plakoglobin causes a dominant form of arrhythmogenic right ventricular cardiomyopathy. *Am J Hum Genet*, Vol.171, No.5, (November2002), pp. 1200–1206, ISSN 1237-3648

Schwartz, PJ.; Periti, M. & Malliani, A. The long Q-T syndrome. *Am Heart J*, Vol.89, No.3, (March1975), pp.37 8-390, ISSN 234-667

Schwartz, PJ.; Southall, DP.; Valdes-Dapena, M. & Eds. The sudden infant death syndrome: cardio-respiratory mechanisms and interventions. *Ann NY Acad Sci*, Vol.533, (March 1988), pp.1-:474, ISSN 3421-616

Schwartz, PJ.; Stramba-Badiale, M.; Segantini, A.; Austoni, P.; Bosi, G.; Giorgetti, R.; Grancini, F.; Marni, ED.; Perticone, F.; Rosti, D. & Salice, P. Prolongation of the QT interval and the sudden infant death syndrome. *N Engl J Med*, Vol.338, No.24, (June1998), pp. 1709-1714, ISSN 9624-190

Schwartz, PJ.; Garson, A, Jr.; Paul, T.; Stramba-Badiale, M.; Vetter, VL. & Wren, C. European Society of Cardiology: Guidelines for the interpretation of the neonatal electrocardiogram. A task force of the European Society of Cardiology. *Eur Heart J*, Vol.23, No.17, (September2002), pp. 1329-1344, ISSN 1226-9267

Schaefer, TJ.; Wolford, RW. Disorders of potassium. *Emerg Med Clin North Am*, Vol.23, No.3, (August2005), pp. 723-747 ISSN 1598-2543

Schwartz, PJ.; Spazzolini, C.; Crotti, L.; Bathen, J.; Amlie, JP.; Timothy, K.; Shkolnikova, M.; Berul, CI.; Bitner-Glindzicz, M.; Toivonen, L.; Horie, M.; Schulze-Bahr, E & Denjoy, I. The Jervell and Lange-Nielsen Syndrome. Natural history, molecular basis, and clinical outcome. *Circulation*, Vol.113, No.6, (February2006), pp. 783-790, ISSN 1646-1811

Snyder, CS.; Lucas, V.; Young, T.; Darling, R.; Dalal, G. & Davis, JE. Minimally invasive implantation of a cardioverter-defibrillator in a small patient. *J Thorac Cardiovasc Surg*, Vol.133, No.2, (May2007), pp. 1375–1376, ISSN 1746-7466

Stefanelli, CB.; Bradley, DJ.; Leroy, S.; Dick, M 2nd.; Serwer, GA. & Fischbach, PS. Implantable cardioverter defibrillator therapy of life-threatening arrhythmias in young patients. *J Interv Card Electrophysiol*, Vol.6, No.3, (July2002), pp. 235–244, ISSN 1215-4326

Storm, C.; Hasper, D.; Nee, J.; Joerres, A.; Schefold, JC.; Kaufmann, J. & Roser, M. Severe QTc prolongation under mild hypothermia treatment and incidence of arrhythmias after cardiac arrest--a prospective study in 34 survivors with continuous Holter ECG. *Resuscitation*. Vol.82, No.7, (July2011), pp. 859-862. ISSN 2148-2009

Stramba-Badiale, M.; Spagnolo, D.; Bosi, G. & Schwartz, PJ. Are gender differences in QTc present at birth? MISNES Investigators. Multicenter Italian Study on Neonatal Electrocardiography and sudden infant death syndrome. *Am J cardiol*, Vol.75, No.17, (June1995), pp. 1277-1278, ISSN 7778-558

Vetter, VL.; and Horowitz, LN. (1982) Electrophysiologic residua and sequelae of surgery from congenital heart defects. *Am J Cardiol* , Vol.50, No.3, (September1982), pp. 588–604, ISSN 7051-800

Wang, Q.; Shen, J.; Splawski, I.; Atkinson, D.; Li, Z.; Robinson, JL.; Moss, AJ.; Towbin, JA. & Keating, MT. SCN5A mutations associated with an inherited cardiac arrhythmia, long QT syndrome. *Cell*, Vol.80, No.2, (March1995), pp. 805-811, ISSN 7889-574

Wang, Q.; Curran, ME.; Splawski, I,.; Burn, TC.; Millholland, JM.; VanRaay, TJ.; Shen, J.; Timothy, KW.; Vincent, GM.; de Jager, T.; Schwartz, PJ.; Towbin, JA.; Moss, AJ.; Atkinson, DL.; Landes, GM.; Connors, TD. & Keating, MT. Positional cloning of a novel potassium channel gene: KVLQT1 mutations cause cardiac arrhythmias. *Nat Genet*, Vol.12, No.1, (Janurary1996), pp. 17-23, ISSN 8528-244

Ward, OC. A new familial cardiac syndrome in children. *J Ir Med Assoc*, Vol.54, (April1964), pp. 103-106, ISSN 1413-6838

Wolfe, RR.; Driscoll, DJ.; Gersony, WM.; Hayes, CJ.; Keane, JF.; Kidd, L.; O'Fallon, WM.; Pieroni, DR. & Weidman, WH. Arrhythmias in patients with valvar aortic stenosis, valvar pulmonary stenosis, and ventricular septal defect. Results of 24-hour ECG monitoring. *Circulation*, Vol.87, No.2, (February1993), pp. I89-101, ISSN 8425-327

Zeppenfeld, K.; Schalij, MJ.; Bartelings, MM.; Tedrow, UB.; Koplan, BA. Soejima, K. & Stevenson, WG. Catheter ablation of ventricular tachycardia after repair of congenital heart disease: electroanatomic identification of the critical right ventricular isthmus. *Circulation*, Vol.116, No.20, (November2007), pp. 2241– 2252, ISSN 1796-7973

14

Psychological Approach to the Cardiac Arrhythmias: A Focus on the Emotions

Ana Myriam Sánchez Bonomo
and Tereza Cristina Cavalcanti Ferreira de Araujo
University of Brasília
Brazil

1. Introduction

This chapter proposes a psychological approach to the cardiac arrhythmias. Initially, psychosocial risk factors highlighted in the specialized literature will be reviewed: socioeconomic status, social support, age, gender, type A behavior pattern, stress and depression. Following this, studies regarding the impact of negative emotions and positive emotions on cardiac rhythm will be reported, with emphasis on the investigation conducted during the Holter monitoring. Finally, prospects for future research will be outlined and the role of the psychologist in Cardiology will be discussed.

2. Psychosocial risk factors

Having the control and prevention of heart disease as their main goal, many researchers, both in Biomedicine and Psychology, have struggled to identify its predisposing elements. Risk factors can be initiators, promoters, potentiators or precipitators, according to the disease stage in which they operate. However, from the psychological point of view, the most interesting distinction is that which distinguishes them as modifiable (e.g. smoking and sedentary lifestyle), partially modifiable (e.g. menopause, and high waist-hip ratio) and non-modifiable (e.g. family history and age).

Today, it has been established that well known organic risk factors - such as hypertension, hypercholesterolemia, obesity and diabetes - explain only 40% of the occurrence of cardiac disease (Kubzansky & Kawachi, 2000). In fact, empirical studies have demonstrated the relationship between cardiovascular diseases and psychosocial factors, such as the accumulation of stress, the type A behavior pattern, hostility and depression. That is, the literature indicates that psychosocial factors act synergistically with biological factors, increasing the predisposition to cardiac events (Frasure-Smith & Lesperance, 1998, Rozanski et al., 1999).

Some of the most widely studied psychosocial factors will be addressed next.

2.1 Socioeconomic status

Low socioeconomic status is associated with an increase in unhealthy behavior and other harmful psychosocial factors, significantly contributing to an increase of risk in healthy people, and with a worse prognosis in people with installed coronary artery disease (Rozanski et al., 1999). Linked to these conditions are the difficulties of: access to health services, adherence to prescribed care, nutritional diet composition and installation of an adequate sanitary network (Gallo & Mathews, 2003; Lotufo, 1996).

Some studies suggest that, on one hand, the lower levels of socio-economic status precede the development of depressive symptoms and disorders, and of anxiety. Conversely, it is believed the socioeconomic status tends to diminish in individuals with impaired physical or emotional health. Therefore, it is increasingly accepted that these factors interact in a dynamic and reciprocal way (Gallo & Mathews, 2003).

2.2 Social support

Population surveys have found relationships between coronary artery disease and simple indicators of social support, such as marital status and the habit of visiting friends (Frasure-Smith & Lesperance, 1998; Rozanski et al., 1999). The effects of the social support depend on both the nature of the receiver and the source of the support. Studies have shown that pessimistic individuals do not benefit from social support and that the support given by friends is more effective than that given by strangers. In general, people with a social support network or that feel less alone live longer and in a healthier way, regardless of gender, because the social support directly affects the physiological responses to stress (Glynn et al., 1999).

In postmortem studies with *cynomolgus* monkeys, it was found that females raised in isolation presented more coronary atherosclerosis than isolated males and than specimens raised in groups. The incidence of atherosclerosis in these females was four times higher than in females raised in social groups and is associated with the weakening of ovarian function, hypercholesterolemia and exaggerated heart rate responses (Rozanski et al., 1999). These results suggest that females are more susceptible to social isolation.

Berkman and Syme (1979, as cited in Eaker, 1998) found that the number of social ties is inversely related to total mortality among women. Regarding mortality from coronary diseases, it was observed that the only significantly related element was the absence of social groups or communities.

High levels of perceived social support confer a lower risk for future cardiac events (Rozanski at al., 1999). Berkman et al. (1992, as cited in Eaker, 1998) found data suggestive, although limited, that social support is related to increased post-myocardial infarction survival. Thus, the probability of the first myocardial infarction being fatal is higher among unmarried men than married ones (Glynn et al., 1999).

Social support facilitates the prognosis of coronary artery disease by predisposal to adherence to treatment and to modification of risk factors, as well as alleviating the emotional and physical responses to environmental stress (Frasure-Smith & Lesperance, 1998). In addition, social support prevents the engagement in risk behaviors such as smoking, consumption of fatty foods and excessive alcohol consumption. Social support reduces the arterial pressure levels and the cardiac response in the face of stressor stimuli in humans, with an inverse relationship between levels of adrenaline in the urine, the degree of social support and resting heart rate (Rozanski et al., 1999).

2.3 Age

Age remains one of the major risk factors for coronary diseases. Hypertension, the coronary artery diseases and cardiac insufficiency are common in the elderly, encouraging the perception that there is a general decline in cardiovascular function associated with aging. Age causes specific changes in the cardiovascular system, such as prolonged duration of the contraction and relaxation and decreased chronotropic response to catecholamines (Schulman, 1981). Fleg and Kennedy (1982, as cited in Carvalho-Filho, 2000) found ventricular arrhythmias in 80% and supraventricular arrhythmias in 88% of a sample of individuals of both sexes, aged between 60 and 85 years. In the sample studied by Chandra et al. (1988, as cited in Carvalho-Filho, 2000), the prevalence was 93.2%, both for ventricular arrhythmias as well as supraventricular arrhythmias.

However, age is only a risk factor for coronary diseases when over 65 years, though not for idiopathic arrhythmias, as demonstrated in the study of Lane et al. (2005). These authors found that patients with idiopathic ventricular fibrillation were significantly younger (36.0 ± 11.6 years) than patients with coronary disease (57.1 ± 8.1 years).

It must be considered that in situations of stress, older individuals manifest less increase in cardiac reactivity than younger people. Despite perceiving them with the same intensity, older adults present less physiological reactivity to the emotions and worry less about inhibiting them. It is possible that the decrease in cardiac reactivity faced with emotions is due to physiological aging, similar to what happens in other biological systems, or that it is the result of changes in the emotional regulation skills, especially in relation to the internalization and externalization of the emotions (Labouvie-Vief et al., 2003). Uchino et al. (2005) found evidence of increased cardiac and vascular reactivity to stress in older individuals and that age predicts an increase in systolic arterial pressure related to stress.

Although physiological aging predisposes for the emergence of cardiac diseases, maturity with respect to the emotions and the changes in social relationships could act as protectors for events or other complications, since this preserved the cognitive resources. The importance of the nature of social relationships also changes as a result of age. Thus, the Alameda County Study found that marital status was more important among the participants under 60 years of age at the beginning of the study, whereas among the participants over 65 years of age, the bonds of friendship and with other family members were more significant to predict mortality (Stansfeld & Fuhrer, 2002).

2.4 Gender

Eaker (1998) suggests that psychosocial risk factors for cardiac disease are the same for both genders. However, the male gender appears as a risk factor because the research has focused on analyzing more men than women. Studies regarding prevalence indicate that the high mortality rates among women were due to the high incidence in this group and not a reflection of a differentiated service (Lotufo, 1996). In other words, hormonal factors, genetic inheritance, differences in cerebral structure and function, and psychosocial factors seem to be associated with the prevalence of coronary disease among women.

Among the psychosocial factors, the psychological style and mechanisms, the social and family role exercised by women, and social and professional changes are increasing highlighted (Perez et al., 2005). The climacteric stage, in turn, is related to various psychological symptoms and complaints, such as irritability, anxiety and depression, and these symptoms are exacerbated in women who have lost their social role and are unable to establish new existential goals (Favarato & Aldrighi, 2001).

Studies also show that the prognosis of coronary diseases is worse in women than in men. Data from the American Angioplasty Registry show that the success rate of myocardial revascularization and coronary angioplasty surgeries are similar, however, the postoperative complications are greater in women. In general, women have a greater age, and a higher prevalence of diabetes mellitus, hypertension, angina and cardiac insufficiency (Lima & Nussmacher, 1996).

Frasure-Smith and Lesperance (1998) suggest that the association between cardiac diseases and depression is similar in men and women. However, the majority of research is performed on men, with a proportion of 2:1, even though the incidence of depression and anxiety is higher in women (Kubzansky & Kawachi, 2000; Perez, 2004). There are also few studies on the effect of hostility in women. The type A behavior pattern did not present an association with the incidence of coronary disease in women (Eaker, 1998). In contrast, Favarato and Aldrighi (2001) compared various aspects related to the quality of life during menopause and concluded that sadness, tearfulness, nervousness and dissatisfaction with life were more commonly reported by women with coronary pathologies than by the control group.

The gender differences in the incidence of coronary artery disease and atherosclerosis are attributed to the effects of estrogen. Pre-menopausal women, or those on hormone replacement therapy, have relative protection from coronary disease, ischemic stroke and atherosclerosis (Lima & Nussmacher, 1996). However, it must be remembered that the curve of incidence of these pathologies in women has a delay of approximately 10 years when compared to men. It is assumed, therefore, that atherosclerosis progresses for years and the clinical symptoms observed in the menopause began years before (Perez, 2004; Rozanski et al., 1999).

There are biological differences between men and women also in relation to platelet aggregation, a factor that predisposes to thrombus formation. *In vitro* studies found that aspirin, the most used drug to inhibit platelet aggregation in the clinical practice, inhibits this phenomenon in men but not in women (Lima & Nussmacher, 1996).

Menopause is also reflected in the incidence of depression, due to estrogens being related to serotonin metabolism, in that, their presence would have a similar effect to antidepressants, with respect to neurotransmission (Almeida & Fráguas Jr., 1996). Evidence suggests that psychosocial stress causes hypothalamic hypogonadism and these ovarian abnormalities reduce levels of estrogen, with manifestations ranging from subclinical luteal phase defects with regular menstrual intervals to irregular cycles of amenorrhea, hypercholesterolemia, and other neuroendocrine and behavioral indicators. Atherosclerosis is therefore accelerated, predisposing to coronary artery disease and possibly ischemic stroke (Rozanski et al., 1999).

The social roles of gender make the reactions different when faced with the same stimulus. Men and women may feel anger in the same proportions and for almost the same reasons. However, men more freely express their negative emotions, experiencing anger more frequently although they repress fear. They express emotions with higher levels of physiological activation. In contrast, women report a greater range of emotions and verbalize more intensely, repressing both the experience and the expression of anger, concern themselves more with the reactions of others. The suppression of anger determined by socialization, in women, causes the feeling or demonstration of this emotion to generate other negative emotions such as guilt, anxiety, shame and depression (Kubzansky & Kawachi, 2000; Lavoiea et al., 2001). This summation of emotions increases physiological reactivity, especially among adolescents and young women, a trend that decreases with age (Labouvie-Vief et al., 2003; Lavoiea et al., 2001).

The studies that have investigated marriage as a source of social support found that, among men, marriage is a protective factor and among women there is little or no relationship between marriage and health. Similarly, divorce or widowhood is more harmful to the health of men (Glynn et al., 1999).

2.5 Type A behavior pattern

The Type A behavior pattern (TABP) corresponds to a set of reactions of a person facing a situation that seems challenging (Laham, 2001). Friedman and Rosenman identified the TABP in the 1950s, and characterized it as a syndrome consisting of hostility, feelings of competition and exaggerated commitment to work (Rozanski et al., 1999). This behavioral pattern is seen to be more evident in the male gender, though easily identified in women when they have to perform competitive professional activities (Almeida & Fráguas Jr., 1996). Among the psychological aspects the following also stand out: hyperactivity, restlessness, rapidity, hurry, impatience, time urgency, hostility, competitiveness, low frustration tolerance, feeling of being under pressure, need to show competence, high sense of responsibility and inattention to symptoms of pain or fatigue. As fatigue is the earliest and most common symptom of an impending heart attack, the individual postpones seeking help by denying or ignoring it (Laham, 2001; Sirois & Burg, 2003).

Interpersonal relationships are problematic, with characteristics of dominance, tension and emotional aggressivity, anger, marital and professional problems, and social mobility and inconsistency (Laham, 2001; Sirois & Burg, 2003).

The physiological manifestations of the TABP are: a) higher cholesterol levels, even in young people; b) increased variability in arterial pressure; c) high levels of frequent and prolonged sympathetic stimulation; d) cardiovascular and biochemical changes harmful to the heart and blood vessels; e) intense discharge of catecholamines; f) greater progression of atherosclerosis; g) less decrease in platelet aggregation after ergometric testing; and h) greater acceleration of blood coagulation under stress (Laham, 2001).

The TABP is two times more related to the increase of coronary artery disease and five times more related to the recurrence of myocardial infarction (Rozanski et al., 1999).

Despite this evidence, several other studies have found no link between the TABP and the risk of coronary diseases (Rozanski et al., 1999). Studies with patients recovering from myocardial infarction suggest that the TABP has a protective effect and population studies have reported increases in the prevalence of the TABP simultaneous with decreases in the rates of coronary artery disease (Frasure-Smith & Lesperance, 1998).

2.6 Stress

Stress, through neurohormonal activation of the hypothalamic-pituitary-adrenal axis, has systemic effects that influence the processes of atherosclerosis and thrombogenesis, also suggesting associations between psychological stress and cardiac infarction in patients with idiopathic ventricular fibrillation. There is evidence that the more stressful events an individual experiences in a given period of time, the greater the possibility of an occurrence of cardiac events (Frasure-Smith & Lesperance, 1998; Lane et al., 2005).

The studies on the subject distinguish three modalities of stress: chronic, subacute and acute. Chronic stress may be associated with decreased vagal tone, which in itself is an established risk factor for cardiac mortality (Lane et al., 2005). The type of chronic stress most studied in relation to coronary artery disease is that associated with work. Work activities with high demands and low pay are recognized as predictors of cardiac events, relating to greater progressions of carotid atherosclerosis and increasing by four times the risk of death (Rozanski et al., 1999).

Subacute stress lasts for some months. Acute stress, in turn, is the type most investigated recently by means of longitudinal studies (Lucini et al., 2005; Rozanski et al., 1999). Epidemiological studies show an increase in cardiac events in situations of public calamity such as earthquakes or war. Thus, during the 1994 earthquake in Los Angeles, rates of mortality due to coronary artery disease increased from an average of 4.6 in the previous week to 24 on the day of the earthquake (Burg et al., 2004; Lampert et al., 2002; Rozanski et al., 1999). During the Korean War autopsies were carried out on soldiers whose average age was 22 years and coronary lesions were found in 77% of the cases analyzed (Giannotti, 2002).

The hypothesis that stress causes myocardial ischemia, increased blood pressure or electrophysiological changes can be investigated in the laboratory by means of exposure to controllable stressors, such as mental arithmetic and verbal fluency tests (Rozanski et al., 1999). Approximately half of the patients with symptomatic coronary artery disease present left ventricular dysfunction when subjected to mental stress tests (Jain et al., 2001). James et al. (2000) found that psychological stress caused by cognitive tests resulted in electrophysiological responses in patients with coronary stenosis, but not in patients with normal coronary arteries.

The mental stress tests caused sympathetic activation, increased cardiac rate and arterial pressure and reduced left ventricular ejection fraction, however did not produce change in the parasympathetic tone (Jain et al., 2001). Even when the cardiac rate increases are small, the increases in arterial pressure are substantial when compared to those resulting from physical exercise (Rozanski et al., 1999). Previous studies had demonstrated that ischemia induced by mental stress is associated with the greatest risk, when compared with ischemia induced by exercise (Blumenthal et al., 2005). The increase of the adrenalin serum levels seems to relate psychological stress to platelet aggregation (Kubzansky & Kawachi, 2000).

Patients who present myocardial ischemia when subjected to physical stress tend to also present it when subjected to mental stress in laboratory tests. However, myocardial ischemia produced by mental stress is not usually perceptible to the conventional electrocardiogram and is clinically silent, usually occurring with low heart rate elevations compared with physical exercise (Rozanski et al., 1999).

The frequency and magnitude of ischemia induced by mental stress vary according to the type of stressor. When the stressor has a greater emotional load, or is personally relevant, such as the task of reporting personal errors or remembering episodes of anger, it results in greater increases in the frequency and magnitude of abnormalities of the left ventricular wall than those caused by non-specific mental stressors, such as mental arithmetic. It was also found that mental stress causes increased coronary vasoconstriction and that the coronary microcirculation does not dilate sufficiently (Rozanski et al., 1999).

Lampert et al. (2002) investigated the occurrence of arrhythmias in situations of daily life. Some activities showed potential association with the occurrence of arrhythmias, such as driving, discussing and receiving bad news. Physical activity was associated with the period preceding the arrhythmia and there was no interaction between physical activity and emotions.

Negative emotions and stress are interconnected, because in determining whether an event is stressful, one must know the interpretation of this event for the individual and its significance (Kubzansky & Kawachi, 2000). The emotional and psychological involvement of the participant is an important component of the mental stress tests. However, studies that use cognitive tests as mental stressors found inconsistent results which were difficult to replicate. Jain et al. (2001) believe that this is due to the attenuation of the responses caused by familiarization, conditioning or adaptation of the participant to the repetition of the tests. Recent experimental findings suggests that sympathetic overstimulation resulting from stress can increase the concentration of protein kinase C in the central cerebral structures, such as the prefrontal lobe, leading to a deregulation of the thinking, mood or behavior (Lucini et al., 2005).

2.6.1 Tako-Tsubo syndrome or broken-heart syndrome

Since the 1990s, the so-called Tako-Tsubo syndrome has been reported in the literature. It is also known as ventricular apical ballooning syndrome, transitional broken heart syndrome and stress cardiomyopathy. Its pathophysiology is still not sufficiently understood, and the syndrome is characterized by chest pain and clinical, electrocardiographic and echocardiographic changes that mimick an acute myocardial infarction. It is different of the latter condition in that the coronary arteries do not show obstructions and there is significant recovery of the ventricle. In general, the syndrome affects women after menopause age, between 60 and 75 years old, although cases in children have also been reported (Finn et al., 2005; Lemos et al. 2008; Merli et al., 2006).
It persists for a few weeks and its onset can be precipitated by intense emotional stress such as death or illness of a family member, distressing events, arguments with relatives or friends, traffic accidents, financial losses, termination of employment and change of residence. There is also an increased incidence after natural disasters, such as the 2004 earthquakes in Japan. Other psychosocial impacts of major events, such as wars and sport matches, are frequently associated. Approximately 1-2% of cases of hospitalization because of signs of acute myocardial infarction account for this syndrome (Núñez Gil et al., 2009).

2.7 Depression

Depression is strongly associated with the neurohormonal imbalance related to the pathogenesis of the cardiac diseases and is considered both a primary and secondary risk factor (Frasure-Smith & Lesperance, 1998; Pinton et al., 2006). It includes feelings of sadness, loneliness, hopelessness, guilt and shame, and has well-defined diagnostic criteria. It occurs frequently associated with some type of loss, characterized by a behavioral inhibition, with decreased mobilization of the physiological resources (Kubzansky & Kawachi, 2000; Rozanski et al., 1999). Depression is twice as common among women (Lavoiea et al., 2001), among single people and those without close friends (Almeida & Fráguas Jr., 1996; Perez et al., 2005).
Even with all the evidence associating depression to the cardiac diseases, cardiologists still have difficulties in making this association, because the somatic symptoms of fatigue, lack of energy, loss or increase in appetite and sleep disturbances are common and can be confused with symptoms of the cardiopathy (Perez et al., 2005).
Not only is depression as a diagnostic entity related to disease. The presence of depressive symptoms is also related to the occurrence of cardiac events (Rozanski et al., 1999) and increases the risk of mortality by between two and four times (Pinton et al., 2006). Depressive symptoms are significantly associated with psychological factors such as hopelessness, despondency, apathy, intolerance to frustration and cognitive distortions (Perez et al., 2005; Shnek et al., 2001; Sirois & Burg, 2003). Several studies have suggested that depression is associated with decreased survival in the short and long term in survivors of myocardial infarction (Pitzalis et al., 2001).
The prevalence of depression is approximately three times higher in patients with coronary disease than in the general population (Rozanski et al. 1999; Sirois & Burg, 2003). It is estimated that the prevalence of clinically significant depressive disorders in cardiac

patients is around 14% to 27%. Psychiatric evaluations showed that 16% of the patients studied by Lane et al. (2005) presented moderate or severe depression in the three months preceding the cardiac episodes.
Depression predicts the occurrence of myocardial infarction, angina, angioplasty and/or myocardial revascularization surgery, as well as presenting itself as an independent risk factor for mortality, with the same prognosis as left ventricular dysfunction and history of previous myocardial infarction (Sirois & Burg, 2003). Longitudinal studies have found between 1.5 and 2.0 times higher risk for coronary events in people diagnosed with depression or with self-reported depressive symptoms (Kubzansky & Kawachi, 2000).

3. Emotions and their effects on cardiac rhythm

3.1 Negative emotions and positive emotions

The conceptual and theoretical description of the emotions has been the subject of much debate. However, most experts agree that the emotions comprise affective, cognitive, behavioral and neurobiological components which sustain the adaptive behavior (Gallo & Mathews, 2003; Kubzansky & Kawachi, 2000). Emotions are perceived as internal phenomena that cause external manifestations or signs, being organic or behavioral. Emotional experiences must be distinguished from emotional disorders, which are psychiatric disorders that encompass diverse symptoms, behavior and cognitive and affective processes, occurring infrequently when compared with the emotional experiences (Gallo & Mathews, 2003).
The emotions can be grouped into the positive and negative, however, the specialists still disagree about whether these groups are two poles of the same dimension, or form distinct dimensions (Gallo & Mathews, 2003). Richman et al. (2005) identified four families of positive emotions: joy, interest, contentment and love. Shaver et al. (1987, as cited in Hupka et al., 1999) defined six categories of emotions subordinate to the general classification of negative and positive emotions: anger, fear, sadness, joy, love and surprise. Within these categories, they distributed the emotional lexicons of the English language in several subcategories: affection, lust, longing, cheerfulness, zest, contentment, pride, optimism, enthrallment, relief, amazement, irritation, exasperation, rage, disgust, envy, torment, suffering, sadness, disappointment, shame, neglect, sympathy, horror and nervousness.
Emotions rarely occur in isolation and there is great variability of expression. Thus, in response to stimuli with the same emotional load, some individuals are more responsive than others and this tendency has been termed emotional reactivity (Carels et al., 1999). The hyperactivity of the sympathetic nervous system leading to exaggerated responses of cardiac rate and arterial pressure in situations of engagement, dispute or aversiveness is called, by some authors, cardiovascular reactivity (Rozanski et al., 1999).
The literature suggests that when the style of regulation is more expressive and externalized, physiological reactivity is lower (Labouvie-Vief et al., 2003). Specialists also suggest that emotional reactivity that deviates from the norm in both directions is related to a risk of hypertension and probably also to arrhythmia (Carels et al., 1999; Kubzansky & Kawachi, 2000).
Several measures and criteria have been used in studies regarding emotions, including clinical diagnoses of pathologies such as, for example, the definition of depression and anxiety (Kubzansky & Kawachi 2000). The majority of studies on emotions use self-reports, although this tends toward inaccuracy, because it involves remembering and reconstructing.

Some adopt methods of inducing emotions in the laboratory, but the generalization of the results cannot be determined (Thomas & Diener, 1990). Longitudinal studies separate the participants into "exposed" and "unexposed" to the risk factor and relate the two groups to the emergence of the target pathology, however, there is no way to determine if a person was exposed or not to a particular emotion (Kubzansky & Kawachi, 2000).

Even with so many limitations, associations have been found between emotions and disease. Emotions can influence the onset of specific diseases or may result from diseases, influencing their prognosis. The relationship between emotions and cardiovascular health is, therefore, bidirectional, with the cumulative effect over time (Kubzansky & Kawachi, 2000). Studies have shown that patients with ambulatory ischemia during routine activities are more likely to have experienced negative emotions in the hours prior to the ischemic episode. Individuals with high emotional reactivity are 2.5 times more likely to show myocardial ischemia in the quotidian, 3.0 times more likely to manifest it in the laboratory and almost 4.0 times more likely to manifest it on two occasions (Carels et al., 1999).

Emotions, especially the negative ones, alter cardiovascular reactivity and neuroendocrine functioning, affecting the autonomic nervous system and hypothalamic-pituitary-adrenal axis acting on the cardiovascular system. These changes cause hypercholesterolemia, elevation of the level of catecholamines in the plasma and urine, impaired platelet functioning favoring platelet aggregation, thrombosis and rupture of existing plaques, impairment in vagal control functioning, increased cardiac rate, alterations in the electrical stability of the heart and reduction of cardiac variability, with a negative impact on the prognosis for coronary disease (Kubzansky & Kawachi, 2000; Perez et al., 2005; Richman et al., 2005; Sirois & Burg, 2003). Excessive or chronic emotional activation increases the levels of adrenalin and noradrenalin, increasing the quantity of free fatty acids, the arterial pressure, the cardiac rate and total peripheral resistance (Kubzansky & Kawachi, 2000).

Sudden death of cardiac origin has been associated with intense and prolonged emotions (Lampert et al., 2002). Furthermore, intense transient emotional states can cause the detachment of atherosclerotic plaques, initiating acute cardiac events, such as sudden death (Kubzansky & Kawachi, 2000).

There is still no consistent evidence of this association in relation to cardiac arrhythmias (Lampert et al., 2002), even knowing that "negative emotions such as anxiety and depression can affect the electrical stability of the heart by altering the autonomic regulation (specifically, reducing the cardiac rate variability)" (Kubzansky & Kawachi, 2000, p. 330) and that behavioral factors cause excessive sympathetic activation, triggering arrhythmias (Rozanski et al., 1999).

The arrhythmias of behavioral origin are caused by the sum of three conditions: a) myocardial electrical instability, usually due to previous coronary disease, b) an acute triggering event, often related to mental stress, and c) a chronic intense psychological state, which often include depression and hopelessness (Rozanski et al., 1999).

There is evidence that different emotions are related to different patterns of cardiac response. Studies show that anger increases the cardiac rate by between 5.0 and 9.0 beats per minute (bpm), fear increases it by between 5.5 and 8.0 bpm, sadness by between 4.0 and 7.0 bpm and joy by between 2.0 to 3.0 bpm (Labouvie-Vief et al., 2003). A study conducted with resident physicians showed an increase of unsustainable atrial and ventricular ectopic arrhythmias due to the stress of receiving an emergency call (Burg et al., 2004; Lampert et al., 2002).

3.1.1 Anger and hostility

Evidence for the association between anger and cardiac disease is still limited, however, suggestive. Studies show that high levels of anger precede the cardiac diseases, while others suggest that both the suppression and expression of anger have cardiac consequences (Kubzansky & Kawachi, 2000).

Anger is an emotional experience that ranges from an irritation or mild annoyance to a full fury (Sirois & Burg, 2003). It occurs in response to events perceived as unfair and accompanies physiological activation, leading to aggressive behavior, being strongly interlinked with hostility (Kubzansky & Kawachi, 2000). Anger, its expression, and hostility may influence the incidence of recurrent depression among women (Lavoiea et al., 2001).

The manifestation of anger and hostility, while stable personality traits, are associated with increased ischemia (Burg et al., 2004). An anger-trait is defined as the disposition to perceive situations as annoying or frustrating and the tendency to respond to these situations with higher frequencies of anger (Spielberger, 1998, as cited in Richman et al., 2005).

Stimuli that generate responses of anger are more likely to provoke abnormalities in the cardiac rhythm (Rozanski et al., 1999), conferring risk for cardiac diseases through the persistence of exaggerated cardiovascular reactivity (Lavoiea et al., 2001). The emotions of anger and anxiety can precipitate arrhythmias due to increased sympathetic activity. It is therefore possible that anger and anxiety, present in a chronic form, increase the risk of arrhythmias due to the influence on the sympathetic-parasympathetic equilibrium (Burg et al., 2004). Not only the expression of anger, but also its inhibition and the inability to discuss feelings of anger are related to cardiac diseases (Kubzansky & Kawachi, 2000).

Anger not only contributes to the development of atherogenesis and to cardiac disease but also triggers acute coronary events (Chang et al., 2002; Kubzansky & Kawachi, 2000). Both anger and physical exercise can cause non-fatal myocardial infarctions and/or transient ischemia (Lampert et al., 2002), however, in the two hours subsequent to episodes of anger, the relative risk of myocardial infarction increases by more than two times (Rozanski et al. 1999; Sirois & Burg, 2003). In the study by Lampert et al. (2002) anger episodes of moderate intensity were reported preceding 15% of the cardiac events studied.

The phenomenon of arrhythmias triggered by anger can be observed both in patients with recurrent episodes as well as those with single episodes, however, the study of the association between anger and cardiac arrhythmias is difficult because in a study it is virtually impossible to select participants with different tendencies (Lampert et al., 2002).

3.1.2 Anxiety

Anxiety is characterized by the perception of the inability to predict, control or obtain results in circumstances evaluated as threatening and covers physiological responses (Carels et al. 1999; Kubzansky & Kawachi, 2000). Patients who presented ventricular arrhythmias associated with emotions obtained scores above the average of the general population in anxiety tests (Burg et al., 2004).

Anxiety has been shown to be related to the occurrence of cardiac events by affecting the autonomic cardiac control, which could increase the risk of fatal ventricular arrhythmias (Sirois & Burg, 2003) and reduce the R-R variability (Rozanski et al., 1999). In addition, acute states of anxiety may lead to hyperventilation, which in turn triggers coronary vasospasm (Kubzansky & Kawachi, 2000).

Initially it was not possible to relate anxiety with cardiac diseases (Kubzansky & Kawachi, 2000). However, more recent studies, which used self-reporting, have suggested that the mere presence of symptoms may be a risk factor, without the need to meet the diagnostic criteria for anxiety. The experience of moderate intensity anxiety can trigger potentially fatal arrhythmias in patients with ischemic cardiac disease. Patients with higher scores in Spielberger's anxiety tests also reported anxiety in the 15 minutes prior to an ischemic event (Burg et al., 2004). Similarly, Denollet and Brutsaert (1998, cited in Sirois & Burg, 2003) found that individuals with high scores in the State-Trait Anxiety Inventory and in the social inhibition scale of the Heart Patients Psychological Questionnaire suffered more cardiac events during the eight years of follow-up, regardless of ventricular function impairment.

Large-scale surveys were conducted to better demonstrate the relationship between anxiety and cardiac events. The Determinants of Myocardial Infarction Onset Study observed an increased relative risk of myocardial infarction in the two hours following an episode of anxiety. Both the Normative Aging Study and the Framingham Heart Study associated symptoms of anxiety with an increased risk of fatal coronary heart diseases (Kubzansky & Kawachi, 2000).

However, the studies that relate anxiety and autonomic control of the heart do not have consistent results, probably due to the different measures used and because anxiety is often associated with depression (Pitzalis et al., 2001).

Few studies have examined the prognostic significance of anxiety in patients diagnosed with cardiac disease.

3.1.3 Positive emotions

The studies regarding emotions has flourished in recent years, however research into positive emotions has not kept pace. Possibly, due to the difficulties in conceptualization and definition and because the positive emotions seem to be more diffuses. In fact, taxonomies of basic emotions only identify one positive emotion for every three or four negative emotions. Thus, there is little consensus about what can be considered a positive emotion. Another factor that certainly complicates the study of positive emotions is to realize that for specific negative emotions there are specific facial expressions and that this does not occur with the positive emotions, which share the facial expression of the smile between them. Furthermore, different autonomic responses were demonstrated related to negative emotions, however, the same was not verified in situations of positive emotion (Fredrickson, 1998).

A form of positive emotion that has received certain attention is curiosity, a term used to describe hypothetical mechanisms that serve to guide or attract an organism in the direction of new stimuli (Swan & Carmelli, 1996). Curiosity is defined as an affective state or trait that appears closely related to interest, being related to wanting to investigate, learn and incorporate new experiences. Thus, Richman et al. (2005) followed, for two years, a population composed of 4,027 men aged between 55 and 69 years to verify the relationship between hope, curiosity and hypertension, diabetes mellitus and respiratory infections. For each unit increase in curiosity test scores, the researchers perceived a 57% decrease in the risk of developing hypertension. This decrease was 40% for the scores of the hope tests in the first year of follow-up. In the second year of follow-up, patients with higher scores in the hope tests had a 48% reduction.

Positive emotions may have the potential to reduce the effects of stress on the cardiovascular system even faced with inevitable negative life events. Concepts such as optimism and positive attitude can cause negative events to be viewed with the confidence that the future holds something positive and better. The internally generated, positive emotional state seems to modify the adverse effects of prolonged exposure to negative emotions (Danner et al., 2001; Richman et al., 2005).

3.2 The Holter Examination: An investigation regarding activities and emotions

Autonomic dysregulation in the context of stress has been investigated both in animals and in laboratory conditions, however, few studies have been conducted in everyday situations, probably due to the difficulty of making accurate measurements in the midst of multiple environmental factors and because of the perceptual variability between subjects (Lucini et al., 2005). It is important to consider that, under experimental conditions, the occurrence is restricted of emotions still little known. Therefore, recognition of the influence of other emotions in the arrhythmogenesis is also restricted. Thus, the study of emotional changes that occur in the quotidian of people with ambulatory electrocardiographic monitoring can better clarify important research questions. Additionally, from the standpoint of diagnostic evaluation, this feature is relatively simple and accessible.

In view of these scientific and clinical interests, a study was conducted with the following objectives: a) to identify emotions simultaneous to arrhythmias at different times of the day; b) to verify that the same activity can be presented simultaneously to arrhythmias at different times of day; c) to verify the occurrence of similar arrhythmias in individuals with similar emotional reports; d) to identify aspects of daily experience that occur simultaneously to arrhythmias, e) to verify whether people that conduct similar activities present similar arrhythmias and f) to describe and analyze the association between emotions and activities reported during the 24-hour Holter Examination (Sánchez, 2007; Bonomo & Araujo, 2009).

A total of 13 men and 17 women participated in the investigation, aged between 48 and 69 years, with complete high school education as the minimum level of schooling, who did not use antiarrhythmic medication, antipsychotics or beta blockers and had the ability to communicate orally and in writing. The data obtained during the examination were first transferred to a memory card, coupled to the Holter device. As usual, after receiving guidance on how to proceed within the 24 hour period, the return was scheduled for the following day with a view to removing the device at the same time. The recorded electrocardiographic information were processed by computer, generating a Tabular Report.

In the Daily Report, in addition to recording the activities performed during period of the examination, the participants were asked to record the concomitant emotions. If different emotions occurred during the same activity, they should register this emotional change, its intensity and the time. After removal of the device and evaluation by a cardiologist, they were interviewed by the psychologist researcher using a previously prepared script. These reports were audio recorded and later transcribed. The Daily Report data were paired, hour by hour, with the Tabular Report data. Those periods which, even after completion of the interview, remained without comment, were registered as "without report".

Initially, the data found in the Daily Reports and Tabular Reports were analyzed by means of descriptive statistics, using the arithmetic mean of the reports. It is worth explaining that the analysis was focused on the waking period, with reports being excluded where patients said they were asleep, since there are limitations for the participant to record this experience. The daily activities and the emotional reports were organized into categories and subcategories. Subsequently, the software Alceste - *Analyse de Lexèmes Concurrents dans les Énnoncés Simples d'un Texte* - was used for content analysis of the interviews.

3.2.1 Distribution of the ventricular and supraventricular arrhythmias

The women presented more arrhythmias, both ventricular (mean = 121.82) and supraventricular (mean = 265.59). The men presented a mean of 68.15 ventricular arrhythmias and 67.69 supraventricular arrhythmias. That is, the women presented more than twice the number of supraventricular than ventricular arrhythmias, however, these arrhythmias were distributed differently throughout the examination period (Bonomo & Araujo, 2009).

3.2.2 Distribution of arrhythmias by activity category

The activities were organized into three categories: a) physical activity, b) mental activity and c) travelling. Figure 1 shows that, among the women, the physical activities were more associated with ventricular arrhythmias and less with supraventricular arrhythmias. In the men, the exact opposite occurred. It can also be seen that in both men and women the mental activities were associated more with supraventricular arrhythmias than with ventricular arrhythmias. Regarding travelling, the association with supraventricular arrhythmias was higher in the female group.

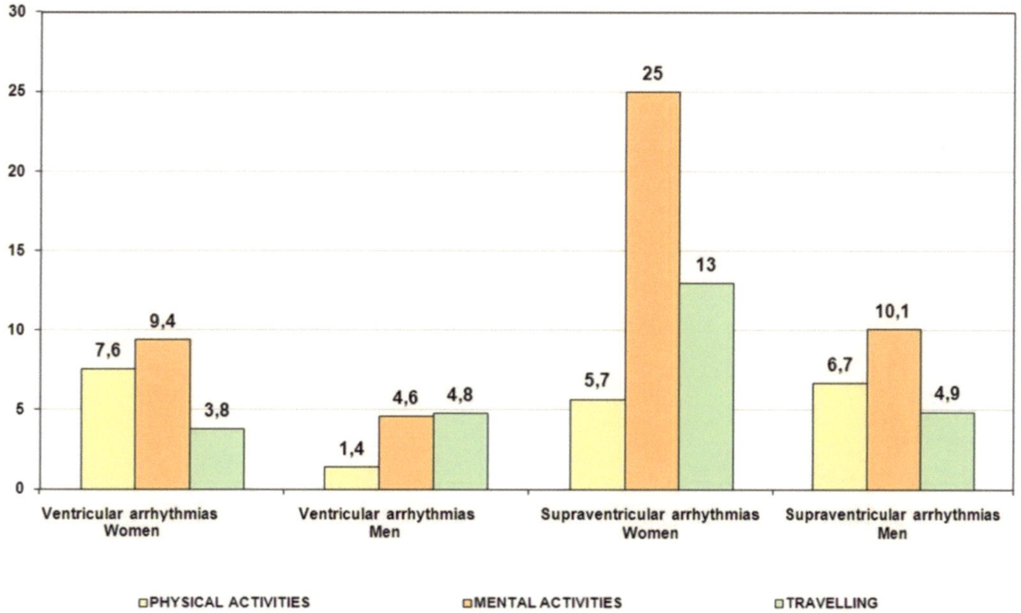

Fig. 1. Distribution of the mean of the reports of ventricular and supraventricular arrhythmias by category of activity.

3.2.3 Distribution of arrhythmias by emotion category

It was verified that only the reports of worry and sadness were similar between the two groups. Joy was the emotion that obtained the highest difference in the means of the reports, being more perceived by the women (see Table 1).

Categories	Subcategories	WOMEN		MEN	
		Total	%	Total	%
Positive	Blessed	5	3.1%	1	0.7%
	Joy	27	17.0%	3	2.2%
	Satisfaction	8	5.0%	-	-
	Security	-	-	3	2.2%
Neutral	Tranquility	68	42.8%	81	60.5%
Negative	Anxiety	14	8.8%	9	6.7%
	Worry	16	10.1%	17	12.7%
	Anger	9	5.7%	12	9.0%
	Surprise	1	0.6%	-	-
	Sadness	11	6.9%	8	6.0%
	Total	159	100%	134	100%

Table 1. Categories and subcategories of emotions reported by the participants

3.2.4 Emotions simultaneous to ventricular arrhythmias

The subcategory feeling blessed was the most frequently associated with ventricular arrhythmias in both genders (Figure 2). In the women, worry was related more with ventricular arrhythmias than anxiety and in the men this relationship was exactly the inverse. Anger was shown to be related to ventricular arrhythmias in the men but not in the women.

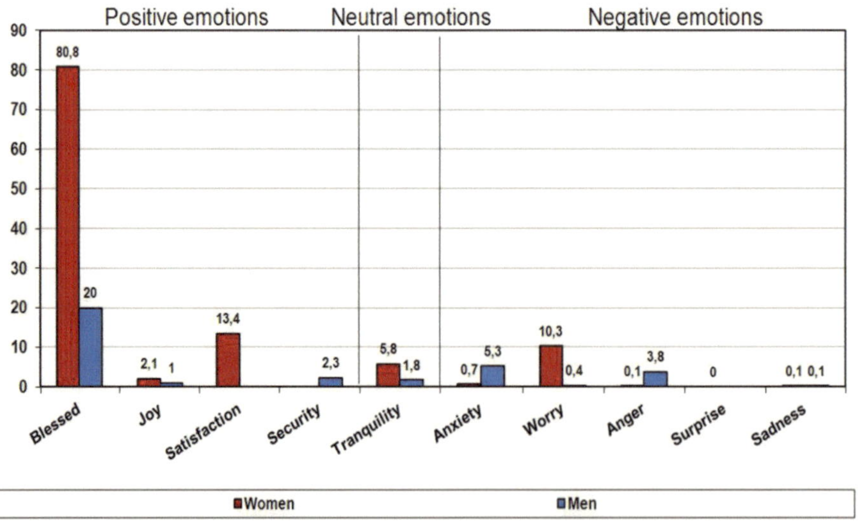

Fig. 2. Mean of ventricular arrhythmias in each subcategory of emotions reported.

Sadness was not simultaneous with ventricular arrhythmias in either gender. In the situations accompanied by reports of tranquility, ventricular arrhythmias were recorded more frequently in the women than in the men, possibly due to the activities that the women were performing.

3.2.5 Emotions simultaneous to supraventricular arrhythmias

Almost all the emotions that were recorded by both genders appeared simultaneously more frequently among women (see Figure 3).

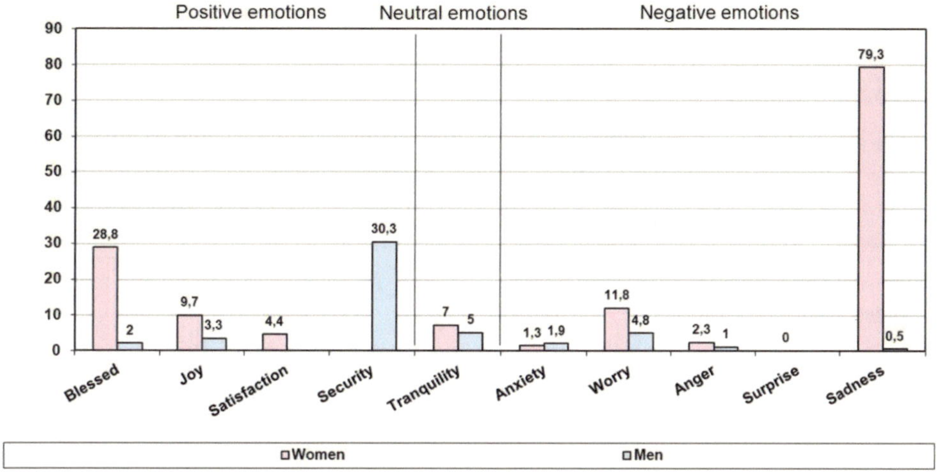

Fig. 3. Mean of supraventricular arrhythmias in each subcategory of emotions reported.

In summary, the majority of the emotions reported by the participants were presented more simultaneously to supraventricular than to ventricular arrhythmias. Both for men and women, the mean of the reports of sorrow concomitant to ventricular arrhythmias were very low. Anger differed from all the other emotions, it was simultaneous to more ventricular arrhythmias in the men and to supraventricular arrhythmias in the women. Surprise was the least identified category. This may reflect the difficulty in conceptualizing it, which indicates the need for more studies.

The analysis of the interviews also revealed the need for recognition of the efforts performed on behalf of the family members. When this recognition was not perceived by the participants, frustration occurred. It is worth mentioning that the majority attributed their organic disorders to external factors, having difficulty linking them clearly to their behavior or emotions. The men and women reported similar emotions in different social situations. The women said they were happy in situations of interaction with the family and the men when they were with friends. In fact, the men reported less interaction with the family, which in most cases, was limited to discussion of problems with the wife.

This study showed that the 24-hour Holter examination enables the identification of the simultaneity between emotions, daily life and cardiac arrhythmias.

4. Conclusions

It is considered that if knowledge about the participation of the emotions in arrhythmogenesis is continually improved, it will be possible to generate support for

psychological guidance based more on, and tailored to, the daily routine of the patients. For example, meditation, which reduces the frequency of premature ventricular contractions (Giannotti-Hallage, 1990), could be recommended at times of circadian peak.
In summary, disease prevention and health promotion depends on knowledge regarding the psychosocial determinants of risk behaviors and of the psychosocial processes that affect the triggering and experience of the chronic diseases. Therefore, to comprehend how the emotional factors trigger the functional imbalance of the heart may contribute to the planning of more effective therapeutic strategies. Certainly, the contribution of Applied Psychology to the area of Cardiology is increasingly promising concerning innovations for the work of the professionals of various categories integrated in interdisciplinary teamwork.

5. Acknowledgments

The National Council of Scientific and Technological Development (CNPq) for support for the research projects linked to the Laboratory of Health and Human Development (Labsaudes) of the University of Brasilia. The professors Angela Almeida and Adriana Giavoni (*in memoriam*) for their collaboration in the data analysis.

6. References

Almeida, O. P. & Fráguas Jr., R. (1996). Depressão e doença cardiovascular. *Revista da Sociedade de Cardiologia do Estado de São Paulo* 6(6): 749-756.

Blumenthal, J. A., Sherwood, A., Babyak, M. A., Watkins, L. L., Waugh, R., Gerorgiades, A., Bacon, S. L., Hayano, J., Coleman, R. E. & Hinderliter, A. (2005). Effects of exercice and stress management training on makers of cardiovascular risk in patient with ischemic heart disease: A randomized controlled trial. *Journal of American Medical Association* 293(13): 1.626-1.634.

Bonomo, A. M. S. & Araujo, T. C. C. F. (2009). Psicologia aplicada à Cardiologia: um estudo sobre emoções relatadas em exame de Holter. *Psicologia: Teoria & Pesquisa* 25(1): 65-74.

Burg, M. M., Lampert, R., Joska, T., Batsford, W. & Jain, D. (2004). Psychological traits and emotion-triggering of ICD shock-terminated arrhythmias. *Psychosomatic Medicine* 66: 898-902.

Carels, R. A., Sherwood, A., Babyak, M., Gullette, E. C., Coleman, R. E., Waugh, R., Jiang, W. & Blumenthal, J. A. (1999). Emotional responsivity and transient myocardial ischemia. *Journal of Consulting and Clinical Psychology* 67(4): 605-610.

Carvalho Filho, E. T. (2000). Como diagnosticar e tratar arritmias cardíacas no idoso. *Revista Brasileira de Medicina* 57(4), URL: www.moreirajr.com.br/revistas.asp?fase=r003&id_materia=330

Chang, P. P., Ford, D. E., Meoni, L. A., Wang, N. Y. & Klag, M. J. (2002). Anger in young men and subsequent premature cardiovascular disease: The precursors study. *Archives of Internal Medicine* 168(8): 901-906.

Danner, D. D., Snowdon, D. A. & Friesen, W. V. (2001). Positive emotions in early life and longevity findings from the nun study. *Journal of Personality and Social Psychology* 80: 804-813.

Eaker, E. D. (1998). Psychosocial risk factors for coronary heart disease in women. *Cardiology Clinics* 16(1): 103-111.

Favarato, M. E. C. S. & Aldrighi, J. M. (2001). A mulher coronariopata no climatério após a menopausa: implicações na qualidade de vida. *Revista da Associação Médica Brasileira* 47(4): 339-345.

Finn, B., Young, P. & Bruetman, J. E. (2005). Takotsubo discinesia apical transitoria: Presentacion de 4 casos y revisión de la literatura. *Medicina.* 65(5): 415-418. URL: www.scielo.org.ar/scielo.php?script=sci_arttext&pid=S0025-76802005000500006&lng=es.

Frasure-Smith, N. & Lesperance, F. (1998). Role of psycho-social factors in CVD. *Evidence-based Cardiovascular Medicine* 2(3): 64-65.

Fredrickson, B. L. (1998). What good are positive emotions?. *Review of General Psychology* 2: 300-319.

Gallo, L. C. & Matthews, K. A. (2003). Understanding the association between socioeconomic status and physical health: Do negative emotions play a role?. *Psychological Bulletin* 129(1): 10-51.

Giannotti-Hallage, A. (1990). Papel das emoções e das situações psicologicamente estressantes na gênese das arritmias cardíacas e morte súbita, In: B. W. R. Lamosa (ed.). *Psicologia aplicada à Cardiologia,* Fundo Editorial BYK, São Paulo, pp. 71-78.

Giannotti, A. (2002) Prevenção da doença coronária: perspectiva psicológica em um programa multiprofissional *Psicologia USP* 13(1): 167-195.

Glynn, L. M., Christenfeld, N. & Gerin, W. (1999). Gender, social support, and cardiovascular responses to stress. *Psychosomatic Medicine* 61(2): 234-242.

Jain, D., Joska, T., Lee, L. F., Burg, M., Lampert, R. & Zaret, B. L. (2001). Day-to-day reproductibility of mental stress-induced abnormal left ventricular function response in patients with coronary artery disease and its relationship to autonomic activation. *Journal of Nuclear Cardiology* 8(3): 347-355.

Hupka, R. B., Lenton, A. P. & Hutchison, K. A. (1999). Universal development of emotion categories in natural language. *Journal of Personality and Social Psychology* 77(2): 247-278.

Laham, M. A. (2001). El patrón de conducta Tipo A, In: M. A. Laham. (Ed.). *Psicocardiologia. Abordaje psicológico al paciente cardíaco,* Ediciones Lumiere, Buenos Aires, pp. 45 -71.

Lane, R. D., Laukes, C., Marcus, F. I., Chesney, M. A., Sechrest, L., Gear, K., Fort, C. L., Priori, S. G., Schwartz, P. J. & Steptoe, A. (2005). Psychological stress preceding idiopathic ventricular fibrillation. *Psychosomatic Medicine* 67(3): 359-365.

Lemos, A. E. T., Araujo, A. L. J. Lemos, M. T., Belém, L. S., Vasconcellos Filho, F. J. & Barros, R. B. (2008). Síndrome do coração partido (síndrome de Takotsubo). *Arquivos Brasileiros de Cardiologia 90*(1): e1-e3.

Lotufo, P. A. (1996). Doenças cardiovasculares no Brasil: Por que altas taxas de mortalidade entre mulheres?. *Revista da Sociedade de Cardiologia do Estado de São Paulo* 6(6): 667-671.

Lucini, D., Di Fede, G., Parati, G. & Pagani, M. (2005). Impact of chronic psychological stress on autonomic cardiovascular regulation in otherwise healthy subjects. *Hypertension* 46(5): 1.201-1.206.

Kubzansky, L. D. & Kawachi, I. (2000). Going to the heart of the matter: Do negative emotions cause coronary heart disease?. *Journal of Psychosomatic Research* 48*:* 323-337.

Labouvie-Vief, G., Lumley, M. A., Jain, E. & Heinze, H. (2003). Age and gender differences in cardiac reactivity and subjective emotion responses to emotional autobiographical memories. *Emotion* 3(2): 115-126.

Lampert, R., Joska, T., Burg, M. M., Batsford, W. P., McPherson, C. A. & Jain, D. (2002). Emotional and physical precipitants of ventricular arrhythmia. *Circulation* 106: 1.800-1.805.

Lavoiea, K. L., Miller, S. B., Conwaya, M. & Fleetb, R. P. (2001). Anger, negative emotions, and cardiovascular reactivity during interpersonal conflict in women. *Journal of Psychosomatic Research* 51(3): 503-512.

Lima, J. A. C. & Nussbacher, A. (1996). O coração da mulher é diferente?. *Revista da Sociedade de Cardiologia do Estado de São Paulo* 6: 704-706.

Merli, E., Sutcliffe, S., Gori, M. & Sutherland, G. G. R. (2006). Tako-Tsubo cardiomyopathy: new insights into the possible underlying pathophysiology. *European Journal of Echocardiography* 7(1):53-61.

Núñez Gil, I. J., Lucas Mendez, M. & García-Rubira, J. C. (2009). Cardiopatía de estrés o síndrome de Tako-Tsubo: conceptos actuales. *Revista Argentina de Cardiologia* 77(3): 218-223. URL: www.scielo.org.ar/scielo.php?script=sci_arttext&pid=S1850-37482009000300011&lng=es.

Perez, G. H. (2004). Fatores de risco da doença arterial coronária em mulheres: Uma visão psicossomática, In: A. L. A. Ribeiro & D. P. Rosa (Eds.), *Mulher & coração: Aspectos psicológicos ligados à cardiopatia,* Papirus, São Paulo, pp. 89-104.

Perez, G. H., Nicolau, J. C., Romano, B. W. & Laranjeira, R. (2005). Depressão e síndromes isquêmicas miocárdicas instáveis: Diferenças entre homens e mulheres. *Arquivos Brasileiros de Cardiologia* 85(5): 319-326.

Pinton, F. A., Carvalho, C. F., Miyazaki, M. C. O. S. & Godoy, M. F. (2006). Depressão como fator de risco de morbidade imediata e tardia pós-revascularização cirúrgica do miocárdio. *Brazilian Journal of Cardiovascular Surgery* 21(1): 68-74.

Pitzalis, M. V., Iacoviello, M., Todarello, O., Fioretti, A., Guida, P., Massari, F., Mastropasqua, F., Russo, G. D. & Rizzon, P. (2001). Depression but not anxiety influences the autonomic control of heart rate after myocardial infarction. *American Heart Journal* 141(5): 765-771.

Richman, L. S., Kubzansky, L., Maselko, J., Kawachi, I., Choo, P. & Bauer, M. (2005). Positive emotion and health: Going beyond the negative. *Health Psychology* 24(4): 422-429.

Rozanski, A., Blumenthal, J. A. & Kaplan, J. (1999). Impact of psychological factors on the pathogenesis of cardiovascular disease and implications for therapy. *Circulation* 99: 2.192-2.217.

Sánchez, A. M. (2007). *Abordagem psicológica das arritmias cardíacas: Uma análise das emoções relatadas em exame de Holter*. University of Brasília.

Schulman, S. P. (1981). Envelhecimento cardiovascular e adaptação à doença, In: J. W. Hurst, B. Logue, R. C. Schlant & Wenger, N. K. (Ed.), *O coração, artérias e veias*. Guanabara Koogan, Rio de Janeiro, pp. 535-539.

Shnek, Z. M. , Irvine, J. , Stewart, D. & Abbey, S. (2001). Psychological factors and depressive symptoms in ischemic heart disease. *Health Psychology* 20(2): 141-145.

Sirois, B. C. & Burg, M. M. (2003). Negative emotion and coronary heart disease. A review. *Behavior Modification* 27(1): 83-102.

Sloan, R. P., Bagiella, E., Shapiro, P. A., Kuhl, J. P. MPhil, D. C., Berg, J. & Myers, M. M. (2001). Hostility, gender, and cardiac autonomic control. *Psychosomatic Medicine* 63(3): 434-440.

Stansfeld, S. & Fuhrer, R. (2002). Social relations and coronary heart disease, In: S. Stansfeld, & M. Marmot (Eds.), *Stress and the heart: Psychosocial pathways to coronary heart disease,* BMJ Books, Londres, pp. 72-85.

Swan, G. E. & Carmelli, D. (1996). Curiosity and mortality in aging adults: A 5-year follow-up of the Western Collaborative Group Study. *Psychological and Aging* 11(3): 449-453.

Thomas, D. L. & Diener, E. (1990). Memory accuracy in the recall of emotions. *Journal of Personality and Social Psychology* 59(2): 291-297.

Uchino, B. N., Holt-Lunstad, J., Bloor, L. E. & Campo, R. A. (2005). Aging and cardiovascular reactivity to stress: Longitudinal evidence for changes in stress reactivity. *Psychology and Aging* 20(1): 134–143.

Part 4

Uncommon Heart Rhythm Disorders

15

The Variations in Electrical Cardiac Systole and Its Impact on Sudden Cardiac Death

F. R. Breijo-Marquez[1] and M. Pardo Ríos[2]
[1]*Clinical and Experimental Cardiology, School of Medicine, Commemorative Hospital, Boston, Massachusetts*
[2]*School of Medicine and Dentistry, University Research Institute on Aging, University of Murcia,*
[1]*USA*
[2]*Spain*

1. Introduction

Before anything else, is essential to define what is the **electrical cardiac systole**. Especially when there are so many discrepancies among different authors.

Includes cardiac electrical systole from the beginning of the P wave (atrial depolarization) to the end of the T wave (ventricular repolarization).

Would cover thus the P wave, PR interval, QRS complex, ST segment, T wave.

For other authors, this one only would include from the beginning of QRS complex to the end of the T wave.

There are several changes, especially in its length, that can cause a sudden death in case that they are not adequately diagnosed and, thus, with the properly treated.

2. Standard values (in length)

P-wave: 0.06-0.09 seconds in length.
PR- interval: 0.12 to 0.20 seconds in length.
QRS- complex: 0.06 to 0.10 seconds in length.
QT- interval (corrected): 0.40 to 0.44 seconds in length.
RR- interval: 0.60-1.00 seconds in length.
Normal duration of cardiac electric systole: 35-45% of total duration of the cardiac cycle (R-R interval)

(The length of cardiac electrical systole is considered normal until reaching 45% of the overall length of cardiac cycle: a greater value is considered as prolonged and lesser is considered as shortened)

The sudden death is defined for most authors as a natural death that happens very instantaneously or within the first hour from the beginning of the symptoms, in a patient with well-known previous disease or without her, but is unexpected totally. Although we do not agree with some nuances of such definition, we will give it as acceptable.

Consequently, any sudden death should be considered either of cardiac origin when the heart is the affected organ, structurally or without macroscopic alterations of its structure.
The cardiac problems are the main cause of unexpected death. It is estimated that occurs about 1 case of sudden death for every 100,000 young athletes each year (under 35). Even though exercise is beneficial for health, sport of competition increases the risk of sudden death [Brignole M, et al 2004].

CARDIAC COMMOTION.
CORONARY ARTERY ANOMALY.
LEFT VENTRICULAR HYPERTROPHY OF UNDETERMINED CAUSE.
MYOCARDITIS.
RUPTURE OF AORTIC ANEURYSM.
ARRHYTHMOGENIC RIGHT VENTRICULAR CARDIOMYOPATHY.
BYPASS CORONARY ARTERY.
AORTIC VALVE STENOSIS.
ATHEROSCLEROTIC DISEASE OF THE CORONARY ARTERY.
DILATED CARDIOMYOPATHY.
MYXOMATOUS MITRAL DEGENERATION.
ASTHMA.
HEATSTROKE.
DRUG ABUSE.
OTHER CARDIOVASCULAR CAUSES.
LONG QT SYNDROME.
RUPTURED BRAIN ANEURYSM.
CARDIAC SARCOIDOSIS.
TRAUMATIC CARDIAC INJURY.

[Thijs, RD., 2005]

Table 1. The most frequent causes of sudden death in overall.

The three most common causes for sudden cardiac death are:

1. Hypertrophic cardiomyopathy (HCM). [Figure 1]:

It is a disease of the myocardium in which a portion of the myocardium is hypertrophied (thickened) without any obvious cause. It is perhaps most well-known as a leading cause of sudden cardiac death in young athletes. The occurrence of Hypertrophic cardiomyopathy is a significant cause of sudden unexpected cardiac death in any age group and as a cause of disabling cardiac symptoms [Richardson P., 1996]. Younger people are likely to have a more severe form of Hypertrophic cardiomyopathy. HCM is frequently asymptomatic until sudden cardiac death, and for this reason, some suggest routinely screening certain populations for this disease [Doerer JJ., 2009].
A cardiomyopathy is a primary disease that affects the muscle of the heart. With Hypertrophic cardiomyopathy (HCM), the sarcomeres (contractile elements) in the heart replicate causing heart muscle cells to increase in size, which results in the thickening of the heart muscle. In addition, the normal alignment of muscle cells is disrupted, a phenomenon known as myocardial disarray. HCM also causes disruptions of the electrical functions of the heart. HCM is most commonly due to a mutation in one of 9 sarcomeric genes that results in a mutated protein in the sarcomere, the primary component of the myocyte (the muscle cell of the heart) [Maron BJ ., 2010].
While most literature so far focuses on European, American, and Japanese populations, HCM appears in all racial groups. The prevalence of HCM is about 0.2% to 0.5% of the general population [Kuller LH., 1980]

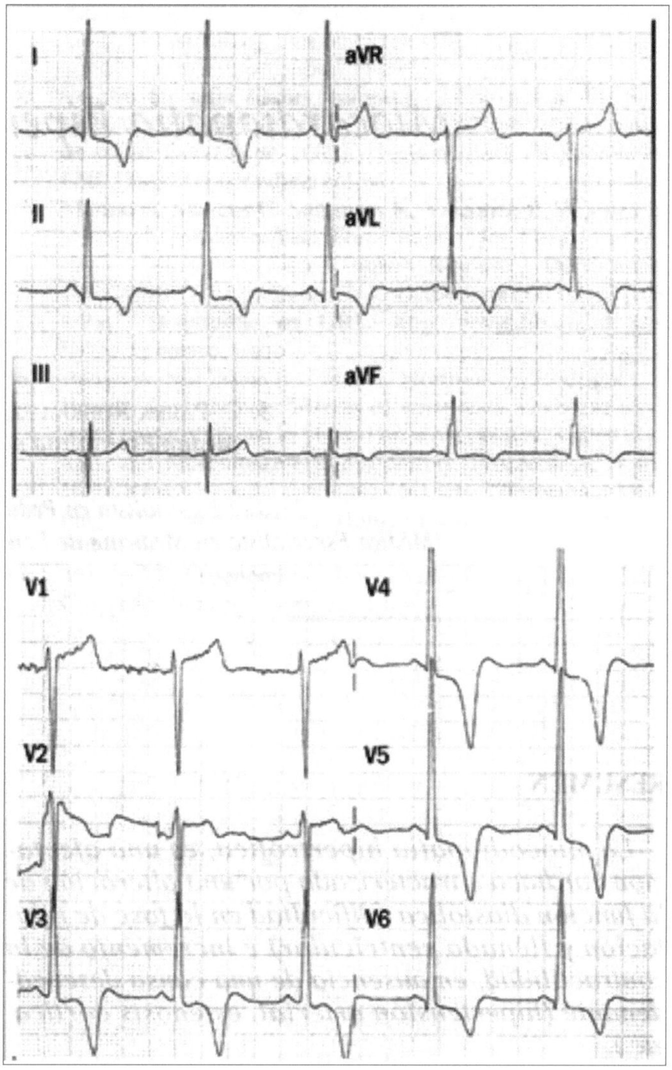

Fig. 1. ECG is abnormal., 80-90% of cases. Abnormal Q-waves in inferior leads. Increasing the voltage in medium or left precordial (V3-V6). ST segment depression, negative T- waves in precordial leads, middle and left. Less often: Increasing in the left atrium, left axis, Giant negative T waves, atrial fibrillation, ventricular extra-systoles, ventricular tachycardia in severe cases.

2. Arrhythmogenic right ventricle cardiomyopathy (ARVD). [Figure 2]

Arrhythmogenic right ventricular dysplasia (ARVD), also called arrhythmogenic right ventricular cardiomyopathy (ARVC) or arrhythmogenic right ventricular dysplasia/cardiomyopathy (ARVD/C), is an inherited heart disease. ARVD is caused by genetic defects of the parts of heart muscle known as desmosomes, areas on the surface of heart muscle cells which link the cells together [Lahtinen, AM., 2011]. The desmosomes are composed of several proteins, and many of those proteins can have harmful mutations. The disease is a type of non-ischemic cardiomyopathy that involves primarily the right ventricle. It is characterized by hypokinetic areas involving the free wall of the right ventricle, with fibro fatty replacement of the right ventricular myocardium, with associated arrhythmias originating in the right ventricle. ARVD is often found in association with diffuse palmo-plantar keratoderma, and woolly hair, because their genes are nearby and often inherited together. ARVC/D is an important cause of ventricular arrhythmias in children and young adults. It is seen predominantly in males, and 30-50% of cases have a familial distribution.

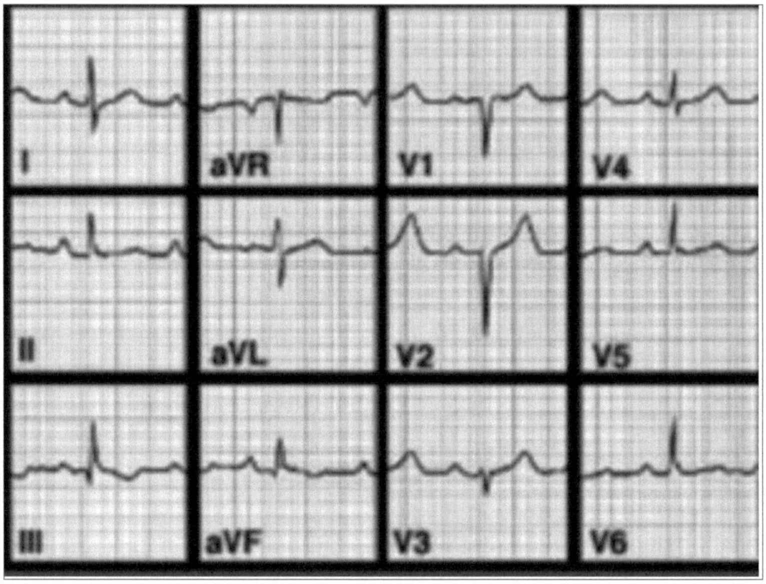

Fig. 2. 90% of individuals with ARVD have some EKG abnormality. The most common EKG abnormality seen in ARVD is T wave inversion in leads V_1 to V_3. However, this is a non-specific finding, and may be considered a normal variant in right bundle branch block (RBBB), women, and children under 12 years old. RBBB itself is seen frequently in individuals with ARVD. This may be due to delayed activation of the right ventricle, rather than any intrinsic abnormality in the right bundle branch. The **epsilon wave** is found in about 50% of those with ARVD. This is described as a terminal notch in the QRS complex. It is due to slowed intraventricular conduction. The epsilon wave may be seen on a surface EKG; however, it is more commonly seen on signal averaged EKGs. Ventricular ectopy seen on a surface EKG in the setting of ARVD is typically of left bundle branch block (LBBB) morphology, with a QRS axis of -90 to +110 degrees. The origin of the ectopic beats is usually from one of the three regions of fatty degeneration (the "triangle of dysplasia"): the RV outflow tract, the RV inflow tract, and the RV apex.

3. Arrhythmogenic sudden death syndrome:

It is a generic name that includes many alterations in cardiac electrical conduction capable of produce instant death.

This syndrome includes all sudden cardiac deaths wherein the cause of death could not be diagnosed, even after the necropsy. It is the cause of more 5% of all sudden cardiac deaths. That is, if we discard the non-cardiac causes and structural heart problems, this problem is denominated as arrhythmogenic sudden death syndrome from a generic form. As the

diagnostic techniques are being more appropriate each day, these numbers grows exponentially [Strickberger SA., 2006].
Here, would be included all events from our chapter proposal : Alterations in electrical cardiac systole and its impact on sudden cardiac death.

3. Other disorders in electrical cardiac systole as cause for sudden cardiac death

As we have said previously, the electrical cardiac systole originates from the beginning of the P wave (atrial depolarization) to the end of the descending branch of the T wave (ventricular repolarization). Are included, therefore, the succession of P-QRS-T and its corresponding intervals and segments: PQ, ST and QT. The mathematical possibilities in the variation on length of electrical systole of the heart may be several. It is well documented and demonstrated that such changes in length can cause that be more vulnerable and unstable all myocardial cells, and can also cause serious cardiac arrhythmias, several syncope episodes and even sudden death for this motive. Even today, many of these disorders are poorly understood and, too many times, its clinical manifestations are categorized as "episodes of epilepsy"; other times (most) are classified within a "common sack" called "channelopathies", when -actually- is the alteration from electrical cardiac systole the true etiology of them.
All these disorders can cause syncopal episodes and a sudden cardiac death.
The measures and lengths of the different components of electrical cardiac systole, considered for most authors as normal are these:
PR-interval: 0.120- 0.200 seconds.
QRS complex: 0.08-0.120 seconds.
QT-interval (corrected): 0.350-0.450 seconds. (Here, there is much disagreement among different authors). The most used methods for QT interval correction, since it is frequency-dependent, are Bazett, Fridericia.
When the PR-interval is lesser than 0.120 seconds, we call it a short PR-interval. In contrast, when is greater than 0,200 seconds, we call it a first-degree AV block. When the QRS complex is lesser than 0.08 seconds, we call it "narrow QRS" but when is greater than 0,120 seconds, we call it "wide QRS". Likewise, when the corrected QT- interval length is lesser than 0,350 seconds, we call it Short QT- interval and when is greater than 0,450 seconds, we call it a Long QTc- interval.
It is clear that there may be, in the same ECG recording, a combination of them all.
Some of these disorders, we will explain briefly below.

3.1 Wolff-Parkinson-White's syndrome (WPWS)

Wolff-Parkinson-White syndrome (WPWS) is a congenital heart disease (PRKAG2. Genetic map 7q36) characterized by a premature ventricular depolarization caused by an abnormal atrioventricular accessory pathway, between the atria and ventricles, known as Kent's bundle. However, even today, is called into question the real cause of Wolff-Parkinson-White, there are some authors who believe that, PRKAG2 mutations, are caused by a glycogen storage cardiomyopathy associated with WPWS, because the overwhelming majority of accessory pathways occur in individuals without structural heart disease, and probably without this mutation. The pathogenesis of accessory pathway formation in PRKAG2 may be completely different, and some authors believe it is due to an inflammation of myocardial cells that occur in the atrial-ventricular connections [L. Wolff., 1930].

In fact, do not even know if the accessory pathways are mediated genetically or due to environmental exposures or randomly.
A short PR interval, a delta wave, a wide QRS complex (greater than 120 ms) and, occasionally, alterations in the ventricular repolarization are its main electrocardiographic characteristics on the ECG. Its incidence varies between 0, 1% and 3% in the general population.
It is essential to achieve the right differential diagnosis between:

•	Wolff-Parkinson-White's syndrome or real ventricular pre-excitation.
•	Lown-Ganong-Levine syndrome or accelerated atrioventricular conduction.
•	Mahaim's syndrome.
•	"Short PR alongside short QT" intervals in the same person. (Breijo's Pattern).

3.1.1 Typical ECG image of the Wolff-Parkinson-White

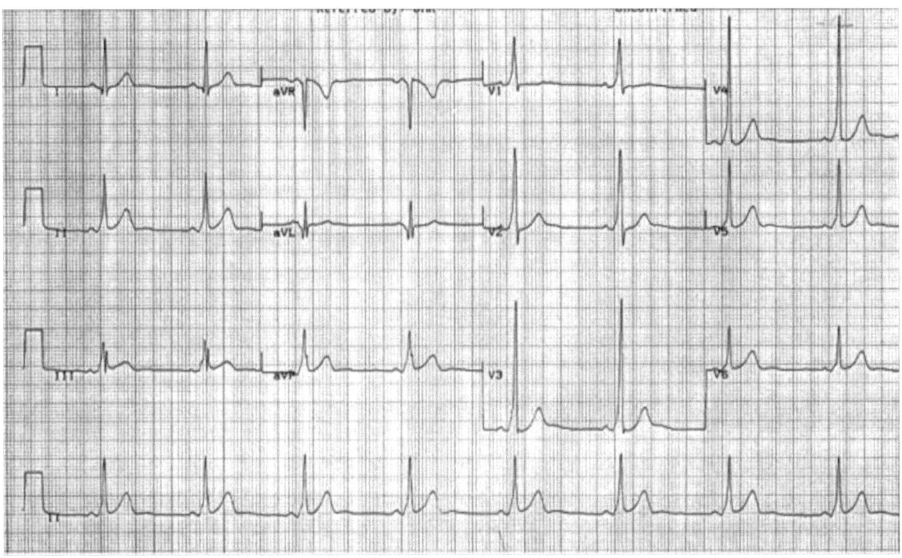

In this context of ECG recording, that has a normal heart rate, a short PR interval, a delta-wave and an early ventricular repolarization can be seen.

3.2 Lown-Ganong-Levine syndrome (LGL)

This syndrome was described in 1952 by Lown, Ganong, and Levine, forming the famous now used to describe it. It is considered a preexcitation syndrome [Lown B, Ganong WF, Levine SA., 1952].
We now know four types of pre-excitation syndrome:

- Wolff-Parkinson-White or ventricular preexcitation true.
- Lown-Ganong-Levine or accelerated atrioventricular conduction.
- Short PR alongside short QT" intervals in the same person. (Breijo's Pattern).
- Mahaim Syndrome.

LGL is a disease entity that is included within the more general condition called Short PR-Interval).

3.2.1 Etiology

- Acquired .
- Congenital :
  - Inherited.
  - Not inherited.

The familial form is inherited, as an autosomal dominant genetic trait has been associated with the PRKAG2 gene that encodes the activated AMP protein kinase, responsible for transport and store energy from the heart. A mutation in this gene could explain the susceptibility of the heart to the crises of tachycardia. Mutation has been identified on the long arm of chromosome 7 (7q34-q36).

The Lown-Ganong-Levine may affect approximately 1 in every 50,000 people.

Several structural abnormalities have been proposed as the possible basis for LGL, including the presence of James's fibbers, Mahaim's fibbers, Brechenmacher and underdeveloped anatomic sinus node (hypoplastic).

Each of these fibbers can only be identified histologically.

Thus, unless other studies demonstrate definitive- structural or functional -abnormalities, the diagnosis of LGL remains a clinical diagnosis.

In the absence of significant structural heart disease, the mortality rate appears to be very low.

Patients may present with an acute episode of tachycardia or a history of symptoms suggestive of paroxysmal tachycardia.

In diagnosis is necessary to make:

1. A standard test for tachycardia, including an ECG to document the rhythm.
2. Serum electrolytes, calcium, magnesium levels, and levels of serum thyroid hormone-stimulating hormone (TSH). Lithemy.
3. History suggestive of recurrent paroxysms of tachycardia,
4. A Holter monitor or event recorder may be useful to document the rhythm during acute symptomatic episodes.
5. An ergometric study.
6. In rare cases, an implantable monitor for pace may be helpful.
7. Family History. (Screening).

3.2.2 Differential diagnosis with Wolf-Parkinson-White

Although apparently similar, there are differences, which, in our opinion, are critical with respect to drug treatment elective. The key differences are:

- The LGL is a PR- interval shortened due to, the presence of accessory pathway, prevents the AV node but normal QRS because the accessory pathway (James fibbers) binds directly to the sinus and depolarizes the ventricles not directly, but does so by typical pathway, by the Hiss-Purkinje system.
- Not displayed "Delta waves -" in D1, aVL, V5 and V6.
- The QRS complexes tend to be narrow because there is usually no interventricular conduction disturbance.
- It is not be as frequent the association of atrial fibrillation during concomitant crisis.

3.2.3 Prognosis

No studies have shown an increased risk of sudden death or reduced survival for patients meeting the criteria for the diagnosis of LGL.

3.2.4 Current therapeutic bases

Rarely, the drug medical therapy can have failures usually, but there are patients in who there is not effective (for patients who continue to have recurrent and intolerable symptoms). In such extreme cases are used:

- Radiofrequency ablation (RF).
- The external pacemaker.
- The Implantable Cardioverter Defibrillators (ICDs).

This destroys the accessory pathway using a catheter (tube) inserted into the body to reach the heart. The success rate of this procedure ranges between 85 and 95% depending on the location of the extra or additional route.

Digoxin, verapamil and beta-blockers (other drugs commonly used to treat other types of tachycardia) can increase the frequency of episodes of tachycardia in some people with this syndrome. Beta-blockers may increase cardiac depression.

We can use drugs such as adenosine (Inpatient), and amiodarone to control or prevent episodes of tachycardia.

For the control of tachycardia is usually proceed according to the severity of the implementation of vagal maneuvers carotid massage type and Valsalva maneuver (forced expiratory made with the nose and mouth closed).

3.2.5 Typical ECG image of the Lown-Ganong-Levine

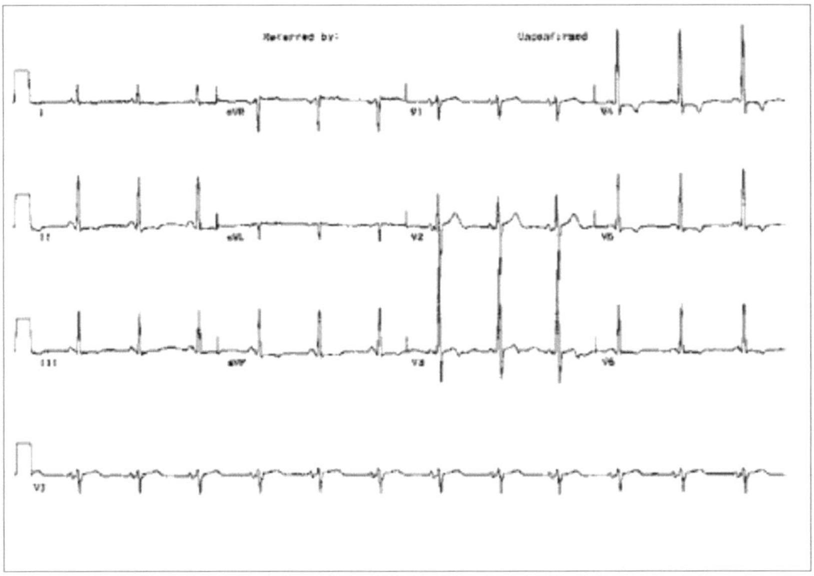

3.3 Short PR-interval alongside short QT-interval on the same person (Breijo's pattern)

In 2006, Breijo-Marquez, Pardo Ríos et al. evaluated a series of young patients, who had had, since childhood, many episodes of nocturnal palpitations, chest pain, full loss of consciousness (syncope), and which were accompanied by tonic-clonic seizures. All had been diagnosed and treated as epileptic episodes. Treatment outcomes were null. They were always considered as normal, in every cardiac studies performed absolutely [Breijo-Marquez, FR., 2008].

However, all these patients had an ECG recording common:

"A PR-interval lesser than 0,120 seconds with a QTc-interval equal to or lesser than 0.350 seconds".

That is, a pattern of short PR and QTc in the same person.

The correct treatment was begun (beta-blockers and, in some cases, an implantable cardio defibrillator, ICD.). Was removed all treatment from epilepsy.

The outcome to date is satisfactory.

Although we don't know, with certainty, the etiology of this pattern of ECG to date, we know that there were two important confusions:

First. - The physicians mistook to syncopal episode, with an epileptic episode.

Second. - The syncopal episodes are due to a cardiac disorder (was a cardiogenic syncope due to a cardiac electrical systole's alteration).

This ECG recording may be easily confused with a Lown-Ganong-Levine, since both have a short PR-interval. Nevertheless, in this type of ECG pattern there is also a short QTc-interval.

Unfortunately, both entities are confused with epileptic episodes too often.

Sudden cardiac death is extremely frequent in this type of event.

3.3.1 Typical ECG image of the "short PR alongside short QT" intervals in the same person (Breijo's Pattern)

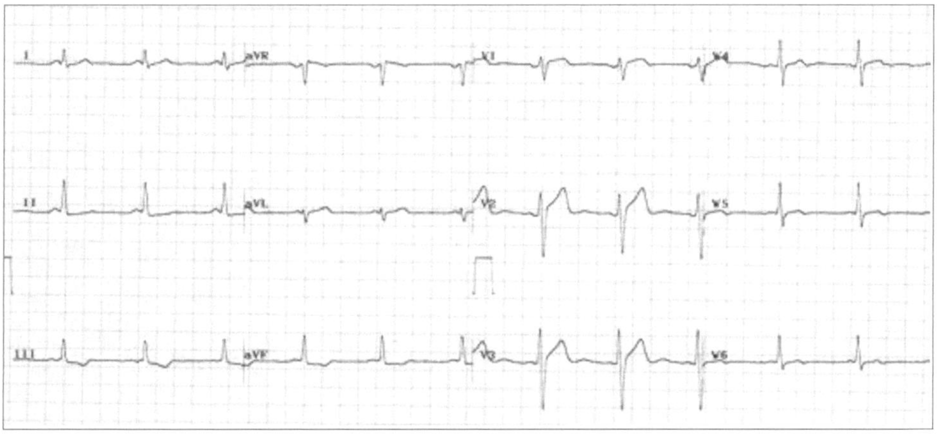

This ECG recording was the first with 12 leads that was obtained from our Hospital from Boston. MA. The patient was a 17 years-old male. We can see a shortening of the PR and QT intervals (Bazett), especially in inferior and left precordial leads. PR-interval length is lesser than 0.120 seconds and QTc length is lesser than 0.350 seconds. Patient had the symptoms exposed previously. He was also diagnosed for epileptic episodes. However, he had syncopal episodes and two cardiac arrests by cardiological disturbances.

3.4 Mahaim syndrome

Mahaim syndrome is characterized by:

The PR- interval with a standard length. Presence of pseudo-delta wave in the initial phase of the QRS complex because the sinus stimulus enters to AV node where physiological suffers a delay and then depolarizes the ventricles by an abnormal way: Mahaim fibers [Mahaim, I., 1937]

That is:

- PR-interval with a normal length.
- Wide QRS complexes.

3.4.1 Typical ECG image of the Mahaim's syndrome

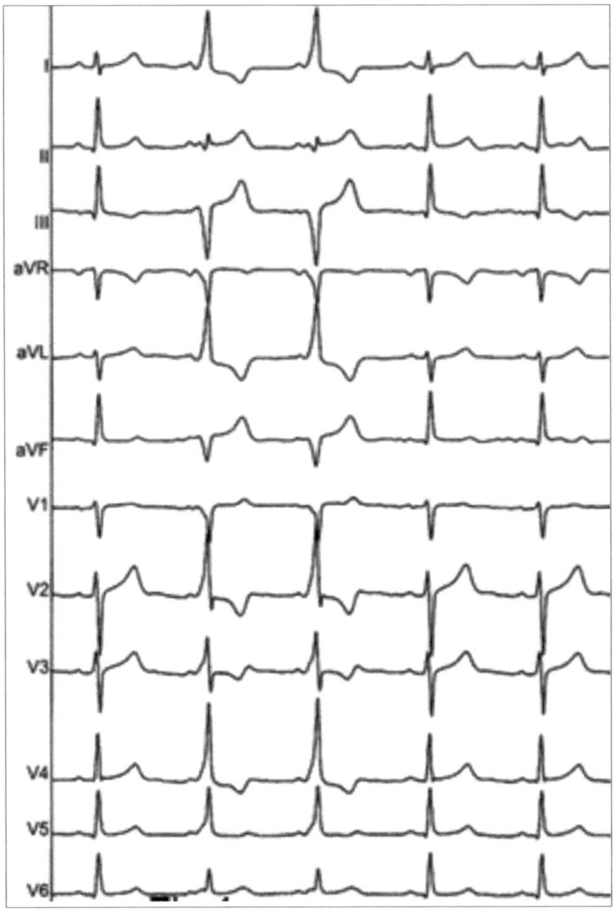

4. Differential diagnosis among various entities with alterations in electrical cardiac systole

ENTITY.	PR-interval	QRS complex	QTc -interval
W.P.W	Short.	Wide (δ-wave)	Normal
L.G.L	Short	Normal	Normal
Mahaim	Normal or Short	Normal or wide	Normal
Breijo's Pattern	Short	Normal	Short

Differential diagnosis, based on the characteristics from the different intervals and complex.

5. Some variations in electrical cardiac systole that can cause sudden death

(All these examples were discovered by Breijo-Marquez, FR. et al. They are still very underdiagnosed).

1. WOLFF-PARKINSON-WHITE AND PROLONGED"Q-T"PATTERNS IN THE SAME ELECTROCARDIOGRAPHIC RECORD [Breijo-Marquez, FR., 2011].

Wolff-Parkinson-White syndrome (WPWS) is a congenital heart disease (PRKAG2. Genetic map 7q36) characterised by a premature ventricular depolarisation caused by an abnormal atrioventricular accessory pathway known as Kent's bundle. Prolonged QT syndrome (PQTS) consists of an abnormal prolongation of the QT interval on the ECG, which can be both inherited and acquired. This anomaly is known to favour the occurrence of malign cardiac arrhythmias, above all polymorphic ventricular tachycardia, ventricular fibrillation and "torsade de pointes".

When taken separately, both syndromes have little incidence, which leads us to expect this incidence to be even lower when they are found on the same electrocardiogram. Incidentally, the current medical literature contains no publications on this topic. This clinical case aims to establish the existence of an electrocardiographic pattern characterised by WPW and a PQTS pattern on an ECG record. With a high susceptibility to crisis of tachycardia, especially at night, several episodes of syncope, even cardiac arrest and sudden cardiac death.

The patient is a 24 old- years man. Since childhood, he has suffered from more than four tachycardia attacks, three documented syncope episodes, as well as two cardiac arrests recovered, for which he was treated with electric discharges. Afterwards, he was treated with radiofrequency ablation of Kent's bundle, with permanent positive results so far.

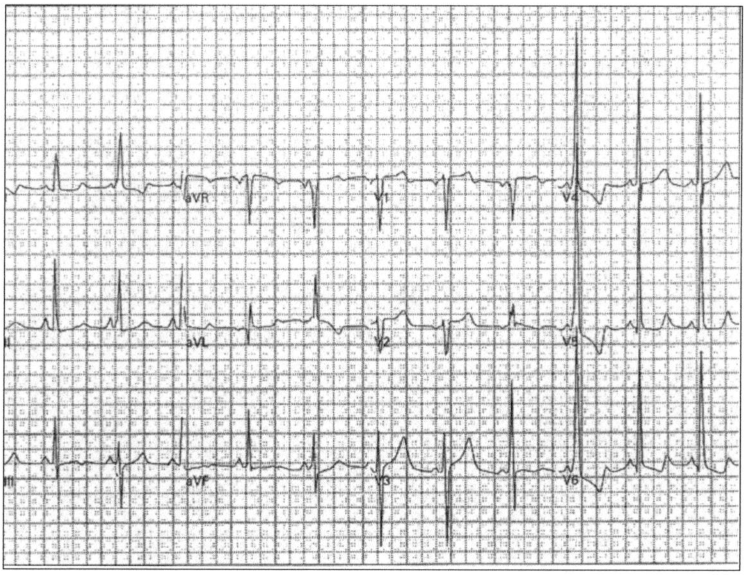

ECG' Image.

We can see a typical ECG recording of an intermittent WPW and a Long QT-interval together in a patient with several syncopal episodes and a recovered cardiac arrest.

2. ECG PATTERNS WITH SHORT PR INTERVAL TOGETHER TO A LONG QT (A) AND FIRST-DEGREE AV BLOCK ALONGSIDE A LONG QT (B: INCREASED OF CARDIAC ELECTRICAL SYSTOLE). [Breijo Marquez, FR., 2009].

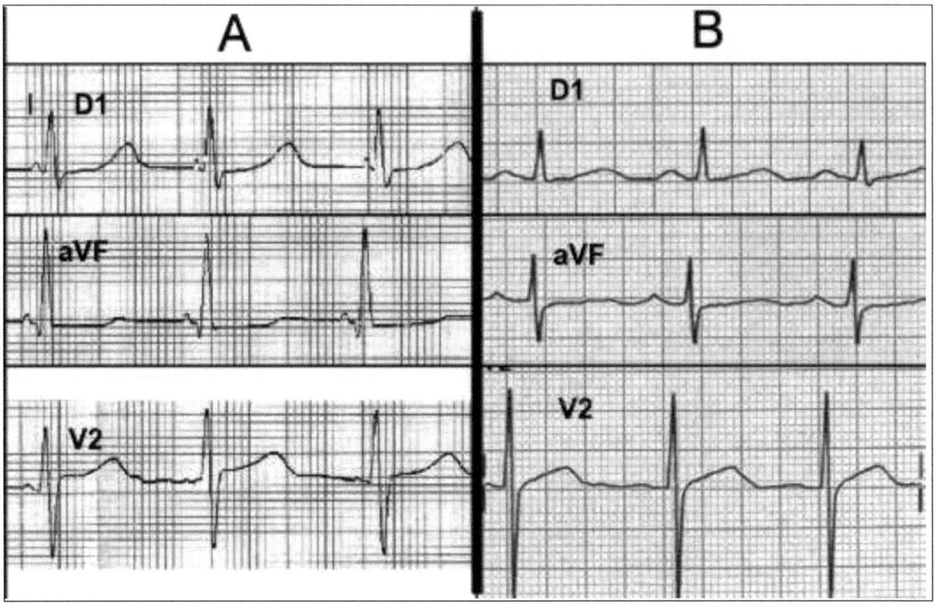

In this exposition, we present the ECG record of two patients with an obvious diversity and variability of alterations in the electrical system of heart. These electrical cardiac disturbances could explain completely the symptomatology from patients: nocturnal palpitations, several syncopal episodes.

In Figure A, we can see the presence of a short PR-interval together to a Long QT-interval. In Figure B, we can also see an ECG recording with a Long PR-interval alongside a Long QT-interval.

3. PRESENCE OF A CRITICAL STENOSIS IN LEFT ANTERIOR DESCENDING CORONARY ARTERY ALONGSIDE A SHORT "P-R" AND "Q-T" PATTERN, IN THE SAME ELECTROCARDIOGRAPHIC RECORD [Breijo-Márquez, FR., 2010].

The knowledge of the heart and its functions is increasing every day. However, many cardiac dysfunctions remain undocumented.

One of them might be the presence of the Wellens' sign, minimally elevated or isoelectric ST segments, and inverted T waves in the precordial leads, without changes in the QRS complex, together with a shortened of "P-R and Q-T intervals" in the same electrocardiographic record. Both patterns are greatly underdiagnosed. The risk implied by the aforementioned underdiagnosis could have lethal consequences because the inherent problems in a short "P-R"-"Q-T" pattern could be added to those inherent in Wellens' sign.

Hereby, we set out to show both the description of the clinical case and the electrocardiogram (ECG) recording of a male having previously mentioned collection of symptoms.

The patient is a 42-year-old single man, previously diagnosed with unstable angina, who is an occasional smoker with arterial hypertension and who was prescribed a felodipine (5 mg/d) and ramipril (5 mg/d) treatment. The patient was complaining about an intense, oppressive, and progressive pain in the chest, which bore no relation to physical effort. The pain radiated toward both jaws and was accompanied by acute autonomic symptoms.

The sublingual administration of nitrates proved to be effective and led to a reduction of the pain as well as an improvement in the alterations the patient was showing. The ECG at presentation showed ST-segment elevations by more than 2 mm in all the precordial leads except lead one. The laboratory tests verified myocardial injury: L-lactate dehydrogenase, 1.220 UI/L (reference range, 230-460 UI/L);creatine kinase, 560 U/L (reference range, 37-290 U/L); creatine kinase], 1.85-14.45 U/L); aspartate transaminase, 376 U/L (reference range, 3-40 UI/L); alanine transaminase, 121 U/L (reference range, 5-37 UI/L); and troponin, 3.5 µg/L (Reference range, 0-0.1 ng/mL).

In spite of the elevated biochemical markers of myocardial injury, the case was classified as an unstable angina variant.

The patient made full recovery as well as radical improvement of the clinical manifestations after the administration of nitrates (b30 minutes). As soon as the patient was clinically stabilized and the enzymatic levels regained their stability, the patient was discharged. He was also given a medical appointment in the hospital 10 days later so that he could be submitted to a new evaluation (We must add that, we do not know why the patient was not studied according to international guidelines during his first cardiac evaluation: angiography study within 24 hours at least). The patient showed no symptoms whatsoever when he returned home.

However, the patient returned to the hospital before his appointment was scheduled, describing similar symptoms to those, he had previously been afflicted by, but complaining, they were more acute and persistent.

That is the reason why the patient was automatically transferred to intensive care, where he was diagnosed with Wellens' sign.

After the patient was clinically and hemodynamically stabilized, he underwent a battery of diagnostic tests, which included an angiographic study, an echocardiogram and a single-photon emission computed tomography (SPECT) study.

Interestingly enough, the patient was reported to have had 3 short syncope attacks, from which he had fully recovered. He also had several nocturnal palpitation episodes, which were diagnosed as idiopathic supraventricular tachycardia.

As far as his family clinical history is concerned, an uncle on his father's side is known to have died of sudden death at the age of 46. His father had a history of acute coronary syndrome with ECG changes confined to the anterolateral leads.

The Wellens' sign represents an evolutionary stage of ST elevation acute coronary syndrome. Today, most of the patients are classified as non-ST elevation myocardial infarction, as they will have elevated troponin levels. Some patients are classified as unstable angina. The patients have similar symptoms: severe oppressive chest pain and radiation of the pain to different segments over a short period, but they usually respond to the administration of nitrates very quickly. Electrocardiographically speaking, the patients have very characteristic patterns: T-wave symmetrical inversion, with occasionally very deep T waves in precordial derivations, especially in V3 to V4, although these characteristics may extend to all the precordial derivations.

The Wellens' sign is associated with a critical stenosis in the left anterior descending coronary artery. Before the widespread implementation of invasive cardiology and effective antithrombotic therapy, 3 of 4 patients with this ECG pattern developed a usually extensive anterior myocardial infarction within a few weeks of admission. Our patient had bypass surgery.

Breijo et al. described the pattern of short "P-R and Q-T" intervals in 2006. It is characterized by the presence of an ECG with a P-R interval lesser than 0.12 seconds and the Q-T interval lesser than 0.350 seconds and, which, in more than 80% of cases, is accompanied by syncope episodes, nocturnal tachycardia, and occasionally, by ventricular fibrillation and even sudden death.

The key to an accurate diagnosis of both dysfunctions must begin with a detailed analysis of all the symptoms reported by the patient. The ECG recording provides an almost definitive confirmation:

- The T-wave characteristics in precordial derivations.
- The duration of P-R and Q-T intervals.

5.1 Typical images of ECG recording (A: Crisis of myocardial infarction. B: Recovered)

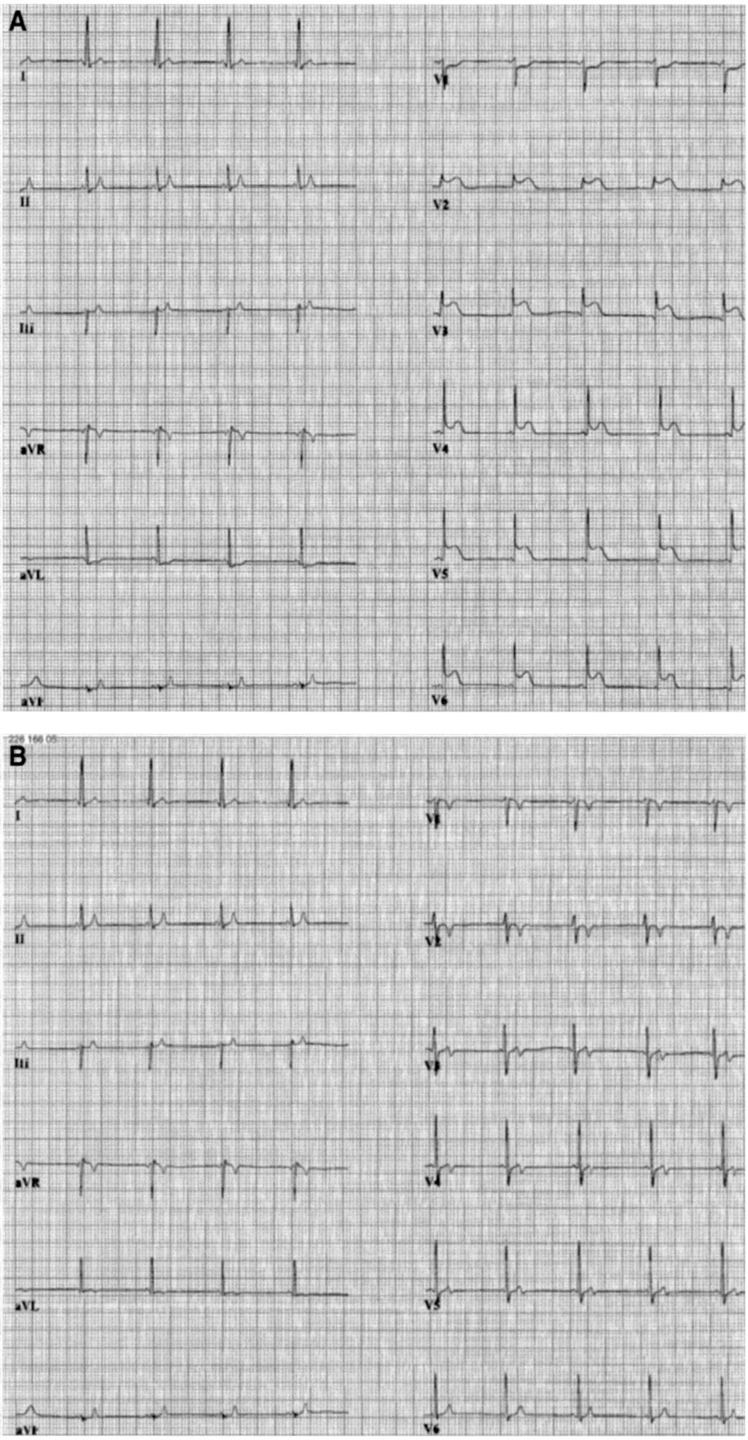

5.2 Thoughts about the patterns described above

All have a clear variation in the electrical cardiac systole.
All have a strong tendency to produce events of tachycardia / ventricular fibrillation.
Hence, all have a great capacity to produce cardiac arrest which, if not adequately diagnosed and treated, will inevitably occur sudden cardiac death.

6. Acknowledgements

To Lourdes and Alejandro Breijo, for their unselfishness collaboration from Miami. Florida. USA.
To Guadalupe Moreno Galisteo, whose smile always encouraged me to work.

7. References

Alboni P, Alboni M, Bertorelle G. (2008) The origin of vasovagal syncope: to protect the heart or to escape predation? *Clin Auton Res*, Vol.18, pp. 170-8.

Breijo Marquez, FR. Pardo Ríos, M. (2009). Variability and diversity of electrical cardiac systole. *BMJ Case Reports,* doi:10.1136/bcr.06.2008.0284.

Breijo Marquez, FR. Pardo Ríos, M. Alcaraz Baños, M. (2010). Association of Short PR Interval, Long QT Interval, and Sudden Cardiac Death in a Young Male. *Rev Esp Cardiol*, Vol. 63, pp. 362-4.

Breijo-Marquez, FR. (2008). Decrease of electrical cardiac systole. *Int J. Cardiol,* Vol. 126, pp. 36-8.

Breijo-Márquez, FR. Pardo Rios, M. (2010). Presence of a critical stenosis in left anterior descending coronary artery alongside a short "P-R" and "Q-T" pattern, in the same electrocardiographic record. *J Electrocardiology* , pp. 422-424.

Breijo-Marquez, FR. Pardo Ríos, M. (2010). Sudden cardiac death in a young adult with diagnosed with Tietze syndrome. *Rev. Esp. Dolor*, Vol. 56, pp. 321-6.

Breijo-Marquez, FR. Pardo Ríos, M. (2011). Wolff-Parkinson-White and Prolonged "Q-T" Patterns in the Same Electrocardiographic Record. *J Clinic Experiment Cardiol*, Vol. 2, pp. 118-20.

Brignole M, Alboni P, Benditt DG, Bergfeldt L, Blanc JJ, Bloch Thomsen PE, et al. (2004) Task Force on Syncope, European Society of Cardiology. Guidelines on management (diagnosis and treatment) of syncope —update 2004, *Europace*, Vol. 6, pp.467-537.

Brignole M, Gianfranchi L, Menozzi C, Raviele A, Oddone D, Lolli G, et al. (1993). Role of autonomic reflexes in syncope associated with paroxysmal atrial fibrillation. J *Am Coll Cardiol*, Vol. 22, pp 1123-9.

Consensus statement on the definition of orthostatic hypotension, pure autonomic failure, and multiple system atrophy. (1996). *J Neurol Sci*, Vol.144, pp. 218-9.

Ebert SN, Liu XK, Woosley RL. (1998). Female gender as a risk factor for drug-induced cardiac arrhythmias: evaluation of clinical and experimental evidence. J Womens Health, Vol.7, pp. 547-57.

Gibbons CH, Freeman R. (2006). Delayed orthostatic hypotension: a frequent cause of orthostatic intolerance. *Neurology*, Vol. 67, pp. 28-32.

Grubb BP, Kosinski DJ, Boehm K, Kip K. (1997). The postural orthostatic tachycardia syndrome: a neurocardiogenic variant identified during head-up tilt table testing. *Pacing Clin Electrophysiol*, Vol. 20, pp. 2205-12.

Hoefnagels WA, Padberg GW, Overweg J, Van der Velde EA, Roos RA. (1991) Transient loss of consciousness: the value of the history for distinguishing seizure from syncope. *J Neuro,* Vol. 238, pp. 39-43.

Leitch JW, Klein GJ, Yee R, Leather RA, Kim YH. (1992). Syncope associated with supraventricular tachycardia: an expression of tachycardia or vasomotor response? *Circulation,* Vol. 85, pp. 1064-71.

Lombroso CT, Lerman P. (1967). Breathholding spells (cyanotic and pallid infantile syncope). *Pediatrics,* Vol. 39, pp. 563-81.

Mathias CJ, Mallipeddi R, Bleasdale-Barr K. (1999). Symptoms associated with orthostatic hypotension in pure autonomic failure and multiple system atrophy. *J Neurol,* Vol. 246, pp. 893-8.

Naschitz J, Rosner I. (2007). Orthostatic hypotension: framework of the syndrome. *Postgrad Med J,* Vol. 83, pp. 568-74.

Podoleanu C, Maggi R, Brignole M, Croci F, Incze A, Solano A, et al. (2006). Lower limb and abdominal compression bandages prevent progressive orthostatic hypotension in the elderly. A randomized placebo-controlled study. *J Am Coll Cardiol,* Vol.48, pp. 1425-32.

Soteriades ES, Evans JC, Larson MG, Chen MH, Chen L, Benjamin EJ, Levy D. (2002). Incidence and prognosis of syncope, *N Engl J Med,* Vol. 347, pp.878-85.

Stephenson J. (1990) Fits and Faints. Oxford: Blackwell Scientific Publications. pp. 41-57.

Strickberger SA, Benson DW, Biaggioni I, Callans DJ, Cohen MI, Ellenbogen KA, et al. (2006). American Heart Association Councils on Clinical Cardiology, Cardiovascular Nursing, Cardiovascular Disease in the Young, and Stroke; Quality of Care and Outcomes Research Interdisciplinary Working Group; American College of Cardiology Foundation; Heart Rhythm Society. AHA/ACCF scientific statement on the evaluation of syncope. *J Am Coll Cardiol,* Vol. 47, pp. 473-84.

Tea SH, Mansourati J, L'Heveder G, Mabin D, Blanc JJ. (1996). New insights into the pathophysiology of carotid sinus syndrome. *Circulation,* Vol. 93, pp. 1411-6.

Thijs RD, Benditt DG, Mathias CJ, Schondorf R, Sutton R, Wieling W, et al. (2005) Unconscious confusion —a literature search for definitions of syncope and related disorders. *Clin Auton Res,* Vol .15, pp. 35-9.

Van Dijk JG, Sheldon R. (2008). Is there any point to vasovagal syncope? *Clin Auton Res,* Vol.18, pp. 167-9.

Verheyden B, Gisolf J, Beckers F, Karemaker JM, Wesseling KH, Aubert A, et al. (2007). Impact of age on the vasovagal response provoked by sublingual nitroglycerine in routine tilt testing. *Clin Sci (Lond),* Vol.113, pp. 329-37.

Wieling W, Ganzeboom KS, Saul JP. (2004). Reflex syncope in children and adolescents. *Heart,* Vol.90, pp. 1094-100.

Wieling W, Krediet P, Van Dijk N, Linzer M, Tschakovsky M. (2007). Initial orthostatic hypotension: review of a forgotten condition. *Clin Sci (Lond),* Vol. 112, pp.1 57-65.

Zareba W, Moss AJ, Le Cessie S, Locati EH, Robinson JL, Hall WJ, Andrews ML. (1995). Risk of cardiac events in family members of patients with Long QT syndrome. *J Am Coll Cardiol,* Vol. 26, pp.1685-91.

16

Bradycardia in Children During General Anaesthesia

Judith A. Lens[1], Jeroen Hermanides[1], Peter L. Houweling[1], Jasper J. Quak[2] and David R. Colnot[2]
[1]*Diakonessenhuis Utrecht, Departments of Anaesthesiology*
[2]*Otolaryngology/Head and Neck Surgery*
The Netherlands

1. Introduction

Bradycardia in association with anaesthesia may lead to insufficient cardiac output and decreased delivery of oxygen to vital organs. In children the heart rate is the dominant factor for cardiac output, since the developing heart is less compliant and contractile and stroke volume cannot increase much. Thus, when bradycardia occurs in children during anaesthesia, cardiac output falls and may lead to serious cardiac arrhythmias and even cardiac arrest. In this chapter, the incidence, causes and risk factors, as well as the consequences and possible treatment of bradycardia in children during general anaesthesia are described and discussed. A focus is made on the incidence and causes of bradycardia in children undergoing adenotonsillectomy under general anaesthesia.

2. Bradycardia and general anaesthesia in children

2.1 Physiology

The normal heart rate decreases with increasing age in children (Figure 1). Therefore, a heart rate less then 100 beats per minute in very young children is a bradycardia by definition. For children 3 years of age, this means a heart rate less then 65 beats per minute. In the first months after birth, the risk for bradycardia is even higher as a result of an autonomic imbalance in the heart innervation (Rothrock, 2004).
Causes for bradycardia can be either intrinsic (e.g. cardiac abnormalities), or extrinsic (e.g. medication). During general anaesthesia children are at an increased risk of bradycardia in case of hypoxemia or hypervagotonia. Hypoxemia can be caused by administration of anaesthetics or other medication. Hypervagotonia can be evoked by oesophageal or nasal stimulation as a consequence of anaesthesia, for example in case of endotracheal intubation. However, surgery can also cause hypervagotonia by manipulation of the head or neck region, which is especially the case in otolaryngology. Among otolaryngology surgical procedures, adenotonsillectomy is a procedure likely to be responsible for direct stimulation of the vagal nerve. This stimulation is caused by placement of the mouth gag and the instruments used during the surgical procedure and the manipulation in the mouth and oropharynx. Together with placement of ventilation tubes, adenotonsillectomy is one of the most frequently performed types of surgery in children worldwide.

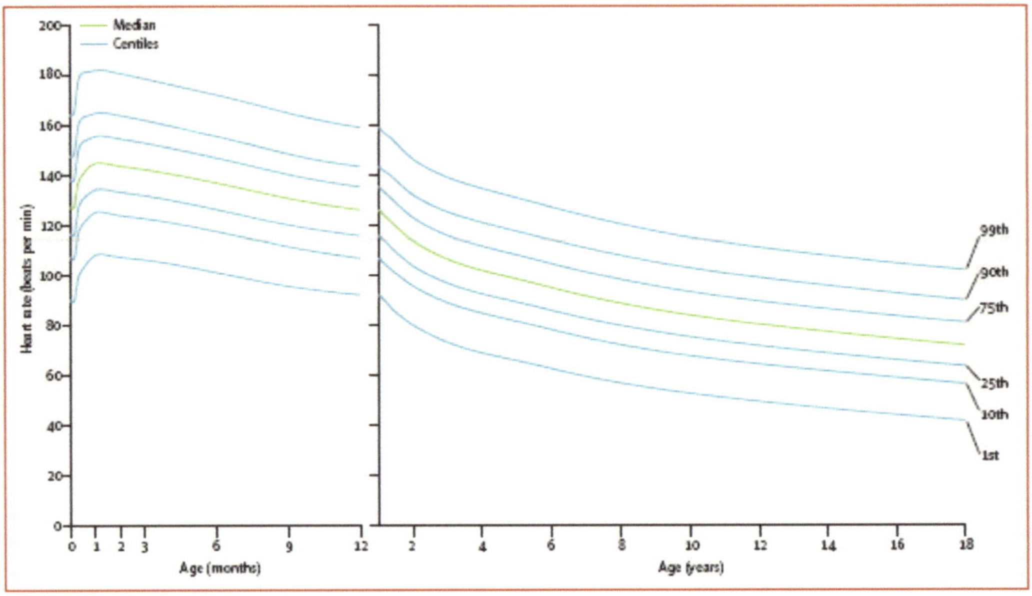

Fig. 1. Heart rate values in centiles from birth to age 18. (Fleming et al, 2011)

2.2 Aetiology

Bradycardia during general anaesthesia can have different causes, and depending on patient characteristics and conditions, the sequelae can be serious. Especially in children, bradycardia can lead to failure of cardiac output and may also lead to serious cardiac arrhythmias and even cardiac arrest. In a study performed by the Australian Patient Safety Foundation, the first 4000 incidents reported to the Australian Incident Monitoring Study (AIMS) were analysed for the incident bradycardia. A total of 265 reports describing bradycardia in both adults and children during anaesthesia were extracted and studied (Watterson et al., 2005). In general, bradycardia was associated with hypotension in 51% of cases, cardiac arrest in 25% of cases and hypertension in one case. In 22% of reports apparent desaturation or an abnormality of ventilation was described. The authors concluded that cardiopulmonary events causing bradycardia are more likely than other causes to be associated with cardiac arrest. The causes of bradycardia were drug events in 28% of cases, airway related events in 16%, autonomic reflexes in 14%, and regional anaesthesia in 9% of the cases. Most episodes of bradycardia occurred during surgery (61%), whereas 20% was observed before and during induction.

In 43 of these 265 reports, bradycardia occurred in children under the age of 14 years. The distribution of ASA grading in children was similar to that of adults, but the haemodynamic profile was different for children as compared to adults. Whereas in adults airway and drug events together were responsible for 44% of causes, in children up to 75% of bradycardias were associated with airway and drug events. Airway events were the predominant cause of bradycardia in children (47%). In 51% of children studied there was no abnormality of blood pressure, which was attributed to the high incidence of airway events, in which hypoxaemia was associated with rapid deterioration in heart rate. Hypotension was present in 21% of the cases, but cardiac arrest was described in 32% of the cases. Whereas a good

outcome was reported in 63% of both adults and children, in only 48% of incidents concerning children a good outcome was reported. This might indicate that an incident during general anaesthesia with bradycardia in children has an important risk of poor outcome.
An epidemiologic study by Keenan and co-workers on bradycardia during anaesthesia concluded from data abstracted from almost 8,000 anaesthetic records of children 0-4 years of age that the frequency of bradycardia was 1.27% in the age group 0-1 years of age. This was considerably less in the older age groups, that is 0.65% and 0.16% in the 3rd and 4th year of age, respectively (Keenan et al., 1994). Causes of bradycardia included disease or surgery in 35%, inhalation anaesthetics in 35%, and hypoxaemia in 22% of children. Hypotension was observed in 10% of patients, whereas asystole of ventricular fibrillation occurred in 10%. All children underwent non-cardiac surgery and brdaycardia was defined as heart rate lower than 100 beats per minute. The study population was considerably younger than in the study described by Watterson. The authors concluded that bradycardia was more frequent in very young children aged 0-1 years undergoing anaesthesia, and that it was associated with substantial morbidity such as hypotension and asystole.

2.3 Airway related

The laryngeal reflex prevents foreign substances from entering into the lower airway and maintaining upper airway integrity. However, in some circumstances the laryngeal reflexes can induce cardiorespiratory events, that can even lead to life-threatening events such as apnea or even death. Gastroesophageal and pharyngolaryngeal refluxes are associated with both bradycardia and apnea, and may play a role in acute life threatening events (ALTE) or sudden infant death syndrome (SIDS). In airway management during general anaesthesia the laryngeal reflex can cause bradycardia by vagal stimulation and apnoea (Reix et al., 2007). In procedures especially during induction of anaesthesia, such as intubation, bradycardia and apnoea can be provoked. Other manoeuvres, like inserting a nasal feeding tube or head manipulation after endotracheal intubation, can induce bradycardia in a later phase of anaesthesia. In newborns and infants the upper airway sensitivity is even increased due to the immaturity of the chemo- and mechanoreceptors in the larynx. The innervation of the larynx is displayed in Figure 2.
In airway management during anaesthesia, the incidence of bradycardia is reported to be 0.5-4.2%, and the risk is increased when children are younger (Keenan et al., 1994, Fastle and Roback, 2004; Gencorelli et al., 2010). In an analysis of bradycardia incidents during anaesthesia, 20% of bradycardia events occurred in the pre-induction or induction phase (Watterson et al. 2005). In a large study population of 1070 children aged 3–12 years who underwent rapid sequence induction for intubation, bradycardia was observed in 5 patients (0.5%). Bradycardia was defined as a heart rate lower than 60 beats per minute. In the same study group, moderate hypoxemia with SaO_2 of 80-89% was observed in 20 patients (1.9%) and 18 patients (1.7%) developed severe hypoxemia with SaO_2 lower than 80%. The risk for hypoxemia was increased when the weight was below 20 kg (Gencorelli et al., 2010). In another group of 163 children undergoing rapid sequence induction for intubation, the incidence of bradycardia was 4%. The median age was 12 months (range 3 months to 19 years), which might explain the higher incidence of bradycardia. Definition of bradycardia was a heart rate falling two standard deviations below normal for age as described by the American Heart Association (Table 1).

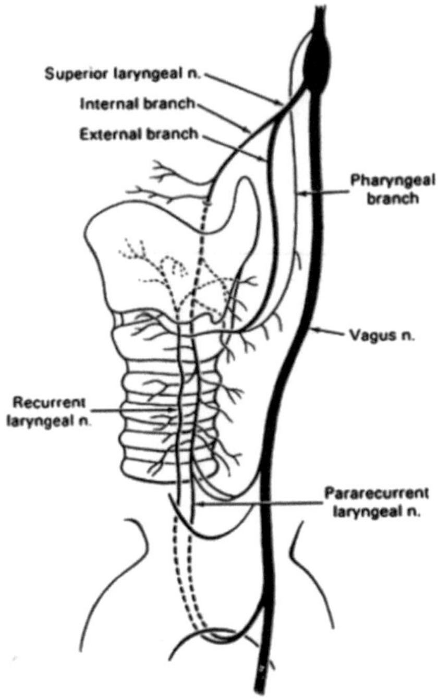

Fig. 2. Innervation of the larynx, reproduced from Reix et al, 2007

Age	Heart Rate
0-3 months	85-205
3 months to 2 years	100-190
2-10 years	60-140
>10 years	60-100

Table 1. The 95% confidence interval for normal heart rates in children (American Heart Association).

Analysis of the children with bradycardia showed hypoxemia prior to the bradycardia in 4 out of 6 patients. Most of the patients were intubated for respiratory disease (45%), trauma (19%), or seizures (12%). All bradycardia episodes resolved with ventilation or after endotracheal intubation (Fastle and Roback, 2004). In a series of 475 children (aged 1–22 years) who underwent operative intervention for post-tonsillectomy haemorrhage, bradycardia during rapid sequence induction was observed in 20 (4.2%) of patients. Bradycardia was defined as a heart rate lower than 60 beats per minute, appearing in at least two consecutive recorded vital signs, 15 seconds apart. In total 9.9% of the studied cohort had a moderate or severe hypoxemic event. Moderate hypoxemia was defined as $SaO_2 < 90\%$, and severe hypoxemia was defined as $SaO_2 < 80\%$. All bradycardia events resolved without pharmacological intervention (Fields et al., 2010).

2.4 Medication related

Many drugs used in the operating theatre can cause bradycardia. Calcium-channel blockers and ß-blockers are specifically used to slow heart rate. Also amiodarone has calcium channel and ß-blocking properties. Most anaesthetics used during general anaesthesia have the potential of inducing bradycardia. In an extensive meta-analysis, propofol was associated with increased risk of bradycardia, also when compared to other anaesthetics (Tramèr et al., 1997), an odds ratio of 2.3 is thereby reported. Although it is difficult to compare the different trials, it seems clear that propofol carries an evident risk of bradycardia. The risk of death after bradycardia during propofol anaesthesia was 1.4/100.000. However, propofol is often administered together with opioids and muscle relaxants, which are also associated with bradycardia. By stimulation of the muscarinic receptors of the heart, suxamethonium (a depolarizing muscle relaxant) can cause bradycardia. Case reports on the occurrence of bradycardia or even asystole with the use of succinylcholine have been published (Delphin et al., 1987). However, incidence numbers are lacking. Also other non-depolarizing muscle relaxants and opioids like fentanyl or remifentanil have been associated with development of bradycardia in a meta-analysis of 85 randomised, controlled trials (Komatsu et al., 2007). Clonidine, an α-2-receptoragonist which is frequently used in addition to local anaesthesia, can also elicit bradycardia (Pöpping et al., 2009). From the vapour anaesthetics, halothane has been associated with the most cardiovascular changes, including bradycardia especially in adenotonsillectomy (van Nouhuys, 1973; Slappendel & Rutten, 1989). Data on bradycardia and the use of sevoflurane, isoflurane and desflurane is scarce. Thus, many drugs used in the perioperative period have been more or less associated with bradycardia. It is however difficult to elucidate which drugs contribute most to this risk, as randomized trials are lacking and most drugs are administered simultaneously.

2.5 Premedication with atropine

As discussed before, children that need endotracheal intubation commonly develop bradycardia. In literature there is discussion about the effect of premedication with atropine in children under the age of 5. Some authors advise atropine as pretreatment in all children under 1 year of age receiving succinylcholine and all patient with profound bradycardia during intubation. As stated earlier, bradycardia during intubation is probably due to combined vagal response and hypoxia. During intubation the vagal nerve is activated and because the parasympathetic-sympathetic imbalance in young children, this reaction is more profound in children. This imbalance disappears at the age of one year (Rothrock and Pagane, 2005). By administrating atropine, or other anticholinergic medication, the incidence of bradycardia could decrease. Atropine inhibits the binding of acetylcholine on the muscarinereceptors, thereby diminishing the vagal response and bradycardia. On the other hand, atropine can induce dysrhythmias, such as tachycardia. It has some side-effects that could be unwanted, such as malignant hyperthermia, seizure and an increased risk of aspiration by relaxation of the lower oesophageal sphincter. In case of underdosing of atropine, there is a chance of provoking bradycardia. In case of overdosing, ventricular dysrhythmias and tachyarrhythmia may occur.

The review of Fleming and co-workers is a good overview of the evidence pro and contra the use of atropine. Most evidence for the use of atropine as a standard in all children under the age of 18 is from before 1990. Halothane and repeated succinylcholine was often used in that period. Therefore there was an increased risk for bradycardia. Nowadays, incidence of bradycardia is decreased because other anaesthetics showing less side-effects are used. Considering the disadvantage of atropine, it can be stated that standard premedication is not advised (Fleming et al., 2005).

2.6 Physical status

Infants with a poor physical status have an increased risk for bradycardia. A higher ASA score is associated with more bradycardia, especially with an ASA score higher than 3. Infants with congenital diseases, especially heart disease may develop bradycardia easier and more prominent. Formally pre-mature infants have considerably more risk for apnoea and bradycardia. This can be associated with cardiac arrest and death. To reduce this risk, elective surgery should be postponed until after 55 weeks of post conceptual age. For explanation of ASA score, see Table 2.

ASA score	
1	A normal healthy patient
2	A patient with mild systemic disease
3	A patient with severe systemic disease
4	A patient with severe systemic disease that is a constant threat to life
5	A moribund patient who is not expected to survive without the operation
6	A declared brain-dead patient whose organs are being removed for donor purposes

Table 2. ASA classification system according to the American Society of Anaesthesiologists.

Children with Down syndrome have an increased risk of developing bradycardia during anaesthesia. Up to 50% of them have congenital cardiac abnormalities. But irrespective of the presence or absence of congenital heart disease, bradycardia as well as hypotension during anaesthetic induction in children with Down syndrome (n=567) occurred more frequently as compared to controls (Kraemer et al., 2010). Although patients with Down syndrome develop bradycardia at the same time after induction, the decrease in heart rate from baseline was greater in patients with Down syndrom as compared to healthy children (Bai et al., 2010).

The presence of obstructive sleep apnea-hyppopnea syndrome (OSAS) can influence the heart rate in children. Bradycardia is a common feature in children with OSAS during overnight sleep (Huang et al., 2008). Children woth OSAS undergoing adenotonsillectomy had more respiratory complications (Sanders et al., 2006).

2.7 Age

Cardiovascular and respiratory factors are the major causes of cardiopulmonary arrest in the pediatric population during anesthesia. Data from the American Society of Anesthesiologist Closed Claims Project showed that cardiopulmonary arrest during anesthesia in the pediatric population was different than in the adult population. In the pediatric population, cardiopulmonary arrest during anesthesia was commonly caused by respiratory events (inadequate ventilation with cyanosis and/or bradycardia proceding the cardiac arrest) and is more likely to result in mortality than in the adult cases. As known from the in 1994 founded Pediatric Perioperative Cardiac Arrest (POCA) registry anesthesia related cardiopulmonary arrest is fortunately an uncommon event, that is 1.4 per 10,000. It must, however, be emphasized that although cardiac arrest is rare significant, bradyarrhythmias must be treated immediately to prevent an irreversible cardiac arrest which occurs in 26% and have a mortality rate of 72% (Morray, 2010). Special precaution measurement should be considered in patients less than 1 year with severe underlying or concurrent disease having emergency surgery as they are the most at risk for a fatal outcome. In patients who are ASA 1 or 2, 64% of the cardiac arrests are medication-related arrests. In these patients conservative management includes removing or reducing the dose of drugs known to inhibit the sinus atrial node or removing the surgical stimulus (i.e oculocardia reflex). If this is not effective or possible, anticholinergics like atropine or sympathicomimetics (i.e. ephedrine, epinephrine, isoproterenol) must be considered. The risk of bradycardia and cardiovascular complications in children is inversely proportional to age.

2.8 Temperature

Lowering temperature is a risk for developing bradycardia, in children as well as in adults. In extreme cases of hypothermia (less than 32 °C), extreme bradycardia with a heart rate of less than 40 beats per minute may occur. In a case report concerning a child with an extreme bradycardia of 30 beats per minute at a temperature of 24.8°C, no serious effects in neurological outcome were observed (Balagna et al., 1999). In adults hypothermia is often deliberately used in patients after cardiac arrest to protect their brain. These patients have a better neurological outcome. In these adults, bradycardia is often monitored. Usually there is no decreased myocardial contractility (Polderman and Herold, 2009).

3. The incidence of bradycardia in children undergoing adenotonsillectomy

3.1 Incidence and surgical technique

Adenotonsillectomy is one of the most frequently performed types of surgery in children worldwide. The surgical rate in United States and England is approximately 50-65 per 10,000, respectively. In the Netherlands the surgical rate in 1998 was 115, and was even higher in the decades before (Van den Akker et al., 2004). In the last decade, the incidence of adenotonsillectomy has decreased to a surgical rate of 110 per 10,000 in 2008 (Prismant, 2010). In The Netherlands, the most frequently used surgical technique for adenotonsillectomy is the guillotine technique as described by Sluder in 1911. One of the advantages of the guillotine technique as compared to traditional dissection is a shorter duration of surgery (Mulder et al., 1995). Moreover, several studies have shown that the guillotine technique is less painful (Homer et al., 2000). Finally, there is less blood loss during surgery, and the incidence of postoperative haemorrhage is lower (Wake et al., 1989; Ünlü et al., 1992; Scheenstra et al., 2007; Lowe et al., 2007). The guillotine technique can be performed intubated and nonintubated under inhalation anaesthesia. A nonintubated adenotonsillectomy can be performed either in supine of sitting position.

Whereas the traditional dissection technique for adenotonsillectomy is the dominant technique worldwide, in The Netherlands guillotine adenotonsillectomy is most frequently performed, and in the majority of patients the surgery is performed nonintubated under inhalation anaesthesia (Tjon Pian Gi et al., 2010). For several years, there has been discussion about the ideal anaesthesia technique for adenotonsillectomy, either intubated or nonintubated. Those in favor of the intubated technique, claim that the most important reason to use endotracheal intubation is that the airway is secured, thus allowing the administration of inhalation anaesthetics and/or oxygen. Moreover, intubation could decrease the incidence of aspiration of blood or tissue, for example of the adenoid or tonsils. However, there is no evidence whether intubation indeed decreases the risk of aspiration of, for example, blood. In the nonintubated child, the short duration of anaesthesia and the fact that no intravenous muscle relaxantia are used, may allow the child to recover more quickly and thus decrease the risk of aspiration of blood, since laryngeal reflexes will be earlier as compared to intubated patients due to the use of more anaesthetics. This, among others, may be in favor of performing adenotonsillectomy nonintubated under inhalation anaesthesia. As already mentioned, the duration of surgery is substantially shorter. Moreover, the amount of inhalated anaesthetics administered to the child is less as compared to children undergoing adenotonsillectomy intubated. Only inhalation anaesthetics (sevoflurane) are necessary, whereas for the intubated technique muscle relaxantia are required. In a Dutch study performed by Mulder, it was found that the incidence of postoperative fever and pain was lower in children undergoing adenotonsillectomy under inhalation anaesthesia and nonintubated as compared to those undergoing the adenotonsillectomy intubated (Mulder et al., 1995). An explanation for this observation could be that intubation through an infection upper airway (tonsils) might facilitate spread of microorganisms to the lower respiratory tract. Another explanation was that the children undergoing adenotonsillectomy nonintubated had better laryngeal and tracheal reflexes, thus allowing a more effective removal of aspirated fluids by coughing direct postoperatively.

3.2 Hypoxemia and bradycardia in children undergoing adenotonsillectomy

Cardiac arrhythmias as a consequence of bradycardia have been described in children undergoing adenotonsillectomy with inhalation anaesthesia (Van Nouhuys, 1973; Slappendel and Rutten, 1989). The inhalation anaesthetics used in these studies were nitrous oxide, halothane and trichloroethylene. Although nitrous oxide is still used nowadays, the used of trichloroethylene and halothane has been decreased significantly. The different types of inhalation anaesthetics, and the specific type of surgery may well contribute to the occurrence of bradycardia. Only few studies have compared different anaesthesia techniques, nonintubated versus intubated, and comparison of the supine versus sitting position. In a prospective, randomised trial three groups of patients were compared (Knape, 1988). The first group of patients (n=42) underwent adenotonsillectomy with Sluder technique nonintubated, in a sitting position. In a second group of patients (n=42), the adenotonsillectomy was performed intubated. The third group (n=38) underwent circumcision nonintubated. Oxygen levels were registered using pletysmography. In this study, the pulse rate was not assessed. The incidence of hypoxemia was measured for each group. Hypoxemia was defined as SaO_2 lower than 90% and severe hypoxemia as SaO_2 lower than 75%. Nitrous oxide was used as inhalation anaesthetic, together with halothane, for all patients including those undergoing adenotonsillectomy intubated. The number of episodes per 100 patients was calculated for hypoxemia. In the nonintubated group undergoing adenotonsillectomy in a sitting position, the number of hypoxemia episodes was 331 per 100 patients, which was significantly higher than the incidence of hypoxemia in the group undergoing adenotonsillectomy with intubation, 29 per 100 patients. The incidence of hypoxemia in the control group undergoing circumcision was 32 per 100 patients. Severe hypoxemia with SaO_2 lower than 75% was only observed in the patients undergoing adenotonsillectomy in a sitting position and nonintubated. The incidence of severe hypoxemia was 117 per 100 patients. Hypoxemia occurred at the end of surgery and direct postoperatively in the nonintubated group undergoing adenotonsillectomy in a sitting position, whereas hypoxemia in the intubated group was seen after extubation. In the control group undergoing circumcision nonintubated hypoxemia was observed at the time the child got awake, indicating laryngospasm. In the study by van der Werff, a total of four groups were compared with different anaesthesia techniques (van der Werff et al., 1991). Children underwent adenotonsillectomy with Sluder technique nonintubated (n=20), adenoidectomy (n=20), adenotonsillectomy with Sluder technique nonintubated with placement of grommets (n=20), or only placement of grommets (n=20). All patients underwent surgery in a supine position. In none of the patient groups severe hypoxemia with SaO_2 lower than 75% was observed. In the group of patients undergoing adenotonsillectomy with Sluder technique nonintubated with placement of grommets, the mean SaO_2 was 94% versus 97% for the other groups. Wagemans performed continuous SaO_2 registration and assessment of pulse rate in 37 children undergoing adenotonsillectomy or placement of grommets under inhalation anaesthesia (Wagemans et al., 1991). Adenotonsillectomy was performed nonintubated, in a sitting position. Both groups received nitrous oxide and halothane as inhalation anaesthetics. Hypoxemia was defined as SaO_2 lower than 90% and bradycardia was defined as a heart frequency under 70 beats per minute. In the patients undergoing adenotonsillectomy, a mean SaO_2 of 94.7% was found, as compared to a mean SaO_2 of 96.5% in the patient group undergoing placements of grommets. This was not significantly different. In only one patient (5.3%) undergoing adenotonsillectomy a single SaO_2 lower than 90% was observed. The time of hypoxemia was 35 seconds and the lowest registration value of SaO_2 was 74%. Bradycardia was not observed in both groups. These findings were considerably different from those described by Knape, who found in 80% of patients hypoxemia with a SaO_2 lower than 90%. The authors concluded that the duration of surgery was increasingly shorter in their study population for adenotonsillectomy: 24 seconds versus 80 seconds in the patients studies by Knape. They concluded that the interaction between the anaesthesiologist and otolaryngologist was of great importance, resulting in a shorter duration of surgery. This leads to their conclusion that performing adenotonsillectomy under inhalation anaesthesia nonintubated in a sitting position, is a safe procedure. Based on these studies the Dutch Association of Otolaryngology and Head & Neck Surgery, in cooperation with the Dutch Institute for Healthcare Improvement (CBO) published the practice guideline 'Adenoid and tonsil disorders in secondary care' in 2008 (CBO, 2008). In this practice guideline, the advice was given to perform adenotonsillectomy using guillotine technique according to Sluder in a supine position if nonintubated inhalation anaesthesia is given.

In a study recently performed by our departments, we retrospectively analysed the incidence of hypoxemia and bradycardia in children undergoing adenotonsillectomy (Kretzschmar et al., 2010). Analysis was performed on a total of 2963 children who underwent adenotonsillectomy nonintubated in a sitting position. Hypoxemia was defined as a SaO_2 lower than 85% with a duration longer than 60 seconds. Incidental desaturation was defined as SaO_2 lower than 90%, with a duration shorter than 60 seconds. Bradycardia was defined as a heart frequency under 60 beats per minute, for longer than 30 seconds. Incidental bradycardia was defined as a heart frequency lower than 60 beats per minute for a duration shorter than 30 seconds. For both incidental desaturation and bradycardia, the incidence per 100 patients was calculated in order to compare our data with earlier studies described above. Sevoflurane was used as inhalation anaesthetic. Hypoxemia occurred in 132 patients (4.5%) and the incidence of incidental desaturations (SaO_2 lower than 90%) was 217 per 100 patients. In 1724 patients no incidental desaturations at all were seen. In 280 patients (9.4%) bradycardia was observed. The incidence of incidental bradycardia, a heart frequency lower than 60 beats per second but shorter than 30 seconds, was 234 per 100 patients. In 2683 patients (90.6%) bradycardia with a heart rate lower than 60 and a duration of more than 30 seconds did not occur. In 25 patients (0.8%) bradycardia and hypoxemia both occurred. The bradycardia was registered at the same moment or directly after hypoxemia in 3 of these 25 patients. All episodes were reversible and in none of the patients peri-operative complications due to hypoxemia or bradycardia were observed.

	No Hypoxemia	Hypoxemia	Total
No Bradycardia	2576 (86.9%)	107 (3.6%)	2683 (90.6%)
Bradycardia	255 (8.6%)	25 (0.8%)	280 (9.4%)
Total	2831 (95.5%)	132 (4.5%)	2963 (100%)

Table 3. Incidence of hypoxemia and bradycardia in patients undergoing adenotonsillectomy. Hypoxemia was defined as a SaO_2 lower than 85% with a duration longer than 60 seconds. Bradycardia was defined as a heart frequency under 60 beats per minute, for longer than 30 seconds.

Different explanations for the occurrence of bradycardia can be given. Bradycardia as a direct consequence of hypoxemia is one of these, and can indicate severe problems during anesthesia. This was only observed in 3 of the patients (0.001%), and was reversible in all of them. It seems that the specific type of surgery is more likely to cause the bradycardia. Due to the placement of the mouth gag and guillotine procedure with manipulation of the tissue of the pharyngeal wall it is likely that the vagus nerve is stimulated leading to a reflex of lowering the heart rate.

We concluded that bradycardia and hypoxemia both occur during adenotonsillectomy nonintubated in a sitting position. Both bradycardia and hypoxemia have shown to be reversible and do not lead to perioperative complications. The incidence of bradycardia directly during or after an episode of hypoxemia is extremely rare, in our study the incidence was 0.001%. However, bradycardia does occur relatively often, that is in 9.5% of patients. One of the most important explanations is the specific kind of surgery, where stimulation of the vagal nerve leads to bradycardia.

4. Discussion

Cardiac output is determined by the product of heart rate and left ventricular stroke volume. Bradycardia may result in an insufficient rate to sustain cardiac output and hence oxygen delivery to tissue beds. This is particularly so in the case of young children in whom cardiac output is more affected by changes in heart rate than stroke volume. A prompt appropriate response to bradycardia under anaesthesia is important as some causes are rare and/or obscure and homeostatic mechanisms may be impaired by anaesthetic agents. Hamilton and co-workers suggest in a recent meta-analysis that a preemptive targeted approach to the management of hemodynamics in the perioperative period may reduce morbidity and mortality for high-risk surgical patients (Hamilton et al., 2011). Flick et al reported that postoperative cardiac arrest occurred most often in children with congenital heart disease as a result of factors not related to anesthesia. While cardiac surgery accounted for only 5% of all procedures, 87.5% of all arrests occurred in patients with congenital heart disease, usually during cardiac surgery as a result of failure to wean from cardiopulmonary bypass. Anesthesia factors were related in only 7.5% of all arrests, with an incidence of 0.65 per 10,000 anesthetics. Only six anesthesia-related arrests occurred in noncardiac cases during the 17-yr study period (Flick et al., 2007).

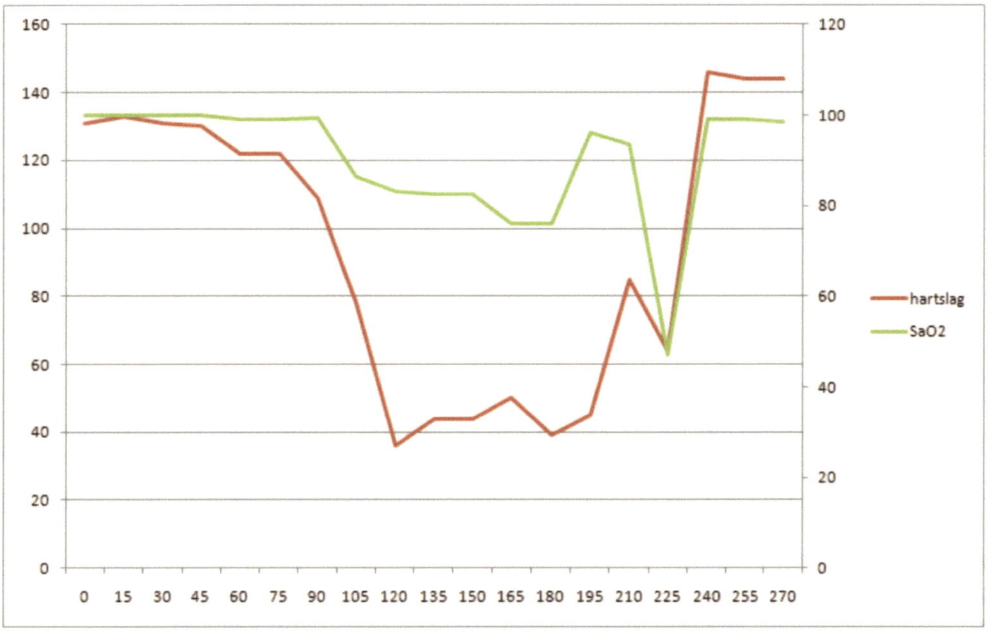

Fig. 3. Registration results of SaO_2 (green line, right axis, SaO_2 in %) and heart rate (red line, left axis, in beats per minute) as measured in time (horizontal-axis, in seconds) during inhalation anaesthesia in a 6-years old child undergoing adenotonsillectomy in sitting position.

During adenotonsillectomy under inhalation anaesthesia, bradycardia and hypoxemia both occur. In our study on children undergoing adenotonsillectomy in a sitting position nonintubated, both bradycardia and hypoxemia have shown to be reversible and do not lead to perioperative complications. The incidence of bradycardia directly during or after an episode of hypoxemia was extremely rare (0.001%). However, bradycardia does occur relatively often, in 9.5% of patients undergoing adenotonsillectomy in a sitting position nonintubated. An explanation might be a combination of study population, relatively young children, as well as the anaesthetics used, and the specific type of surgery leading to stimulation of the vagal nerve. Further research is necessary to compare different anesthesia techniques for adenotonsillectomy, with and without intubation.

5. Conclusion

Both bradycardia and hypoxemia occur relatively often during adenotonsillectomy, performed nonintubated in a sitting position under inhalation anaesthesia. The incidence of bradycardia in these children is 9.5%. Both bradycardia and hypoxemia are reversible and do not lead to perioperative complications. The incidence of bradycardia directly during or after an episode of hypoxemia is extremely rare. In general, in the pediatric population cardiovascular and respiratory factors are the major causes of cardiopulmonary arrest during anesthesia. The major causes of anesthesia-related cardiac arrest in the pediatric population are hypovolemia, preoperative anemia, pharmacological toxicity, hypoventilation and airway obstruction. Cardiopulmonary arrest during anesthesia in the pediatric population is different as compared to the adult population. In children, cardiopulmonary arrest during anesthesia is commonly caused by respiratory events and is more likely to result in mortality than in the adults. Anesthesia related cardiopulmonary arrest is fortunately an uncommon event, but it must be emphasized that significant bradyarrhythmias must be treated immediately to prevent an irreversible cardiac arrest. Special precaution measurement should be considered in patients less than 1 year with severe underlying or concurrent disease having emergency surgery as they are the most at risk for a fatal outcome. Finally, it must be clear that children should be cared for in facilities with adequate skilled medical and nursing staff and appropriately sized equipment.

6. References

Bai W., Voepel-Lewis, T., Malviya S. (2010) Hemodynamic changes in children with Down syndrome during and following inhalation induction of anesthesia with sevoflurane. *Journal of Clinical Anesthesia,* Vol 22, pp. 592-597

Balagna, R., Abbo, D., Ferrero, F., Valori, A., Peruzzi, L. (1999) Accidental hypothermia in a child. *Paediatric Anaesthesia,* Vol. 9: 342-244

CBO Kwaliteitsinstituut voor de gezondheidszorg (2008) Richtlijn Ziekten van Adenoïd en Tonsillen in de Tweede lijn. Utrecht: http://www.cbo.nl/thema/Richtlijnen/Overzicht-richtlijnen/KNO

Fastle, R.K. and Roback, M.G. (2004) Pediatric rapid sequence intubation. Incidence of reflex bradycardia and effects of pretreatment with atropine. *Pediatric Emergency Care,* Vol. 20 (10), pp. 651-655

Field, R.G., Gencorelli F.J., Litman, R.S. (2010) Anesthetic management of the pediatric bleeding tonsil. *Pediatric Anaesthesia,* Vol. 20, pp. 982-986

Fleming, B., McCollough, M., Henderson, S.O. (2005) Myth: atropine should be administered before succinylcholine for neonatal and pediatric intubation. Can J Emerg Med, Vol. 7 (2), pp. 114-117

Flick R.P., Sprung J., Harrison T.E., Gleich S.J., Schroeder D.R., Hanson A.C., Buenvenida S.L., Warner D.O. (2007) Perioperative cardiac arrests in children between 1988 and 2005 at a tertiary referral center: A study of 92,881 patients. *Anesthesiology,* Vol. 106, pp. 226–237

Gencorelli F.J., Fields, R.G., Litman, R.S. (2010) Complications during rapid sequence induction of general anaesthesia in children: a benchmark study. *Pediatric Anaesthesia,* Vol. 20, pp. 421-424

Hamilton, M.A., Cecconi, M., Rhodes, A. (2011) A Systematic Review and Meta-Analysis on the Use of Preemptive Hemodynamic Intervention to Improve Postoperative Outcomes in Moderate and High-Risk Surgical Patients. *Anesth & Analg,* Vol. 112(6), pp. 1259-1521

Homer, J.J., Williams, B.T., Semple, P., Swanepoel, A. en Knight, L.C. (2000) Tonsillectomy by guillotine is less painful than by dissection. *Int J Pediatr Otorhinolaryngol,* Vol 52, pp. 25-29

Huang, Z., Liu, D., Zhong, J., Chen, Q., Zhou, L., Sun, C., Wang, J. (2008) *Lin Chung Er Bi Yan Hou Jing Wai Ke Za Zhi,* Vol 22 (21), pp. 984-986

Keenan, R.L., Shapiro, J.H., Kane, F.R., Simpson, P.M. (1994) Bradycardia during Anesthesia in Infants. An Epidemiologic Study. *Anesthesiology*, Vol 80, pp. 976-982

Kalkman, C.J., Peelen, L., Moons, K.G., Veenhuizen, M., Bruens, M., Sinnema, G., De Jong, T.P. (2009) Behavior and Development in Children and Age at the Time of First Anaesthetic Exposure. *Anesthesiology,* Vol 110, pp. 805-812

Knape, J.T.A. (1989) Het verloop van de arteriële zuurstofsaturatie bij twee anesthesietechnieken voor (adeno)tonsillectomie bij kinderen. *Ned Tijdschr Geneeskd,* Vol 132, pp. 919-922

Komatsu, R., Turan, A.M., Orhan-Sungur, M., McGuire, J., Radke, O.C., Apfel, C.C. (2007) Remifentanyl for general anaesthesia: a systematic review. *Anesthesiology,* Vol. 62 (12), pp. 1266-1280

Kraemer, F.W., Stricker, P.A., Gumaney, H.G., McClung, H., Meador, M.R., Sussman, E., Burgess, B.J., Ciampa, B., Mendelsohn, J., Rehman, M.A., Watcha, M.F. (2010) Bradycardia During Induction of Anaesthesia with Sevoflurane in Children with Down Syndrome. *Anesth Analg,* Vol. 111, pp. 1259-1263

Kretzschmar, M.J., Siccama, I., Houweling, P.L., Quak, J.J., Colnot, D.R. (2010) Hypoxemia and bradycardia in children during adenotonsillectomy without intubation. *Ned Tijdschr Geneesk,* Vol. 154, pp. 1715-1719

Lowe, D., van der Meulen, J., Cromwell, D., Lewsey, J., Copley, L., Browne, J., Yung, M., Brown, P. (2007) Key messages from the National Tonsillectomy Audit. *Laryngoscope,* Vol 117, pp. 717-724

Morray, J.P. (2010) Cardiac arrest in anesthetized children: recent advances and challenges for future. Pediatric Anesthesia, doi:10.1111/j.1460-9592.2010.03440.x

Mulder, J.J.S., Mönnink, J.P., De Grood, P.M.R.M. (1995) Adenotonsillectomie volgens Sluder: met of zonder endotracheale intubatie? *Ned Tijdschr Geneeskd,* Vol 139, pp. 2730-2732

O'Connell T. Update in paediatric cardiopulmonary resuscitation. In: Keneally J, ed. Australasian anaesthesia. Melbourne: ANZCA, 1994:27–37

Polderman, K.H., Herold, I. (2009) Therapeutic hypothermia and controlled normothermia in the intensive care unit: practical considerations, side effects, and cooling methods. *Crit Care Med,* Vol. 37 (3), pp. 1101-1120

Pöpping, D.M., Alia, N., Marret, E., Wenk, M., Tramèr, M.R. (2009) Clonidine as an adjuvant to local anaesthetics for peripheral nerve and plexus blocks: a meta-analysis of randomized trials. *Anesthesiology,* Vol. 111(2), pp. 406-415

Prismant (2010), Informatie-expertise, ziekenhuisstatistieken, verrichtingen. Available from: www.prismant.nl

Scheenstra, R.J., Hilgevoord, A.A.J. en Van Rijn, P.M. (2007) Ernstige nabloeding na klassieke (adeno)tonsillectomie: zeldzaam en meestal op de dag van de ingreep. *Ned Tijdschr Geneeskd,* Vol 151, pp. 598-601

Reix, P., St-Hilaire, M., Praud, J-P. (2007) Laryngeal sensitivity in the neonatal period: from bench to bedside. *Pediatric Pulmonology,* Vol. 42, pp. 674-682

Rothrock, S.G. and Pagane, J. (2005) Letter to the Editors. *Pediatric Emergency Medicine,* Vol. 21 (9), pp. 637-638

Sanders, J.C., King, M., Mitchell, M.A., Kelly, J.P. (2006) Perioperative complications of adenotonsillectomy in children with obstructive sleep apnea syndrome. *Anesth Analg,* Vol 103 (5), pp. 1115-1121

Slappendel, R. & Rutten, J.M.J. (1989) Hartritmestoornissen tijdens adenotomie en adenotonsillectomie. *Ned Tijdschr Anesthesiol,* Vol2, pp. 11-13

Tjon Pian Gi, R., Bliek, V., Borgstein, J. (2010) The Sluder method in the Netherlands and the incidence of postoperative haemorrhage in a pediatric hospital. *Int J Ped Otorhinolaryngol,* Vol 74, pp. 56-59

Tramèr, M.R., Moore, R.A., McQuay, H.J.M. (1997) Propofol and bradycardia: causation, frequency and severity. *Brit J Anaesthesia,* Vol. 78, pp. 642-651

Ünlü, Y, Tekalan, S.A, Cemiloglu, R., Ketenci, I., Kutluhan, A. (1992) Guillotine and Dissection Tonsillectomy in Children. *J Laryngol Otol,* Vol. 106, pp. 817-820

Van den Akker, E.H., Hoes, A.W., Burton, M.J., Schilder, A.G.M. (2004) Large International Differences in (adeno)tonsillectomy rates. *Clin Otolarynol,* Vol. 29, pp. 161-164

Van der Meulen, J. (2004) Tonsillectomy technique as a risk factor for postoperative haemorrhage. *Lancet,* Vol 364, pp. 697-702

Van Nouhuys, F. (1973) Afwijkingen in het elektrocardiogram tijdens adenotonsillectomie onder narcose. *Ned Tijdschr Geneeskd,* Vol 117, pp. 137-141

Wagemans, M.F.M., van Dijk, B., Bakker, N.C., Ten Voorde, B.J., Faes, Th.J.C., Zuurmond, W.W.A., van der Werff, D.B.M., Scheffer, G.J. (1991). Continue SaO_2-meting en ECG-registratie onder inhalatieanesthesie voor adenotonsillectomie bij kinderen in zittende houding. *Ned Tijdschr Anesth,* Vol 4, pp. 61-61

Wake, M. & Glossop, P. (1989). Guillotine and dissection tonsillectomy compared. *J Laryngol Otol,* Vol. 103, pp. 588-591

Watterson, L.M., Morris, R.W., Westhorpe, R.N., Williamson, J.A. (2005) Crisis management during anaesthesia: bradycardia. *Qual Saf Health Care,* Vol. 14: e7

17

Spiral Waves, Obstacles and Cardiac Arrhythmias

Daniel Olmos-Liceaga
University of Sonora
México

1. Introduction

The propagation of electrical waves through cardiac tissue is a very important phenomenon to study since those waves activate the mechanisms for cardiac contraction, responsible to pump blood to the body. An electrical wave of excitation, called also an action potential wave, is initiated periodically at a place called the sinoatrial node, the natural pacemaker of the heart. This wave, propagates throughout the atria where it arrives at the atrioventricular node, where after some time delay, it propagates to the ventricles via the Purkinje fibers (Zaret et al., 1992). In normal conditions, this process is repeated approximately 70 to 100 times each minute and is commonly referred to as a heartbeat. The condition at which abnormal generation or propagation of excitation waves during the process described above, is termed as arrhythmia.

One of the proposed mechanisms involved in the development of certain type of arrhythmias, are spiral waves, a particular form of functional reentry (Fenton et al., 2002; Veenhuyzen et al., 2004). Spiral waves, are self sustained waves of excitation that rotate freely or around an obstacle, reactivating the same area of tissue at a higher frequency than the normal SA node would do, increasing the normal heartbeat rate. In the worst scenario, a spiral wave might break up into smaller spiral waves giving uncoordinated contractions of the heart in a phenomenon known as fibrillation. When this phenomenon occurs in the ventricles, the heart quivers and looses its strength to pump blood to the body leading to immediate cardiac arrest (Fenton et al., 2002; Zaret et al., 1992). Fibrillation, is the main cause of death in industrialized countries (Fenton et al., 2002; Priori et al., 2002; Tang et al., 2005; Zipes, 2005).

An important research area is the study of the interaction of spiral waves in cardiac tissue with obstacles. Obstacles in cardiac tissue can be partially excitable or non excitable. Examples of partially excitable obstacles are scar tissue (Starobin et al., 1996) or ionic heterogeneities (Starobin et al., 1996; Tusscher & Panfilov, 2002; Valderrábano et al., 2000), whereas examples of non excitable obstacles are arteries (Valderrábano et al., 2000) or the natural orifices in the atria (Azene et al., 2001).

It has been observed that an obstacle in cardiac tissue might act as a stabilizer of spiral wave dynamics (Davidenko et al., 1992; Ikeda et al., 1997; Kim et al., 1999; Lim et al., 2006; Pertsov et al., 1993; Valderrábano et al., 2000), as it provides a transition between meandering spiral waves (Ikeda et al., 1997) or multiple spiral waves (Shajahan et al., 2007; Valderrábano et al., 2000) into a simple rotation spiral, which is attached to the obstacle. This transition is clinically important because as it has been shown, fibrillation like activity changes to a tachycardia regime (Kim et al., 1999).

The interaction of spiral waves with obstacles and its relationship with the transition between different arrhythmic regimes has been experimentally and computationally studied by different researchers (Azene et al., 2001; Comtois & Vinet, 2005; Ikeda et al., 1997; Shajahan et al., 2007; 2009; Valderrábano et al., 2000). Valderrabano et al. (Valderrábano et al., 2000) studied in a cardiac tissue preparation the transition between ventricular fibrillation and ventricular tachycardia due to the presence of obstacles; Ikeda et al. (Ikeda et al., 1997), also considered the transition of different arrhythmic regimes due to the attachment of a spiral wave to an obstacle of minimum size. Shajahan et al. (Shajahan et al., 2007) used the Luo-Rudy and Panfilov models to study the transition of spiral turbulence to a simple rotating spiral wave due to the presence of an obstacle, which again provides a transition between different arrhythmic regimes; Xie et al. (Xie et al., 2001) presented a computational study of the effects of regional ischemia on the stability of a spiral wave; Azene et al. (Azene et al., 2001) carried out a computational study of the attachment and detachment of wavefronts to obstacles based on the Luo-Rudy model; Olmos (Olmos, 2010) studied the interaction of spiral waves in a particular case of the meandering regime, with rectangular obstacles. The aim in that work was to understand better necessary conditions in order to obtain attachment of the meandering spiral wave to the obstacle.

However, the interaction of spiral waves with obstacles and its relationship with transitions between different arrhythmic regimes, is a topic that has not been completely understood. For example, the interaction of a spiral wave in the meandering regime with an obstacle, has not previously being considered. Such interactions can be very complex (Olmos & Shizgal, 2008; Yermakova & Pertsov, 1986), and the determination of the conditions for which a meandering spiral wave attaches to an obstacle is an important endeavor. On the other hand, it has been considered that the presence of obstacles can be only of a stabilizing nature, which is not always the case. Therefore, the main objective of this work is to present a numerical study of the interaction of spiral waves with obstacles and to show the existence of different transitions due to the presence of obstacles.

By considering non-excitable and partially excitable obstacles we will show that obstacles cannot only stabilize the dynamics as shown in (Ikeda et al., 1997; Kim et al., 1999; Lim et al., 2006), but also, they can act as destabilizers. In both cases and by different mechanisms, the obstacle might act as a switch between two arrhythmic regimes, in which one is less dangerous than the other. In the case of non-excitable obstacles, it is shown that under certain conditions like the size of the obstacle, a more complex arrhythmia might appear.

To this end, this work will consist in the following sections. We start by presenting a general background about generation and propagation of action potentials (Section 2). In Section 3, we describe the model equations considered in the simulations. Then, in Section 4 the formation of a spiral wave is discussed. In the same section, we discuss the concepts of meandering and drift of spirals, which will be essential in explaining the results in this work. We follow this section by presenting the results obtained with partially excitable obstacles and non-excitable obstacles (Sections 5 and 6). We finish this work with Section 7 by presenting some conclusions, limitations and open questions in this topic.

2. Generation and propagation of an action potential

An important electrical property of atrial and ventricular cells is excitability. At rest, a ventricular cell has a transmembrane potential of about $u = -84mV$ (Beeler & Reuter, 1977), which is called the resting membrane potential (RMP). If a short time pulse of current is applied such that the new potential is below $-60mV$, the value of u will return to the RMP immediately. However, if the potential is raised above $u = -60mV$, the transmembrane potential will undergo a large excursion raising its value approximately to $28mV$, generating a peak, then a plateau and finally return to the RMP (Fig. 1). This phenomenon is called an action potential (AP) and cells with this property are called excitable cells. The value of u above which an AP is elicited, which in this case is $u \approx -60mV$, is called the threshold potential value u_{th}.

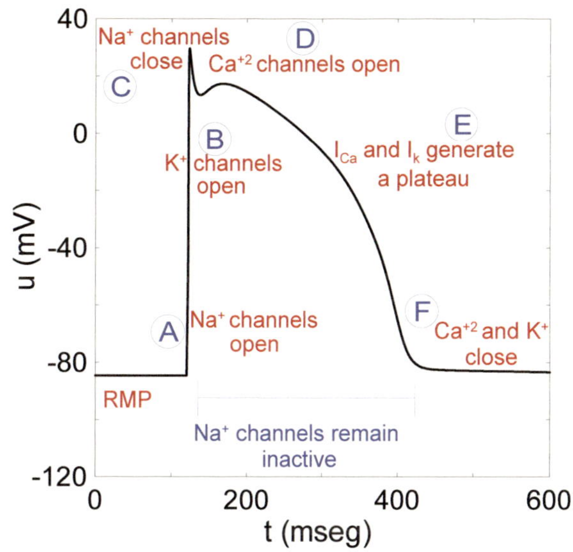

Fig. 1. Membrane potential u versus time during an AP. Representative mechanisms involved in the generation of an AP in a cardiac cell.

Changes in the membrane potential are due mainly to the passage of Na^+, K^+ and Ca^{++} ions via ion channels and other mechanisms through the cell membrane. The ion channels are membrane proteins which allow the passage across the membrane of specific type of ions between the interior and exterior of the cell. An essential part of the work by Hodgkin and Huxley (Hodgkin & Huxley, 1952) was to establish that the *Na*, *K* and *Ca* channels can be opened or closed, and that state depends on the membrane potential at a given time.

The general mechanism by which an AP is generated is as follows: Initially the cell is at rest i.e. the potential across the cell membrane is at the RMP value. When the current is applied such that the new potential is above u_{th}, *Na* channels open in a fast time scale and a flux of Na^+ inside the cell, follows (Fig. 1A). The *Na* current is responsible for the rapid change in u, which changes dramatically from $-60mV$ to $28mV$ in a phenomenon called depolarization. In Fig. 1B, *K* channels open in a slow time scale compared to the time scale of the *Na* channels opening, and K^+ flow outside the cell. In Fig. 1C, the *Na* channels close and the K^+ current lowers the membrane potential generating a peak in the AP. After that, *Ca* channels open in a slow time scale and a flow of Ca^{++} from outside to inside the cell occurs (Fig. 1D). During this stage, *K* and *Ca* currents move in the opposite direction, generating what is called a plateau (Fig. 1E). Finally, both channels close and the membrane potential returns to the RMP value (Fig. 1F).

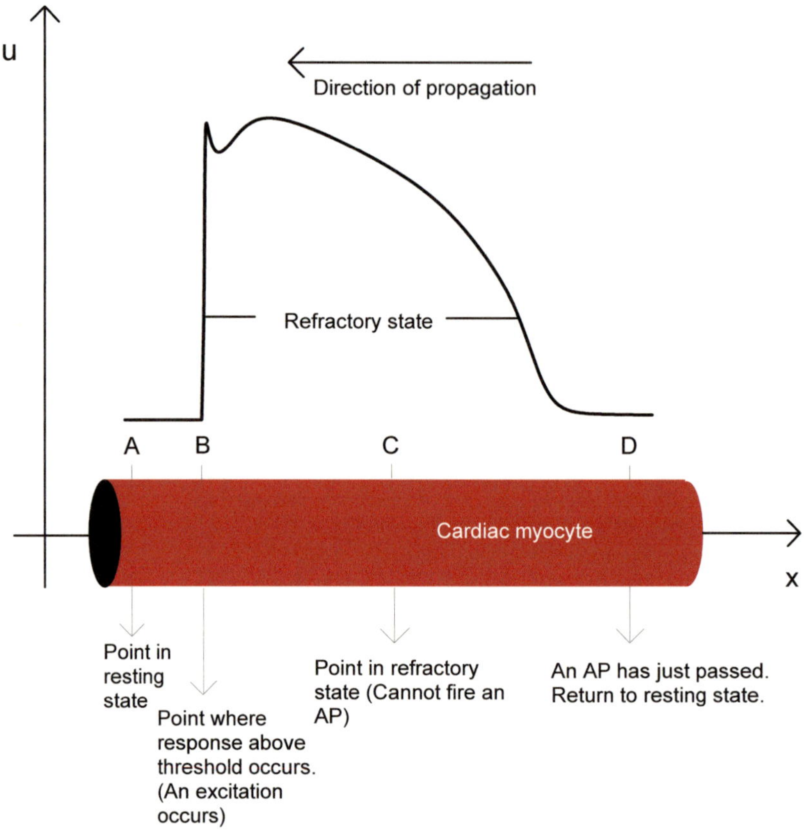

Fig. 2. Propagation of an AP. The propagation is taken over a hypothetical large myocyte.

Each location of the cell membrane, once it has a response above u_{th}, will experience an AP. The AP generated in a cell location, with the proper conditions (Kléber & Rudy, 2004), will propagate through the rest of the cell and through the cardiac tissue. The general mechanism by which an AP travels through cardiac muscle can be explained by considering a large single cell as shown in Fig. 2. In Fig. 2, it is considered that an AP is propagating only in the x direction and from right to left. At location A, the membrane potential is at the RMP value and it is ready to accept an AP. At point B, an AP has just been elicited. At point C, an AP is in process and at this location the cell is in refractory state and another AP cannot be generated. Durig this stage the Na channels, responsible for the depolarization of the cell, are closed and remain inactive for a time called the refractory period. Finally, at location D, an AP has just passed and at this location the membrane potential has almost returned to the RMP value.
Therefore, the propagation of the AP is as follows. At location B, where the AP has just been elicited, Na ions are entering to the cell. These ions generate a current in the x direction due to the concentration gradient in a neighborhood of point B. These ions move to location A, increasing its corresponding u value until it reaches u_{th}. Then, an AP is elicited at location A and the AP advances in space. Therefore, propagation of the AP follows.

3. The model equations

In order to make simulations we consider equations of the reaction-diffusion type given by

$$\frac{\partial u}{\partial t} = \nabla \cdot (D \nabla u) - \frac{1}{C_m}(I_{ion}) \tag{1}$$

where, u is the transmembrane potential, D is the conductivity tensor, C_m is the capacitance and I_{ion} is the sum of the different ionic currents. There are different forms in which I_{ion} can be chosen, depending on which cell type is considered. For example the Luo-Rudy (Luo & Rudy, 1994) or the Priebe-Beuckelmann (Priebe & Beuckelmann, 1998) models are considered for ventricular cells, whereas the Courtemanche (Courtemanche et al., 1998) and the Nygren (Nygren et al., 1998) models were developed for atrial cells. Other models are the Yanagihara model for the sinoatrial node (Yanagihara et al., 1980), and the DiFrancesco- Noble model for the Purkinje cells (DiFrancesco & Noble, 1985). A complete list of models can be found in (Fenton & Cherry, 2008).

In this work, we consider the ionic currents given by Fenton and Karma (Fenton & Karma, 1998). This set of equations is a minimal model and was designed to mimic the behavior of complex models with a minimum number of variables. The Fenton-Karma (FK) equations are of the reaction diffusion type. They are given by

$$\begin{aligned} \frac{\partial u}{\partial t} &= \nabla \cdot (D \nabla u) - \frac{1}{C_m}(I_{fi} + I_{so} + I_{si}) \\ \frac{\partial v}{\partial t} &= \frac{1}{\tau_v^-}\Theta(u_c - u)(1 - v) - \frac{1}{\tau_v^+}\Theta(u_c - u)v \\ \frac{\partial w}{\partial t} &= \frac{1}{\tau_w^-}\Theta(u_c - u)(1 - w) - \frac{1}{\tau_w^+}\Theta(u_c - u)w \end{aligned} \tag{2}$$

where

$$\begin{aligned} I_{fi} &= -\frac{v}{\tau_d}\Theta(u - u_c)(1 - u)(u - u_c) \\ I_{so} &= \frac{u}{\tau_o}\Theta(u_c - u) + \frac{1}{\tau_r}\Theta(u - u_c) \\ I_{si} &= -\frac{w}{2\tau_{si}}(1 + \tanh[k(u - u_c^{si})]) \\ \tau_v^-(u) &= \Theta(u - u_v)\tau_{v1}^- + \Theta(u_v - u)\tau_{v2}^- \end{aligned} \tag{3}$$

In this case, $u = u(x,t)$ measures the membrane potential at a location x and time t, whereas v and w are gate variables. I_{fi}, I_{so} and I_{si} denote fast inward, slow outward and slow inward currents, respectively. Also $D = 0.001$, $C_m = 1, \tau_d = 0.403, \tau_r = 50.0, \tau_{si} = 44.84, \tau_o = 8.3, \tau_v^+ = 3.33, \tau_{v1}^- = 1000.0, \tau_{v2}^- = 19.2, \tau_w^+ = 667.0, \tau_w^- = 11, u_c = 0.13, u_v = 0.055, u_c^{si} = 0.85$. $\Theta(x)$ is the Heaviside step function. Numerically, we consider $\Theta(x)$ as

$$\Theta(x) = \frac{1}{2}(1 + \tanh(50x))$$

Equations (2) are solved in a rectangular domain $\Omega = [-7,7] \times [-7,7]$ using finite differences with $N = 512$ points in each dimension. Advancing in time is done with Euler as in (Fenton & Karma, 1998) with $dt = 0.125$. At the domain boundary and at the boundary of non-excitable obstacles (Section 6), no-flux boundary conditions were imposed. Boundary conditions at obstacles were implemented as done in (Morton & Mayers, 2005).

4. Generation of a spiral wave

Spiral waves have been observed to occur in cardiac tissue (Ikeda et al., 1997; Isomura et al., 2008; Pertsov et al., 1993) and in computer models (Isomura et al., 2008; Olmos, 2010; Otani,

2000). There are different ways in which a spiral wave might be generated. For example, spiral waves arise when an unexcitable obstacle is stimulated with high frequency of AP (Panfilov & Kenner, 1993); they can also be generated by using the method of cross-field stimulation (Pertsov et al., 1993); and they might arise due to the appearance of ectopic beats (Otani, 2000). Ectopic beats can arise due to abnormal calcium cycling (Benson & Holden, 2005) or by overload of calcium inside the cell (Luo & Rudy, 1994).

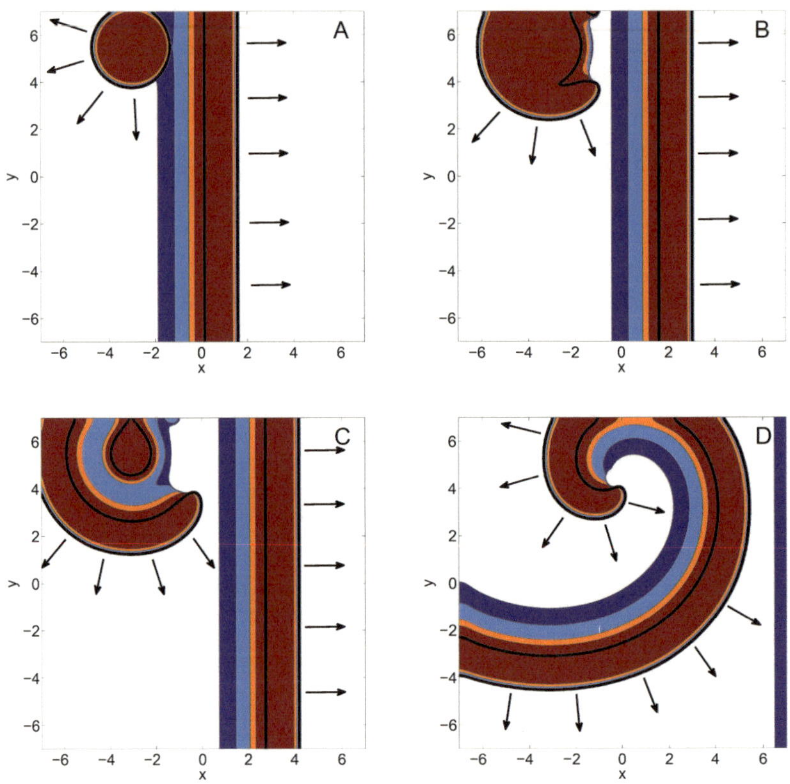

Fig. 3. Generation of a spiral wave due to ectopic activity. See text for details. The black bold line is the contour plot $u(x, y, t^*) = 0.1$. The different colored regions represent different levels of refractoriness of the medium. The region in white represents the medium completely recovered and an AP can be elicited. The region in red is a completely unexcitable region as an AP is occurring. The regions in orange and clear blue have a very low excitability level. The region in dark blue is more excitable and an AP might propagate in this region. The arrows point the direction of wave propagation. (x and y are in cm)

A particular and simple way in which the formation of a spiral wave can be explained, is shown in Fig. 3, where a solution of Eq. (2) is shown for four different integration times. In Fig. 3A, a pulse travels from left to right as shown by the direction of the arrows. After the pulse has passed, an ectopic firing appears at the back of the pulse. The ectopic firing starts propagating in all directions except at the back of the front where the region is still in refractory state (Fig. 3B). The abnormal firing generates a curved front with a free end that propagate downwards (Fig. 3C). The original AP moves to the right, disappears at the right boundary and the region that was initially in refractory state is now ready to accept another AP. Then, the free end can propagate on the recovered region generating a spiral wave (Fig. 3D). After a spiral wave has been generated, if its rotation frequency is faster than the stimulation frequency from the sinoatrial node, then the spiral wave becomes the new pacemaker of the heart (Lee, 1997).

4.1 Meandering and drift of a spiral wave

When a spiral wave evolves in excitable media in general, its dynamics are ruled by (i) the local conducting mechanisms, and; (ii) the heterogeneities of the medium. The former gives rise to a phenomenon called meandering, whereas the later to a phenomenon referred to as drift of a spiral wave.

One way to get a better understanding of meandering and drift of a spiral wave, is by studying the evolution of the position of its tip. The tip of a spiral wave can be defined in a variety of ways and a resume can be found in (Fenton et al., 2002). In this work it is considered the tip of the spiral wave as the point over the level curve $u = 0.5$ with zero normal velocity (Fenton et al., 2002).

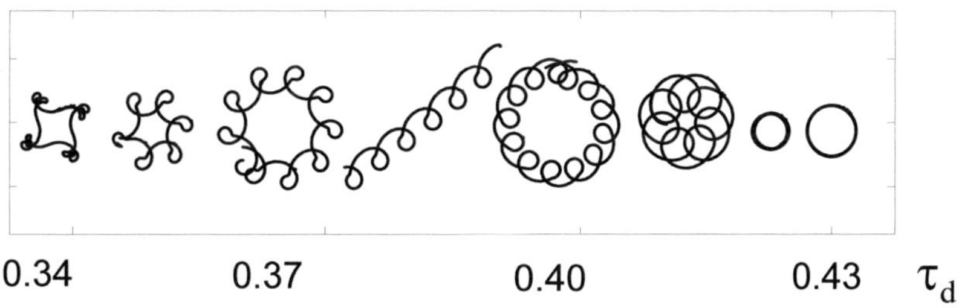

Fig. 4. Tip trajectories of the spiral waves obtained with Eqns. (2), with $u_c = 0.13$ and varying the parameter τ_d from 0.34 to 0.43. An increase in the value τ_d implies a reduction in the excitability of the medium.

4.1.1 Meandering of a spiral wave

In Fig. 4, different tip trajectories of spiral waves corresponding to different values of τ_d are shown. The value τ_d controls the speed at which the depolarizing ions enter to the cell and is a measure of the excitability of the cell (Efimov et al., 1995; Fenton et al., 2002). An increase in the value τ_d implies a reduction in the excitability of the medium. When $\tau_d = 0.43$ the tip of the spiral wave traces a circumference. When the value of τ_d is reduced to 0.425 the radius of the circular trajectory is reduced. However, when the value of τ_d is reduced to about 0.415 the trajectory is no longer circular but a curve that resembles an epitrochoid (Fig. 5B). Decreasing the value of τ_d increases the radius R (Fig. 5B) of the epitrochoidal trajectory. For $\tau_d = 0.3965$ the value of R tends to infinity obtaining a trochoidal trajectory (Epitrochoid with $R = \infty$). For smaller values of τ_d the tip trajectory resembles an hypotrochoid of radius R (Fig. 5A). For values less than $\tau_d = 0.34$ deformations of hypotrochoidal trajectories are obtained (Fig. 4).

The phenomenon shown in Fig. 4, is called meandering of the tip trajectory or meandering. In order to understand the mechanisms behind meandering it is necessary to study the recovery regions when the spiral wave is propagating in the medium. In Fig. 6, it is shown the contour of the variable $u(x, y, t^*) = 0.1$ for a particular time t^* (Labeled bold line in Fig. 6B); Also, are shown different regions corresponding to the level of recovery of the medium, given by the variable v in Eqns. 2, plotted also for the time t^*. The region in black means that the region is

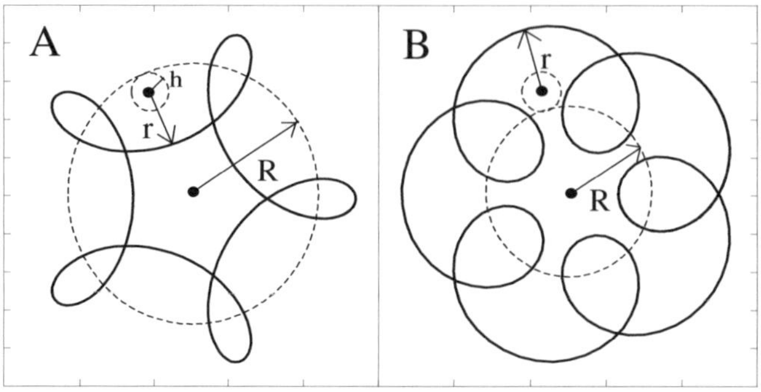

Fig. 5. (A) An hypotrochoid and; (B) an epitrochoid. From (Olmos, 2007)

completely unexcitable (v in this case is close to zero); As the region becomes clearer, the value of v gets closer to 1 and therefore the region is able to accept more easily another AP. The line in blue is the trajectory followed by the tip for a time interval around t^*.

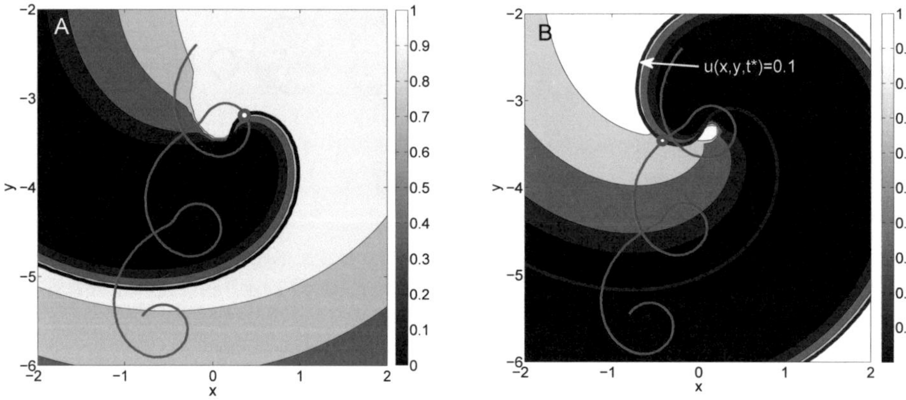

Fig. 6. Propagation of a spiral wave generated with Eqns. (2) with $\tau_d = 0.3965$. The line in blue represents the trajectory of the tip. The different coloured regions represents different levels of refractoriness given by the v variable. For v close to 0 (black), the region is in its maximum level of refractoriness and an AP cannot be elicited here. For $v \approx 1$ (white), the region is almost or totally recovered and an AP can be elicited in this region. (A) Formation of a petal; (B) Formation of an arc. The blue dot filled in white, is the location of the tip of the spiral.

In Figures 4 and 6, it is shown that the trajectory of the tip of the spiral wave has high and low curvature in an alternate and periodic fashion. The part with high curvature is referred to as a petal, whereas the part with low curvature, an arc. In Fig. 6A, the tip is tracing a petal, whereas in Fig. 6B, an arc.

In Fig. 6A, it is shown the spiral wave at the time where the tip is tracing a petal. In this case, the front that is close to the tip (blue dot filled in white) of the wave, propagates through a region that is almost completely recovered giving a maximum in the curvature of the trajectory. A different scenario occurs in Fig. 6B, where the tip is tracing an arc. Here, it is clear that the front close to the tip of the spiral propagates through a region that is not

completely recovered. This causes the front to propagate in another direction, where the medium is more excitable. This deviation generates the low curvature part of the trajectory or the arc. This process occurs periodically and the trajectory shown in Fig. 6 is obtained.
In order to give an explanation about the occurrence of the different trajectories obtained in Fig. 4, we use the information of the previous paragraph and the facts that (i) $1/\tau_d$ is the speed at which the Na ions enter to the cell to depolarize it. For shorter τ_d the ions enter faster to the cell, and; (ii) from Eqns. (2), changing the value of τ_d does not affect the threshold value u_{th}. Consider the case shown in Fig. 6, where $\tau_d = 0.3965$, ie, when the tip trajectory is trochoidal. In Fig. 6A, a petal is being traced. When the value of τ_d is reduced then the flux of Na ions (In Eqns. (2), I_{fi} is carried by Na ions) is increased. Therefore, the larger amount per time unit of ions with a constant diffusion coefficient, makes that the spiral wave will trace a petal with larger curvature than in the case with $\tau_d = 0.3965$. In the same way, it will follow that the front of the spiral wave will reach its own tail before than the case with $\tau_d = 0.3965$. Therefore, it is obtained an hypotrochoidal trajectory like the one shown in Fig. 4 with $\tau_d = 0.37$. A similar argument follows for epitrochoidal trajectories.

4.1.2 Drift of a spiral wave

Drift of a spiral wave is a directed change of its location with time in response to perturbations (Biktashev, 2007). There are different ways in which drift might occur and an complete list can be found in (Biktashev, 2007). In this work we focus on two different ways in which drift occurs (Fig. 7). In Fig. 7A, it is shown the drift of a spiral wave due to the presence of inhomogeneities. Initially, we considered a spiral wave with $\tau_d = 0.43$. With this choice of τ_d, the tip of the spiral wave traces a circumference. After some integration time, we changed the value of τ_d to 0.39 for $y < 0$. The result of this change in the value of τ_d is shown in Fig. 7A. In the figure, it is observed that the tip trajectory no longer traces a circumference but a trajectory that resembles a spring. When the tip is far from the interphase $y = 0$, the trajectory traces the usual circumference. However, when the tip hits the region above $y = 0$, the curvature generated is higher than the curvature below $y = 0$ due to the decrease in τ_d. This causes a drift of the position of the center of the circumference. It follows that the trajectory moves along the line $y = 0$ where there is a difference in τ_d between the two phases.

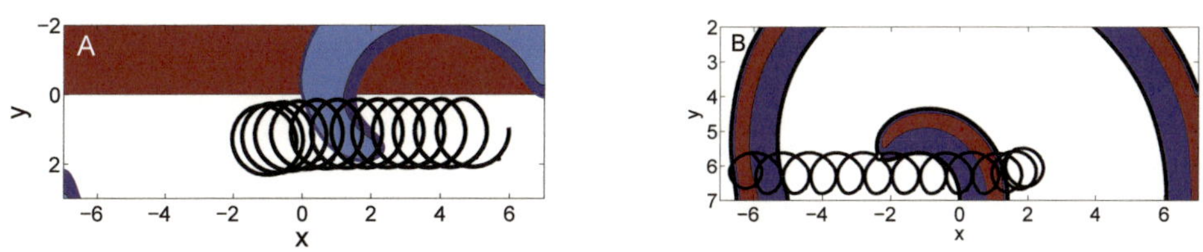

Fig. 7. Drift of a spiral wave due to (A) Inhomogeneities in the medium, and; (B) Interaction with a boundary. In (A) $\tau_d = 0.43$ for $y \geq 0$ and $\tau_d = 0.39$ for $y < 0$.

In Fig. 7B, it is shown the drift of a spiral wave due to the presence of a boundary. In this case, when a spiral wave with a circular tip trajectory gets close enough to a boundary, there is an increase in the curvature of the trajectory giving as a consequence drift of the center of the circular trajectory. Therefore, the trajectory drifts along the boundary. The physical mechanism by which the gain in curvature of the trajectory is observed, is apparently as follows: The impermeable boundary prevents the spread of the current produced by the spreading wavefront, which is equivalent to local rise in the excitability of the medium close to the boundary (Yermakova & Pertsov, 1986), and therefore an increase in the curvature of the trajectory (Subsection 4.1.1).

5. Partially excitable obstacles

Partially excitable obstacles are inhomogeneities in the tissue that originate from changes in single-cell properties such as the conductance of ion channels (Shajahan et al., 2009). Such inhomogeneities can arise from damaged or scar tissue (Starobin et al., 1996), when a lesion is created via ablation (Azene et al., 2001) or by regional hyperkalemia (Xie et al., 2001). These changes affect the propagation speed of the pulse (Kléber & Rudy, 2004), the action potential duration (Beeler & Reuter, 1977; Efimov et al., 1995; Shajahan et al., 2009) and prolongs recovery of excitability after the occurrence of an action potential (Xie et al., 2001).

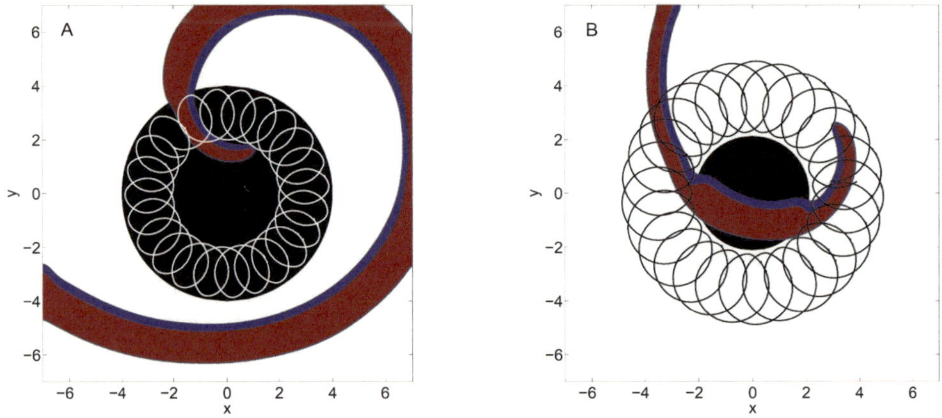

Fig. 8. Tip trajectories of spiral waves obtained with Equations (2) with a partially excitable circular obstacle (A) $\tau_d = 0.38$ outside the circular obstacle and $\tau_d = 0.43$ inside, $r = 4$; (B) $\tau_d = 0.43$ outside the obstacle and $\tau_d = 0.38$ inside, $r = \sqrt{4.5}$.

The stability of spiral waves depending on inhomogeneities in the medium has been studied by Shajahan (Shajahan et al., 2009) and Xie (Xie et al., 2001). In this work, we focus on partially excitable obstacles of circular shape. A pair of simulations are shown in Fig. 8. In Figure 8A, $\tau_d = 0.38$ outside the circular obstacle and $\tau_d = 0.43$ inside. The radius of the obstacle is $r = 4$. In the previous section, the tip of the spiral wave followed the boundary between the two regions. In Figure 8A, it is shown that the trajectory also follows such boundary, which corresponds to the boundary of the inhomogeneity. In this case, it is shown that the tip traces a curve that resembles an hypotrochoid. In the case where the value of τ_d is inverted, i.e. $\tau_d = 0.43$ outside the inhomogeneity and $\tau_d = 0.38$ inside, with a radius $r = \sqrt{4.5}$, we obtain the trajectory shown in Fig. 8B. Here, the trajectory obtained resembles an epitrochoid. This last result has been presented in (Biktashev, 2007) within a frame of drift due to inhomogeneities where inside the obstacle the refractory period is longer than outside.

Now, consider varying the radius of the obstacle. In Fig. 9 we present the results of considering the two cases presented in Fig. 8. In the top row, we show the case when the trajectory resembles a hypotrochoid. In order to obtain these trajectories, we took $\tau_d = 0.43$ inside the obstacle, such that inside the obstacle the trajectory is circular. Outside the obstacle τ_d was taken as 0.38, such that the trajectory outside is hypotrochoidal. The radius of the obstacle is increased from left to right. When the radius of the obstacle is less than the radius of the circumference traced by the tip trajectory, the trajectory is circular. As the radius of the obstacle is increased, the trajectory changes from circular to hypotrochoidal. Then, by considering an increase in the radius of the obstacle, the circular trajectory experiences a bifurcation as the one periodic rotation changes to a two period rotation. This result was reported by Mikhailov et al. (Mikhailov et al., 1994) where a circular domain with no flux boundary conditions was considered.

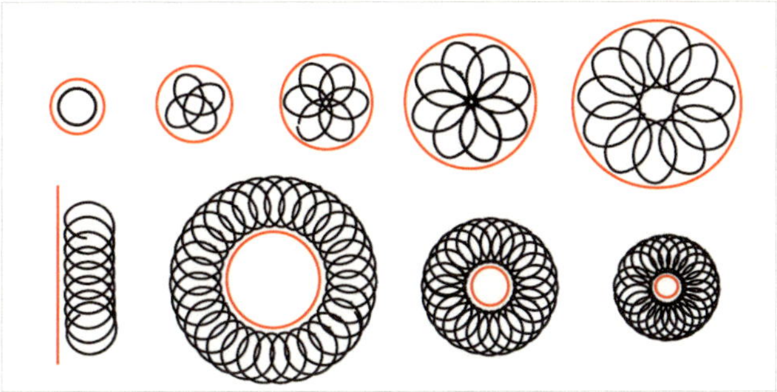

Fig. 9. Trajectories obtained with Eqns. (2) with a partially excitable circular obstacle and different radii. The red circle in each case, represents the boundary of the obstacle. Top row: $\tau_d = 0.38$ outside the circular obstacle and $\tau_d = 0.43$ inside. Circular and hypotrochoidal trajectories are obtained; Bottom row $\tau_d = 0.43$ outside the obstacle and $\tau_d = 0.38$. Epitrochoidal trajectories are obtained

In the bottom row of Fig. 9 is shown the case when the trajectory traces an epitrochoid. In this case, if we take a smaller radius, an epitrochoidal trajectory remains even by taking R tending to zero. Additionally to this result, it is also clear that by considering partially excitable obstacles it is possible to obtain the case of an epitrochoidal trajectory with $R = \infty$ and therefore a transition between the hypotrochoidal and epitrochoidal cases. Just like the case of meandering discussed in subsection 4.1.1.

The results presented in the top row of Figure 9, have a completely different meaning from those presented in (Mikhailov et al., 1994). As an example, consider the tip trajectory shown in Fig. 10, which corresponds to the upper left case shown in Fig. 9. Initially, the tip of the spiral wave is located outside of the obstacle. Because $\tau_d = 0.38$ outside the obstacle, an hypotrochoid is obtained. However, as soon as the trajectory hits the obstacle, the tip of the spiral wave gets trapped by the obstacle and the trajectory becomes circular (Fig. 10).

Therefore, in this section we have shown that heterogeneities in the conducting properties of the medium can give different results. (i) If inside the obstacle we take a value of τ_d^1 such that the tip trajectory is a circumference of radius r_1 and outside the obstacle the value of τ_d is less than $\tau_d^2 < \tau_d^1$, where τ_d^2 gives a circular trajectory with radius $r_2 < r_1$, then if the radius of the obstacle is $r \in [r_2, r_1]$ then a circular tip trajectory due to the interaction between the tip of the spiral wave and the obstacle is obtained. Clearly, this case includes the situation of having an epitrochoidal or hypotrochiodal trajectory outside the obstacle (with the values of τ_d given in Fig. 4). (ii) Under the same conditions as above but the radius r of the obstacle larger than r_1, then the trapped trajectory will trace a hypotrochoid. Observe that in this regime, we can obtain a transition from epitrochoidal (given by meandering) to hypotrochoidal trajectory

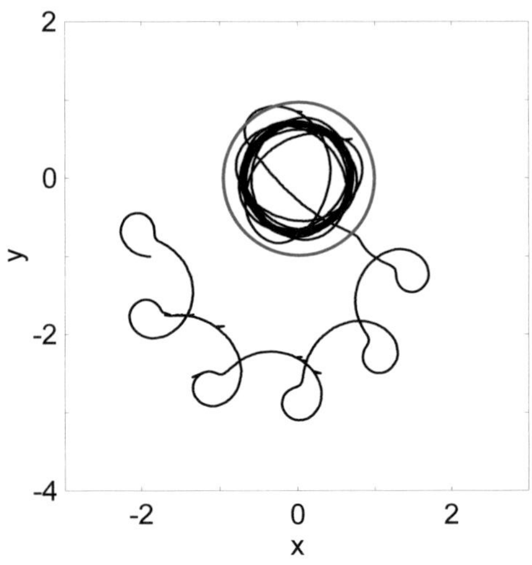

Fig. 10. $\tau_d = 0.38$ outside $\tau_d = 0.43$ inside the obstacle. The radius of the obstacle is $r = 1$. The simulation was done in the domain $\Omega = [-7,7] \times [-7,7]$, but a zoom of the region of interest is shown. x and y in cm.

(given by drift of the spiral wave). (iii) Finally, when the values of τ_d inside and outside the obstacle are reverted, what is obtained is an epitrochoidal trajectory.
It is important to observe that two periodic rotations, named epitrochoidal and hypotrochoidal trajectories, and transitions from circular to hypotrochoidal regimes, are also obtained through drift. Therefore, the presence of partially excitable obstacles in cardiac tissue may induce the existence of trajectories that mimic the meandering behavior.

6. Non-excitable obstacles

Obstacles in cardiac tissue have been modeled with regions where the zero flux condition is imposed (Azene et al., 2001; Isomura et al., 2008; Panfilov & Kenner, 1993; Shajahan et al., 2009; Starobin et al., 1996; Valderrábano et al., 2000). Arteries (Valderrábano et al., 2000) and the natural orifices in the atria, (Azene et al., 2001) are examples of this type of obstacles. Also, these obstacles can be artificially generated in experimental preparations by making cuts in the tissue (Cabo et al., 1996; Ikeda et al., 1997).
The interaction of spiral waves with non excitable obstacles has been considered by different authors (Azene et al., 2001; Ikeda et al., 1997; Isomura et al., 2008; Panfilov & Kenner, 1993; Shajahan et al., 2009; Starobin et al., 1996; Valderrábano et al., 2000). Of particular interest is the work by Ikeda (Ikeda et al., 1997), where it is observed that when a spiral wave attaches to an obstacle, a transition between two different classes of arrhythmias is observed.
In the present section we extend the results observed by Ikeda (Ikeda et al., 1997) and show that the presence of non excitable obstacles, just as the partially excitable ones, can stabilize or destabilize spiral wave dynamics. Initially, it is considered a spiral wave in the circular regime ($\tau_d = 0.426$), with a circular obstacle with radius $r = 1.7$ and center in the origin. In this regime, we placed the tip of the spiral wave near the obstacle. The result is shown in Fig. 11. In this situation, it is observed that the spiral rotates and at the same time starts moving around the obstacle. Due to the drift at an impermeable boundary plus the circular shape of the obstacle, it is observed that the tip of the spiral traces a curve very similar to an

epitrochoid. Therefore, the presence of a circular obstacle, has changed the simple rotation of the spiral wave into a two periodic rotation. This phenomenon, was observed for obstacles of all sizes above mesh partition. The speed of the drift was a decreasing function of the radius.

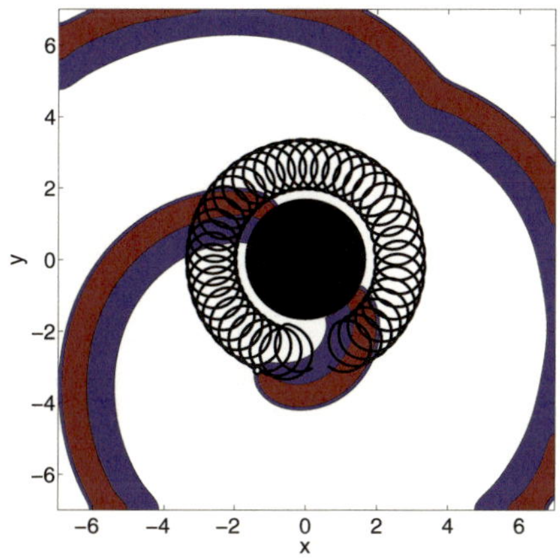

Fig. 11. Drift of a spiral wave around a circular obstacle. $\tau_d = 0.426$, radius $r = 1.7$.

In our second experiment, we considered a spiral wave in the epitrochoidal regime ($\tau_d = 0.405$). In the same way, we placed the spiral wave in such way that the tip of the spiral interacts with the obstacle. The results are shown in Fig. 12. In the figure, it is shown a spiral wave in the epitrochoidal regime interacting with the circular obstacle at different integration times. In Figs. 12A,B, it is shown that the spiral wave traces an epitrochoid. As soon as the spiral wave hits the boundary, the tip trajectory changes its direction due to the boundary effects (Olmos & Shizgal, 2008; Yermakova & Pertsov, 1986). In the figure, it is shown that the tip of the spiral wave hits the boundary four times. In the first three interactions, it is observed that the spiral bounces at the obstacle. However, in the fourth interaction it is observed that the spiral wave attaches to the obstacle (Fig. 12C). A major consequence obtained is that the two frequency rotation given by the epitrochoidal regime, changes after a transient, to a simple rotation given by the circular regime.
The change from the two rotation period to simple rotation was due to attachment of the spiral wave to the obstacle (Olmos, 2010). However, this experiment raises different questions. When the tip of the spiral hits the obstacle, why in some cases bouncing is observed and then attachment?, Does attachment always occur? Does attachment depend on the size of the radius of the obstacle?, How long it takes to a spiral to attach to the obstacle? To answer these questions is a very difficult task.
In order to show the complexity of this problem, we consider a previous analysis done in (Olmos & Shizgal, 2008). We interact the tip of spiral waves in the trochoidal regime ($R = \infty$ in Fig.5) with a flat boundary. With these settings we remove the effect of the curvature of the obstacle and the curvature of the epitrochoidal and hypotrochoidal regimes. We took initial conditions such that the trajectory had an incident angle θ_i with respect to the boundary (Fig. 13A).
When the tip of a spiral wave interacts with a boundary, there are two possible outcomes. The tip of the spiral wave bounces at the boundary as in Fig. 13A, or disappears at the boundary, in which case the spiral wave also disappears from the domain (Olmos & Shizgal, 2008). When

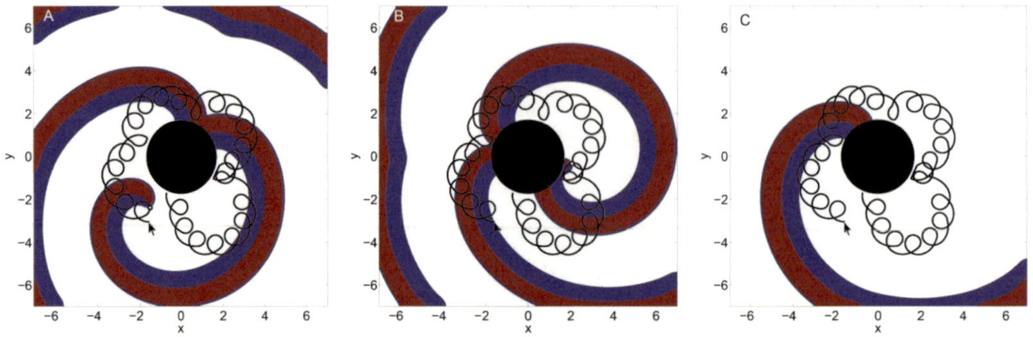

Fig. 12. Interaction of a spiral wave in the epirtrochoidal regime with a circular obstacle for different integration times. The arrow points at the place where the trajectory starts. (A) shows the trajectory of the spiral wave meandering; (B) the spiral wave hits the obstacle and bounces, and; (C) the spiral wave hits the obstacle and gets anchored. Note the difference in the frequency of excitation between (A)-(B) and (C).

considering obstacles, the effect of bouncing is the same for a boundary and for the obstacle. However, the effect of annihilation at a boundary becomes attachment of the spiral wave to the obstacle (Olmos, 2010). In Fig. 13B, we show the probability of annihilation of a spiral wave at the boundary as a function of the incident angle, following the procedure in (Olmos & Shizgal, 2008). From the figure, it is clear that for $\theta_i \in [0^o, 60^o] \bigcup [160^o, 180^o]$ the tip of the spiral wave bounces at the boundary. For $\theta_i \in (60^o, 160^o)$ in some cases, there was observed bouncing but also annihilation. As we increase the value of θ_i from 60° to 140°, there is an increase in the proportion of spiral waves that annihilate at the boundary. For $\theta_i = 140^o$ all the trajectories considered in the simulations disappeared at the boundary giving annihilation. From there, as the value of θ_i is increased up to $\theta_i = 160^o$, the proportion of spirals that bounced at the boundary increased again.

Based on the previous information, we run several examples in the epitrochoidal regime ($\tau_d = 0.405$) as the one shown in Fig. 12. We considered obstacles with three different radius, $r = 0.8$, $r = 1.1$ and $r = 1.7$. From there, we took all the cases where attachment of the spiral wave to the obstacle was obtained. It was observed from this numerical experiment that the angles at which attachment occurred, ranged from 10° to 100°. From this observation and from Fig. 13B, it is shown that for incident angles $\theta_i \in [10^o, 60^o]$, annihilation at the flat boundary is not possible, but attachment to the circular obstacle is possible.

The phenomenon of obtaining attachment for angles θ_i that in the flat boundary gave bouncing might be expected from the studies in (Leal-Soto, 2011; Olmos, 2010), where a spiral wave in the trochoidal regime interacted with the face of a square shaped obstacle. In these studies, it is shown that a spiral wave that would experience bouncing in a flat boundary, will experience attachment to the obstacle, as the interaction of the spiral wave takes place near a corner of the obstacle. Therefore, when we consider a circular obstacle, the interactions of the tip of the spiral wave with the obstacle can be thought as the interaction of the tip of a spiral with a smoothed corner of a square shaped obstacle. This explains why attachment is observed for angles less than $\theta_i = 60^o$ observed in the simulations.

Attachment to the circular obstacle was observed to happen with angles θ_i between 10° to 100°. This does not imply that attachment is not possible for θ_i outside this range of values. In fact, from the simulations, the interaction of the spiral wave with the obstacle rarely

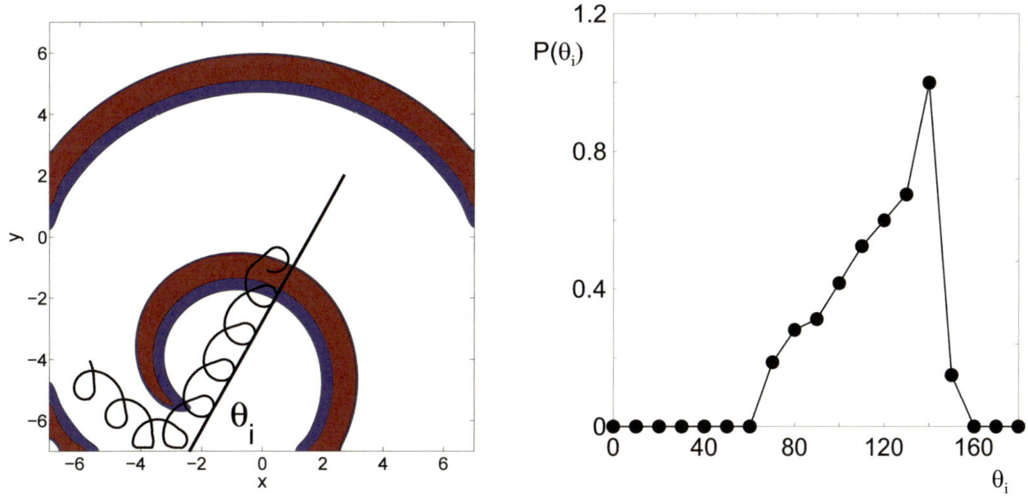

Fig. 13. (A) Interaction of a spiral wave in the trochoidal regime ($R = \infty$ in Fig. 5, $\tau_d = 0.3965$) with a boundary. θ_i is the angle of incidence. In the figure, the tip of the spiral wave bounces at the boundary. (B) Probability of annihilation of the spiral wave at the boundary for a particular angle of incidence θ_i.

occurs with angles greater than 100°. This basically happens because we are considering epitrochoidal trajectories. If we consider hypotrochoidal trajectories, then interactions will take place mostly with angles above 90°.

6.1 More complex dynamics

The interaction of a meandering spiral wave with an obstacle has different outcomes. In Fig. 14A, we show how complex dynamics can be. We took a spiral wave in the epitrochoidal regime such that the tip touches the obstacle and bounces at it. The dynamics of the tip trajectory are shown in Fig. 14A. From the figure it is clear that the trajectory hits the obstacle repeatedly following no visible pattern. As seen in the figure, there is no attachment of the spiral to the obstacle for large time integrations. Clearly, the activation of the tissue is completely irregular and might be considered as being in a fibrillatory regime.

When we consider an obstacle of a very small size, and an epitrochoidal trajectory, it is observed that the trajectory follows a more stable pattern (Fig. 14B). In this case, the trajectory gets close to the obstacle periodically and it can be said that it happens each time the trajectory traces an epitrochoid. As soon as the tip of the trajectory gets close to the obstacle, the boundary effects induce an increase in the curvature of the trajectory, producing drift of the spiral wave. It is important to note that the increase in the curvature is very small as the size of the obstacle is also very small. This small perturbation in the tip trajectory allows the trajectory to preserve the epitrochoidal trajectory as opposed in what is shown in Fig. 14A.

In this section, we have shown that obstacles might act as a switch between the one and two periodic rotations. Therefore, it follows that the presence of obstacles does not necessarily induce a more stable regime in the spiral wave. Moreover, if the spiral wave is in the epitrochoidal regime, the result might be (i) A transition to a simple rotation scheme; (ii)

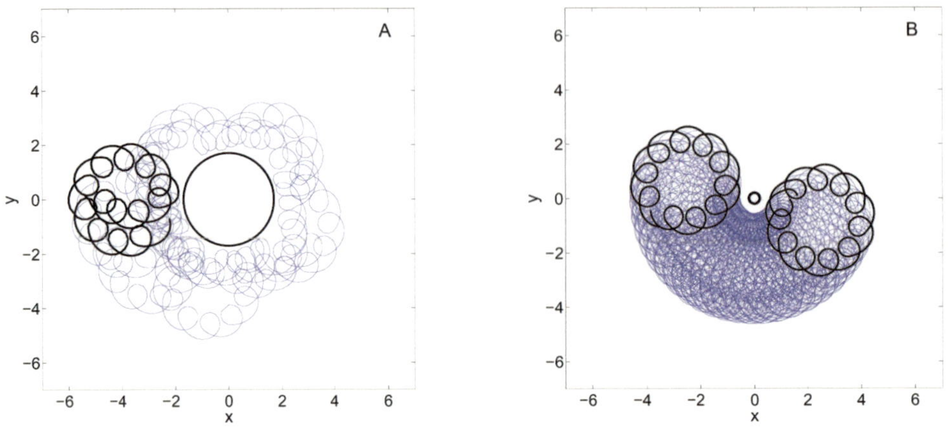

Fig. 14. Tip trajectories traced by a spiral wave solutions of Eqns. (2) when a circular obstacle is imposed. (A) The trajectory does not follow a regular pattern; (B) When the size of the obstacle is small enough a three periodic trajectory is obtained.

A transition to a more complex pattern, and; (*iii*) if the radius of the obstacle is sufficiently small, a transition to a three period rotation [1].

7. Conclusions, limitations and open questions

In this work, it was considered the interaction of spiral waves in the circular and meandering regime with partially and non excitable obstacles of circular shape. The aim was to understand the transitions that occur between three different regimes: the circular, the epitrochoidal and the hypotrochoidal. The presence of a spiral wave in the circular regime, provides a periodic stimulation of the tissue in a more stable fashion than the other two regimes, as only one excitation frequency is present. When a spiral wave attaches to an obstacle the arrhythmic regime is the same as is the tip of a spiral wave were tracing a circle.

When partially excitable obstacles were considered (Section 5), it was shown that the presence of such inhomogeneities induced the appearance of epitrochoidal and hypotrochoidal trajectories, commonly associated to meandering. This implies that epitrochoidal and hypotrochoidal trajectories might arise due to meandering or drift. It is important to point out that tip trajectories obtained with meandering, like linear trajectories (Fenton et al., 2002), were not obtained with drift. Nonetheless it is important to understand the nature of these trajectories to apply the proper procedure to remove them.

Transitions between different spiral wave regimes were obtained when an obstacle was placed in the medium (Sections 5 and 6). In Section 5, tip trajectories changed from epitrochoidal or hypotrochoidal to circular ones. Also, the reversed process might be obtained, i.e. circular trajectories can switch to epitrochoidal or hypotrochoidal trajectories. Finally, transitions from epitrochoidal to hypotrochoidal might also be obtained. On the other hand, in Section 6, it was shown that the presence of an obstacle, might act as a switch between two different arrhythmic regimes. (*i*) Simple rotating spirals changed to a two period meandering spiral wave; (*ii*) Two periodic meandering spiral waves changed to (*a*) simple rotating spiral; (*b*) Three periodic meandering spiral wave and; (*c*) More complex trajectory with no regular pattern associated.

[1] Strictly speaking, the trajectory is not three periodic, but there are three frequencies associated to the tip motion.

In general, it was shown that the presence of inhomogeneities in the medium not only stabilizes the spiral wave dynamics as shown in (Ikeda et al., 1997; Kim et al., 1999; Shajahan et al., 2007) but also might generate more complex dynamics, which implies that the presence of obstacles might induce a more dangerous arrhythmic regime than the one without the obstacle.

Drift of a spiral wave had been considered only for planar boundaries (Yermakova & Pertsov, 1986) and inside circular domains (Mikhailov et al., 1994). In this work, it was presented the drift of a spiral wave around a circular obstacle which was not previously reported. Up to now, there are still missing conditions for general shape obstacles that allow drift of the spiral wave around the obstacle, when the spiral tip traces a circle. A similar analysis for partially excitable obstacles is missing. i.e. which geometric properties must have an obstacle such that the tip trajectory of a spiral wave will follow its boundary?

The study of attachment of meandering spiral waves to non-excitable obstacles is a very difficult task, as there is not a clear a pattern that relates the radius of the obstacle and the radius of the epitrochoid. Also, it is still the question of studying which type of trajectory, epitrochoidal or hypotrochoidal, will attach more easily to an obstacle of a given size. In this work it was not considered the study of hypotrochoidal trajectories and non-excitable obstacles as the original study was to establish conditions to consider an obstacle as a switch between the circular and epitrochoidal regime.

8. Acknowledgements

The author would like to acknowledge ACARUS at the University of Sonora, for their facilities for the numerical computations. This work was supported by PROMEP.

9. References

Azene, E. M.; Trayanova, N. A. & Warman, E. (2001). Wave Front-obstacle interactions in cardiac tissue: a computational study. *Ann. Biomed. Eng.*, Vol. 29, No. 1, (January 2001) (35-46), 0090-6964

Beeler, G. W. & Reuter, H. (1977). Reconstruction of the action potential of ventricular myocardial fibres. *J. Physiol.*, Vol. 268, No. 1, (June 1977) (177-210) 0022-3751

Benson, A. P. & Holden, A. V. (2005). Calcium oscillations and ectopic beats in virtual ventricular myocytes and tissues: bifurcations, autorhythmicity and propagation, In: *Lecture Notes in Computer Science*, Frangi, F; Radeva P. I.; Santos A. & Hernandez, Springer, (895-897), Springer-Verlag Berlin, 3-540-26161-3, Berlin, Germany

Biktashev V. N. (2007). Drift of spiral waves. *Scholarpedia*, Vol. 2, No. 4, (2007) (1836), 1941-6016

Cabo, C.; Pertsov, A. M.; Davidenko, J. M.; Baxter, W. T.; Gray, R. A. & Jalife J. (1996). Vortex shedding as a precursor of turbulent electrical activity in cardiac muscle. *Biophys. J.*, Vol 70, No. 3, (March 1996) (1105-1111), 0006-3495

Comtois, P. & Vinet, A. (2005). Multistability of reentrant rhythms in an ionic model of a two-dimensional annulus of cardiac tissue. *Phys. Rev. E*, Vol. 72, No. 5, (November 2005) 051927(1-11), 1539-3755

Courtemanche, M.; Ramirez, R. J. & Nattel S. (1998). Ionic mechanisms underlying human atrial action potential properties: insights from a mathematical model. *Am. J. Physiol. and Heart Circ. Physiol.*, Vol. 275, No. 1, (July 1998) (H301-H321), 0363-6135

Davidenko, J. M.; Pertsov, A. V.; Salomonsz, R.; Baxter, W. & Jalife, J. (1992). Stationary and drifting spiral waves of excitation in isolated cardiac muscle. *Nature*, Vol. 355, No. 6358, (January 1992) (349-351), 0028-0836

DiFrancesco, D. & Noble, D. (1985). A model of cardiac electrical activity incorporating ionic pumps and concentration changes. *Phil. Trans. R. Soc. Lond.*, Vol. 307, No. 1133, (January 1985), (353-398), 0962-8436

Efimov, I. R.; Krinsky, V. I.; & Jalife, J. (1995). Dynamics of rotating vortices in the Beeler-Reuter model of cardiac tissue. *Chaos, Sol. and Frac.*, Vol. 5, No.3-4 (March-April 1995) (513-526), 0960-0779

Fenton, F. H. & Cherry, E. M. (2008). Models of cardiac cell. *Scholarpedia*, Vol. 3, No. 8, (2008) (1858), 1941-6016

Fenton, F. H. & Karma, A. (1998). Vortex dynamics in three-dimensional continuous myocardium with fiber rotation: Filament instability and fibrillation. *CHAOS*, Vol. 8, No. 1, (March 1998) (20-47), 1054-1500

Fenton, F. H.; Cherry, E.; Hastings, H. M. & Evans, S. J. (2002). Multiple mechanisms of spiral wave breakup in a model of cardiac electrical activity. *CHAOS*, Vol. 12, No. 3, (September 2002) (852-892), 1054-1500

Hodgkin, A. L. & Huxley, A. F. (1952). A quantitative description of membrane current and its application to conduction and excitation in nerve. *J. Physiol*, Vol. 117, (August 1952), (500-544), 0022-3751

Ikeda, T.; Yashima, M.; Uchida, T.; Hough, D.; Fishbein, M. C.; Mandel, W. J.; Chen, P. S. Karagueuzian, H. (1997). Attachment of meandering reentrant wave fronts to anatomic obstacles in the atrium - Role of the obstacle size. *Circ. Res.*, Vol. 81, No. 5, (November 1997) (753-764), 0009-7330

Isomura, A.; Hörning, M.; Agladze, K. & Yoshikawa, K. (2008). Eliminating spiral waves pinned to an anatomical obstacle in cardiac myocytes by high-frequency stimuli. *Phys. Rev. E.* Vol. 78, No. 6, (December 2008) 066216(1-6), 1539-3755

Kim, Y.; Xie, F.; Yashima, M.; Wu, T.; Valderrábano, M.; Lee, M.; Ohara, T.; Voroshilovsky, O.; Doshi, R. N.; Fishbein, M. C.; Qu, Z.; Garfinkel, A.; Weiss, J. N.; Karagueuzian, H. S. & Chen, P. (1999). Role of papillary muscle in the generation and maintenance of reentry during ventricular tachycardia and fibrillation in isolated swine right ventricle. *Circulation*, Vol. 100, No. 13, (September 1999), 1450-1459, 0009-7322

Kléber, A. G. & Rudy, Y. (2004). Basic Mechanisms of cardiac impulse propagation and associated arrhythmias. *Physiol. Rev.*, Vol. 84, No. 2, (April 2004) (431-488), 0031-9333

Leal-Soto, D. A. (2011). M. Sc. Thesis: Interacción de ondas en espiral y obstáculos en medios excitables con la ecuación de Fitzhugh-Nagumo (In Spanish). Universidad de Sonora, México.

Lee K.J. (1997) Wave Pattern Selection in an Excitable System. *Phys. Rev. Lett.* Vol. 79, No. 15, (October 1997) (2907-2910) 0031-9007

Lim, Z. Y.; Maskara, B.; Aguel, F.; Emokpae R. & Tung, L. (2006). Spiral wave attachment to millimeter-sized obstacles. *Circulation*, Vol 114, No. 20 (November 2006) (2113-2121), 0009-7322

Luo, C.-S. & Rudy, Y. (1994). A Dynamic Model of the Cardiac Ventricular Action Potential.I. Simulations of ionic currents and concentration changes. *Circ. Res.*, Vol. 74, No. 8, (June 1994) (1071-1096), 0009-7330

Luo, C.-S. & Rudy, Y. (1994). A Dynamic Model of the Cardiac Ventricular Action Potential.II. Afterdepolarizations, triggered activity, and potentiation. *Circ. Res.*, Vol. 74, No. 8, (June 1994) (1097-1113), 0009-7330

Mikhailov, A. S.; Davydov, V. A.; Zykov, V. S. (1994). Complex dynamics of spiral waves and motion of curves. *Physica D*, Vol 70, No. 1-2, (January 1994) (pages 1-39) 0167-2789

Morton K. W. & Mayers D. F. (2005). *Numerical Solution of Partial Differential Equations*, Cambridge University Press, 978-0-521-60793-0, Cambridge.

Nygren, A.; Fiset, C; Firek, L.; Clark, J. W.; Lindblad, D.S.; Clark, R. B.; Giles W. R. (1998). Mathematical Model of an Adult Human Atrial Cell: The Role of K^+ Currents in Repolarization *Circ. Res.*, Vol 82, No. 1, (January 1998) (63-81), 0009-7330

Olmos, D. (2007). Ph. D. Thesis: Pseudospectral solutions of reaction-diffusion equations that model excitable media: convergence of solutions and Applications. University of British Columbia, Canada.

Olmos, D. & Shizgal B. D. (2008). Annihilation and reflection of spiral waves at a boundary for the Beeler-Reuter model. *Phys. Rev. E*, Vol. 77, No. 3, (March 2008) (031918 1-14), 1539-3755

Olmos, D. (2010). Reflection and attachment of spirals at obstacles for the Fitzhugh-Nagumo and Beeler-Reuter models. *Phys. Rev. E*, Vol. 81, No. 4, (April 2010) 041924(1-9), 1539-3755

Otani, N. F. (2000). Mini Review: Computer Modeling in Cardiac Electrophysiology. *J. Comput. Phys.*, Vol. 161, No. 1, (June 2000) (21-34), 0021-9991

Panfilov, A. V. & Keener, J. P. (1993). Effects of high frequency stimulation on cardiac tissue with an inexcitable obstacle, *J. Theor. Biol*, Vol. 163, No. 4, (August 1993) (439-448), 0022-5193

Pertsov, A. M.; Davidenko, J. M.; Salomonsz, R.; Baxter, W. T. & Jalife, J. (1993). Spiral waves of excitation underlie reentrant activity in isolated cardiac muscle. *Circ. Res.*, Vol. 72, No. 3, (March 1993) 631-650, 0009-7330

Priebe, L. & Beuckelmann, D. J. (1998). Simulation Study of Cellular Electric Properties in Heart Failure. *Circ. Res.*, Vol. 82, No. 11 (June 1998) (1206-1223) 0009-7330

Priori, S. G.; Aliot, E.; Blømstrom-Lundqvist, C.; Bossaert, L.; Breithardt, G.; Brugada, P.; Camm, J. A.; Cappato, R.; Cobbe, S. M.; Di Mario, C.; Maron, B. J.; McKenna, W. J.; Pedersen, A. K.; Ravens U.; Schwartz, P. J.; Trusz-Gluza, M.; Vardas, P.; Wellens, H. J. J. & Zipes, D. P. (2002). Task Force on Sudden Cardiac Death, European Society of Cardiology. *Europace*, Vol. 4 (January 2002) (3-18), 1099-5129

Shajahan, T. K.; Sinha, S. & Pandit, R. (2007). Spiral-wave dynamics depend sensitively on inhomogeneities in mathematical models of ventricular tissue. *Phys. Rev. E*, Vol. 75, No. 1, (January 2007) 011929(1-8), 1539-3755

Shajahan, T. K.; Nayak, A. R. & Pandit, R. (2009) Spiral-Wave Turbulence and its Control in the Presence of Inhomogeneities in Four Mathematical Models of Cardiac Tissue. *Plos One*, Vol. 4, No. 3, (March 2009) (1-21), 1932-6203

Starobin, J. F.; Zilberter, Y. I.; Rusnak, E. M. & Starmer, C. F. (1996). Wavelet formation in excitable cardiac tissue: the role of wavefront-obstacle interactions in initiating high-frequency fibrillatory-like arrhythmias. *Biophys. J.*, Vol. 70, No. 2, (February 1996) (581-594), 0006-3495

Tang, A. S.; Ross, H.; Simpson, C. S.; Mitchell, L. B.; Dorian, P.; Goeree, R.; Hoffmaster, B.; Arnold M. & Talajic, M. (2005). Canadian cardiovascular society / Canadian heart rhythm society position paper on implantable cardioverter defibrillator use in Canada. *Can J. Cardiol*, Vol. 21, Suppl A, (May 2005) (11A-18A), 0828-282X

Ten Tusscher, K. H. W. J. & Panfilov, A. V. (2002). Reentry in heterogeneous cardiac tissue described by the Luo-Rudy ventricular action potential model. *Am J. Physiol. Heart Circ. Physiol.*, Vol. 284, No. 2, (February 2002) (H542-H548), 0363-6135

Valderrábano, M.; Kim, Y.-H.; Yashima, M.; Wu, T.-J.; Karagueuzian, H. S. & Chen, P.-S. (2000). Obstacle-induced transition from ventricular fibrillation to tachycardia in isolated swine right ventricles: Insights into the transition dynamics and implications for the critical mass. *J. Am. Col. Cardiol.*, Vol. 36, No. 6, (November 2000) (2000-2008), 0735-1097

Veenhuyzen, G. D.; Simpson, C. S. & Abdollah, H. (2004). Atrial Fibrillation. *CMAJ*, Vol. 171, No. 7, (September 2004) (755-760), 0820-3946

Xie, F.; Qu, Z.;Garfinkel A. & Weiss J. N. (2001). Effects of simulated ischemia on spiral wave stability. *Am. J. Heart Circ. Physiol.*, Vol. 280, No. 4, (April 2001) (H1667-H1673). 0363-6135

Yanagihara, K.; Noma, A. & Irisawa, H. (1980). Reconstruction of sino-atrial node pacemaker potential based on the voltage clamp experiments. *Jap. J. Physiology*, Vol. 30, No. 6, (1980) (841-857), 0021-521X

Yermakova, Y. A. & Pertsov, A. M. (1986). Interaction of rotating spiral waves with a boundary. *Biophysics*, Vol. 31, No. 5,(932-940) 0006-3509

Zaret, B. L.; Moser, M. & Cohen, L. S. (1992). *Yale University School of Medicine Heart Book*, Hearst books, 0-688-09719-7, New York.

Zipes, D. P. (2005). Epidemiology and mechanisms of sudden cardiac death. *Can J. Cardiol*, Vol. 21, Suppl A, (May 2005) (37A-40A), 0828-282X

18

Electrical Storm

Federico Guerra, Matilda Shkoza, Marco Flori and Alessandro Capucci
Cardiology Clinic, Marche Polytechnic University
Italy

1. Introduction

Electrical storm (ES) is usually defined as a clustering of destabilizing episodes of ventricular tachycardia or ventricular fibrillation in a short period of time, requiring multiple cardioversions or defibrillations. Many criteria have been proposed to define ES since the early 1990s, when the term was first introduced to indicate a state of electrical instability with several ventricular tachycardias (VT) or ventricular fibrillations (VF) over a few hours. At present an official and widespread definition of ES is not available. ES has been defined differently, from two or more to twenty or more episodes within 24 hours. Some definitions were based on number of hemodynamically unstabilizing episodes, others relied on number of shocks needed (or just delivered, whether appropriate or not), and some others on time between each single episode. More imaginative definitions include "VT recurring immediately after termination", "VT for an half of each of three days" and "VT resulting in more total ventricular ectopic beats than sinus beats in 24 hours" (Israel et al, 2007). Fortunately, nowadays most cardiologists define ES as recurrent VT or VF, at least 3 in a 24 hours period, as this is probably the most appropriate and solid definition. This definition does not include the presence of haemodynamic instability, since the intervention of modern implanted cardioverter-defibrillator (ICD) usually terminates the arrhythmia before its clinical and hemodynamical consequences.

Similarly to definitions, many names have been used as synonymous to ES, such as arrhythmic storm, recurrent short-term ventricular arrhythmia, VT clusters and electrical instability. In this chapter we will use the term ES, as the most used and widespread in clinical practice.

ES is more frequently seen as an acute complication of myocardial infarction, as a not-so-uncommon adverse event in ischemic and non ischemic dilated cardiomyopathy and in genetic arrhythmia syndromes, such as congenital long QT syndrome and Brugada syndrome. However, the highest incidence of ES is reported in heart failure patients with ICD. This incidence, which ranges from 4% to 60% according to different studies, is mainly due to two factors. First, ICD can detect the VT of VF underlying a clinical episode of dizziness, syncope or even aborted sudden cardiac death, thus making the diagnosis far easier. Second, and most important, it can effectively treat the first and second VT or VF, thus saving the patient from sudden cardiac death and making him able to withstand more arrhythmic episodes.

The current chapter will summarize the current epidemiology and diagnosis of electrical storm, as well as give some insight on current recommendation regarding pharmacological and non pharmacological treatment.

2. Epidemiology of electrical storm

2.1 Incidence of electrical storm and its different causative arrhythmias

In the last twenty years, several studies were carried out to determine the incidence of ES (table 1).

Author	Year	Definition	Population	%
Wood	1995	≥3 VT/VF ≤24 h	ICD (secondary prevention)	10
Kowey	1996	≥2 VT/VF ≤24 h	All ES patients	-
Villacastin	1996	≥2 shocks for VT	ICD (secondary prevention)	20
Fries	1997	>2 VT ≤ 1 h	ICD (secondary prevention)	60
Credner	1998	≥3 VT/VF ≤24 h	ICD (secondary prevention)	10
Nademanee	2000	≥20 VT/VF ≤24 h ≥4 VT/VF ≤1 h	All ES patients	-
Greene	2000	≥3 VT/VF ≤24 h	ICD (secondary prevention)	18
Bansch	2000	≥3 VT/VF ≤24 h	ICD (secondary prevention)	28
Exner	2001	≥3 VT/VF ≤24 h	ICD (secondary prevention)	20
Verma	2004	≥2 VT/VF ≤24 h	ICD (secondary prevention)	10
Arya	2005	≥3 VT/VF ≤24 h	ICD (30% primary prevention)	13
Brigadeau	2006	≥2 VT/VF ≤24 h	ICD (secondary prevention)	58
Honhloser	2006	≥3 VT/VF ≤24 h	ICD (secondary prevention)	23
Sesselberg	2007	≥3 VT/VF ≤24 h	ICD (primary prevention)	4
Nordbeck	2010	≥3 VT/VF ≤24 h	ICD (55% primary prevention)	7
Streinert	2011	≥3 VT/VF ≤24 h	ICD (81% primary prevention)	7

Table 1. Incidence of electrical storm according to different definitions and populations.

However, due to different definitions of ES and different populations, results vary widely. Most of the evidences come from ICD populations implanted after sustained ventricular arrhythmias, in which ES incidence ranges from 10 to 60 %. ICD recipients implanted for primary prevention, either with underlying ischemic or idiopathic dilated cardiomyopathy, have a lower incidence of ES (from 4 to 7%).

Little is known about incidence after acute myocardial injury, except that is more common in acute ST-elevation myocardial infarction (STEMI), when STEMI is associated with an important left ventricular dysfunction and when reperfusion therapy (either fibrinolysis or percutaneous angioplasty) is late or ineffective.
Similarly, exact incidence and prevalence of ES in genetic arrhythmic syndromes such as Brugada syndrome, familiar long QT syndrome, short-coupled variant of torsade de pointes and right ventricular arrhytmogenic cardiomyopathy is still unknown. Albeit they are all rare conditions, patients afflicted by genetic arrhythmic syndromes are tipically young and otherwise healthy subjects, therefore in immediate need for ES primary prevention.
More than 8 out of 10 arrhythmic episodes constituting ES are monomorphic VT (mVT), with polymorphic VT (pVT) and VF far behind in prevalence (Table 2).

Author	Year	mVT (%)	pVT+VF (%)
Credner	1998	71	29
Greene	2000	97	3
Bansch	2000	91	8
Exner	2001	86	14
Verma	2004	52	48
Brigadeau	2006	90	10
Honhloser	2006	91	9
Sesselberg	2007	78	22
Nordbeck	2010	85	15
Streinert	2011	73	27

Table 2. Prevalence of different ventricular arrhythmia types in ES.

Sustained monomorphic VT is usually related to structural heart disease. Monomorphic VT self-propagation is made possible by a reentry mechanism around a fixed anatomic barrier, which is often represented by a myocardial scar from a previous MI. The same ischemic cardiomyopathy, as it progresses, leads to fibrosis which in turn leads to conduction slowdowns, creating the perfect pathway for reentrant VT. In this particular setting an otherwise harmless trigger such as a premature ventricular contraction is necessary to start monomorphic VT. Monomorphic reentrant VT does not require active ischemia as a trigger, and is an uncommon cause of ES in acute myocardial infarction.
VF and pVT are due to different mechanisms, comprehending multiple activation of different ventricular foci (pVT) or chaotic activation of the whole endocardial ventricular surface (VF). These two arrhythmias are more common in acute myocardial infraction or

when a long QT interval is present. Therefore QT interval should be assessed in all patients with ES due to pVT or VF as soon as sinus rhythm has been restored. Acquired causes of long QT, such as hypokalemia, hypocalcemia, hypomagnesemia, hypothyroidism and medication known to prolong QT interval, should be corrected as soon as possible. Inherited causes of long QT should be suspected whether an acquired cause cannot be found.

2.2 Short and long-term prognosis of electrical storm

Available data strongly suggest that patients who experience an ES have a poor outcome. Only a few trials were inconclusive regarding the role of ES as a mortality marker, and those usually had a wider definition of ES or a shorter follow-up. In secondary prevention populations such as the one of the AVID trial (Exner et al, 2001), patients with ES had a higher risk for non-sudden cardiac death (OR 2.4). In a substudy of the MADIT-II trial, which enrolled primary prevention patients, the risk of death was even higher (OR 7.4). Consistent findings suggest that the increase in mortality is mainly due to the worsening of ventricular dysfunction leading to end stage heart failure, with only a small proportion of sudden cardiac or other deaths (Gatzoulis et al, 2005). This hypothesis is also supported by the fact that risk of death after ES reaches its peak around 2-3 months after the acute event.

Another main clinical consequence of ES is hospitalization, which is required for a proper treatment in approximately 80% of patients (Bänsch et al, 2000). Hospitalization rates grow higher with each shock delivered, reaching 100% if 3 or more shocks are needed. Hospitalization is in turn associated with a poorer quality of life and higher costs.

Patients who experience an ES are more likely to have multiple ES over time. Recent data showed that recurrence of ES happens in more than half of all patients with ES, and is more common within the first year after the original ES episode (Streitner et al, 2011).

2.3 Pseudo-storm

Sometimes multiple recurrent ICD discharges are not associated with ES but are due to device malfunctioning. Pseudo-storm is defined as recurrent inappropriate ICD discharges over 24 hours. Far from being a minor complication, pseudo-storm is usually physical and psychological harmful and potentially lethal. The most common causes of inappropriate ICD shock include supraventricular tachycardia with high ventricular response and oversening of peaked T waves, myopotentials or electrical noise (Gradaus et al, 2003).

Recurrent ICD shocks can cause myocardial injury by direct electrocution cell injury and by activation of signaling pathways in the molecular cascade of HF, the most important of all being adrenergic neurohormonal system. Adrenergic iperactivity may then synergize with recurrent ventricular arrhythmias in exacerbating ventricular dysfunction and worsening heart failure. In a recent paper on a typical ICD population, Sweeney et al. demonstrated that electrical shocks were associated with an increased risk of death independently of underlying ventricular arrhythmia (Sweeney et al, 2010). Authors esteemed that for every delivered shock, whether appropriate or not, the risk of death increases by 20%. On the other hand, no increased risk was associated with anti-tachycardia pacing (ATP) therapies. Pseudo-storm does not only cause myocardial damage, but can deplete a full device battery within hours, potentially leaving the patient unprotected from life-threatening arrhythmic events. Although a very rare complication, fatal arrhythmias actively caused by pseudo-storm are possible. Messali and coworkers described a patient who, three months after an ICD replacement, received six consecutive shocks related to detection of noise interpreted as VF. Unfortunately, the sixth shock triggered a true VF, which was not treated due to the end of the therapeutic sequence, and which led to the patient's death (Messali et al, 2004).

Pseudo-storm should be treated by immediate intervention to suppress ICD shocks. Moreover, inappropriate discharges from ICD should be avoided at all cost by an optimal device programming. ATP therapy should be preferred over shock in the therapeutic sequence, due to its more favorable risk profile.

3. Clinical presentation of electrical storm

3.1 Electrical storm in acute myocardial infarction

Electrical storm, when present, is often the initial manifestation of ischemia and usually starts in the first 48 hours of an ST-elevation MI. In that case, pVT is almost always the ventricular arrhythmia underlying ES. Ischemia and adrenergic activation increase Purkinje cell automaticity, thus letting multiple spontaneous firing. Necrosis, altered myocite membrane potential, electrolytic imbalance and even reperfusion damage can all contribute to increase dispersion of refractory periods between epicardium and endocardium, thus facilitating the propagation of multiple reentry waves.

ES is a strong negative prognostic factor in acute myocardial infarction. In one study where ES was defined as ≥20 VT or VF episodes/day or ≥4 VT/VF episodes/hour, one-week incidence of non-sudden death was as high as 50%. The majority of patients who survived the acute phase, however, have a prognosis relatively comparable with other ES populations. Along with pharmacological therapy, swift and effective reperfusion is crucial to end arrhythmic episodes. Retrospective studies and registry data suggest the hypothesis that, with modern reperfusion therapy currently available, the incidence of ES could be associated with reperfusion time.

3.2 Electrical storm in heart failure

Heart failure is an important risk factor for ES. Most of the times, idiopathic dilated cardiomyopathy is the structural heart disease underlying heart failure in ES patients, followed in prevalence by ischemic cardiomyopathy (Gasparini et al, 2008). Hypertrophic cardiomyopathy and valvular cardiomyopathy, albeit uncommon, has been associated with heart failure worsening leading to ES (Credner et al, 1998).

Left ventricular ejection fraction (LVEF) is the most widespread and easy to obtain marker of systolic dysfunction and has been used to test the association between heart failure and ES. Several studies have found an altered LVEF as an independent risk factor for ES, along with older age, chronic renal failure, causative arrhythmia and electrolytic imbalances (Exner et al, 2001 and Brigadeau et al, 2006). On the other hand, Streitner and coworkers found that a LVEF lower than 30% was not predictive for the initial ES event, but brought a 2.2-fold increased risk for ES recurrence (Streitner et al, 2011).

Current evidence suggests that, more than the presence or absence of heart failure by itself, it is the progression of heart failure and structural cardiomyopathy the real factor in promoting ES and ES recurrence. Therefore, prevention of further systolic function deterioration after an initial ES is mandatory and must be achieved through optimization of medical and resynchronization therapy.

3.3 Electrical storm in patients with congenital pro-arrhythmic diseases

Genetic arrhythmic syndromes or inherited arrhythmic disorders comprise a group of syndromes with unique genetic abnormalities and presentations but with very similar clinical outcomes, the most terrifying of which are life-threatening arrhythmias and sudden cardiac death. Some of them, such as Brugada syndrome and long QT syndrome, affect structural normal hearts, whereas others, such as arrhythmogenic right ventricular cardiomyopathy and left ventricular non-compaction affect deeply the myocardial tissue, and are included in the cardiomyopathies classification. ES has been described in the Brugada syndrome, in the familiar long QT syndrome, in the short-coupled variant of torsade de pointes, in catecholaminergic polymorphic ventricular tachycardia, in arrhythmogenic right ventricular cardiomyopathy and in myocardial non-compaction. Overall, these syndromes are quite rare, being Brugada syndrome the most prevalent with 5 cases out of 10.000, and association with ES in even rarer. However, patients affected by these syndromes are typically young and otherwise completely healthy, making diagnosis and treatment of these conditions challenging.

4. Laboratory and electrical storm

Although electrolytic imbalances, such as hypokalemia, hyperkalemia and hypomagnesemia are a well known risk factors for ventricular arrhythmias and hence ES, many papers report that an evident trigger in a majority of patients cannot be identified by laboratory alone. Credner et al. underlined the presence of hypokalemia, along with acute coronary syndrome and worsening heart failure as potential triggers in 26% of the patients in his case-records (Credner et al, 1998). Similarly, Bänsch et al. found hypokalemia as a potential cause of ES in 20% of their cohort. According to the SHIELD trial, electrolytic imbalance was responsible for storm triggering in only 4% of patients (Hohnloser et al, 2006).
In 2006 for the first time Brigadeau et al. highlighted a possible role of creatinine in predicting ES, identifying a storm trigger in 36% of the whole cohort. Among most common triggers (such as acute coronary syndrome, high body temperature, hypokalemia or hyperkalemia, hyperthyroidism and acute heart failure) chronic renal failure, identified as a creatinine clearance lower than 60 ml/min, was independently associated with ES occurrence. Thus, this study concluded that the patients with a defibrillator who are likely to undergo electrical storm are those who have both low left ventricular ejection fraction and chronic renal failure (Brigadeau et al, 2006). In a recent MADIT II chronic kidney disease was associated with a 2.1-fold increase in risk for ES in both primary and secondary prevention patient (Sesselberg et al., 2007).
Thyroid disorders (both hypothyroidism and hyperthyroidism) have been suggested as a trigger for ES. However, at present there is scarce evidence of an important role of thyroid hormones in ventricular arrhythmias pathogenesis. In one case report ES was attributed to amiodarone-induced thyrotoxicosis (Marketou et al, 2001). The patient was unresponsive to medical therapy and the ES was successfully terminated by thyroidectomy.
In conclusion, in an ES setting laboratory could play an important role. Electrolytic abnormalities such as hypokalemia, hyperkalemia and hypomagnesemia should be promptly diagnosed and corrected, as potential triggers of arrhythmic events. High serum levels of BNP, creatinine and PCR are valid markers for respectively decompensated heart failure, chronic renal insufficiency and pro-inflammatory state, and should be assessed in every patients experiencing ES as useful stratification tools.

5. Electrical storm therapy

5.1 Pharmacological therapy

5.1.1 Amiodarone

Amiodarone is widely used in the treatment of ventricular arrhythmias. Intravenous amiodarone appears to be the most effective agent for ES, and may even suppress ventricular tachycardia that recurs despite chronic oral amiodarone therapy. In acute ES, a rapid intravenous amiodarone administration (300 mg or 5 mg/kg rapid push followed by repeated boluses at half the above doses for breakthrough episodes) blocks fast sodium channels in a use-dependent fashion (producing more channel blockade at faster heart rates), inhibits norepinephrine release, and blocks L-type calcium channels without prolonging ventricular refractoriness. On the other hand, prolonged ventricular refractory periods are seen in oral amiodarone therapy over periods ranging from days to weeks. Amiodarone has few negative inotropic effects and is safe in patients who have depressed systolic function. It is in fact the only anti-arrhythmic drug with solid safety evidences in patients with NYHA class III and IV or recently decompensated heart failure. Moreover, the incidence of torsades de pointes is low in such patients despite the potential significant prolongation of the QT interval. Amiodarone efficacy in terminating ES is approximately 60%. When compared with placebo in the ARREST trial, amiodarone improved survival to hospital admission in patients who had a cardiac arrest that involved VF or pulseless VT (Kudenchuk et al, 1999). Amiodarone can be effective even when other agents have been ineffective. Levine and colleagues examined 273 hospitalized patients who had electrical storm that was refractory to lidocaine, procainamide, and bretylium therapy (Levine et al, 1996). When amiodarone was given, 46% of the patients survived for 24 hours without another episode of VT, and another 12% improved after taking amiodarone plus lidocaine or procainamide. Side effects of short-term amiodarone intravenous use are rare. A combination of intravenous amiodarone and propranolol improves survival rates and should be the mainstay of therapy in acute management of ES.

Oral amiodarone is effective as adjunctive therapy to prevent recurrent ICD shocks. The OPTIC (Optimal Pharmacological Therapy in Implantable Cardioverter) study compared amiodarone (200 mg maintenance dose following 6 weeks of loading) plus β-blocker with sotalol (240 mg adjusted for renal function) or β-blocker alone (Connolly et al, 2006). Appropriate shocks were reduced by amiodarone compared with β-blocker therapy only by 70%, inappropriate shocks were reduced by 78%, appropriate shocks and ATP were reduced by 70%, and all-cause shocks excluding the first 21 days were reduced by 82%. The mean number of shocks per year was 4.32 in the beta-blocker only group, 0.93 in the sotalol group, and 0.51 in the amiodarone group. Although long-term amiodarone therapy is usually successful, substantial side effects include pulmonary fibrosis, hypothyroidism, liver toxicity, and corneal deposits. In addition, amiodarone may increase the energy required for successful defibrillation, so patients with ICDs should undergo repeated defibrillation threshold testing. Patients who have episodes of electrical storm despite amiodarone therapy may benefit from β-blockers adjunctive therapy or undergo RF ablation.

5.1.2 β-blockers

β-blockers play a key role in the management of electrical storm. Their effects were discovered in the 1970s, when they were studied as therapy for acute MI. First evidences regarding a possible role as anti-arrhythmic drugs come from canine models (Anderson et al, 1983). All β-blockers increased 6-fold the fibrillation threshold and made the animals less susceptible to fibrillation under ischemic and non-ischemic conditions. The improvement was greater with the use of more potent β-blockers and with those that antagonized both β1 and β2 receptors. Although several β-blockers decrease susceptibility to VF, most of the studies have focused on propranolol. Propranolol consistently decreases the incidences of fatal VF during acute MI and sudden cardiac death after MI (Tsagalou et al, 2005). In patients with congestive heart failure, propranolol decreases sympathetic outflow more than does metoprolol, perhaps because β2 receptors prevail in failing hearts (Newton et al, 1996). The lipophilic nature of propranolol enables active penetration of the central nervous system and the blockade of central and prejunctional receptors in addition to peripheral β receptors. Propranolol may effectively suppress an electrical storm even when metoprolol has failed (Tsagalou et al, 2005). Therefore, propranolol, given at a dose of 0.15 mg/kg intravenous bolus over 10 minutes followed by a 3-5 mg dose every 6 hours, is a first line therapy in emergency ES setting. Nademanee and coworkers investigated the efficacy of sympathetic blockade in electrical storm comparing propranolol, esmolol, and left stellate ganglionic blockade to combined lidocaine, procainamide, and bretylium therapy (Nademanee et al, 2000). All their patients have experienced a recent MI and more than 20 episodes of VT within 24 hours or more than 4 episodes per hour. Sympathetic blockade provided a marked survival advantage (78% versus 18% at one week, and 67% versus 5% at one year). Despite the high doses of propranolol, an increase in heart failure progression was not reported in this study, although it is known from previous studies that propranolol can exacerbate heart failure in patients with poor systolic function and use in these patients should be carefully monitored. The short acting intravenous esmolol may also be used but its dosing and titration are somewhat more complicated. Miwa et al. have demonstrated that landiolol, an ultra-short acting β1-selective blocker is useful as a life-saving drug for amiodarone-resistant ES (Miwa et al, 2010). Landiolol in ES is used intravenously with an initial dose of 2.5 μg/kg*min, which can be doubled every 10 minutes if first dose is ineffective, up to a maximum dose of 80 μg/kg*min. Landiolol has a shorter plasma half-life (4 minutes) than esmolol (9 minutes) or propanolol (2 hours) and higher β1 selectivity. These properties suggest that adverse respiratory effects, such as bronchial asma, are less likely to develop and to persist with landiolol, which make it more suitable for emergency medical care. When amiodarone was ineffective, landiolol inhibited ES in 33 patients (79%) at a mean dose of 7.5 μg/kg*min. All patients in whom landiolol was ineffective died of arrhythmia. Of the 33 patients in whom landiolol was effective, 25 survived and were discharged (60% of all patients). At present, landiolol is not available in most European countries and its safety profile in ES still needs to be assessed, making this drug a promising alternative to propranolol when amiodarone alone is ineffective.

5.1.3 Lidocaine

Intravenous sodium-channel blockers (lidocaine, procainamide) are minimally effective in suppressing shock-resistant VT/VF and ES (Credner et al, 1996 and Nademanee et al, 2000). Lidocaine binds to fast sodium channels in a use-dependent fashion. Binding increases under cellular conditions that are common in ischemic VT, such as reduced pH, faster stimulation rate and reduced membrane potential. However, lidocaine has relatively weak antiarrhythmic properties outside the ischemic setting: conversion rates from VT to sinus rhythm range from 8% to 30%. In one study enrolling patients with out-of-hospital, shock-resistant VT or VF, only 12% of those randomized to lidocaine survived to hospital admission, versus 23% who received amiodarone. On the basis of this and other findings, amiodarone has replaced lidocaine as first line therapy for refractory VT and VF. Actual recommendations suggest intravenous lidocaine only in the treatment of polymorphic VT associated with acute ischemia. If lidocaine is used, it should be administered as an intravenous bolus of 0.5 to 0.75 mg/kg that is repeated every 5 to 10 min as needed. A continuous intravenous infusion of 1 to 4 mg/min maintains therapeutic levels. The maximum total dose is 3 mg/kg over 1 hr.

5.1.4 Procainamide

Procainamide blocks fast sodium channels in a use-dependent fashion and is metabolized to N-acetylprocainamide, which in turn blocks potassium channels and accounts for much of the antiarrhythmic effect in vivo. When given as a loading dose of 100 mg over 5 min, procainamide is a reasonable choice for terminating monomorphic VT. In patients with depressed systolic function procainamide can cause hypotension or prolong QRS width by more than 50%, either of which would necessitate discontinuation of the drug. Procainamide prolongs the QT interval and therefore could cause torsade de pointes. Its use is contraindicated in patients with impaired renal function, because N-acetylprocainamide is excreted by the kidneys.

5.1.5 Azimilide

Azimilide is an experimental class III antiarrhythmic drug that blocks calcium channels and prolongs the energy potential and refractory periods. The recently published SHIELD trial showed that azimilide is effective and helps to reduce the number of ICD discharges, though not mortality (Stefan et al, 2006). A secondary analysis of the SHIELD data found that during a prospective one-year follow up azimilide significantly reduced the incidence of ES in comparison with placebo. Azimilide could become an alternative for the treatment of ES whenever it becomes commercially available.

5.1.6 Polypharmacological approach

Optimization of β-blocker therapy is the first important step, particularly when the electrical storm is triggered by ischemia or increased sympathetic tone. The next step is initiating anti-arrhythmic therapy if patient still experiences ES. In the absence of contraindications (such as QT lengthening or polymorphic ventricular tachycardia), amiodarone is generally the antiarrhythmic drug of choice and has been validated in numerous clinical trials (Kowey et al, 1995 and Wood et al, 1995). Most of the time, optimized β-blocker therapy plus intravenous amiodarone will control the electrical storm within 24 to 48 hours. This appears to be the most effective therapy for electrical storm. If the intravenous combination of amiodarone and β-blockers proves inefficacious, the addition of lidocaine is a reasonable option. Although controlled data are not available, combination of anti-arrhythmic drug allows lower and better tolerated doses of individual drugs, and offers the potential of synergistic effects.

5.1.7 Sedation

The physical and emotional stress that patients experience in association with electrical storm and multiple electrical cardioversions increases adrenergic tone and often perpetuates arrhythmias. All patients who have electrical storm should be sedated. Sedation or general anesthesia are needed in resistant cases where repeated shocks or anti-tachicardia transthoracic pacing are needed. Short-acting anesthetics such as propofol, benzodiazepines, and some agents of general anesthesia have been associated with the conversion and suppression of VT (Burjorjee & Milne, 2002). Left stellate ganglion blockade and thoracic epidural anesthesia have also suppressed electrical storms that were refractory to multiple antiarrhythmic agents and β blockade (Nademanee et al, 2000). These therapeutic approaches directly target nerve fibers that innervate the myocardium, and a reduced adrenergic tone is most likely responsible for the reported efficacy. Is currently unknown whether sedative and anesthetic agents may have direct antiarrhythmic effects.

5.2 Implantable defibrillators: First-line therapy and first-line diagnostic?

ES is quite common in ICD recipients. In different studies the incidence of ES in patients with an ICD ranges from 10 to 60% when ICDs are implanted for secondary prevention (Arya A et al, 2005) and 4% to 7% when ICDs are implanted for primary prevention (Sesselberg et al, 2007). A higher incidence of ES in ICD patients is related to an higher cardiovascular mortality and morbidity among ICD recipients. As previously said the presence of ICD allows the physician to recognize more arrhythmias and the patient to survive the arrhythmia and hence manifest more episodes.

Occurrence of ES after ICD implant has changed over time. A paper from the late 1990s reported the peak of incidence of ES between 4 and 5 months after implant (Credner et al, 1998). On the other hand recent evidences pushed the onset of ES to 26 months after implant (Streitner et al, 2011). Total number of episodes varied over time too: as much as 55 mean episodes per patient have been reported (Greene et al, 2000), whereas more recent papers describe far less VT/VF per single patient (Streitner et al, 2011). Both these findings could be explained by changes in antiarrhythmic therapy and ICD technology occurred in this last decade which in turn led to fewer total arrhythmic episodes and improved overall prognosis.

There is a multitude of etiologies of ES in ICD patients: hypokalemia or other electrolytic imbalance, drugs (diuretics, b-adrenergic drugs, alcohol), ischemia, medication noncompliance and less common causes such as fever or stress (Huang et al, 2005 and Israel et al, 2007). The most common cause of ES in ICD patients is exacerbation of heart failure, as underlying ischemic or idiopathic dilated cardiomyopathy could progress despite medical therapy and arrhythmic prevention. Nevertheless, most ES have no clear etiology and even an exhaustive search for acute cause may prove fruitless.

Clinical presentation can vary dramatically depending on arrhythmias typology (monomorphic VT, polymorphic VT or VF) and patient's characteristics (EF, NYHA class, comorbidities). The presence of syncope associated with arrhythmia depends both on hemodynamic factors and on ICD settings (mostly shock charging time). The most important acute consequence related to ES is hospitalization that is required in more than 80% of patients, particularly when shocks are delivered (Bansch et al, 2000). ICD patients presenting ES have higher morbidity and mortality, hence determination of predictors is needed to identify high risk patients.

Data on risk factors of ES are far from comprehensive or conclusive but most studies consider low EF and secondary prevention as major risk factors for developing ES in ICD recipients. High NT-proBNP and hs-CRP, history of atrial fibrillation before implant or single/dual chamber pacing over CRT are also described as predisposing to ES (Streitner et al, 2011).

ICD patients who experienced a first ES are also more likely to experience one or more ES recurrence. Recurrence rate is as high as 80% within 12 months after the first episode, according to Steinert, who described LVEF < 30%, age > 65 years, chronic obstructive pulmonary disease and lack of ACE inhibitors therapy as independent predictors of ES recurrence (Steinert et al, 2011).
Most authors report poor prognosis associated whit ES with a risk of death increased from 1.9 to 17.8 fold. Death rate is usually low during hospitalization and acute episode but increases afterward, particularly during the first year after ES.
Lately, new tools have become available to detect and manage ES in ICD patients. All major ICD companies now offer some sort of home or remote monitoring along with their devices. Home monitoring offers the physician reports for arrhythmic events, device battery and parameters status in real-time. Asymptomatic or lightly symptomatic ES could be then promptly recognized and the patient immediately called in for a check-up without the need to wait for the next programmed ambulatory visit. Figure 1 shows how an ES looks like on auto-generated home monitoring report: the patient experienced 37 arrhythmic episodes in less than 24 hours, 36 VT terminated with a shock after ATP sequence was ineffective and 1 VF episode terminated with ATP.
Figure 2 shows how EGM can be seen and interpreted via remote monitoring. In this EGM VT has been correctly detected and treated by ICD shock.

5.3 Is cardiac resynchronization therapy useful in preventing electrical storm?

Cardiac resynchronization therapy (CRT) is a well established therapy for treatment of moderate to severe heart failure. Several studies assessed benefits from biventricular pacing resulting in prevention of left ventricular remodeling and improvement of hemodynamic, ejection fraction, NYHA class, quality of life, morbidity and mortality (Cleeland et al, 2005). Effects of CRT on ventricular arrhythmias are less well established. Some evidence suggests that pacing itself might cause arrhythmias and some authors reported an increase in incidence of atrial fibrillations, ventricular arrhythmias or even electrical storms after biventricular pacing (Kantharia et al, 2006). However, currently available large-scale trials showed no significant proarrhythmic effects of CRT. On the other hand, there is no strong evidence of a direct antiarrhythmic effect of CRT over single or dual chamber pacing either. Nordbeck et al. compared incidence of ES in 168 CRT and 561 ICD patients. They found significant lower incidence of ES in CRT group (0.6% versus 7%), suggesting that, beside the well known hemodynamic improvements, cardiac resynchronization therapy may reduce the arrhythmia burden in heart failure patients (Nordbeck et al, 2010). An Italian group found a higher incidence of ES (11.3% vs 5.3%) in patients non responder to CRT therapy, defined as minor improvement in NYHA class and ejection fraction (Gasparini et al, 2008). These data support the hypothesis that CRT may have an indirect antiarrhythmic effect, due to factors which are still unclear. Nordbeck suggests that the reduction of arrhythmic burden could be due to improvement of cardiac output and ejection fraction from CRT, as ejection fraction is a known risk factor for ventricular arrhythmias. Another hypothesis by Kowal found some evidences in clinical cases reporting a specific role of cardiac pacing site in development or suppression of VT. He hypothesized that the mechanism of arrhythmia suppression under biventricular pacing could be ascribed to preexcitation of the area of slow conduction responsible for the reentrant arrhythmia (Kowal et al, 2004).
Nevertheless, electrophysiologic effects of CRT are still poorly understood. Biventricular pacing remains a major therapeutic tool in the treatment of heart failure but additional data are required to assess its efficacy as antiarrhythmic therapy.

To:		
Report from 28-Jul-2011 11:45	Patient ID: **S** **P**	
	Device / Device SN: **Lumax 300 HF-T / 60462319**	Patient device SN: **46817123**

Recordings

Recordings - Episode list:

No.	Detection time	Type	Details	Predetection PP/RR	Pretermination PP/RR
84	29-Apr-2011 10:41:41	VT1	ATP: 3; Shocks delivered: 1	772 / 390	835 / 668
83	29-Apr-2011 10:37:42	VT1	ATP: 3; Shocks delivered: 1	772 / 387	816 / 719
82	29-Apr-2011 10:14:07	VT1	ATP: 3; Shocks delivered: 1	773 / 387	845 / 763
81	29-Apr-2011 10:06:14	VT1	ATP: 3; Shocks delivered: 1	770 / 387	922 / 998
80	29-Apr-2011 10:01:45	VT1	ATP: 3; Shocks delivered: 1	787 / 394	795 / 785
79	29-Apr-2011 09:51:22	VT1	ATP: 3; Shocks delivered: 1	787 / 393	801 / 823
78	29-Apr-2011 09:49:28	VF	ATP: 1; ATP One Shot: YES; Shocks aborted: 1	> 1998 / 271	599 / 553
77	29-Apr-2011 09:47:14	VT1	ATP: 3; Shocks delivered: 1	889 / 390	663 / 646
76	29-Apr-2011 09:41:47	VT1	ATP: 3; Shocks delivered: 1	784 / 383	695 / 880
75	29-Apr-2011 09:34:03	VT1	ATP: 3; Shocks delivered: 1	662 / 383	1409 / 917
74	29-Apr-2011 09:20:11	VT1	ATP: 3; Shocks delivered: 1	853 / 379	437 / 654
73	29-Apr-2011 09:04:47	VT1	ATP: 3; Shocks delivered: 1	582 / 387	1049 / 797
72	29-Apr-2011 08:50:27	VT1	ATP: 3; Shocks delivered: 1	786 / 393	> 1998 / 922
71	29-Apr-2011 08:27:16	VT1	ATP: 3; Shocks delivered: 1	672 / 390	555 / 898
70	29-Apr-2011 08:23:31	VT1	ATP: 3; Shocks delivered: 1	638 / 392	1244 / 915
69	29-Apr-2011 08:10:59	VT1	ATP: 3; Shocks delivered: 1	685 / 395	601 / 554
68	29-Apr-2011 06:46:20	VT1	ATP: 3; Shocks delivered: 1	751 / 374	931 / 804
67	29-Apr-2011 06:00:11	VT1	ATP: 3; Shocks delivered: 1	1008 / 405	1225 / 976
66	29-Apr-2011 05:30:13	VT1	ATP: 3; Shocks delivered: 1	784 / 390	566 / 851
65	29-Apr-2011 05:19:23	VT1	ATP: 3; Shocks delivered: 1	690 / 384	727 / 856
63	29-Apr-2011 04:52:44	VT1	ATP: 3; Shocks delivered: 1	766 / 383	1310 / 842
62	28-Apr-2011 23:59:30	VT1	ATP: 3; Shocks delivered: 1	588 / 386	584 / 598
61	28-Apr-2011 22:08:25	VT1	ATP: 3; Shocks delivered: 1	525 / 387	> 1998 / 747
60	28-Apr-2011 20:56:48	VT1	ATP: 3; Shocks delivered: 1	872 / 387	> 1998 / 868
59	28-Apr-2011 19:44:17	VT1	ATP: 3; Shocks delivered: 1	649 / 396	754 / 703
58	28-Apr-2011 19:16:43	VT1	ATP: 3; Shocks delivered: 1	677 / 387	655 / 740
57	28-Apr-2011 19:10:38	VT1	ATP: 3; Shocks delivered: 1	758 / 397	475 / 896
56	28-Apr-2011 19:06:48	VT1	ATP: 3; Shocks delivered: 1	671 / 382	610 / 536
55	28-Apr-2011 19:03:33	VT1	ATP: 3; Shocks delivered: 1	801 / 392	670 / 804
	28-Apr-2011 17:11:56	Follow-up			
54	28-Apr-2011 16:53:24	VT1	ATP: 3; Shocks delivered: 1	873 / 389	508 / 728
53	28-Apr-2011 16:43:14	VT1	ATP: 3; Shocks delivered: 1	1101 / 390	827 / 680
52	28-Apr-2011 16:31:38	VT1	ATP: 3; Shocks delivered: 1	1267 / 390	> 1998 / 878
51	28-Apr-2011 16:15:21	VT1	ATP: 3; Shocks delivered: 1	> 1998 / 385	> 1998 / 783
50	28-Apr-2011 15:49:35	VT1	ATP: 3; Shocks delivered: 1	> 1998 / 394	774 / 768
49	28-Apr-2011 15:34:34	VT1	ATP: 3; Shocks delivered: 1	885 / 396	538 / 760

Fig. 1. 78 year-old patient with dilated idiopathic cardiomyopathy. In this report the patient experienced 37 arrhythmic episodes in less than 24 hours. Physicians can check the report directly online in real time, allowing fast diagnosis of ES and, hence, immediate treatment of ES.

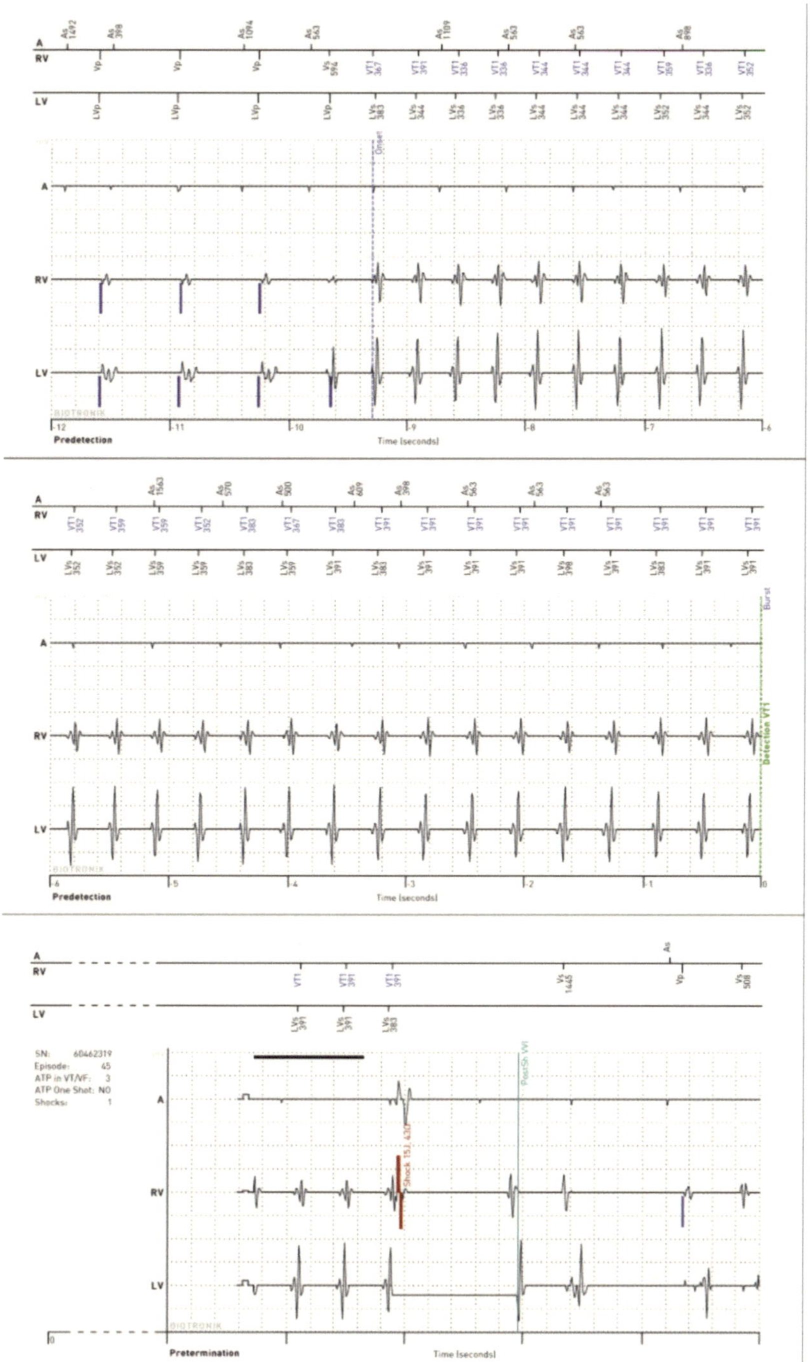

Fig. 2. One of the arrhythmic episodes reported in Fig.1. In this EGM a ventricular tachycardia in VT zone starts abruptly following a premature ventricular contraction. Atrio-venticular dissociation is easily visible. ATP was ineffective whereas 15J delivered shock successfully terminated VT.

5.4 Specific therapy in congenital pro-arrhythmic diseases

Although electrical storm associated with Brugada syndrome is exceptional, it is a major and life threatening event that requires rapid and effective treatment. In most cases presented to date, infusion of isoproterenol (as a 1-2 μg bolus injection followed by continuous infusion at 0.15 μg/min, or at a rate of about 0.003 μg/kg/min tritated to result in a 20% increase in heart rate), was used to terminate electrical storm. Other cases reported intravenous orciprenaline infusion or quinidine as effective in terminating ES. Direct β adrenergic stimulation by isoproterenol and orciprenaline increases the L-type calcium current, which restores the epicardial action potential dome, normalizes ST segment elevations and suppresses ventricular arrhythmias. It should be emphasized that orciprenaline or quinidine use as last resort approach in ES is limited to cases of confirmed Brugada syndrome, while in the majority of ES associated with ischemic or dilated cardiomyopathy, orciprenaline or quinidine application may result in fatal outcome.

In the congenital long QT syndrome, high dose β-blockers can suppress the occurrence of ES and frequent ICD discharges. In refractory cases, left cardiac sympathetic denervation results in marked reduction in ES incidence.

In the ES associated with the short-coupled variant of torsade de pointes ventricular tachycardia, verapamil or the combination of verapamil and mexiletine is somewhat effective. Intravenous magnesium and overdrive pacing are the treatment of choice for drug-induced torsade de pointes.

Arrhythmogenic right ventricular cardiomyopathy and myocardial non-compaction deeply modify heart structure, and ES associated with these conditions is usually resistant to medical therapy. Heart transplantation represents nowadays the only viable option for terminating recurrent, haemodynamically destabilizing arrhythmias in these patients.

5.5 Last resource therapies. Radio-frequency ablation and heart transplantation

5.5.1 Radio-frequency ablation

Although radiofrequency catheter ablation (CA) has an established role in the treatment of recurrent VT, only recently it has been suggested as a method of choice in management of ES, especially when pharmacological and ICD therapies fail. The best candidates for CA are those ventricular arrhythmias in which the initiating beat or premature ventricular contractions morphologically identical to the initiating beat can be localized with electroanatomical mapping. In patients affected with ischemic cardiomyopathy the typical site of the initiating beat is around the border zone of the scar tissue. The procedure can be performed under light anesthesia or deep sedation, according to the hemodynamic state of the patient. If the VT is not incessant, a stimulation protocol from right and left ventricle and up to three extrastimuli is usually applied to induce clinical VT and determine its characteristics. Mapping and ablation is usually performed by an irrigated-tip catheter introduced into the right ventricle or left ventricle by direct femoral vein approach or retrograde transaortic or transseptal approach, respectively. Electroanatomical mapping is nowadays the standard of care, being safe and effective.

The largest series of patients undergoing CA for refractory ES has been described by Carbucicchio and coworkers. Solid electrophysiological evidence of the effective treatment of the presenting VT was achieved in 89% of patients, whereas a transient effect of CA causing short-term stabilization but ineffective in long-term ES prevention was observed in the remaining 11% of patients (Carbucicchio et al, 2008). In this latter group, CA acted only as a temporary bailout, with no impact on ES recurrence. In a recent Czech study RF ablation proved effective in suppression of ES in 84% of cases; however, repeated procedures were necessary in 1 out of 4 patients (Kozeluhova et al, 2011). Severely depressed left ventricular ejection fraction, highly-dilated left ventricle, renal insufficiency, and ES recurrence after previous ablation procedure were independently associated with adverse outcome within the first 6 months after the procedure. Is it still unclear whether inducibility testing of the VT at the end of the study is predictive of mortality and arrhythmic recurrences, as currently available data are controversial.

Successful CA of refractory ES in the absence of a detectable trigger has also been described. Schreieck and colleagues reported a case series of 5 ischemic patients with unmappable recurrent VTs, in which CA was attempted targeting delayed local potentials guided by voltage mapping and pace mapping (Schreieck et al, 2004). These isolated delayed potentials are found exclusively in areas of dense scar, making this kind of technique ineffective in idiopathic dilated cardiomyopathy.

On a side note, patients with pseudo-storm due to inappropriate ICD shocks induced by atrial tachyarrhythmias can benefit from CA of atrial flutter, atrial fibrillation or even AV node ablation.

5.5.2 Heart transplantation

Patients with no significant comorbidities except for recurrent ES who experienced no improvements from pharmacological, device-related and surgical treatment should be considered for cardiac transplantation. Patients with refractory ES associated with a genetic arrhythmia syndromes may also be reasonable candidates for heart transplantation as these patients are typically young, otherwise healthy individuals with good quality of life and prognosis.

In haemodynamically instable patients, intraaortic balloon pump and cardiac assist devices should be used as bridge-to-transplant, as potentially lifesaving.

6. References

Anderson JL, Rodier HE, Green LS. (1983) Comparative effects of beta-adrenergic blocking drugs on experimental ventricular fibrillation threshold. *American Journal of Cardiology*, 51, 1196-1202.

Arya A, Haghjoo M, Dehghani MR, et al. (2005) Prevalence and predictors of electrical storm in patients with implantable cardioverter-defibrillator. *American Journal of Cardiology*, 97, 389–392.

Bansch D, Bocker D, Brunn J. (2000) Clusters of ventricular tachycardias signify impaired survival in patients with idiopathic dilated cardiomyopaty and implantable cardioverter defibrillators. *Journal of the American College of Cardiology*, 36, 566-573.

Brigadeau F, Kouakam C, Klug D, et al. (2006) Clinical predictors and prognostic significance of electrical storm in patients with implantable cardioverter defibrillators. *European Heart Journal*, 27, 700–707.

Burjorjee JE, Milne B. (2002) Propofol for electrical storm; a case report of cardioversion and suppression of ventricular tachycardia by propofol. *Canadian Journal of Anesthesia*, 49, 973-977.

Carbucicchio C, Santamaria M, Trevisi N, et al. (2008) Catheter ablation for the treatment of electrical storm in patients with implantable cardioverter-defibrillators: short- and long-term outcomes in a prospective single-center study. *Circulation*, 29, 117, 462-469.

Cleeland JGF, Daubert JC, Erdman E, et al. (2005) The effect of cardiac resynchronization on morbidity and mortality in heart failure. *New England Journal of Medicine*, 352, 1539-1549.

Connolly SJ, Dorian P, Roberts RS, et al. (2006) Comparison of beta-blockers, amiodarone plus beta-blockers, or sotalol for prevention of shocks from implantable cardioverter defibrillators: the OPTIC Study: a randomized trial. *Journal of the American Medical Association*, 295, 165-171.

Credner SC, Klingenheben T, Mauss O, et al. (1998) Electrical storm in patients with transvenous implantable cardioverter-defibrillators: incidence, management and prognostic implications. *Journal of the American College of Cardiology*, 32, 1909–1915.

Exner DV, Pinski SL, Wyse DG, et al. (2001) Electrical storm presages nonsudden death: the antiarrhythmics versus implantable defibrillators (AVID) trial. *Circulation*, 103, 2066–2071.

Gasparini M, Lunati M, Landolina M et al. (2008) Electrical storm in patients with biventricular implantable cardioverter defibrillator: Incidence, predictors and prognostic implications. *American Heart Journal*, 156, 847-854.

Gatzoulis KA, Andrikopoulos G, Apostolopoulos T, et al. (2005) Electrical storm is an independent predictor of adverse longterm outcome in the era of implantable defibrillator therapy. *Europace*, 7, 184-192.

Gradaus R, Block M, Brachmann J, et al. (2003) Mortality, morbidity, and complications in 3,344 patients with implantable cardioverter defibrillators: results from the German ICD registry EURID. *Pacing and Clinical Electrophysiology*, 26, 1511-1518.

Greene M, Newman D, Geist M, et al. (2000) Is electrical storm in ICD patients the sign of a dying heart? Outcome of patients with clusters of ventricular tachyarrhythmias. *Europace*, 2, 263–269.

Huang DT, Traub D. (2008) Recurrent ventricular arrhythmia storms in the age of implantable cardioverter defibrillator therapy: a comprehensive review. *Progress in Cardiovascular Diseases*, 51, :229-236.

Hohnloser SH, Al-Khalidi HR, Pratt CM, et al. (2006) Electrical storm in patients with an implantable defibrillator: incidence, features, and preventive therapy: insights from a randomized trial. *European Heart Journal*, 27, 3027-3032.

Israel CW, Barold SS. (2007) Electrical storm in patient with implanted defibrillator: a matter of definition. *Annals of Noninvasive Electrocardiology*, 12, 375-82.

Kantharia BK, Patel JA, Nagra BS, et al. (2006) Electrical storm of monomorphic ventricular tachycardia after a cardiac resynchronization therapy defibrillator upgrade. *Europace*, 8, 625-628.

Kowal RC, Wasmund SL, Smith ML, et al. (2004) Biventricular pacing reduces the induction of monomorphic ventricular tachycardia: a potential mechanism for arrhythmia suppression. *Heart Rhythm*, 1:295–300.

Kowey PR, Levine JH, Herre JM, et al. (1995) Randomized, double-blind comparison of intravenous amiodarone and bretylium in the treatment of patients with recurrent, hemodynamically destabilizing ventricular tachycardia or fibrillation. The

Intravenous Amiodarone Multicenter Investigators Group. *Circulation*, 92, 3255-3263.

Kozeluhova M, Peichl P, Cihak R, et al. (2011) Catheter ablation of electrical storm in patients with structural heart disease. *Europace*, 13, 109-13.

Kudenchuk PJ, Cobb LA, Copass MK, et al. (1999) Amiodarone for resuscitation after out-of-hospital cardiac arrest due to ventricular fibrillation. *New England Journal of Medicine*, 341, 871-878.

Levine JH, Massumi A, Scheinman MM, et al. (1996) Intravenous amiodarone for recurrent sustained hypotensive ventricular tachyarrhythmias. Intravenous Amiodarone Multicenter Trial Group. *Journal of the American College of Cardiology*, 27, 67-75.

Marketou ME, Simantirakis EN, Manios EG, et al. (2001) Electrical storm due to amiodarone induced thyrotoxicosis in a young adult with dilated cardiomyopathy: thyroidectomy as the treatment of choice. *Pacing and Clinical Electrophysiology*, 24, 1827-1828.

Messali A, Thomas O, Chauvin M, et al. (2004) Death due to an implantable cardioverter defibrillator. *Journal of Cardiovascular Electrophysiology*, 15, 953-956.

Miwa Y, Ikeda T, Mera H, et al. (2010) Effects of landiolol, an ultra-short-acting beta1-selective blocker, on electrical storm refractory to class III antiarrhythmic drugs. *Circulation Journal*, 74, 856-863.

Newton GE, Parker JD. (1996) Acute effects of beta 1-selective and nonselective beta-adrenergic receptor blockade on cardiac sympathetic activity in congestive heart failure. *Circulation*, 94, 353-358.

Nordbeck P, Seidl B, Fey B et al. (2010) Effect of cardiac resynchronization therapy on the incidence of electrical storm. *International Journal of Cardiology*, 143, 330-336.

Schreieck J, Zrenner B, Deisenhofer I, et al. (2004) Rescue ablation of electrical storm in patients with ischemic cardiomyopathy: a potential-guided ablation approach by modifying substrate of intractable, unmappable ventricular tachycardias. *Heart Rhythm*, 2, 10-14.

Sesselberg HW, Moss AJ, McNitt S, et al. (2007) Ventricular arrhythmia storms in postinfarction patients with implantable defibrillators for primary prevention indications: a MADIT-II substudy. *Heart Rhythm*, 4, 1395–1402.

Stefan H, Hussein R, Craig M, et al. (2006) Electrical storm in patients with an implantable defibrillator:incidence, features, and preventive therapy: insights from a randomized trial. *European Heart Journal*, 27, 3027-3032.

Streitner F, Kuschyk J, Veltmann C et al. (2009) Role of proinflammatory markers and NT-proBNP in patients with and implanted cardioverter defibrillator and an electrical storm. *Cytokine*, 47, 166-172.

Streitner F, Kuschyk J, Veltmann C, et al. (2011) Predictors of electrical storm recurrences in patients with implantable cardioverter-defibrillators. *Europace*, 13, 668-674.

Sweeney MO, Sherfesee L, DeGroot PJ, et al. (2010) Differences in effects of electrical therapy type for ventricular arrhythmias on mortality in implantable cardioverter-defibrillator patients. *Heart Rhythm*, 7, 353-360.

Tsagalou EP, Kanakakis J, Rokas S, et al. (2005) Suppression by propranolol and amiodarone of an electrical storm refractory to metoprolol and amiodarone. *American Journal of Cardiology*, 99, 341-342.

Wood MA, Simpson PM, Stambler BS, et al. (1995) Long-term temporal patterns of ventricular tachyarrhythmias. *Circulation*, 91, 2371-2377.

19

Bradycardia Secondary to Cervical Spinal Cord Injury

Farid Sadaka and Christopher Veremakis
St John's Mercy Medical Center, St Louis University
USA

1. Introduction

Acute spinal cord injury (SCI) is most commonly traumatic in origin but may also result from degenerative spine disease, ischemia, demyelination, inflammation, or rapidly expanding neoplastic, hemorrhagic, or pyogenic masses (Ghezzi et al, 2001). In the United States, traumatic SCI with or without bony injury has an annual incidence of 28 to 55 per million, with an average of 10,000 new cases a year and a prevalence of 200,000 (Sekhon & Fehlings, 2001). The average age at the time of injury is 32 years and the male/female ratio is 4:1. More than half (55%) of traumatic SCI involves the cervical cord. The most common causes of SCI are traffic accidents (motor vehicle, bicycle, pedestrian) (40%- 50%), assault (10%-25%), falls (20%), work-related injuries (10%-25%), and sports/recreation-related injuries (10%-25%) (Cheung et al, 2002; Surkhin et al, 2000). In traumatic cervical SCI, 3-month mortality is 20% to 21%. The independent predictors of mortality are level of cord injury, Glasgow Coma Scale, respiratory failure, and age. Principal causes of death are respiratory disorders, cardiovascular disorders, pulmonary embolism, infections, and suicide (Claxton et al, 1998; DeVivo et al, 1999, Yeo et al, 1998). Cardiovascular disorders are responsible for 40.5% of deaths, being the most common cause of mortality in patients with SCI (Garshick et al, 2005).

2. Cardiovascular instability

Cardiovascular instability is a frequent complication of SCI, especially when the upper thoracic or cervical cord is involved (Figure 1). Peripheral sympathetic denervation results in arteriolar dilation and pooling of blood in the venous compartment, while interruption of cardiac sympathetic innervation (T1- T4) promotes bradycardia (Figure 2) and reduces myocardial contractility. The autonomic nervous system modulates cardiac electrophysiology, and, consequently, autonomic dysfunction can lead to ventricular arrhythmias. Concomitantly, parasympathetic input to the heart (from the vagus nerve, cranial nerve [CN] X) remains intact and may frequently result in bradycardia, especially with cervical SCI. Less commonly, cardiac arrest has been documented. Bradycardia is often precipitated by tracheal stimulation (for example, during suctioning) and hypoxia (Mathias et al, 1976; Piepmeier et al, 1985). Reflex bradycardia and cardiac arrest occur due to a vago-vagal reflex. Under normal circumstances, this reflex is opposed by sympathetic activity. As a compensatory response to hypoxia, a pulmonary-vagal reflex occurs, designed to increase respiratory rate and pulmonary inflation. However, in patients with SCI, compensatory sympathetic activity is eliminated, leaving parasympathetic activity unopposed, leading to severe bradycardia and potentially cardiac arrest. Studies of cardiovascular abnormalities after SCI show that as many as 100% of patients with motor complete cervical injuries (American Spinal Injury Association [ASIA] grades A and B) develop bradycardia, 68% are hypotensive, 35% require pressors, and 16% have primary cardiac arrest. Of persons with motor incomplete cervical injuries (ASIA grades C and D), 35-71% develop bradycardia, but few have hypotension or require pressors. Among patients with thoracolumbar injuries, 13-35% have bradycardia (Lehmann et al, 1987; Wirth et al, 2007). Bradycardia is more frequently encountered in the acute phase, and is more severe in the first 2–6 weeks after trauma (Krassioukov et al, 2007; McKinley et al, 2006). Cardiovascular dysfunctions improve in time. The reasons are not well understood, but synaptic reorganization or hyperresponsiveness of alpha receptors may play a role (Gondim et al, 2004).

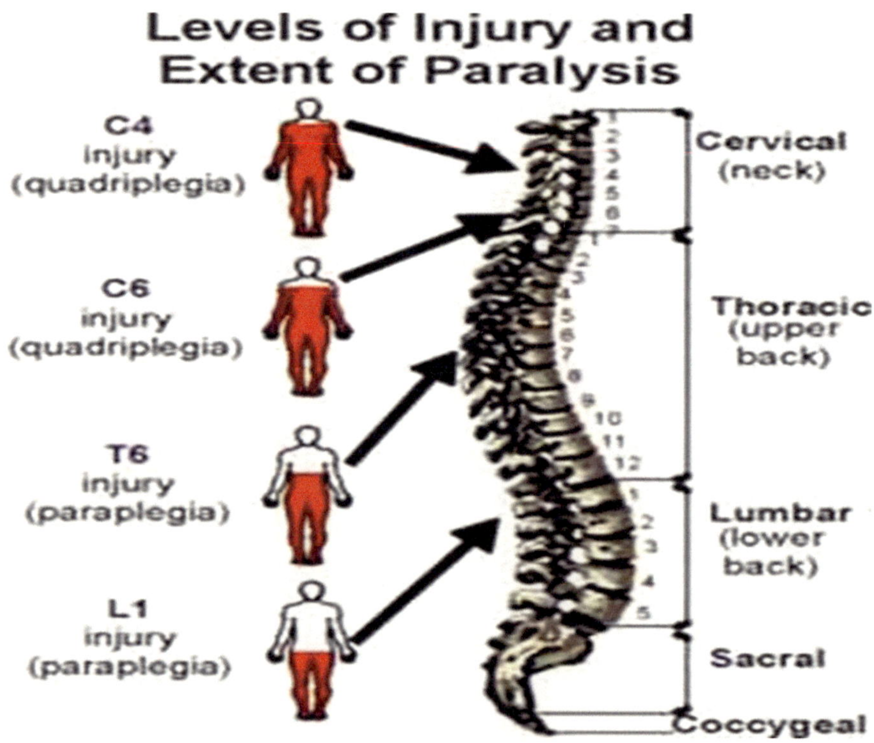

Fig. 1. Spinal cord and level of injury.

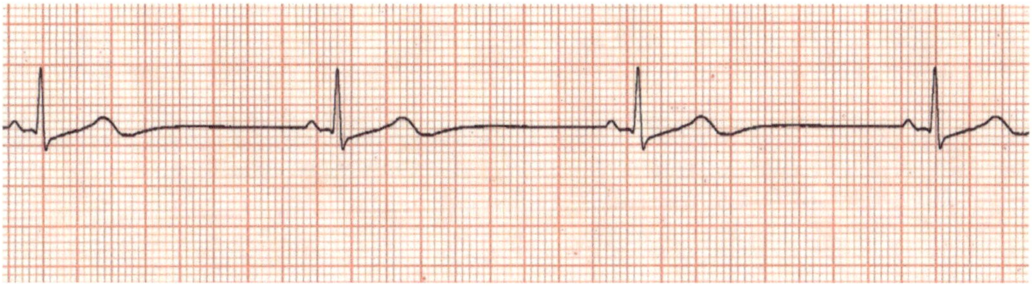

Fig. 2. Sinus Bradycardia during cervical SCI.

Cardiovascular control in acute and chronic SCI has been investigated by measuring the response to a variety of cardiovascular markers (blood pressure, heart rate, and plasma levels of norepinephrine and epinephrine) before ,during and after application of noxious stimuli below the level of the lesion. In acute SCI, noxious stimuli (eg. bladder stimulation) caused minimal changes in heart rate and plasma norepinephrine and epinephrine levels. In chronic SCI, noxious stimuli induced bradycardia and elevation in plasma norepinephrine but not in epinephrine levels. Resting plasma norepinephrine and epinephrine levels in both the acute and chronic SCI were lower than in normal subjects (Mathias et al, 1979).

The tilt test has been used to evaluate and delineate alterations in sympathetic cardiovascular compensation, which reflect the degree of autonomic dysfunction. Autonomic and cardiovascular responses to tilt test are blunted in persons with quadriplegia or paraplegia (Welch et al, 2005). Such tests could be used to noninvasively assess autonomic dysfunction in persons with SCI, determine the degree of sympathetic disruption, and assess the risk of developing cardiac arrhythmias, especially bradycardia. However, there are very few studies on these bedside tests upon which to solidly base conclusions and recommendations.

3. Treatment

3.1 Pharmacotherapy

Although bradycardia after cervical SCI usually resolves within 6 to 8 weeks after injury, it may progress to complete heart block and cardiac arrest. As such, the acute management and maintenance of cardiovascular stability in these patients may range from a practical clinical chore to a potentially lifesaving responsibility. There is limited data available regarding the optimal and best treatment available for symptomatic bradycardia in this patient population (Table 1). All data on therapeutic management of bradycardia secondary to cervical spinal cord injury is based on case reports, case series and observational studies.

Atropine, an anticholinergic agent, is generally recommended as the first-line agent for bradycardia after cervical spinal cord injury. Atropine improves conduction through the atrioventricular (AV) node by reducing vagal tone through muscarinic receptor blockade. The dose ranges from 0.4 to 0.6 mg, administered intravenously every 4 hours for short-term therapy (Abd & Braun, 1989; Pansoori & Leesar, 2004; Piepmeier et al, 1985; Sadaka et al,

2010; Sakamoto et al, 2007; Schulz-Stubner, 2005; Weant et al, 2007; Whitman et al, 2008; Winslow et al, 1986). Atropine should be kept readily available at the bedside at all times with this patient population, as acute episodes of bradycardia and hypotension may occur suddenly and without warning in the immediate few hours and days following injury.

Modality	Route of administration	Mechanism of action
Atropine	IV	reduces vagal tone by muscarinic receptor blockade
Dopamine	IV infusion	$Beta_1$ receptors on the heart
Epinephrine	IV infusion	$Beta_1$ receptors on the heart
Aminophylline	IV	inhibition of PDE enzyme thus increasing c-AMP with subsequent rise in catecholamines
Theophylline	Enteral or parenteral	inhibition of PDE enzyme thus increasing c-AMP with subsequent rise in catecholamines
Propantheline	Enteral	postganglionic parasympathetic acetylcholine receptor blocker
Permanent Pacemeker	invasive	

Table 1. Therapeutic modalities for bradycardia secondary to cervical SCI.

Another frequently utilized category of intravenous medications includes sympathomimetic agents such as Dopamine or Epinephrine which increase heart rate through action on $Beta_1$ receptors in the heart. Continuous infusions of dopamine at a rate of 2 to 10 mcg/kg/min or epinephrine at a rate of 0.01 to 0.1 mcg/kg/min has been used in the acute setting (Abd & Braun, 1989; Piepmeier et al, 1985; Sadaka et al, 2010; Winslow et al, 1986). Complications include tachyarrythmias, angina pain, palpitations, vasoconstriction, nausea, vomiting and headache.

When intermittent boluses of atropine or continuous infusions of sympathomimetic drugs have failed to prevent recurrent symptomatic bradycardia, or reverse high or complete heart block , permanent pacemaker placement has often been used as the next therapeutic alternative (Franga et al, 2006; Ruiz-Arango et al, 2006). Cardiac pacemaker implantation is advocated for patients with high cervical spinal cord injuries with persistent bradycardia not responding to medical management (Giloff et al,1991). However, specific criteria for placement of a pacemaker are not well defined. The reported number of SCI patients requiring a pacemaker varies from 9 to 17% (Abd & Braun, 1989; Lehmann et al, 1987). Complications of permanent pacemakers include infection, lead malfunction, death during attempted insertion, and death associated with failure to capture.

The methylxanthine agents, including aminophylline and theophylline, have been used effectively for the management of refractory symptomatic bradycardia when other agents have failed (Pansoori & Leesar, 2004; Sadaka et al, 2010; Sakamoto et al, 2007; Schulz-Stubner, 2005; Weant et al, 2007; Whitman et al, 2008). In addition, there are recent reports of methylxanthines used specifically as a successful first line treatment for bradycardia associated with cervical spinal cord injury. None of the patients in the case series needed a pacemaker placement and none of the patients developed drug related side effects (Sadaka et al, 2010). The proposed mechanism for the chronotropic effect of these drugs is via inhibition of phosphodiesterase (PDE) enzyme thus increasing the cyclic adenosine monophosphate with subsequent rise in catecholamines. A clear benefit of these agents is that they may be administered on a fixed schedule as an enteral preparation. An oral (or intravenous) loading dose between 200 and 300 mg was administered in most cases with maintenance doses starting at 100 mg three times daily and continued for up to 12 weeks. Drug serum levels were variable and differed widely among patients. The effective dose of theophylline resulted in serum levels that were below the therapeutic range defined in the literature (10-20 mcg/ml), and ofcourse below the toxic range (>25 mcg/ml). Since no therapeutic index for symptomatic bradycardia has been established, the methylxanthine dose was titrated according to clinical response. The main side effects of these agents are nausea, vomiting, tremor, headache, and seizures. However, No adverse effects were noted in any of the reports. Nonetheless until more experience is gained with this modality, careful attention should be made to monitor drug levels and avoid toxicity. Methylxanthine has also been associated with diaphragmatic strengthening in animal models, another potential beneficial effect to consider in spinal cord injury patients (Whitman et al, 2008).

In patients requiring long-term therapy, there are case reports of successful treatment with propantheline 7.5 to 30 mg every 4 to 6 hours (Abd & Braun, 1989; Winslow et al, 1986). Propantheline competitively blocks the action of acetylcholine at postganglionic parasympathetic receptors. The main side effect reported from chronic propantheline therapy is a reduction in gastrointestinal motility due to its anticholinergic effects.

3.2 Anticipation, prevention & positioning

Bradycardia and potential for cardiac arrest should be anticipated in any patient with spinal cord injury. Bedside care providers should be alerted to the fact that life threatening events occur more frequently with high spinal cord lesions. Personnel should anticipate and document triggers for serious bradycardic episodes. Hyperoxygenation and ambu "bagging" may be helpful prior to tracheal suctioning. Prophylactic atropine administration before tracheal suction, laryngoscopy, or oral intubation has been shown to minimize severity of events (Frankel et al, 1974; Mathias ,1976;Welphy et al, 1975). Theophylline may also be started at the first indication of bradycardia. Particular attention should be paid to other potential exacerbating factors, including rapid changes in positioning, prolonged recumbency, drug adverse effects, underlying infection, and hypovolemia.

Before moving the patient out of supine position, abdominal binder, thigh-high stockings, and elastic bandages to the lower extremities can be applied. These measures decrease venous pooling in the lower extremities and splanchnic vasculature. The patient can be moved slowly, from a supine position to a relatively upright position. A tilt table can be used to slowly bring the patient to the upright position.

3.3 Rehabilitation measures

Active arm exercises can be used to maintain blood pressure while the patient is on the tilt table (Mckinley et al, 2006). Bilaterally functional electric stimulation to lower-limb muscles, quadriceps, hamstrings, tibialis anterior and gastrocnemius during tilting improves orthostatic tolerance in patients with cervical SCI. Functional electric muscle stimulation during tilting maneuver, significantly increases heart rate (Chao et al, 2005).

4. Conclusion

Spinal cord injury is a very common and devastating disease process that can occur as a consequence of motor vehicle collisions, falls or other traumatic injuries. Cardiac disorders are common consequences following SCI. Cardiovascular disturbances are the leading causes of morbidity and mortality in both acute and chronic phases of SCI. Disruption of descendent pathways from superior centers to spinal sympathetic neurons, originating into the intermediolateral nuclei of T1- L2 spinal cord segments results in a reduced overall sympathetic activity and unopposed parasympathetic activity. As a result, the most common cardiac dysrrhythmia is bradycardia. There are a few well established therapeutic modalities (Table 1) for the treatment of bradycardia associated with cervical SCI. All therapeutic options are based on anecdotal reports and small retrospective reviews. Atropine should be kept readily available at the bedside at all times. Based on recent evidence with methylxanthines, we recommend further studies to establish the role of these agents as a first line therapy in this specific patient population. Optimal dose and duration of therapy need to be established. Theophylline's use via entral route as a first line therapy for spinal cord injury-related bradycardia can help avoid the long term use of inotropic and chronotropic infusions and their associated risks and complications, as well as prevent and/or decrease the use of cardiac pacemaker placement and its associated procedural risks and complications. We further recommend the study of xanthine derivates as prophylactic treatment for the first 2-6 weeks of the injury based on the frequency of bradycardia in patients with cervical SCI which is reported to be 100%. Currently, there are no established guidelines regarding permanent pacemaker placement in this patient population. Permanent pacemaker should still be considered in patients with refractory or recurrent bradycardia more than two weeks after the injury. In addition, the incidence of bradycardia after cervical SCI may be decreased by proper prophylactic measures, cardiac exercises and appropriate rehabilitation.

5. References

Abd AG & Braun NM. Management of life-threatening bradycardia in spinal cord injury. Chest.; 95(3):701-702.

Chao CY & Cheing GL. The effects of lower-extremity functional electric stimulation on the orthostatic responses of people with tetraplegia. Arch Phys Med Rehabil. 2005; 86(7):1427-33.

Cheung AT, Weiss SJ, McGarvey ML, Stecker MM, Hogan MS, Escherich A, & Bavaria JE. Interventions for reversing delayed-onset postoperative paraplegia after thoracic aortic reconstruction. Ann Thorac Surg. 2002; 74:413–9.

Claxton AR, Wong DT, Chung F, et al. Predictors of hospital mortality and mechanical ventilation in patients with cervical spinal cord injury. Can J Anaesth. 1998; 45:144–9.

DeVivo MJ, Krause JS, & Lammertse DP. Recent trends in mortality and causes of death among persons with spinal cord injury. Arch Phys Med Rehabil. 1999; 80:1411–9.

Franga DL, Hawkins ML, Medeiros RS, & Adewumi D. Recurrent asystole resulting from high cervical spinal cord injuries. Am Surg. 2006 ; 72(6):525-9.

Frankel HL, Mathias CJ, & Spalding JM. Mechanisms of reflex cardiac arrest in tetraplegic patients. Lancet. 1975; 2(7946):1183-5.

Garshick E, Kelly A, Cohen SA, Garrison A, Tun CG, Gagnon D, & Brown R. A prospective assessment of mortality in chronic spinal cord injury . Spinal Cord. 2005;43[7]:408–416.

Ghezzi A, Baldini SM, & Zaffaroni M. Differential diagnosis of acute myelopathies. Neurol Sci. 2001; 22(suppl 2):60–4.

Giloff IS, Ward SL, & Hohn AR. Cardiac pacemaker in high spinal cord injury. Arch Phys Med Rehab 1991; 72(8):601-3.

Gondim FA, Lopes AC Jr, Oliveira GR, Rodrigues CL, Leal PR, Santos AA, & Rola FH. Cardiovascular control after spinal cord injury. Curr Vasc Pharmacol. 2004; 2(1):71–79.

Krassioukov AV, Karlsson AK, Wecht JM, Wuermser LA, Mathias CJ, & Marino RJ. Assessment of autonomic dysfunction following spinal cord injury: rationale for additions to international standards for neurological assessment . JRRD. 2007; 44(1):103–112.

Lehmann KG, Lane JG, Piepmeier JM, & Batsford WP.Cardiovascular abnormalities accompanying acute spinal cord injury in humans: incidence, time course and severity. J Am Coll Cardiol. Jul 1987; 10(1):46-52.

Mathias CJ. Bradycardia and cardiac arrest during tracheal suction—mechanisms in tetraplegic patients. Eur J Intensive Care Med. 1976; 2(4):147-56.

Mathias CJ, Christensen NJ, Frankel HL, & Spalding JM. Cardiovascular control in recently injured tetraplegics in spinal shock. Q J Med. 1979; 48(100):273–287.

McKinley W, Garstang SV, Wieting JM, Talavera F, Foye PM, Allen KL, & Campagnolo DI. Cardiovascular concerns in spinal cord injury. Cord Injury: eMedicine Specialties/Physical Medicine and Rehabilitation/Spinal; 2006.

Pasnoori VR & Leesar MA. Use of aminophylline in the treatment of severe symptomatic bradycardia resistant to atropine. Cardiol Rev. 2004; 12(2):65-68.

Piepmeier JM, Lehmann KB, & Lane JG. Cardiovascular instability following acute cervical spinal cord trauma. Cent Nerv Syst Trauma. 1985; 2(3):153-60.

Ruiz-Arango AF, Robinson VJ, & Sharma GK. Characteristics of patients with cervical spinal injury requiring permanent pacemaker implantation. Cardiol Rev. 2006; 14(4):e8-e11.

Sadaka F, Naydenov SK, & Ponzillo JJ. Theophylline for bradycardia secondary to cervical spinal cord injury. Neurocrit Care. 2010 Dec;13(3):389-92.

Sakamoto T, Sadanaga T, & Okazaki T. Sequential use of aminophylline and theophylline for the treatment of atropine-resistant bradycardia after spinal cord injury: a case report. J Cardiol. 2007; 49(2):91-96.

Schulz-Stubner S. The use of small-dose theophylline for the treatment of bradycardia in patients with spinal cord injury. Anesth Analg. 2005; 101(6):1809-1811.

Sekhon LHS & Fehlings MG. Epidemiology, demographics, and pathophysiology of acute spinal cord injury. Spine. 2001;26(suppl 24):2–12.

Surkin J, Gilbert BJ, Harkey HL 3rd, Sniezek J, & Currier M. Spinal cord injury in Mississippi: findings and evaluation, 1992–1994. Spine. 2000; 25: 716–21.

Weant KA, Kilpatrick M, & Jaikumar S. Aminophylline for the treatment of symptomatic bradycardia and asystole secondary to cervical spine injury. Neurocrit Care. 2007; 7(3):250-252.

Welch JM, Radulovic M, Weir JP, Lesser J, Spungen AM, & Bauman WA. Partial angiotensin-converting enzyme inhibition during acute orthostatic stress in persons with tetraplegia. . J Spinal Cord Med. 2005; 28(2):103–105.

Welphy NC, Mathias CJ, & Frankel HL. Circulatory reflexes in tetraplegics during artificial ventilation and general anaesthesia. Paraplegia. 1975; 13(3):172-82.

Whitman CB, Schroeder WS, Ploch PJ, & Raghavendran K. Efficacy of aminophylline for treatment of recurrent symptomatic bradycardia after spinal cord injury. Pharmacotherapy. 2008; 28(1):131-135.

Winslow EB, Lesch M, Talano JV, & Meyer PR Jr. Spinal cord injuries associated with cardiopulmonary complications. Spine. 1986; 11(8):809-812.

Wirth B, van Hedel HJ, Kometer B, Dietz V, & Curt A. Changes in activity after a complete spinal cord injury as measured by the Spinal Cord Independence Measure II (SCIM II). Neurorehabil Neural Repair. Aug 30 2007.

Yeo JD, Walsh J, Rutkowski S, Soden R, Craven M, 7 Middleton J .Mortality following spinal cord injury. Spinal Cord. 1998; 36:329–36.

Part 5

Electrophysiology Study of the Heart: Mapping Procedure

20

Electromagnetic Mapping During Complex RF Ablations

Shimon Rosenheck, Jeffrey Banker, Alexey Weiss and Zehava Sharon
Hadassah Hebrew University Medical Center, Jerusalem, Israel

1. Introduction

Electromagnetic mapping has made possible the routine approach to complex arrhythmia mapping. Originally, it was developed to facilitate accessory pathway location, but it only complicated solitary pathway ablation. Especially, with the introduction of atrial fibrillation ablation, the electromagnetic mapping has become an irreplaceable component of this procedure. Latter, this 3-dimentional mapping method facilitated ventricular foci ablation in patients with ventricular tachycardia. During the last decade, the application of this mapping method is continuously extended and applied to a large number of complex arrhythmia cases.
The electromagnetic mapping is based on minimal magnetic field generation around the tip of the catheter and several antennas, located in a special hardware, called location pad, detect this field. In the near future the location pad will be replaced by an intracardiac detection system. As multiple antennas record the signal, the location pad precisely localizes the catheter tip. By apposition of a location on the endocardial surface and the catheter tip, a virtual map of the cardiac chamber is obtained. Multiple points are represented in space and finally, a continuous wall is completed. Moreover, the catheter records the electrical activity in its vicinity, and the electrical flow can be superimposed on the location in the space. A color-coding localizes the starting point of the arrhythmia and the current flow from it.
As of today, an advanced generation is used and data from other imaging systems are merged with the electromagnetic picture. First, magnetic resonance data was merged with the electroanatomic mapping, but today cardiac computed tomography and echo picture might also be merged. Using these merged pictures the anatomical presentation more accurately represents the anatomical structure.

2. A brief history of catheter ablation

The first type of energy used for catheter ablation to cure cardiac arrhythmias was the direct current (DC) shock delivered through the catheter tip in apposition to the desired site of ablation. By ablating the AV junction in supraventricular tachycardia, a reasonable rate control was achieved (Scheinman MM et al, 1982). The ablation of well-defined positioned accessory pathways could also be achieved by DC ablation (Morady F & Scheinman MM, 1984). The DC shock can be adjusted by delivering different amplitude of shocks, but as soon as it was delivered there was no more way to titrate or cancel it. To achieve a titratable energy, a different source is needed and the radiofrequency energy has fulfilled this condition. At the end of 1980's the radiofrequency energy has been introduced into the clinical electrophysiology. With the advent of specific pathways ablation, the clinical electrophysiology has become a continuously extending brunch of the cardiology. The radiofrequency energy in opposite to the direct current shock, can be titrated, limited, suddenly discontinued and reapplied. For this reason, the RF energy is easily applied in clinical practice. The first accessory pathways ablations and AV Nodal pathways ablations were performed during the late 1980's and published for the first time in 1991 (Jackman WM et al, 1991: Calkins H et al, 1991). Since than, a vast amount of literature was published on this subject and almost all type of arrhythmia has become feasible for ablation. In Table 2.1 a list of ablatable arrhythmic substrates is presented.

Arrhythmia Type	Fist performed	Publication
WPW	1989	Jackman WM et al 1991; Clakins H at al, 1991
ANRT	1989	Lee MA at al, 1991
A Flutter	1992	Feld GK et al, 1992; Cosio FG et al, 1993
A Tachycardia	1992	Kall JG& Wilber DJ, 1992; Walsh EP et al, 1992
VT idiopathic	1991-1992	Kuck KH et al, 1991; Klein LS et al, 1992
VT in Heart Disease	1992	Morady F et al, 1993
A Fibrillation	1996	Haissaguerre M et al, 1998
VF idiopathic	2001	Takatsuki S et al, 2001, Haissaguerre M et al, 2002

Abbreviations: WPW-Wolf Parkinson White Syndrome; AVNRT- AV Nodal Reentrant Tachycardia; A Flutter-Atrial Flutter; A Tachycardia-Atrial Tachycardia; VT-Ventricular Tachycardia; A Fibrillation-Atrial fibrillation; VF- Ventricular Fibrillation

Table 2.1. The table summarizes the types of arrhythmia treated with catheter ablation.

In accessory pathway ablation, the presumed location is meticulously mapped with a special developed steerable tip catheter. The pathways are located on the mitral or tricuspid rings, or in the septum separating the left and right heart. When the recoding from this site is satisfactory, RF energy is delivered for certain duration. If the accessory pathway conducts electricity in both directions, or at least, in the antegrade direction (from the atrium to the ventricle), the resting ECG shows a typical preexcitation pattern. Short PR interval and a widening of the QRS characterize this preexcitation. A typical delta wave is preceding the QRS and its direction depends on the location of the pathway. Wolf, Parkinson and White described this type of ECG in 1930 and if it is associated with palpitation is called Wolff-Parkinson-White syndrome (Wolff L et al, 1930). During the RF energy delivery the preexcitation disappears and the ECG becomes normal. After the ablation, during temporary blockage of the AV node with intravenous adenosine injection, AB block is achieved, demonstrating the remaining conduction only through the AV junction.
However, in 50% of the patients the resting ECG is normal, but still the patient can develop supraventricular tachycardia. In this case, the accessory pathway conducts the electricity only in the retrograde direction (from the ventricle to the atrium) and is called concealed Wolff-Parkinson-White syndrome. The mapping is completed either during tachycardia or ventricular pacing. RF energy application eliminates the retrograde conduction without affecting the resting ECG.
Patients with dual AV Nodal conduction may develop supraventricular tachycardia based on reentry circuit in the AV Node. One of the pathways has slow conduction of the electricity and

the other has fast conduction. If the refractoriness of these pathways and the conduction times are appropriate, the electric impulse may be conducted in a circuit constituted by this two pathways and the clinical expression will be supraventricular tachycardia with short VA time. A premature beat during unidirectional block in one of the pathways initiates the tachycardia. Different duration of refractoriness of these pathways creates the unidirectional block. Blocking one of these pathways will prevent induction of the tachycardia. RF ablation is based on the same principle: selective elimination of the conduction on one of these pathways. In the late 1980's the fast pathway was ablated (Lee MA et al, 1991). These fast pathways are located in the anterior site of the AV node very near to the proximal His Bundle. Although the success rate was very high, special attention was needed to avoid complete AV Block. After a year, the slow pathway ablation was described (Jackman WM et al, 1992). The slow pathway is located in the posterior AV nodal area, relatively far from the His Bundle. The ablation of these slow pathways is safer and today is routinely performed in most of the electrophysiology laboratories. After the ablation, the AV refractoriness prolongs and the AH interval (atrial-His conduction time) remains short immediately before the blocking.
The third classical ablation is that of typical atrial flutter (Feld GK et al, 1992, Cosio FG et al, 1993). In typical atrial flutter, a single electrical wavefront circulates in the perimeter of the right atrium. The area between the lower pole of the tricuspid valve and the inferior vena cava is called isthmus. A multipolar catheter on the lateral wall of the right atrium demonstrates the counter-clockwise or clockwise rotation during the flutter. Complete blocking of the isthmus, terminates the flutter. After the successful ablation, pacing at the coronary sinus osteum demonstrates the block, by conduction to the lateral wall only from above the tricuspid annulus.
In atrial tachycardia, idiopathic or peri-scar, and idiopathic ventricular tachycardia from right outflow tract or the basal left ventricle (fascicular), the atrial or the ventricular foci are ablated. The first three ablations, the accessory pathway (WPW) ablation, the selective or non selective AV Nodal pathways ablation and typical atrial flutter ablation are the classical ablations, which rarely if at all need other mapping methods, like the three-dimensional mapping methods. The atrial and ventricular tachycardia foci ablation is feasible in the majority of cases with "simple" electrophysiology mapping, like early activity, bracketing, entrainment, pace mapping, multi-pole catheter mapping, etc. However, occasionally, this mapping is not sufficient and three-dimensional mapping is needed (Marchlinski FE et al, 1998; Leonelli FM et al, 2001; Peichl P et al, 2003; Dong J et al, 2005). As we can notice, in the classical ablations, both the diagnostic test and the ablation procedure are focused on electrophysiology parameters. In atrial and ventricular tachycardia, although there are well defined electrophysiology maneuvers as previously mentioned, the more exact location of the focus and the demonstration of the ablation results demands the advanced electroanatomic mapping.

3. The development of the electroanatomic mapping and the electroanatomic mapping guided ablation

In the early 1990's, Ben Haim and his colleagues developed a new method of three-dimensional mapping of a tubular or spherical organ. First it was presented in the NASPE meeting in 1996 (Smeets J et al, 1996; Ben-Haim SA et al, 1996a; Hayam G et al, 1996; Gepstein L et al, 1996), than published as a new method evaluated in animal model and human subjects (Ben-Haim SA et al, 1996b; Gepstein L et al, 1997, Shpun S et al, 1997; Gepstein L et al, 1998). In this method, the locator pads, located beneath the operating table, generate a week magnetic field. The magnetic field strength is between $5x10^{-6}$ and $5x10^{-5}$ tesla. A miniature sensor embedded in the body of the distal catheter collects these magnetic fields. As the fields vectors have different directions, computer integration of the data resolves the location and orientation of the sensor in space. During the same time, the distal electrodes, located on the catheter tip, record the electrical activity behind it. By collecting multiple points, the heart chamber anatomy and the local electrical impulse in amplitude and timing are superimposed. With higher number of points added, higher precision is achieved. The resolution of the sensor location in space is < 1 mm. Finally, the electrical field propagation is presented on the virtual reconstruction of the heart chamber anatomy. If the amplitude is expressed, scar anatomy is obtained based on very low electrical activity on the scar. Moreover, a transitional region with increasing amplitude will interpose between the scar and normal tissue. In this type of mapping, invagination of conducting tissue in the scar, gaps and marginal zones may present the substrate of arrhythmias. Early in the development of the electroanatomic mapping, the scar mapping contributed to the understanding of the arrhythmia substrate and made possible non-specific scar ablation (Stevenson WG et al, 1998a; Stevenson WG et al, 1998b; Marchlinski FE et al, 2000; Sra J et al, 2001). However, the main development of the electroanatomic mapping happened with the use in atrial fibrillation ablation. After discovery of the triggers in the pulmonary veins, focal ablation was suggested, but the application of this ablation is limited and associated with an increased incidence of complication (Haissaguerre M et al, 1998). The use of electro-anatomic guided ablation offered ablation lines in the antrum of the veins and in this way the ablation is far from the vein itself and also significant debalking is added (Pappone C et al, 1999; Pappone C et al, 2000; Oral H et al, 2003). The ablation was extended to persistent atrial fibrillation and even to long-standing persistent cases (Nademanee K et al, 2004; Oral H et al, 2006; Takahashi Y et al, 2007). This addition contributed to development of this mapping. Additional mapping methods were developed and promoted in parallel with the original electromagnetic mapping, the CARTO mapping. Finally, the list of ablatable substrates has continuously increased and today includes beside atrial fibrillation and ventricular tachycardia in patients with or without structural heart disease, also atrial tachycardia, recurrent and refractory atrial flutter, idiopathic ventricular fibrillation (Knecht S et al, 2009) and more recently, the substrate of Brugada syndrome (Nademanee K et al, 2011). The following sections will describe in details the use of the mapping in each of these indications.

4. Right atrial tachycardia

The mechanism of right atrial tachycardia may be an autonomic focus or reentry around a physical obstacle, most commonly an iatrogenic scar or a post-infectious scar.

4.1 Right atrial tachycardia-reentrant type

For mapping the scar, bipolar voltage mapping is needed. Figure 4.1 shows two views obtained during atrial tachycardia ablation in a 32 year old man, who had a remote atrial septal closure surgery. During the surgery the lateral wall in the right atrium was opened and the septal defect was closed. On a recent echo, no interatrial shunt could be seen demonstrating lack of atrial septal defect and late success of the surgery. However the patient developed incessant and persistent atrial tachycardia. During the electrophysiology study, the right atrium was mapped using bipolar voltage mapping. This technique allows determination of the scar, as on the scar the electrical activity is practically non-existent. We defined everything bellow 0.04V as scar and assigned with red color. The normal tissue is defined everything above 0.47V and assigned with purple. The tissue in between them is the transition zone. As evident from the picture, the two red areas were connected with a continuous ablation line obtained with a point-by-point ablation.

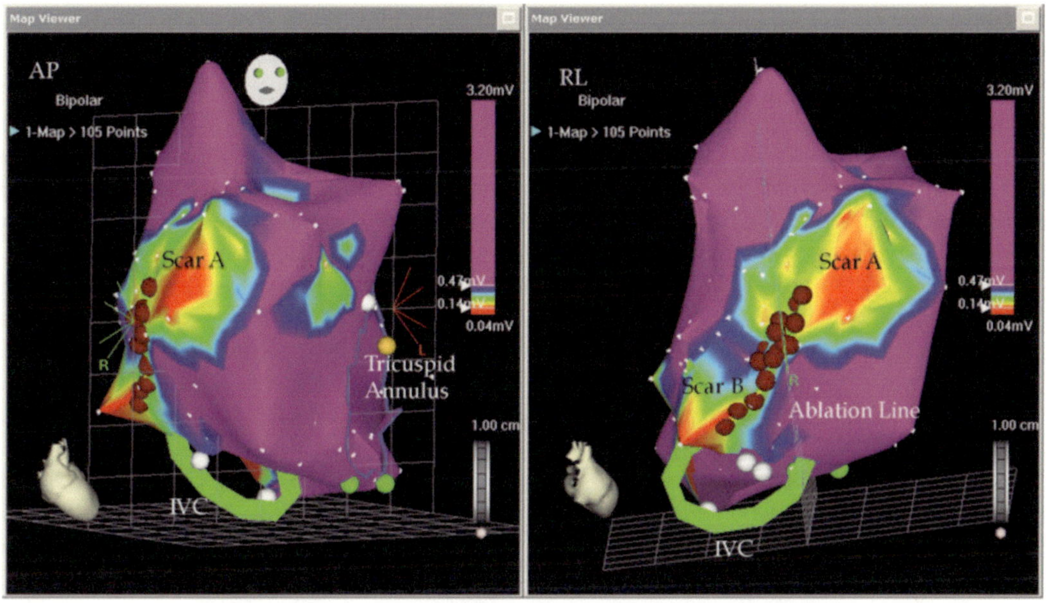

Fig. 4.1. The picture shows the voltage mapping of the right atrium with two scars on the lateral wall, a large (Scar A) and a small one (Scar B). The small one (Scar B) is connected to the Inferior Vena Cava. A small strip on normal myocardium separates the scars and this strip was transected with the ablation line. Annotations: AP- antero-posterior (the left picture); RL- Right lateral (the right picture). For further explanation see the text.

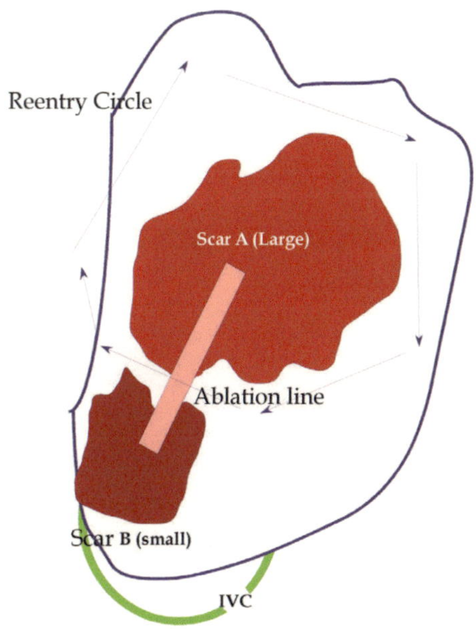

Fig. 4.2. Schematic presentation of picture 4.1; the picture shows the two scars, a large and a small one. The IVC ring limits the small one. To interrupt to reentry circle the ablation line connects the two scars.

During two-year follow-up the patients is free of any arrhythmia. This case demonstrates the of electro-anatomic mapping used for scar dependent atrial tachycardia ablation.

4.2 Right atrial tachycardia-automatic focus type

The next case will exemplify the ablation of automatic paroxysmal atrial tachycardia. The patient is a 17-year-old male patient with a history of palpitation and documented supraventricular tachycardia. Electrophysiology study demonstrated supraventricular tachycardia with long VA time and the ventricular rate was dictated by the atrial rate. Occasionally 2:1 AV conduction and even Wenkebach conduction was documented. The final diagnosis was right atrial tachycardia originating in the inferior third of the crista terminalis. Ablation was focused on the earliest atrial activity using a duodecapolar catheter. The tachycardia terminated during the RF application and has become noninducible. However, after 2 weeks the patient again experienced palpitation and again a similar arrhythmia was documented. The patient was referred for a second ablation this time CARTO guided. The tachycardia was again easily induced with atrial overdrive pacing, but not with atrial premature beats. Figure 4.3 shows the CARTO mapping.

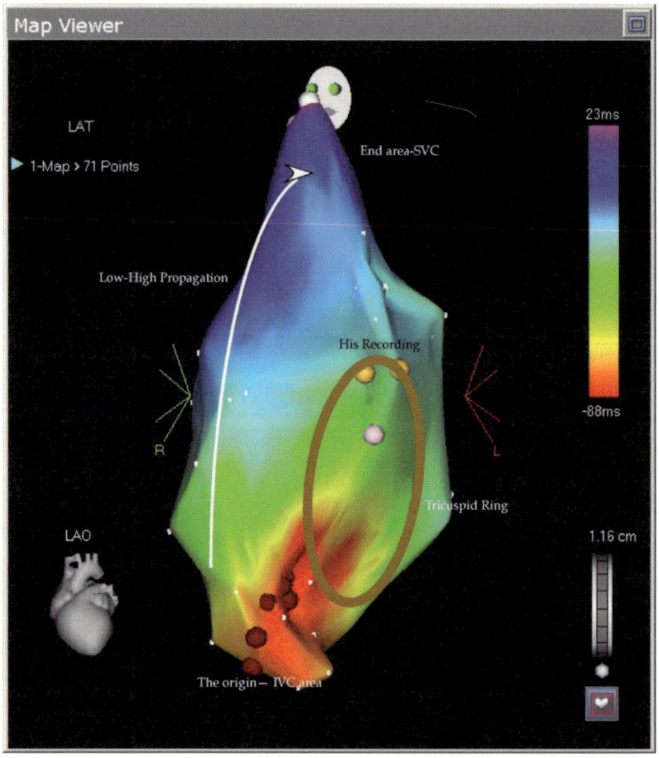

Fig. 4.3. Right Atria Tachycardia with the origin at the Inferior Vena Cava (IVC) area and the activation terminating at the Superior Vena Cava (SVC) area. This is a propagation map and the colors define the timing at each area. The red is the earliest time (-88 msec) and the purple the latest time (+23 msec) compared to the reference catheter. The white line with the arrow shows the activation direction. The red points in the origin area show the Radiofrequency application sites, which terminated the tachycardia rendering it non-inducible.

In this case, voltage mapping cannot be used as no scar could be mapped and the patient had no any previous cardiac procedure except the ablation procedure. For this reason, a propagation mapping was used. During this mapping the virtual reconstruction of the right atrium is completed parallel with accurate timing detection by comparing the activation time with the timing on a reference catheter, in this case in the coronary sinus osteum. The timing of the points located with the mapping catheter is compared with the reference catheter and is assigned with red color if it is early and purple if it is late. In between are the other colors like yellow, green and blue. Finally, a cine presentation shows the flow of the electrical activity, starting at the red point and terminating at the blue points. The red points are the area focused for ablation. As evident in Figure 4.3, the origin is well determined and ablation at this point again terminated the tachycardia leaving it noninducible. During the follow-up the patient is asymptomatic, practicing non-professional sportive activity.
These two cases exemplify not only two types of right atrial tachycardia, but also two methods of mapping. If a scar is to be mapped, the amplitude of the electrical activity will discriminate it from the normal tissue with clear demarcation. The reentry can be completed around a scar and by connecting the scar to a non-conducting tissue will prevent the reentry. This map is called, voltage-map, or scar mapping. In contrary, if the tachycardia is generated by an automatic focus, the earliest activation will reveal the origin of the tachycardia and the ablation may be focused to it. This is achieved by determining the timing at each point and the map is called, flow-map.
These two cases are presenting the classical types of atrial tachycardias. However, occasionally the diagnosis is not so simple and the first impression may be misleading. The electro anatomic mapping may elucidate the diagnosis and make possible the correct ablation. In the next subsection such a complex case is presented.

4.3 Atrial flutter or not flutter that is the question

A 28-year-old man presented with an ECG showing typical atrial flutter and was referred to radiofrequency ablation. He was in sinus rhythm when admitted for the ablation and the inferior isthmus (between the tricuspid ring and the inferior vena cava) was ablated using a 10 mm tip ablation catheter, a duodeca mapping catheter on the lateral wall and a quadripolar pacing-mapping catheter in the proximal coronary sinus. The ablation was performed during coronary sinus pacing and the original collision on the lateral wall was abolished demonstrating the block bellow the valve. Pacing from the coronary sinus and from above the inferior vena cava approved the block in the isthmus. Although the bidirectional block was persistent the patient had additional episode of "typical atrial flutter". In a second electrophysiology study the block in the isthmus was persistent and the patient had still inducible arrhythmia (Figures 4.4 and 4.5). Although the diagnosis of atrial flutter was attempting the duodeca catheter recording showed a big delay in the isthmus area during the tachycardia. This is not acceptable in typical atrial flutter or at least during an isthmus dependent flutter. Figure 4.5 shows details of the duodeca catheter recording during the atrial tachycardia-the last 10 tracings on Figure 4.4. The earliest point on the lateral wall is on pole D5-6. Pole D1-2 records from the median site of the isthmus block and pole D3-4 from the lateral site. The double arrow shows the big delay demonstrating the isthmus block during the tachycardia and non-isthmus dependent tachycardia. For this reason, CARTO mapping was initiated.

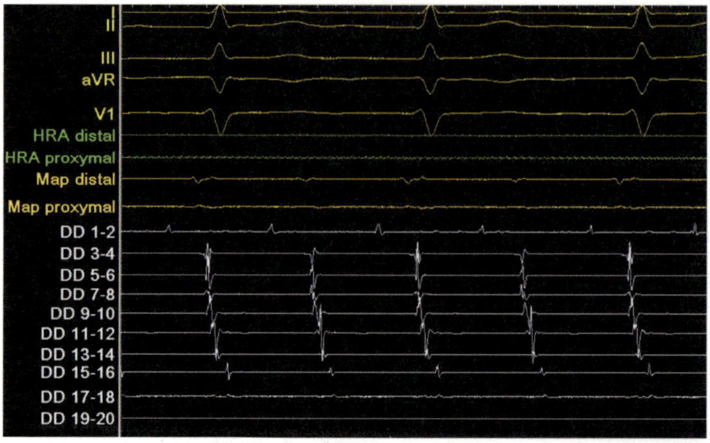

Fig. 4.4. The tracing shows a regular tachycardia, recorded at 100 mm/sec. The first 5 tracing are surface electrograms L_1, L_2, L_3, AVR and V_1. The next two belong to the right atrial tracing as reference for the CARTO mapping (not recording temporarily), than the mapping catheter and finally 10 tracings from the duodeca catheter deployed on the right lateral wall of the right atrium. The tracing on the duodeca catheter reveals unidirectional conduction suggesting atrial flutter. However, the tracing at DD1-2 is extremely delayed. As DD1-2 is medial to the isthmus block line and DD3-4 lateral, this delay demonstrates isthmus block during the tachycardia (See also Fig 4.5)

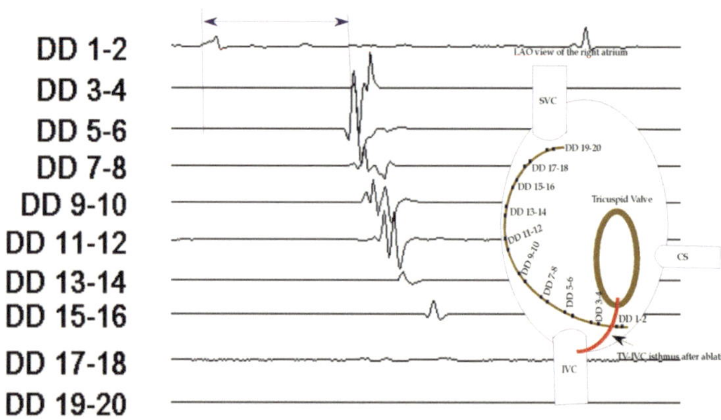

Fig. 4.5. The figure shows the tracing on the duodeca catheter at 200 ms/min recording speed. The cartoon inserted on the tracing shows the right atrium, IVC, SVC and CS. The isthmus block line is also depicted. The position of 10 bipolar poles is also shown. DD 1-2 is medial to the block line and all the other 9 poles are lateral to the line. On the tracing, a long delay is between DD 1-2 and 3-4 demonstrating the persistence of the block during the tachycardia, which is not compatible with typical atrial flutter.

A CARTO mapping demonstrated tachycardia originating from the lateral border of the block line in the isthmus (Figure 4.6) and was abolished by focal ablation using the area determined by the flow-map (Figure 4.7 and 4.8). The surface ECG was misleading and the real arrhythmia was atrial tachycardia and not atrial flutter! The electro-anatomic mapping made possible the correct diagnosis and finally the appropriate treatment.

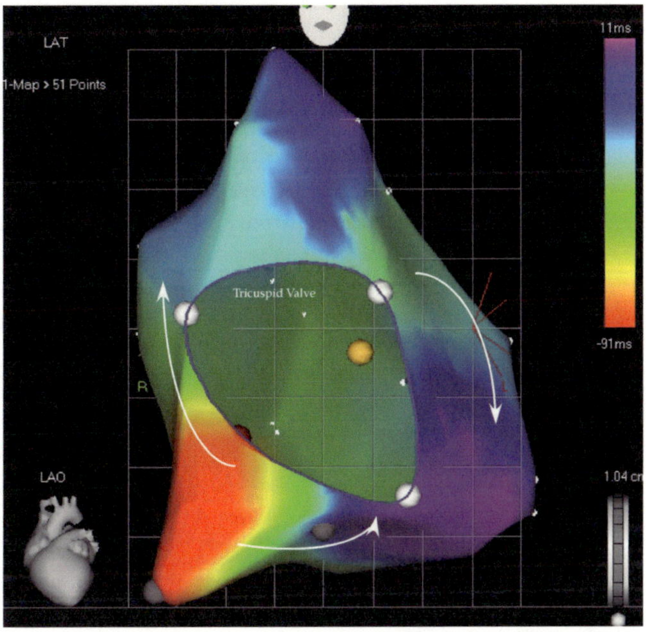

Fig. 4.6. Flow map during the tachycardia showing the early activation lateral to the isthmus line (purple color). The white arrows depict the current flow, simulating the flutter activation pattern except in the area between the origin (red color) and isthmus line (purple color) where a slow conduction in the opposite direction is clearly revealed. The isthmus is invaded from both sites.

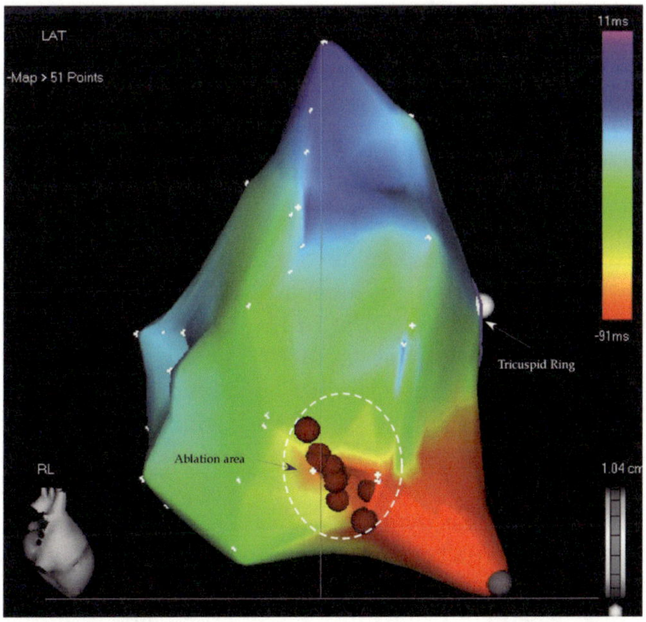

Fig. 4.7. The flow map from right lateral view is superimposed with the ablation mark signs. During the applications in this area the tachycardia terminated as shown in Figure 4.8.

This is an illustration of the importance of electro-anatomic mapping in this case as the surface ECG suggested typical atrial flutter and apparent recurrence after successful ablation of the cavo-tricuspid isthmus. At the first glance, the recording suggests atrial flutter, but there is a sudden delay between DD 3-4 and DD 1-2. This is possible only if the isthmus block is persistent and the catheter is laid over the block line with the tip over the line and the rest of poles before the block line. If the tachycardia can continue despite the block in the isthmus, it cannot be isthmus-dependent flutter. The electro-anatomic mapping revealed the correct diagnosis and made possible the appropriate ablation.

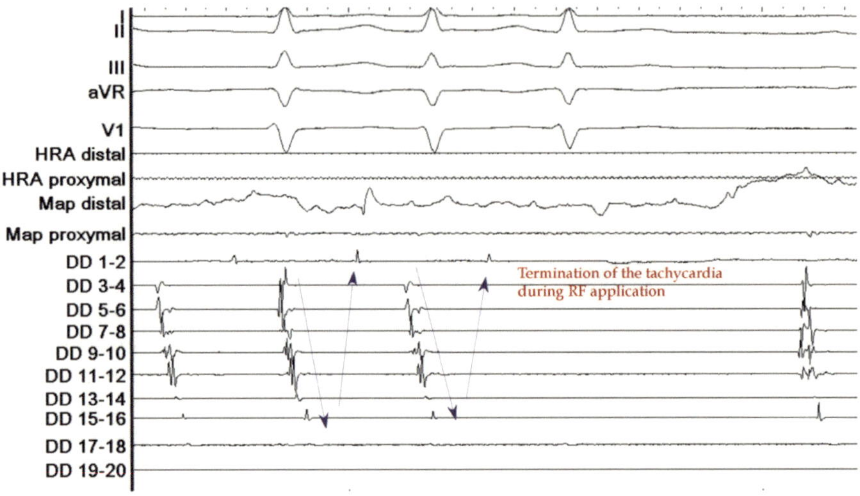

Fig. 4.8. In this tracing during the radiofrequency energy application, the tachycardia terminates and at the right side of the tracing the first sinus beat is seen. Of note, the tachycardia termination is sudden and not caused by ectopic activity, but only by the ablation. During the termination the last recording is from DD 1-2, demonstrating that the origin was between DD 3-4 and 5-6 and the last activation is on DD 1-2 (See Figure 4.6).

5. Left atrial tachycardia

Left atrial tachycardia may be of the same origin like the right atrial tachycardia. The automatic form mostly originates in the pulmonary veins, but the reentry forms originate in the atrial tissue like the reentry tachycardia in the right atrium. The most common form today is related to catheter ablation of atrial fibrillation, which will be discussed and presented within a next section on atrial fibrillation ablation. A rare form is the para-septal atrial tachycardia, which interestingly is associated with patent foramen ovale. For this reason, to map and ablate it, the septum is easily passed and the left atrium is easily mapped. The next presentation will exemplify it and will present the use of electro-anatomic mapping to determine the earliest activation point.

A 48 year old woman was referred because a persistent form of atrial tachycardia. First right atrium was mapped and the earliest activation was on the septal area. The activation time was at about zero time when compared to the reference catheter located in the coronary sinus osteum. By mapping the septum at the fosa ovalis, the catheter passed to the left atrium without need for standard septal puncture. The left atrium was mapped. A fast map was obtained, than the activation was superimposed on it. An early activation was mapped on the anterior wall, immediately above the mitral ring (Figure 5.1). At this point the ablation terminated the incessant atrial tachycardia.

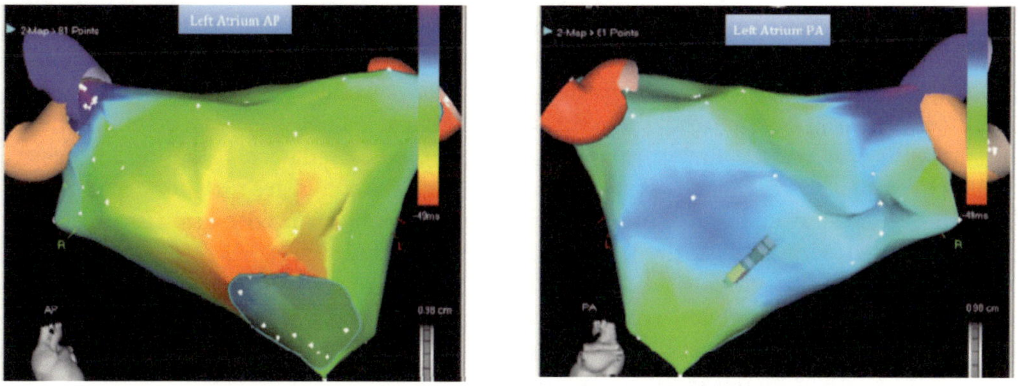

Fig. 5.1. The picture shows the left atrial flow map during incessant tachycardia. The activation time in the anterior wall and above the mitral ring was -43 msec (red color). On the posterior wall the activation times were all longer than 0 msec (compared to the reference catheter at the coronary sinus osteum. The area above the right pulmonary vein is as late as 53 msec after the activation on the reference catheter (purple color).

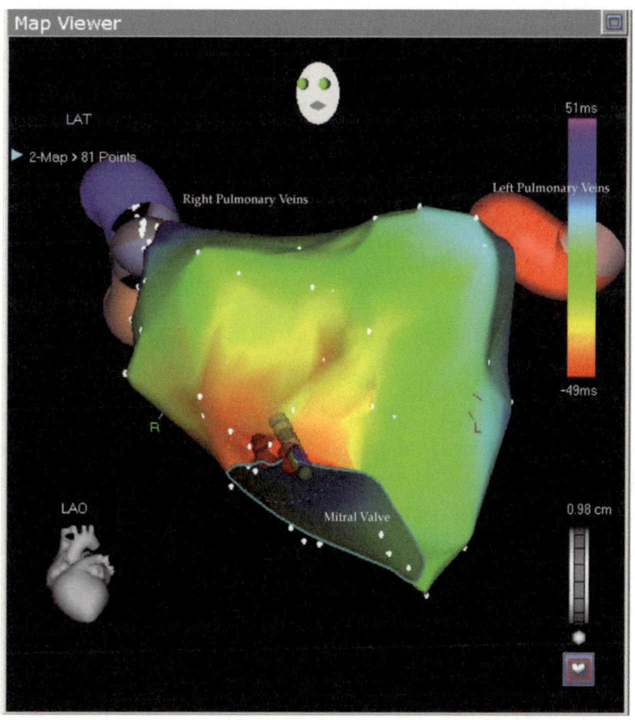

Fig. 5.2. The figure shows the virtual reconstruction of the left atrium during the tachycardia with the earliest point in red color. The catheter tip is pointing to that area. The ablation sites are shown. The tachycardia terminated with these ablation points.

As of today, the published information on electro-anatomic mapping during atrial tachycardia ablation is scars and limited. However, the clinical application is well known and rich and the accumulated and published knowledge is worth to mention. Atrial tachycardia is encounter in both pediatric and adult patients. We have information on the use of electro-magnetic mapping in both groups. In right atrial tachycardia, the use of this mapping adds a significant degree of accuracy and, just like in our patient described in subsection 4.3, rarely the electro-magnetic mapping adds to the correct diagnosis. In patients with incessant focal tachycardia, the electrophysiological maneuvers may be enough but in patients with scar related tachycardia, this mapping has irreplaceable value. In incessant focal tachycardia, the earliest activation in the Crista Terminalis area or along the tricuspid ring will reveal the origin and radiofrequency energy application will terminate it and total cure is achieved. However, if the tachycardia persists or reoccurs, 3D mapping is justified (Subsection 4.2). As previously mentioned, the activation map helps to localize the origin of the tachycardia. In scar related reentrant tachycardia, the scar is delineated and a narrow isthmus in between them is ablated (Subsection 4.1). Voltage mapping delineates the scar, and amplitude lower than 0.14 mV suggests scar.
The published studies involved a limited number of patients, 7 to 120. Focal tachycardias in the right atrium are ablatable with success rate >90% (Kottkamp H et al, 1997; Marchlinski F et al, 1998; Iwai S et al, 2002). The same success rate may be achieved in macroreentrant atrial tachycardia related to post-surgical scar (Iwai S et al, 2002). In the left atrium, focal tachycardias were localized to mitral annulus, roof, posterior wall, appendage and septum (Dong J et al, 2005). Left septal atrial tachycardia is rare and the electroanatomic mapping facilitates its ablation (Marrouche NF et al, 2002). Atrial tachycardia originating in the mitral annulus is also rare and the electro-anatomic mapping also facilitates its ablation (Kistler PM et al, 2003). Our patient presented in section 5 had also tachycardia originating from the mitral annulus (Figures 5.1 and 5.2). In pediatric patients, the acute success is significantly higher with the electro-anatomic mapping compared to standard electrophysiological mapping and the recurrence rate was lower (Cummings RM, 2008).
In all these conditions, the electroanatomic mapping for ablation of all types of atrial tachycardia in the clinical practice is firmly established.

6. Atrial fibrillation ablation

Atrial fibrillation is the most common arrhythmia an presents a great challenge for any cardiologist and even more for the clinical electrophysiologist. This arrhythmia has a very erratic response to antiarrhythmic treatment and for this reasons a non-medical treatment is demanded. Device therapy did not prove to be an effective alternative to the mediocre medical treatment. For this reason, the ablative opinion is an attractive alternative.
Haissaguerre and his colleagues, by investigating the mode of initiation of paroxysmal atrial fibrillation, discovered that the trigger for this type of arrhythmia originates, in the majority of the cases, in the pulmonary veins (Haissaguerre M et al, 1998). Focal ablation of these foci, as a logical next step, turned to be complicated with damage to the vein, narrowing with significant and symptomatic increase in the pulmonary pressure. The electrical connection between the pulmonary vein and left atrium is through distinct pathways (Ehrlich JR et al, J Physiol 2003). Electrical disconnection of these veins avoided this damage and offered the same result. However, the recurrence and occasional pulmonary stenosis were still encountered. In 1999, Pappone and his colleagues suggested

a different approach to disconnect electrically the pulmonary veins (Pappone C et al, 1999; Pappone C et al, 2000; Pappone et al, 2004). This method is based on electroanatomic mapping. The left atrium is approached by passing the inter atrial septum using the Brockenbrough method and the left atrial mapping is completed by virtual reconstruction of the atrial walls and tagging the veins and the mitral annulus. The ablation includes circles around the pulmonary veins and lines connecting the mitral annulus with the ablation line around the left lower pulmonary vein and lines connecting the left and right ablation rings around the veins. In patients with paroxysmal atrial fibrillation, this type of ablation was superior to the pulmonary vein disconnection, with higher success rate and lower recurrence rate after one year (Oral H et al, 2003). Moreover, in patients with persistent atrial fibrillation, circumferential pulmonary vein ablation was superior to amiodarone treatment in preventing recurrence of the fibrillation (Oral H et al, 2006; Pappone C et al, 2006). Multiple escalated methods exemplify the problematicity of the ablation in patients with long persistent atrial fibrillation (Oral H et al, 2006; Takahashi Y et al, 2007; Satomi K et al, 2008). However, consensus was achieved on the necessity of catheter ablation of atrial fibrillation (Calkins H at al, 2007).

Following we will present several patients with atrial fibrillation and electro-anatomic guided ablation.

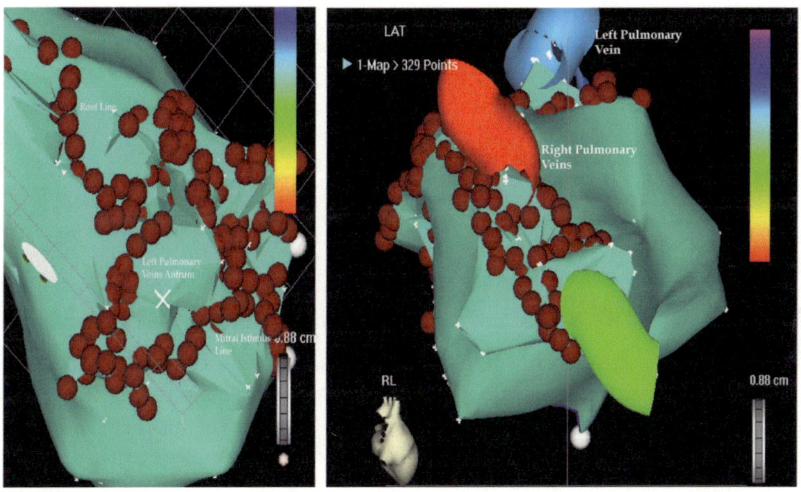

Fig. 6.1. The picture shows the ablation lines around the common left entrance and the two right veins. The lines are continuous.

SB 74 year old woman with a long history of paroxysmal atrial fibrillation on multiple antiarrhythmic medication including beat blockers, calcium channel blockers, Propafenon, Flecainide, Amiodarone all turned to be ineffective. The etiology of the atrial fibrillation was hypertension treated with multiple drugs. Finally she was referred to catheter ablation of atrial fibrillation. In the mean time the fibrillation converted to persistent. An ECHO showed normal systolic left ventricular function with decreased diastolic function, enlarged left ventricle with minimal mitral regurgitation. Patten Foramen Ovale with small left to right shunt was demonstrated. During the ablation, the septum was easily passed and the left atrium was reconstructed using anatomical map as she was in atrial fibrillation. The veins were tagged and the mitral annulus was reconstructed. The veins were circumvented with ablation points and the roofline and mitral isthmus lines were completed. When the radiofrequency was delivered in the junction between the roofline and right superior pulmonary vein the patient converted to sinus rhythm after 2 months of atrial fibrillation. Figure 6.1 shows the ring around the left veins and the right veins; Figure 6.2 shows the posterior view of the left atrium after the ablation. The mapping and ablation were done with CARTO EXP 7. She was in sinus rhythm 5 years after the ablation and during her last follow-up 3 years ago.

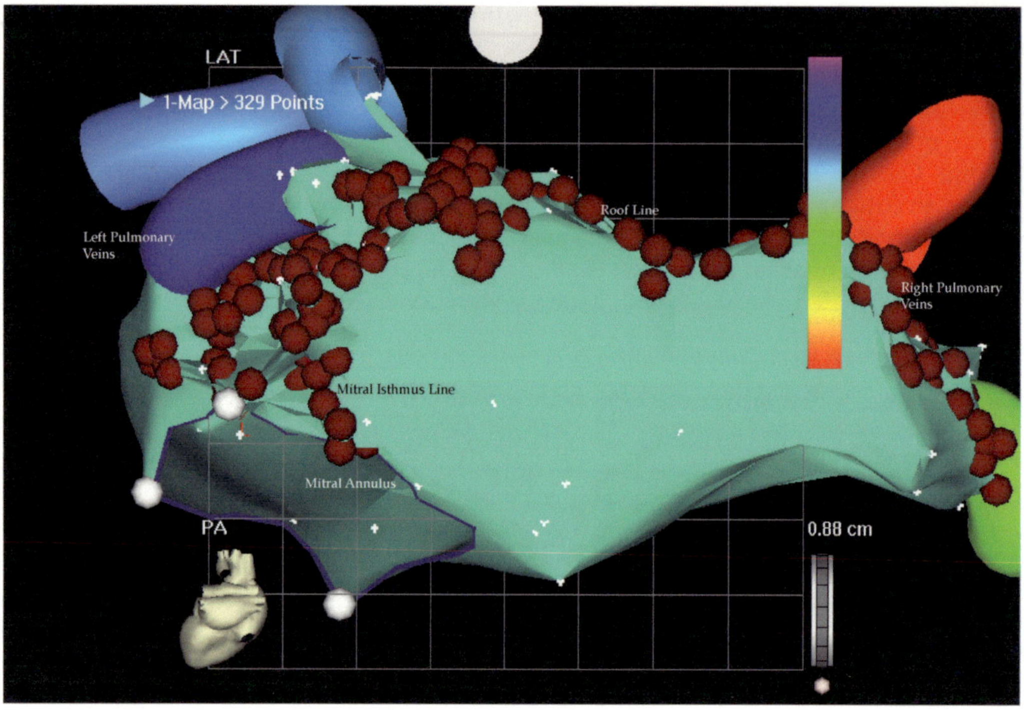

Fig. 6.2. The enlarged left atrium in a posterior view shows the rings around the pulmonary veins, the roofline and the mitral isthmus line. At least two lines connect the peri venous ring to the mitral annulus. There are 3 large left veins with a common entrance to the left atrium. The mapping is an anatomical map different from the mappings in atrial tachycardia ablation (Sections 4 and 5).

MD is 81-year-old man with persistent atrial fibrillation failing multiple medical treatments. He had long history of supraventricular tachycardia and had a successful slow pathway ablation 8 years ago. Two years ago presented with symptomatic atrial fibrillation. Medical treatment with beta-blockers, Propafenon, Flecainide were not effective and Amiodarone was discontinued because hyperthyroidism. As medical treatment had to discontinued because lack of efficacy or side effects he was referred to catheter ablation. At the admission he was in persistent atrial fibrillation for 3 months and without antiarrhythmic treatment. The transseptal catheterization was performed safely under intra cardiac echo guidance. After the ablation he converted to sinus bradycardia. Figure 6.3 shows the ablations lines in the left atrium and presents new modes of mapping (fast map).

SS is a 68-year-old man with long history of atrial flutter and fibrillation and hypertension. In 2002 he had a successful atrial flutter ablation. In 2004 he had catheter ablation of atrial fibrillation using the point-by-point method. Until recently he was in stable sinus rhythm when 3 months ago presented in the follow-up clinic with atrial fibrillation. Anticoagulation was started and referred for a second ablation. In the new mapping there was no electrical activity in the veins, on the posterior wall, but at several points around the veins was a low amplitude regular activity and all this places were ablated again. In the next figures the two mappings will be compared in the same patients emphasizing the advance in the mapping methods. The patient has common entrance of both left and right pulmonary veins. The intracardiac echo used during the second ablation in 2011 approved this anatomical variance.

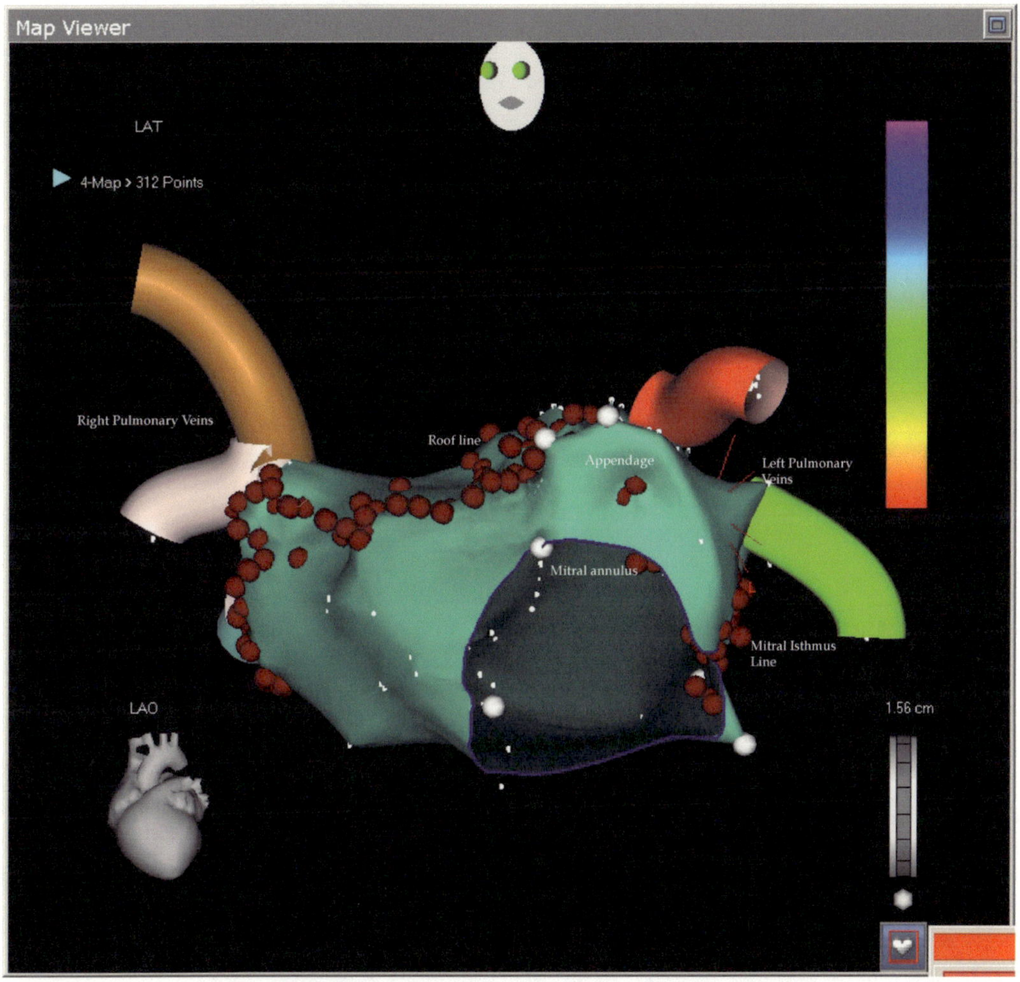

Fig. 6.3. The figure shows 20 degree left anterior view of the left atrium. The appendage covers the ablation ring around the left veins. The atrium is minimally enlarged. There is a common right entrance and two separate left veins. This map was performed using the fast map mode, a new future of the electro-anatomic mapping. The atrial anatomy much more resembles the other imaging models. The lines are continuous and the veins are completely isolated with no residual electrical activity in the veins or posterior wall. The mode is new and for this reason the follow up after the ablation is only 3 months, however the patient is in sinus rhythm.

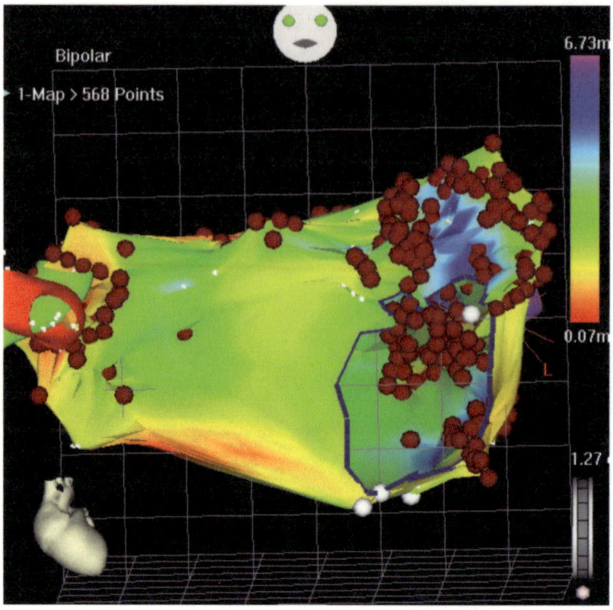

Fig. 6.4. The figure shows the anterior view of the left atrium recorded in 2004 using the point-by point method. The patient was in sinus rhythm during the procedure. A large number of ablation sites are seen through the mitral valve from inside the atrium. The left atrium is not enlarged. The left ablation lines are heavy and the right ablation lines are discrete. The roofline is slightly posterior an not present in this picture.

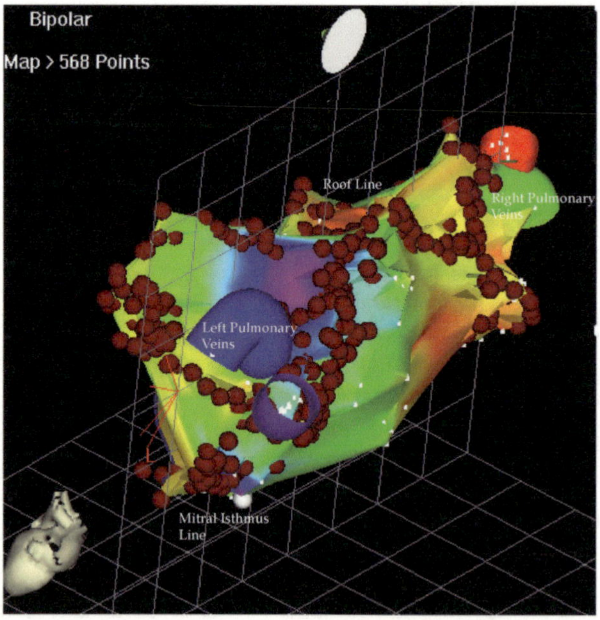

Fig. 6.5. This is a posterior view recorded during the first ablation procedure. The ablation lines are clearly seen and are heavy in the left side and discrete in the right side. The voltage amplitude in the posterior wall is low (red color).

The next figure (6.5) shows the ablation lines in the posterior view and also the roofline not seen in Figure 6.4. Following the ablation the atrial fibrillation was not inducible. The areas around the veins were quiescent from any electrical activity. As the patient had a previous cavo-tricuspid isthmus line ablation, atrial flutter could also not be induced. As mentioned above, after 7 years the patient developed again atrial fibrillation, this time persistent and not paroxysmal. The following pictures will exemplify the second ablation procedure, with a more advanced electro-anatomic mapping system (Figures 6.6 and 6.7).

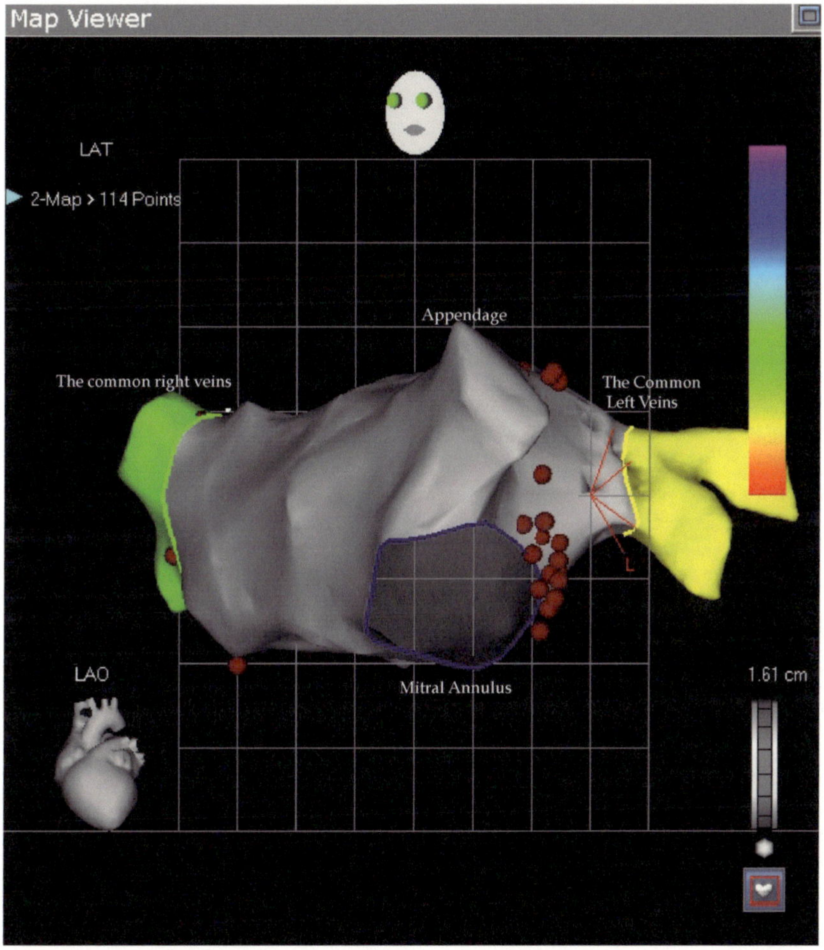

Fig. 6.6. The picture shows the left atrium using the fast map technique. This is the same left atrium like in Figures 6.4 and 6.5, just obtained 7 years latter and using more advanced method of mapping. The veins with common entrance are in colors, left with yellow and right with green. The mitral isthmus was reinforced with several ablation points and the left upper vein is also reinforced at the junction with the roofline were low amplitude relatively slow and regular activity was recorded. The ablation canceled this activity and the entire vein was free of any electrical activity. The next figure will show the areas with residual activity on the right side.

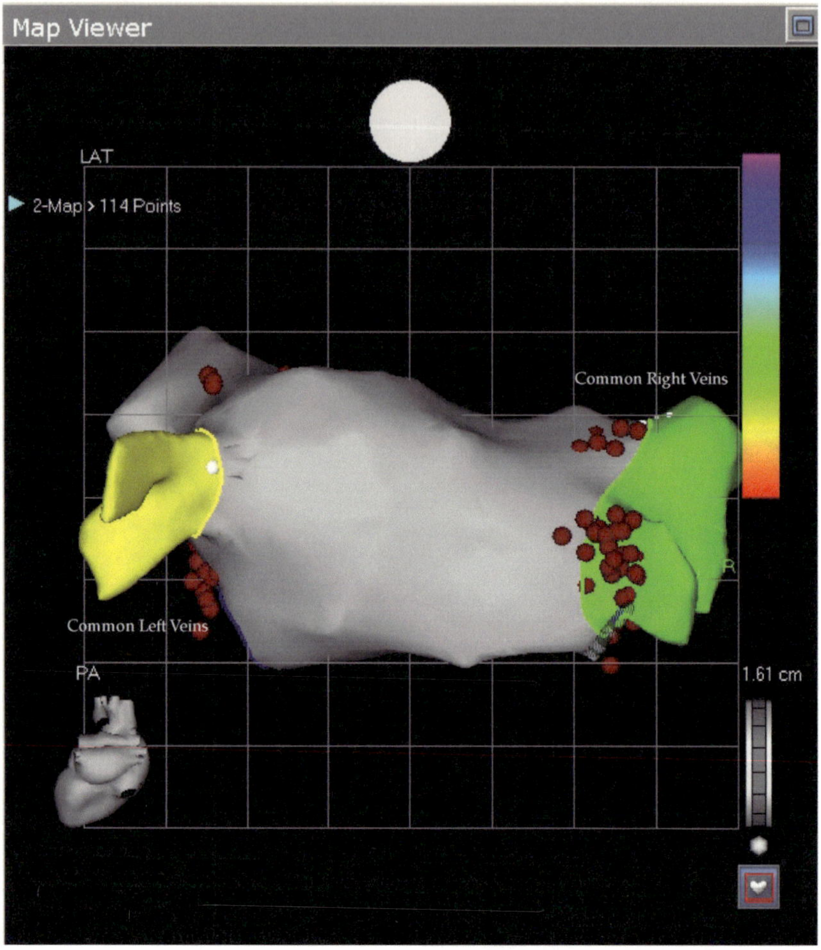

Fig. 6.7. The figure shows the posterior wall recoded with the fast map method. In the lower-posterior border of the right vein and on the junction point with the roofline additional application eliminated the activity and left the entire vein free of any electrical activity. The right vein different from the left, had multiple brunches and with common entrance into the left atrium. The anatomy was approved with the intra-cardiac echo recorded simultaneously with CARTO mapping. The posterior wall also free of electrical activity like in box-ablation (lines anterior to the veins completed with roofline and another line in the low atrium on the posterior wall).

7. Ventricular tachycardia ablation

A vast amount of information was accumulated during the last decades of the 20th Century supporting the superiority of implantable defibrillators (ICD) over any medical treatment in saving patients with high risk for sudden cardiac death (Ezekowitz JA et al, 2003). However, the defibrillator cannot guaranty the quality of life especially in patients with frequent ICD therapy. Moreover, patients may develop clusters of ventricular fibrillation, called VT storm. Some studies even suggest that repeated shock is associated with increased death rate

(Exner DV et al, 2001; Poole JE et al, 2008; Daubert JP et al, 2008; van Rees JB et al, 2011). It is still not clarified if the presence of high number of VT or the shocks signals the imminent death. When both the ICD and adjuvant antiarrhythmic treatment (mainly Sotalol or Amiodarone) cannot prevent frequent recurrence of VT, the only option is the ablation (Sra J et al, 2001). The next step in the strategy is ablation before the storm or frequent recurrence of VT (Reddy V et al, 2007; Stevenson WG et al, 2008; Tung R et al, 2010; Kuck KH et al, 2010; Natale A et al, 2010). The main problem is that patients with structural heart disease have multiple VT foci, large scars with many possible reentry circles. For this reason, focal ablation may be only a temporary step. Occasionally, these patients with reduced left ventricular function may not tolerate hemodynamically the VT and focal ablation may not be feasible. To resolve this problem, scar ablation was suggested (Marchlinski FE et al, 2000; Sra J et al, 2001). The following 4 patients will exemplify these methods in different types of structural heart disease.

AA is a 60-year-old patient with coronary artery disease, large anterior myocardial infarction in the recent past, and ventricular tachycardia. A cardioverter-defibrillator was implanted. As the tachycardia reoccurred, amiodarone treatment was added. Amiodarone did not control the tachycardia and the symptomatic cardioverter-defibrillator therapy and the patient was frequently re-hospitalized.

For this reason, the patient was brought to the electrophysiology laboratory in purpose to study the ventricular tachycardia and to attempt an ablation procedure. The tachycardia was easily and reproducible induced with two premature beats. Although the tachycardia, on chronic amiodarone treatment, was relatively slow, the patient did not tolerate it hemodynamically. Propagation mapping was not applicable and the only option remained the scar/voltage mapping. Interestingly, the mapping revealed two scars, a large one and a small one with a small and narrow strip of myocardium between them. The small scar extended until the mitral annulus and no continuous myocardium surrounded it. The only reentry circuit for the slow tachycardia could be the large scar and by blocking the narrow myocardial strip between the scars necessarily will interfere with the current wave passage around the large scar, too.

The flowing pictures exemplify the scars and the ablation (Figures 7.1, 7.2 and 7.3)

The tachycardia has become not inducible after the ablation and during the 1 year follow-up since the ablation the patient was free of ICD therapies. As we can see, in this case a clear delineation of the reentry circle was revealed by the scar mapping without an intend to map the activation. Scar mapping is the option when the patient cannot tolerate the tachycardia (Marchlinski FE et al, 2000; Sra J et al, 2001). A narrow conduction tissue in the scar serves the tachycardia (Figure 7.2 and 7.3). The strategy is to block this tissue, however it is important to connect the scar to a non-conducting structure like valve annulus, otherwise the ablation will only increase the reentry circle and may render the tachycardia more incessant. In our patient the smaller scar was already connected to the mitral annulus (Figure 7.3) leaving the only possible reentry circle around the large scar and the target of the ablation the narrow myocardial strip in between them. This patient presents an ideal ablatable reentry circle. Eliminating the conduction only on a single possible pathway eliminates also the VT substrates and the patient continues to be without ICD therapy for one year. Identification of the channel was crucial in this procedure and is discussed in recent published literature (Arenal A et al, 2004; Hsia HH et al, 2006).

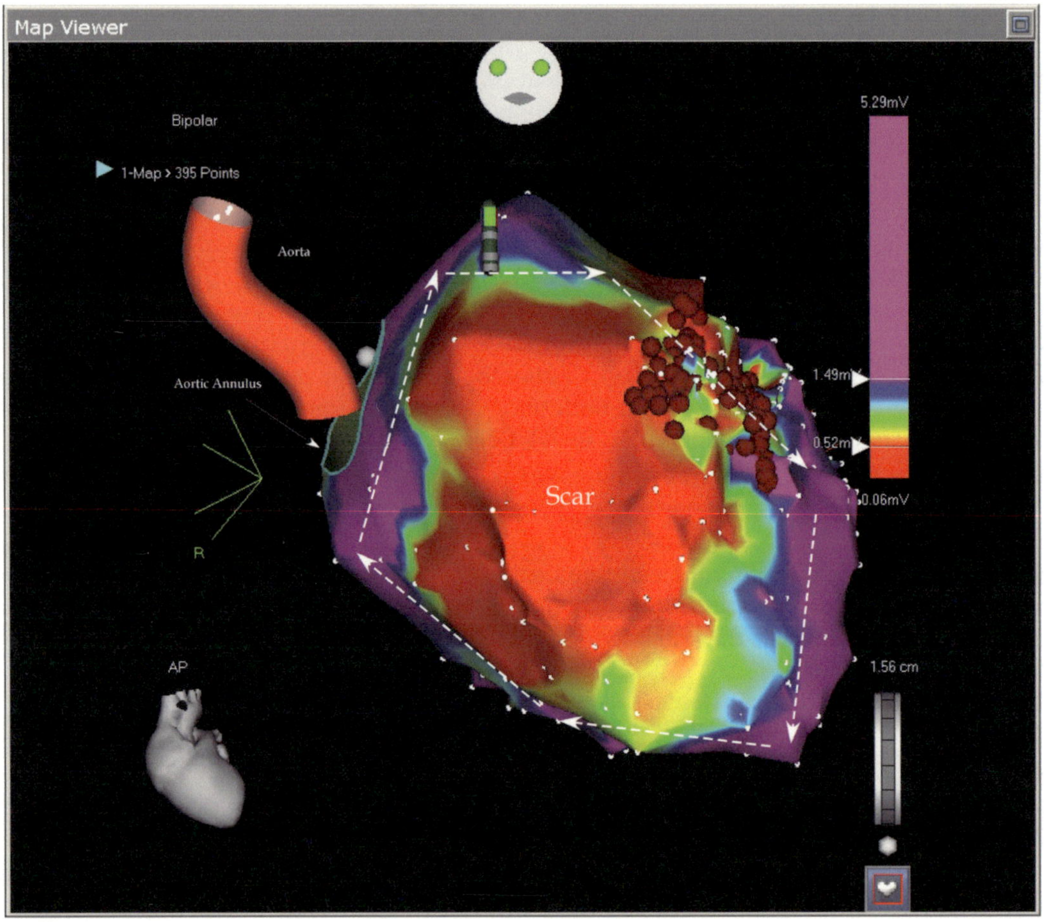

Fig. 7.1. The picture shows the antero-posterior projection of the enlarged left ventricle with a large scar on almost all the anterior wall. Any voltage bellow 0.5 mV (red color) was considered scar and any voltage above 1.5 mV were considered normal myocardium (purple color). In between them three transitional tissues are collared in yellow, green and blue. No tissue penetrated the scar and no central pathways could be mapped. The arrows show the large reentry cycle around the scar. Normal myocardium is around the scar and constitutes the reentry circle. The ablation points (red dots) block the isthmus between two scars (see Figure 6.2)

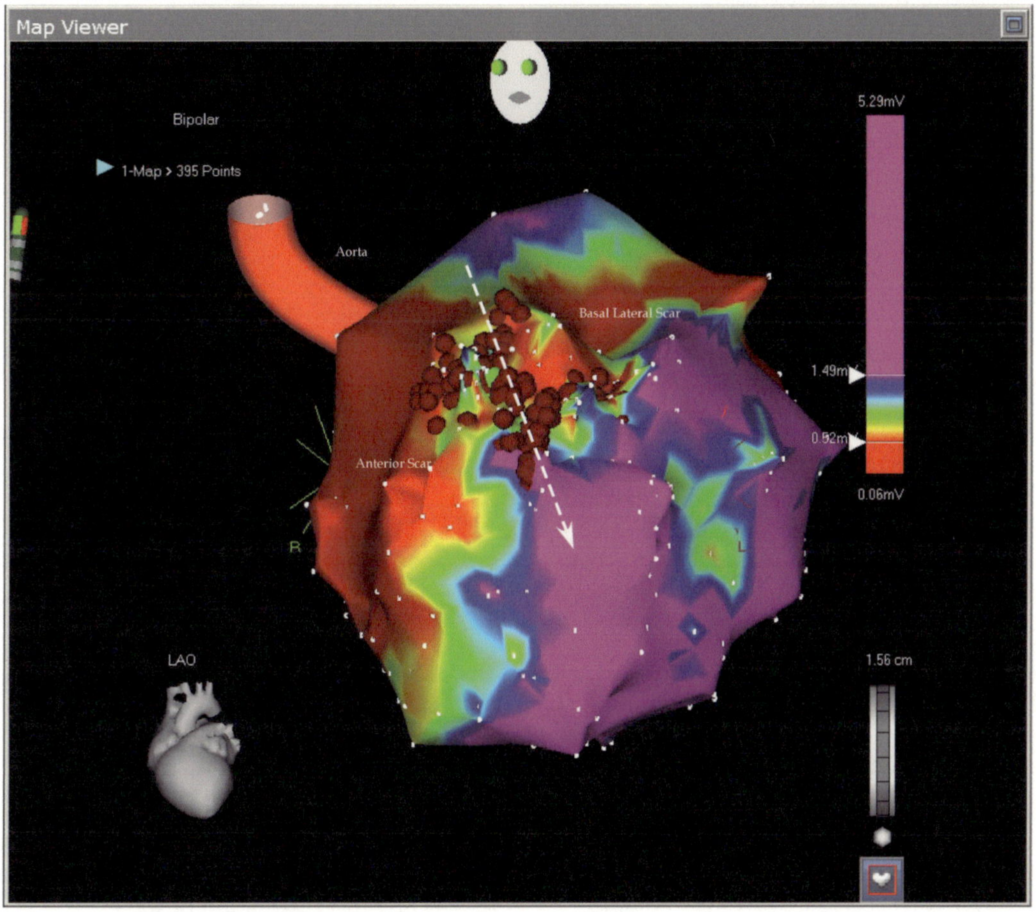

Fig. 7.2. The picture shows the antero-lateral projection of the left ventricle. In this voltage mapping two scars are evident: the large anterior scar and a smaller basal lateral scar. The scars delineate in between them a slowly conducting myocardial tissue called isthmus (arrow). The isthmus is blocked by the ablation points. As we will see in the next picture, the basal scar is extending until the mitral annulus the reason why the reentry could not be closed around it.

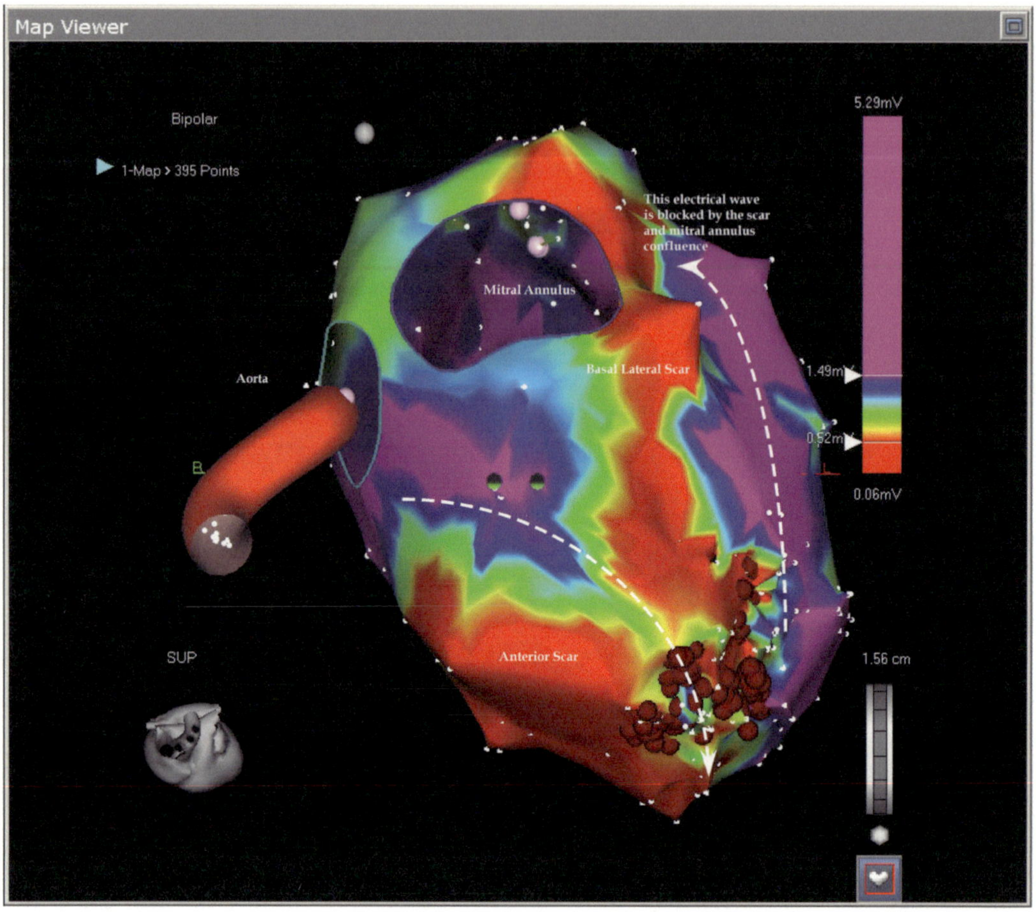

Fig. 7.3. This picture shows the superior projection of the left ventricle with the aortic and mitral annuli. The basal lateral scar is confluent with the mitral ring and this confluence prevents closure of the reentry around this lateral scar leaving only the anterior scar open to permit the reentry. The ablation blocked the isthmus leaving the tachycardia non inducible.

Scar ablation is an accepted approach to ablate ventricular tachycardia. Electromagnetic mapping is indispensable in delineating the scar and magnetic resonance imaging (MRI), three-dimensional computer topographies (CT) and positron emission topographies combined with CT (PET/CT) pictures may enhance it and makes possible evaluation of the exact trans-mural dispersion (Codreanu A et al, 2008; Dickfeld T et al, 2008, Tian J et al. 2010).

The second patient is AG; 61-year-old man with dilated cardiomyopathy, sustained ventricular tachycardia and was referred for CRTD (cardiac resynchronization therapy-defibrillator) implantation. Interestingly, during the implantation, at the left lead pacing threshold measurement, the patient developed ventricular tachycardia. This suggested a tachycardia focus near the pacing area in the left basal posterior-lateral wall.

After the implantation he developed frequent episodes of VT not suppressed by adjuvant medical treatment with amiodarone and mexiletine (Figure 7.4). For this reason he was taken to the electrophysiology laboratory and the left ventricle was mapped during ventricular tachycardia (Figure 7.5 and 7.6). Only a partial mapping was needed (overall 27 points) and the tachycardia origin was located on the basal posterior wall (Figure 7.6), just like suggested by the induction during the implantation. After 4 radiofrequency application on this site the tachycardia terminated and has become non inducible. Of note, the ECG (Figure 7.4 and 7.5) suggested the basal posterior location of the origin and the QRS during the tachycardia had RBBB (Right Bundle Brunch Block), inferior and rightward axis (Figure 7.4 and 7.5).

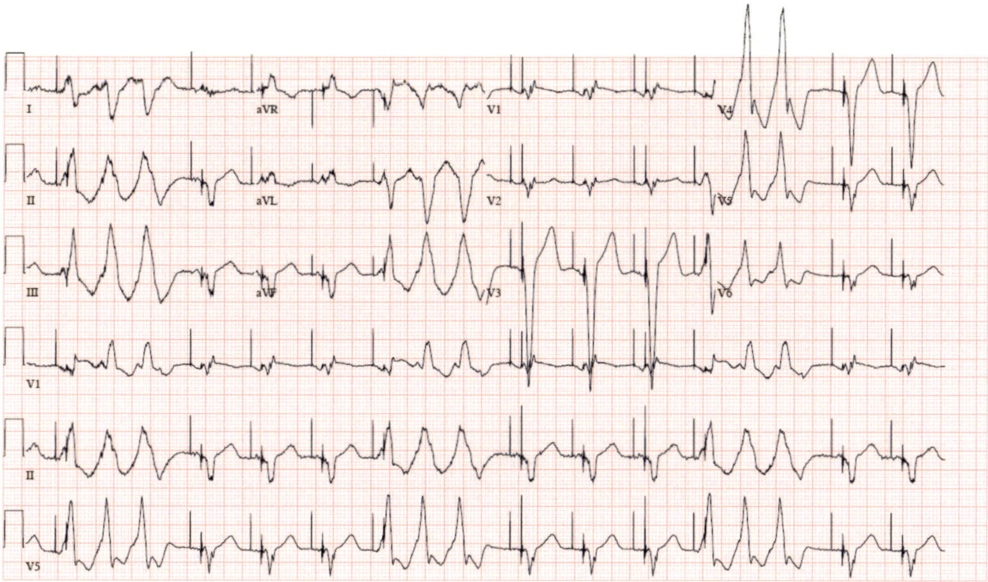

Fig. 7.4. The clinical VT in non-sustained form, but with the same morphology of RBBB, inferior and rightward axis

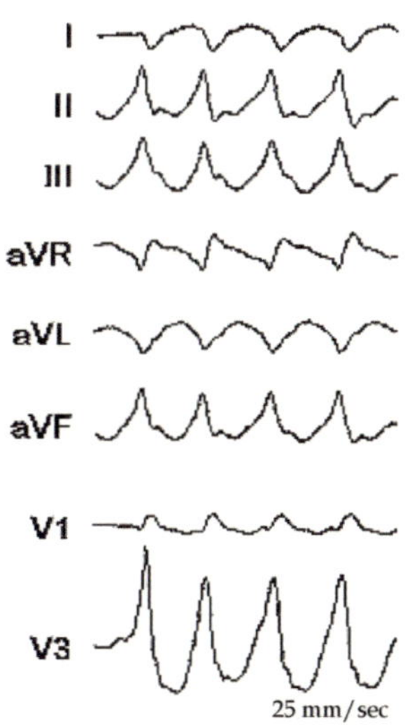

Fig. 7.5. The figure shows the ECG of the VT during the ablation. This VT had RBBB configuration and inferior and rightward axis. This configuration is suggesting a left ventricular VT with the origin in the basal area.

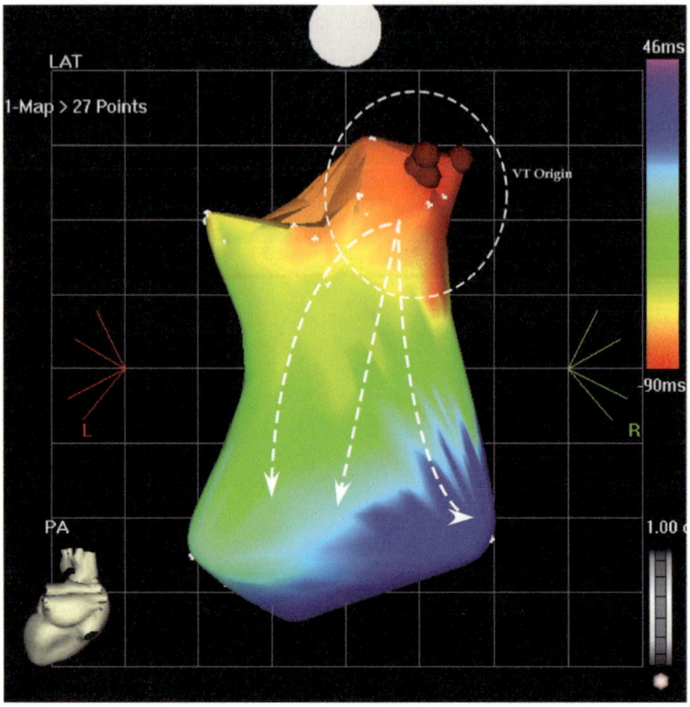

Fig. 7.6. The picture shows the potero-anterior projection of a part of the left ventricle during the VT. The earliest points are located on the basal posterior wall (red area) and the VT is propagated to the apical are as shown by the arrows (blue area). Ablation in this area terminated the VT and rendered it non-inducible.

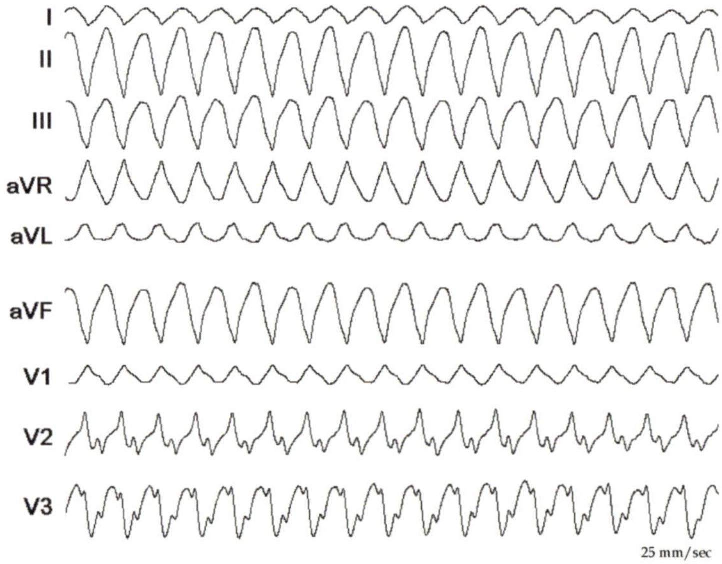

Fig. 7.7. The figure shows the ECG of the second VT during the ablation two weeks after the first one. The QRS has an RBBB configuration and superior axis. When compared with the

first VT (Figure 7.5), the rightward axis is less expressed (L1 compared in the two ECGs, and AVL in the first ECG is negative and in the second is positive). There are also differences in the chest leads available (V3 is strongly positive in the first VT and clearly negative in the second VT). The rates of the VTs are similar.

Although the ablation was successful as exemplified by the previous pictures, the patient presented after two weeks with a second VT (Figure 7.7). He was taken again to the electrophysiology laboratory and the VT was mapped, again with CARTO (Figure 7.8). This time the VT had an RBBB configuration and superior axis! (Figure 7.7)
It was evident that the two VTs are not coming from the same area and again a limited map was completed (to avoid hemodynamic compromise during prolonged mapping). As Figure 7.8 exemplifies, the second VT originated from the apical septum. This are was ablated (Figure 7.9) and interestingly, after the ablation at the earliest point the tachycardia terminated, but was reinduced. This time the second ablation site at this procedure was more inferior, but after termination of the VT by the ablation, it has become noninducible.

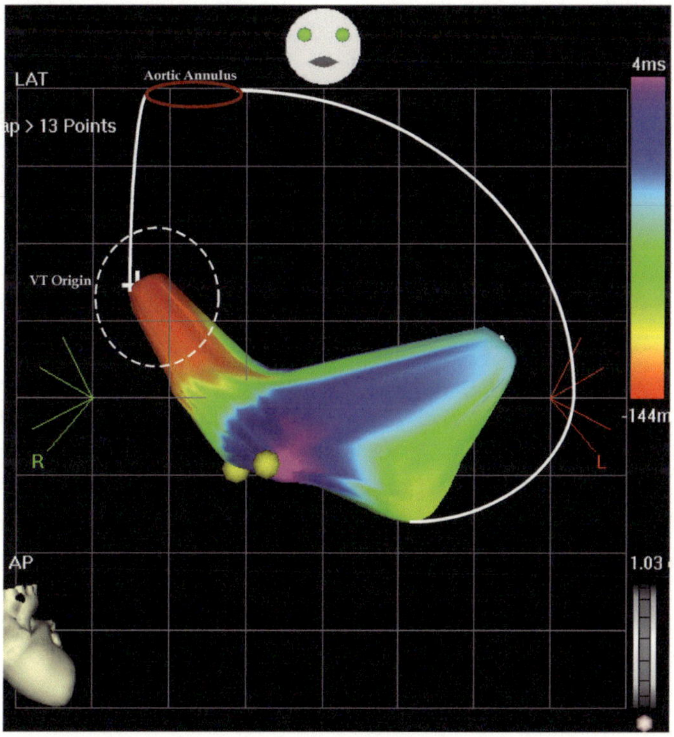

Fig. 7.8. The picture shows an antero-posterior projection of the left ventricular flow map during VT at the second ablation procedure. The left ventricular perimeter is shown with the white lines, including the aortic annulus. The earliest points are originating on the septal area and propagate in the anterior and posterior wall. There is collision on the inferior wall (pink color) and is tagged. The earliest points are -144 msec before the reference catheter in the right ventricle and the collision is 4 msec after the reference catheter.

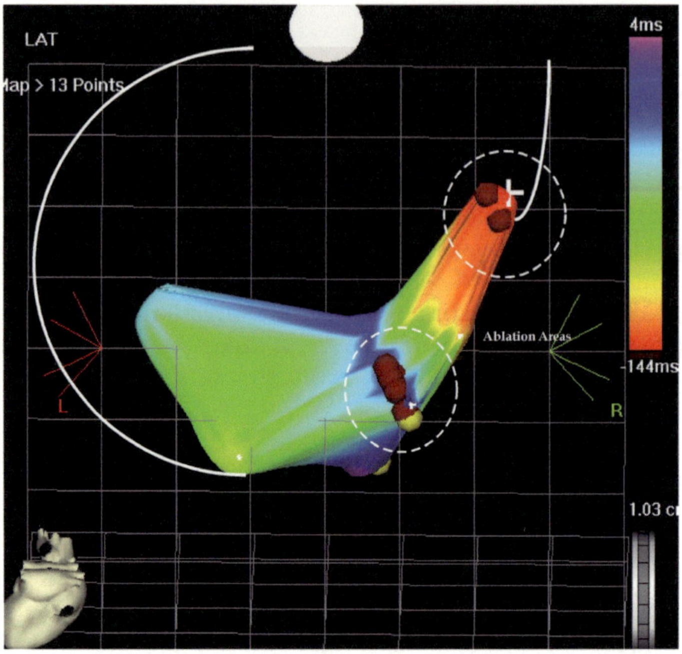

Fig. 7.9. The picture shows the flow map of the left ventricle in postero-anterior projection. Two areas had to be ablated to terminate the VT, first the higher area and earliest one was ablated than the second more inferior are which has become early (not shown) and finally terminated the VT and left it non-inducible.

At the end of the second ablation procedure a very fast VT (200 msec cycle length) was induced requiring DC shock termination (through the implanted ICD which was immediately activated). Two years after the second ablation the patient was free of any ICD therapy. Only rare non-sustained VT was stored by the ICD. In this patient we made several clinical decisions and observations during and around the ablation procedures:

1. The left ventricle mapping was not completed, was quickly achieved and culminated with ablation
2. Propagation mapping was done as this patient has dilated cardiomyopathy and no discrete scar can be mapped
3. Although the ICD was deactivated during the procedure to prevent early termination of the VT during the mapping, it was immediately activated with the induction of the rapid VT (200 msec cycle length- ventricular flutter)
4. The rapid VT-ventricular flutter was not clinical as was not recorded by the ICD during the long follow-up.
5. The proarrhythmic effect of biventricular pacing, well known from the current literature (Nayak HM et al, 2008; Gasparini M et al, 2008, Nordbeck P et al, 2010)

CH was a 59-year-old patient with a large anterior wall myocardial infarction, ventricular tachycardia and implantable defibrillator.

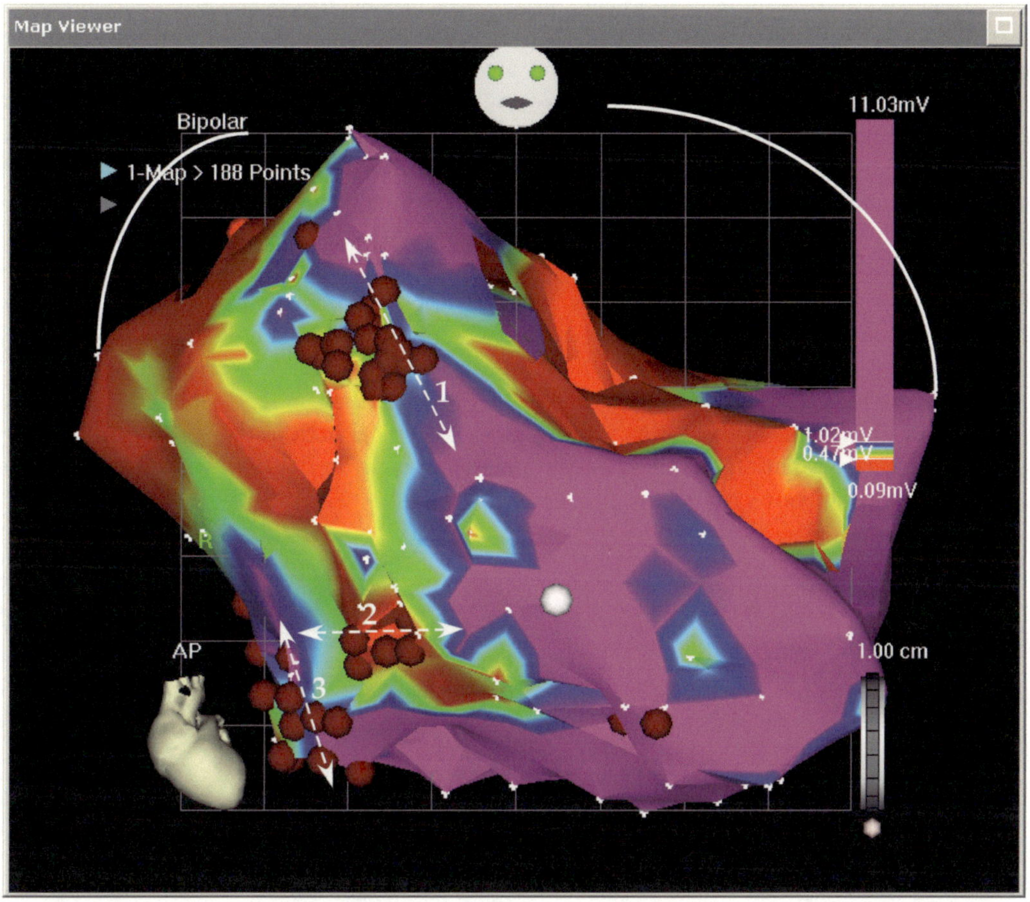

Fig. 7.10. The picture shows the extremely enlarged left ventricle, scar mapping and multiple isthmuses ablation (3 shown on this antero-posterior projection). All the procedure was completed during sinus rhythm, without ventricular pacing. The defibrillator was deactivated during the procedure.

The defibrillator was upgraded to CRTD. Two years after the upgrading, he presented with "VT storm" (more than 150 episodes of VT, majority treated with overdrive pacing and two of them with ICD shock). As medical treatment was not effective and the tachycardia has become resistant to overdrive pacing (including pacing from the RV lead, LV lead and biventricular), he was taken to the electrophysiology laboratory for catheter ablation. It was understood that no mapping during the VT can be completed because the hemodynamic imbalance. Scar mapping was attempted. The left ventricle was extremely enlarged and no catheter was available to complete to basal area mapping. After the ablation the VT frequency was significantly reduced, but not completely abolished and the patient had ventricular assist device implantation, but not survived until appropriate donor heart was available for him.

BN is a 75 year-old-man with a history of a large anterior infarction at the end of 1980's. He was treated with intravenous Streptokinase and despite apparent reperfusion the laboratory tests suggested a large infarction. In the early 1990's he developed aborted sudden cardiac death and a defibrillator was implanted. Occasionally, he had successfully treated episodes of ventricular tachycardia and was resolved with adjuvant amiodarone treatment. In 2008 the defibrillator was upgraded to cardiac resynchronization therapy-defibrillator (CRT-D). Recently he was admitted with incessant tachycardia with a rate between 135-140 beats per minute with relative hemodynamic stability. No medical treatment could suppress the tachycardia, including amiodarone reloading, additional mexiletine, beta-blockers and carvedilol. A coronary angiogram revealed no new coronary lesions and no target for revascularization. As the tachycardia was still incessant, the patient was taken to the electrophysiology laboratory for an ablation attempt. The left ventricle was approached through the aortic valve and the left ventricle was mapped using the fast map technique. The patient was all this time in his slow ventricular tachycardia. As evident in Figure 7.11, the left ventricle is enlarged with a large apical aneurysm and a large scar on the antero-lateral wall. The origin of the tachycardia was in the apical area at the border of the large scar (Figure 7.11). Ablation in this site terminated the tachycardia and was returned to the Cardiology Ward in sinus rhythm.

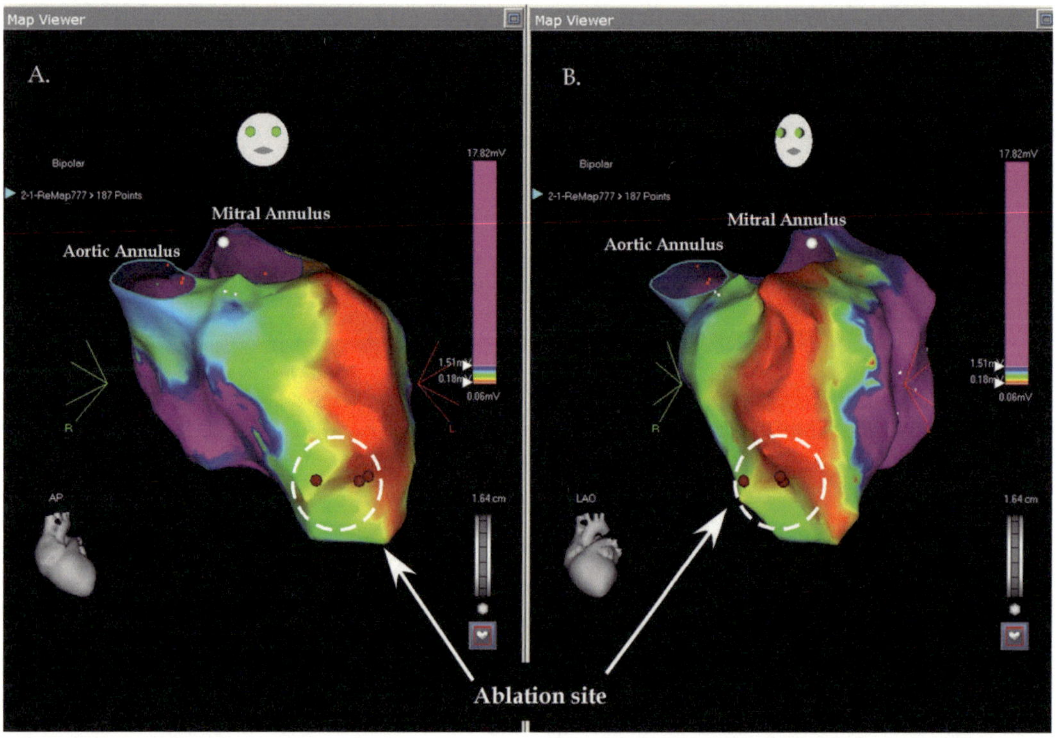

Fig. 7.11. The picture shows the voltage mapping of the left ventricle in two projections: A. antero-posterior; B. left anterior oblique; the ventricle is enlarged with a large apical aneurysm and a large antero-lateral scar. The ablation site is shown in both projections and the ablation was completed during incessant ventricular tachycardia (135 BPM) and propagation mapping. With the two lateral applications the tachycardia terminated spontaneously.

Although the tachycardia was not anymore incessant, the patient still had episodes of tachycardia at a faster rate (150-160 beats per minute). As this tachycardia was not tolerated, he was returned to the electrophysiology laboratory for a “scar ablation”. This time the tachycardia was not induced and the mapping was completed in sinus rhythm (paced rhythm). Using slightly different definitions (scar in the first mapping was defined as <0.18 mV and during the second mapping as <0.54 mV), a large golf of myocardial tissue was revealed in the anterior basal area (Figure 7.12). This area was isolated from the surrounding normal tissue and the ablation area was continued until the mitral annulus to avoid any possible large reentry around the whole scar. Although the endocardial surface was completely blocked, the tachycardia was still inducible with impression of multiple breakthrough points suggesting epicardial origin. However, no real mapping could be completed because the hemodynamic instability during the VT. For this reason, he was scheduled for an epicardial ablation. During the epicardial mapping the origin of the VT was on the apical area and wide area ablation terminated the tachycardia. This epicardial site was almost the same with the successful site during the first mapping. During 3 months follow up the defibrillator recorded and stored only 4 episodes of VT successfully treated with overdrive pacing and not recalled by the patient. He continued the combination of amiodarone and carvedilol treatment. This patient also exemplifies the presence of multiple VT foci in a patient with ischemic cardiomyopathy and a large post myocardial infarction scar.

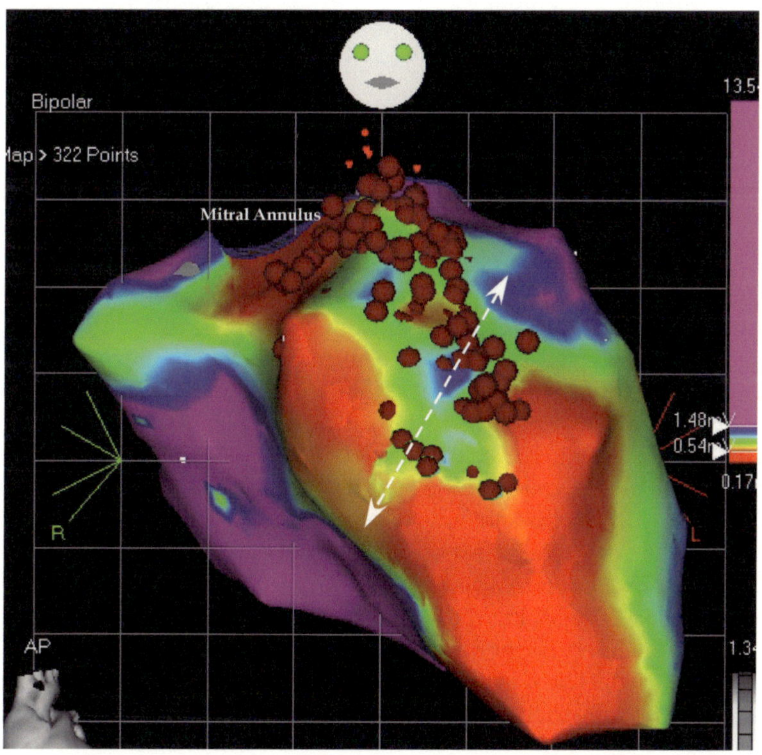

Fig. 7.12. The picture shows the mapping during the second ablation attempt. This is an antero-posterior projection of the left ventricular voltage mapping. The normal tissue was defined as >1.5 mV (like in Figure 6.11), but the scar was defined as <0.5 mV. A large invagination of myocardium into the basal scar was revealed and ablated (see text).

In this patient, with poor left ventricular function and resynchronization therapy, a combined endocardial focal ablation, scar ablation and finally epicardial ablation completed the procedure and achieved an acceptable clinical outcome. The electro-anatomic mapping exemplifies the complexity of the ablation in this patient, and it was possible only using this advanced mapping.

Four patients were presented, each one with a different condition and different mapping. The first patient had a well-defined scar with a clear narrow strip of myocardium dividing it into a large scar and a smaller basal scar limited by the mitral annulus. The second patient has dilated cardiomyopathy without discrete scar and two different foci ablated in two consecutive procedures. The third patient had an extreme ischemic cardiomyopathy, with uncontrollable ventricular tachycardia storm and labile hemodynamic condition. Only scar ablation was possible, because the extremely dilated left ventricle. The fours patient had an enlarged left ventricle, with a large apical aneurysm. The same patient has endocardial focal ablation, scar ablation and finally epicardial ablation.

8. Theoretical aspects

As mentioned in the introduction, first DC shock ablations than RF ablation of solitary pathways in the AV Node or outside it is practiced in clinical electrophysiology. However, DC was used for the first AV Nodal ablation, well-defined origin of WPW and ventricular tachycardia foci. Radiofrequency replaced the DC shock. During 2-3 years first the AV Nodal and AV pathways were ablated. Subsequently, idiopathic VT foci and atrial flutter and focal tachycardia were ablated. In the early 1990's, ventricular tachycardia in structural heart disease, atrial fibrillation and idiopathic ventricular fibrillation were not considered candidates for ablation. Electro-anatomic mapping open the possibility to ablate this complex arrhythmia foci. (Exception was atrial fibrillation where first focal ablation than point ablation guided by special catheters- lasso- preceded the electro-anatomic mapping).

8.1 Atrial tachycardia ablation

In large branching scar, the ablation requires electroanatomic mapping. Patients after corrective surgery of congenital heart disease may develop large scars in the atrium and frequently develop incisional reentry tachycardia. As early as in 2001, several institutions reported small groups or case reports describing the use of electroanatomic mapping (Leonelli FM et al, 2001; Peichl P et al, 2003). Before the use of this mapping, electrophysiological definition of the slow isthmus, called central pathway, was needed. This was a long procedure with limited success. The electro-anatomic mapping delineates the scar, and delineates the isthmus in between scars or in the scar itself. Blocking these pathways, or as occasional called, channels, will prevent induction or spontaneous recurrence of the tachycardia. Interestingly, the number of publication describing the use of electroanatomic mapping for ablation of focal tachycardia ablation is much larger (Kottkamp H et al, 1997; Marchlinski FE et al, 1998; Cummings RM et al, 2008). There is also ample of information on the use of this mapping in the ablation of different left atrial tachycardias (Iwai S et al, 2002; Marrouche NF et al, 2002; Kistler PM et al, 2003; Dong J et al, 2005). Left atrial tachycardias may originate on the septum, along the mitral annulus and from the pulmonary veins. Correct mapping may localize the origin and ensure successful ablation.

Two arrhythmias were extensively discussed in the literature: atrial fibrillation ablation and ablation of ventricular tachycardia in patients with structural heart disease.

8.2 Atrial fibrillation ablation

After the description of the pulmonary vein as trigger in atrial fibrillation, ablation was attempted, first focal, than pulmonary vein isolation (Haissaguerre M et al, 1998). A special catheter was developed- the lasso catheter- to permit mapping of the pulmonary vein osteum and to localize the pathway connecting electrically the vein with the left atrium. This site was ablated and pacing from the coronary sinus could prove the electrical disconnection of the veins (Takahashi Y et al, 2007). This treatment was indicated for patients with paroxysmal atrial fibrillation and not for the other forms of chronic atrial fibrillation, like persistent and permanent. Atrial fibrillation ablation based on electro-anatomic mapping has become an accepted alternative to the pulmonary vein disconnection (Pappone C et al 1999; Pappone C et al, 2000; Pappone C et al 2004; Oral H et al 2006, pappone et al, 2006). Developed at the beginning of this century, this approach offered already at the beginning of its implementation, a possible ablation also for persistent atrial fibrillation and even for long standing persistent type (more then 1 year). The pulmonary vein isolation is achieved by circle ablation in the antrum of the veins. Line ablations in the roof and in the mitral isthmus (between the mitral annulus and the left lower pulmonary vein) completes the procedure and are necessary to avoid left atrial flutter/tachycardia around the ablation rings in the pulmonary vein antrum. One first advantage of the left atrial ablation is the sparing of the vein and by this to reduce to minimum the possible damage to the vessel. This damage may result in pulmonary vein stenosis/occlusion, pulmonary hypertension and symptomatic shortness of breath. The correct and exact reconstruction of the left atrium and its appendages is a prerequisite not only for successful isolation of the pulmonary veins, but also for preventing the above-mentioned damage. Following the original introduction of the electro-anatomic approach to atrial fibrillation ablation, this method was compared with the original pulmonary vein disconnection and both the acute success and the recurrence rate after 1 year was in advantage of the left atrial ablation (Oral H et al, 2003). Moreover, the method was evaluated in patients with long-persistent atrial fibrillation and a significantly higher number of patient in the ablation group was in sinus rhythm after 1 year-77% versus 53% (Oral H et al, 2006a). A large percent of the control group moved to the ablation group and the symptomatic improvement was significantly higher in the ablation group. An additional approach to atrial fibrillation ablation was targeted to complex atrial electrograms. This method is accepted as adjuvant to the left atrial ablation. Finally, even if the first method is use to disconnect the pulmonary veins, the procedure is escalated and elements of the second and third procedure are added (Oral H et al, 2006b; Takahashi Y et al, 2007). Although, we are still not at the end of the way in the development of atrial fibrillation ablation methods, the place of the electroanatomic mapping is well established.
The most complex ablation is probably that of ventricular tachycardia in patients with structural heart disease.

8.3 Ventricular tachycardia ablation

Ventricular tachycardia ablation is going back to 1983 when DC shock was delivered to the ablation site (Hartzler GO, 1983). Soon after the presentation of ablation using radiofrequency energy, it was applied to patients with idiopathic ventricular tachycardia (Kuck KH et al, 1991; Klein LS et al, 1992) and subsequently to ventricular tachycardia in structural heart disease (Morady F et al, 1993). Different methods of pacing helped to localize a critical area in the tachycardia circle or focus pending on the type of heart disease. Although this method was successful, the procedure was prolonged, required a long time to be in ventricular tachycardia and the recurrence rate or new tachycardias generation were high. It has become accepted as an adjuvant to other treatments and focused to the tachycardia causing repeated defibrillator therapy, ventricular tachycardia storm or intolerable shock therapy. The electroanatomic mapping opened to possibility to delineate the scar and reveal any narrow strips of myocardium bridging through the scar. These strips are targeted in the ablation and they are necessary parts of the tachycardia circle. In patients with tolerated tachycardia, the propagation map points to the tachycardia origin. This origin may be the exit point of the reentry circle or the other non-reentry focus (like in patients with dilated or hypertrophic cardiomyopathy). The ablation may be targeted to this early point. There is no need to hold the patient in prolonged tachycardia and no need for the pacing techniques. Moreover, in patients with non-tolerated tachycardia the scar is mapped and is isolated and connected to the valve annulus. Ablation, before defibrillation implantation, may reduce significantly the defibrillator therapy, when compared to non-ablation control group. This approach was called SMASH-VT (Reddy V et al, 2007, Kuck KH et al, 2010). Finally, endocardial ablation may be completed with epicardial ablation (Tedrow U & Stevenson WG, 2009; Sacher F et al, 2010). In patients with post myocardial infarction scars, most of the tachycardia reentry circle is endocardial, but in patients with dilated cardiomyopathy it may be epicardial (Nakahara S et al, 2010).

8.4 Future ablations

There are several other ablation targets recently added to the electrophysiology treatment armamentarium. The first arrhythmia is the idiopathic ventricular fibrillation. Patient with idiopathic ventricular fibrillation may need daily shock therapies and no medical treatment can suppress it. For these patients ablation of the initiating beats origin may reduce the number of treatments needed. These sites are characterized by high density of Purkinje fibers. Clinically, fascicular spikes may be recorded at the successful site in the ventricle (Knecht S et al, 2009; Natale A et al, 2010). If this approach will be applicable in patients with aborted sudden cardiac death and structural heart disease is still on evaluation. The second group with possible future application of electro-anatomic mapping is in patients with Brugada Syndrome. Epicardial fractionated electrograms in the RV outflow may be targeted and after the ablation, the ECG normalizes (Nademanee K et al, 2011). Occasionally, the site may be approached from the endocardium. Of note, the ventricular wall in the RV outflow is relatively thin.

If these two ablations will be implemented in routine practice, the future years will let us know.

9. Conclusions

Complex ablation has become routine in the clinical electrophysiology. Although these arrhythmias originally were approached with classical electrophysiology methods, the electroanatomic mapping simplified them and opened these ablations before rapidly increasing number of electrophysiology centers.

10. References

Arenal A, del Castillo S, Gonzalez-Torrecilla E, Atienza F, Ortiz M, Jimenez J, Puchol A, Garrcia J 7 Almedral J. (2004). Tachycardia-related channel in the scar tissue in patients wuth sustained monomorphic ventricular tachycardia: Influence of the voltage scar definition. *Circulation* Vol. 110:2568-2574

Ben Haim SA, Gepstein L, Hayam G, Ben David J & Josephson MM. (1996a). A new nonfluoroscopic Electroanatomic mapping system. Pacing Clin Electroanatomic mapping system. *Pacing Clin Electrophysiol* Vol. 19:709

Ben-Haim SA, Osadchy D, Schuster I, Gepstein L, Hayam G & Josephson MM. (1996b). Nonfluoropscopic, in vivo navigation and mapping technology. *Nature Med* Vol. 2:1393-1395

Codreanu A, Odille F, Aliot E, Marie PY, Angnin-Poull I, Andonache M, Mandry D, Djaballah W, Regent D, Felblinger J & de Chillou C. (2008). Electroanatomic characterization of post-infarction scars. Comparison with 3-dimensional myocardial scar reconstruction based on magnetic resonance imaging. *J Am Coll Cardiol* Vol. 52:839-42

Cosio FG, Lopez-Gil M, Goicolea A, Arribas F & Barroso JL. (1993). Radiofrequency ablation of the inferior vena cava-tricuspid valve isthmus in common atrial flutter. *Am J Cardiol* Vol. 71:705-709

Cummings RM, Mahle WT, Stieper MJ, Cambell RM, Costelo L, Balfour V, Burchfeld A, Frias PA. (2008). Outcome following electroanatomic mapping and ablation for the treatment of ectopic tachycardia in the pediatric population. *Pediatr Cardiol* Vol. 29:393-397

Daubert JP, Zareba W, Cannom DS, McNit S, Rosero SZ, Wang P, Schuger C, Steinberg JS, Higgins SL Wilber DJ, Klein H, Andrews ML, Hall J, Moss AJ & the MADIT II investigators. (2008). Inappropriate implantable cardioverter defibrillator shock in MADIT II. Frequency, mechanism, predictors, and survival impact. *J Am Coll Cardiol* Vol. 51:1357-1365

Dickfeld T, Lei P, Dilsizian V, Jeudy J, Dong J, Voudouris A, Peters R, Saba M, Shekhar R & Shorofsky S. (2008). Integration of three-dimensional scar maps for ventricular tachycardia ablation with positron emission tomography-computer tomography. *JACC: Cardiovascular Imaging* Vol. 1:73-82

Dong J, Zrenner B, Schreieck J, Deisenhofer I, Karch M, Schneider M, Von Bary C, Weyerbrock S, Yin Y & Schmitt C. (2005). Catheter ablation of left focal atrial tachycardia guided by electroanatomic mapping and new insights into interatrial electrical conduction. *Heart Rhythm* Vol. 2:578-591

Ehrlich JR, Cha TJ, Zhang L, Chartier D, Melnyk P, Hohnloser S & Nattel S. (2003). Cellular electrophysiology of canine pulmonary vein cardiomyocytes: action potential and ionic current properties. *J Physiol* Vol. 551:801-813

ExnerDV, Pinski SI, Wyse G, Renftoe EG, Follman D, Gold M, Beckman KJ, Coromilas J, Lancester S, Hallstrom AP & the AVID investigators. (2001). Electrical storm presages nonsudden death: The Antiarrhythmic Versus Implantable Defibrillators (AVID) Trial. *Circulation* Vol. 103:2066-2071

Ezekowitz JA, Amstrong PW & McAlister FA. (2003). Implantable cardioverter defobrillators in primary and secondary prevention: a systematic review of randomized trials. *Ann Intern Med* Vol. 138:445-452

Feld GK, Fleck P, Chen PS, Boyce K, Bahnson TD, Stein JB, Calisi CM & Ibarra M. (1992) Radiofrequency catheter ablation for the treatment of human type 1 atrial flutter. *Circulation* Vol. 86:1233-1240

Gasparini M, Lunati M, Landolina M, Santini M, Padaletti L, Perego G, Vincenti A, Curnis A, Carboni A, Denaro A, Spotti A, Grammatico A, Regoli F, Boriani G & on behalph of the InSync ICD Italian Registry Investigators. (2008). Electrical storm in patients with biventricular implantable cardioverter defibrillator: incidence, predictors, and prognostic implications. *Am Heart J* Vol. 156:847-854

Gepstein L, Hayam G, Josephson ME & Ben-Haim SA. (1996). A new method for cardiovolumetric measurement based on nonfluoroscopic electrophysiological electroanatomic. *Pacing Clin Electrophysiol* Vol. 19:724

Gepstein L, Hayam G & Ben Haim SA. (1997). A novel model for nonfluoroscopic catheter-based electroanatomic mapping of the heart: in vitro and in vivo accuracy results. *Circulation* Vol. 95:1611-1622

Gepstein L, Goldin A, Lessick J, Hayam G, Shpun S, Schwartz Y, Hakim G, Shofty Turgeman A. Kirshenbaum D & Ben Haim SA. (1998). Electromechanical characterization of chronic myocardial infarction in the canine coronary occlusion model. *Circulation* Vol. 98:2055-2064

Hassaguerre M, Shoda M, Jais P, Nogami A, Shah DC, Kautzner J, Arentz TKalushe D, Lamaison D, Griffith M, Cruz F, de Paola A, Gaita F, Hicini M, Garrigue S, Macle L, Weerasooriya R & Clementi J. (2002). Mapping and ablation of idiopathic ventricular fibrillation. *Circulation* Vol. 106:962-967

Haissaguerre M, Jais P, Shah DC, Takahashi A, Hocini M, Quinou G, Garrigue S, Le Mouroux A, Le Metayer P & Clementy J. (1998). Spontaneous initiation of atrial fibrillation by ectopic beats originating in the pulmonary veins. *N Engl J Med* Vol. 339:659-666

Hartzler GO. (1983). Electrode catheter ablation of refractory focal ventricular tachycardia. *J Am Coll Cardiol* Vol. 2:1107-1113

Hayam G, Gepstein L & Ben-Haym. SA. (1996). Accuracy of the In Vivo Deternination of location using non fluoroscopic electroanatoamical mapping system. *Pacing Clin Electrophysiol* Vol. 19:712

Hsia HH, Lin D, Sayer WH, Callans DJ & Marchlinski FE. (2006). Anatomic characteristics of endocardial substrate for hemodynamic stable reentrant ventricular tachycardia: identification of endocardial conducting channels. *Heart Rhythm* Vol. 3:503-512

Iwai S, Markowitz SM, Stein KM, Mittal S, Slotwiner DJ, Das MK, Cohen JD, Hao SC & Lerman BB. (2002). Response to adenosine differentiates focal from macroreentrant atrial tachycardia. Validation using three-dimensional electroanatomic mapping. *Circulation* Vol. 106:2793-2799

Jackman WM, Beckman KJ, NcClelland JH, Wang X, Friday KJ, Roman CA, Moulton KP, Twidale N, Hazlitt HA, Prior MI, Oren J, Overholt ED, Lazzara R. (1992). Treatment of supraventricular tachycardia due to atrioventricular nodal reentry, by radiofrequency catheter ablation of slow-pathway conduction. N Engl J Med Vol. 327:313-318

Kistler PM, Saders PB, Hussin A, Morton JB, Vohra JK, Sparks PB & Kalman JM. (2003). Focal atrial tachycardia arising from the mitral annulus. Eelctrocardiographic and electrophysiologic characterization. *J Am Coll Cardiol* Vol. 41:2212-2219

Klein LS, Shih HT, Hackett K, Zipes DP & Miles WM. (1992). Radiofrequency catheter ablation of ventricular tachycardia in patients without structural heart disease. *Circulation* Vol. 85:1666-1674

Knecht S, Sacher F, Wright M, Hocini M, Nogami A, Arentz T, Petit B, Frank R, De Chillou C, Lamison D, Farre J, Lavergne L, Weerasooriya R, Cauchemez B, Lellouche N, Derval N, Narayan SM, Jais P & Clementy J, Haissaguerre M. (2009). Long-term follow-up of idiopathic ventricular fibrillation ablation: a multicenter study. *J Am Coll Cardiol* Vol. 54:522-528

Kottkamp H, Hindricks G, Breithardt G & Borggrefe M. (1997). Three-dimentional electromagnetic catheter technology: Elecroanatomical mapping of the right atrium and ablation of ectopic tachycardia. *Pacing Clin Electrophysiol* Vol. 8:1332-1337

Kuck KH, Schluter M, Geiger M & Siebels J. (1991). Successful catheter ablation of human ventricular tachycardia with radiofrequency current guided by an endocardial map of the area of slow conduction. *Pacing Clin Electrophysiol* Vol. 14:1060-1071

Kuck KH, Schamann A, Eckhardt L, Willems S, Ventura R, Delacretaz E, Pitcschner HF, Kautzner J, Schumacher B, Hansen PS & for the VTACH study group. (2010). Catheter ablation of stable ventricular tachycardia before defibrillator implantation in patients with coronary artery disease (VTACH): a multicenter randomized controlled trial. *Lancet* Vol. 375:31-40

Kumagai K, Muraoka S, Mitsutake C, Takashima H & Nakashima H. (2007). A new approach for complete isolation of the posterior left atrium including pulmonary veins for atrial fibrillation. *J Cardiovasc Electrophysiol* Vol. 18:1047-1052

Lee MA, Morady F, Kadish A, Schamp DJ, Chin MC, Scheinman MM, Griffin JC, Pederson D, Goldberger J, Calkins H, deBuitleir M, Kou WH, Rosenheck S, Sousa J & Langberg J. (1991). Catheter modification of the atrioventricular junction with radiofrequency energy for control of atrioventricular nodal reentry tachycardia. *Circulation* Vol. 83:827-835

Leonelli FM, Tomassoni G, Richey M & Natale A. (2001). Ablation of incisional atrial tachycardias using three-dimensional nonfluoroscopic mapping system. *Pacing Clin Electrophysiol* Vol. 24:1653-1659

Marchlinski F, Callans D, Gottlieb C, Rodriguez E, Coyne R & Kleinman D. (1998). Magnetic electroanatomic mapping for ablation of focal atrial tachycardias. *Pacing Clin Electrophysiol* Vol. 21:1621-1635

Marchlinski FE, Callans DJ, Gottlieb CD & Zado E. (2000). Linear ablation lesions of unmappable ventricular tachycardia in patients with ischemic and nonischemic cardiomyopathy. *Circulation* Vol. 101:1288-1296

Marrouche NF, Groenewegen AS, Yang Y, Dibs S & Scheinman MM. (2002). Clinical and electrophysiologic characteristics of left septal atrial tachycardia. *J Am Coll Cardiol* Vol. 40:1133-1139

Morady F & Scheinman MM. (1984). Transvenous catheter ablation of posteroseptal accessory pathway in patients with Wolff-Parkinson-White syndrome. *N Engl J Med* Vol. 310:705-707

Morady F, Harvey M, Kalbfleisch SJ, El-Atassi R, Calkins H & Langberg JJ. (1993) Radiofrequency catheter ablation of ventricular tachycardia in patients with coronary artery disease. *Circulation* Vol. 87:363-372

Nademanee K, McKenzie J, Kosar E, Schwab M, Sunsaneewitayakul B, Vasavakul T, Khunnawat C & Ngarmukos T. (2004). A new approach for catheter ablation of atrial fibrillation: mapping of the electrophysiologic substrate. *J Am Coll Cardiol* Vol. 43:2044 –2053

Nademanee K, Veerakul G, Chandanamattha P, Chaothawee L, Ariyachaipanich A, Jirasirirojanakorn K, Likittanasombat K, Bhuripanyo K & Ngarmukos T. (2011). Prevention of ventricular fibrillation episodes in Brugada Syndrome by catheter ablation over the anterior right ventricular outflow epicardium. *Circulation* Vol. 123:1270-1279

Nakahara S, Tung R, Ramirez RJ, Michowitz Y, Vasedhi M, Buch E, Gima J, Wiener I, Mahajan A, Boyle NG & Shivkumar K. (2010). Characterization of the arrhythmogenic substrate in ischemic and nonischemic cardiomyopathy. Implications for catheter ablation of hemodynamically unstable ventricular tachycardia. *J Am Coll Cardiol* Vol. 55:2355-2365

Natale A, Raviele A, Al-Ahmad A et al. (2010). Venice Chart international consensus document on ventricular tachycardia/fibrillation ablation. *J Cardiovasc Electrophysiol* Vol. 21:339-379

Nayak HM, Verdino RJ, Russo AM, Gerstenfeld EP, Hsia HH, Lin D, Dixit S, Cooper JM, Callans D & Marchlinski FE. (2008). Ventricular tachycardia storm after initiation of biventricular pacing: incidence, clinical characteristics, management, and outcome. *J Cardiovasc Electrophysiol* Vol. 19:708-715

Nordbeck P, Seidl B, Fey B, Bauer WR & Titter O. (2010). Effect of cardiac resynchronization therapy on the incidence of electrical storm. *Int J Cardiol* Vol. 143:330-336

Oral H, Scharf C, Chugh A, Hall B, Cheung P, Good E, Veerareddy S, Pelosi F & Morady F. (2003). Catheter ablation for paroxysmal atrial fibrillation. Segmental pulmonary vein ostial ablation versus left atrial ablation. *Circulation* Vol. 108:2355-2360

Oral H, Pappone, Chugh A, Good E, Bogun F, Pelosi F, Bates ER, Lehmann MH, Vicedomini G, Augello G, Agricola E, Sala S, Santinelli V & Morady F. (2006a). Circumferential pulmonary-vein ablation for chronic atrial fibrillation. *N Engl J Med* Vol. 354:934-941

Oral H, Chugh A, Good E, Sankaran S, Reich SS, Igic P, Elmouchi D, Tschopp D, Crawford T, Dey S, Wimmer A, Lemola K, Jongnarangsin K, Bogun F, Pelosi F & Morady F. (2006b). A tailored approach to catheter ablation of paroxysmal atrial fibrillation. *Circulation* Vol. 113:1824-1831

Pappone C, Oreto G, Lamberti F, Vicedomini G, Loricchio ML, Shpun S, Rillo M, Calabro MP, Conversano A, Ben-Haim SA, Cappato R & Chierchia S. (1999). Catheter ablation of paroxysmal atrial fibrillation using a 3D mapping system. *Circulation* Vol. 100:1203–1208

Pappone C, Rosanio S, Oreto G, Tocchi M, Gugliotta F, Vicedomini G, Sakvati A, Dicandia C, Mazzone P, Santinelli V, Gulletta S & Chiechia S. (2000). Circumferentia radiofrequency ablation of PV ostia. *Circulation* Vol. 102:2619 –28

Pappone C, Manguso F, Vicedomini G, Gugliotta F, Santinelli O, Ferro A, Gulletta S, Sala S, Sora N, Paglino G, Augello G, Agricola E, Zngrillo A, Alfieri O & Santinelli V. (2004). Prevention of iatrogenic atrial tachycardia after ablation of atrial fibrillation: a prospective randomized study comparing circumferential pulmonary vein ablation with a modified approach. *Circulation* Vol. 110:3036-3042

Pappone C, Augello G Sala S, Gugliotta F, Vicedomini G, Gulletta S, Paglino G, Mazzone P, Sora N, Greiss I, Santagostino A, LiVolsi L, Pappone N, Radinovic A, Manguso F & Santinelli V. (2006). A randomized trial of circumferential pulmonary vein ablation versus antiarrhythmic drug therapy in paroxysmal atrial fibrillation. The APAF Study. *J Am Coll Cardiol* Vol. 48:2340-2347

Peichl P, Kautzner J, Cihak R, Vancura V & Bytesnik J. (2003). Clinical application of electroanatomic mapping of "incisional" atrial tachycardia. *Pacing Clin Electrophysiol* Vol. 26:420-425

Poole JE, Johnson GW, Hellkamp AS, Anderson J, Callans DJ, Raitt MH, Reddy RK, Marchlinski FE, Yee R, Guarnieri T, Talajic M, Wilber DJ, Fishbein DP, Oacker DL, Matk DB, Lee KL & Bardy GH. (2008). Prognostic importance of defibrillation shocks in patients with heart failure. *N Engl J Med* Vol. 259:1009-1017

Reddy V, Reynolds MR, Neuzil P, Richardson AW, Taborsky M, Jongnarangsin K, Kralovec S, Sediva L, Ruskin JN & Josephson ME. (2007). Prophylactic catheter ablation for the prevention of defibrillator therapy. *N Engl J Med* Vol. 357:2657-2665

van Rees JB, Borleff JW, de Bie MK, Stijnen T, van Erven L, Bax JJ & Schlij MJ. (2011). Inappropriate Implantable cardioverter-defibrllator shocks. Incidence, predictors, and impact on mortality. *J Am Coll Cardiol* Vol. 57:556-562

Sacher F, Roberts-Thomson K, Maury P, Tedrow U, Nault I, Steven D, Hocini M, Koplan B, Leroux L, Derval N, Seiler J, Wright MJ, Epstein L & Haisaaguerre M. (2010). Epicardial ventricular tachycardia ablation. A multicenter safety study. *J Am Coll Cardiol* Vol. 55:2366-2376

Scheinman MM, Morady F, Hess DS & Gonzalez R. (1982). Catheter-induced ablation of the atrioventricular junction to control refractory supraventricular arrhythmias. *JAMA* Vol. 248:851-855

Shpun S, Gepstein L, Hayam G & Ben Haim SA. (1997). Guidance of radiofrequency endocardial ablation with real-time three-dimentional magnetic navigation system. *Circulation* Vol. 96:2016-2021

Smeets J, Ben Haim S, Ben David J, Gepstein L & Josephson MM. (1996). Non-fluoroscopic endocardial mapping: first experience in patients. *Pacing Clin Electrophysiol* Vol. 9:627

Sra J, Bhatia A, Dhala A, Blanck Z, Deshpande S, Cooley R & Akhtar M. (2001). Electroanatomically guided catheter ablation of ventricular tachycardia causing multiple defibrillation shocks. *Pacing Clin Electrophysiol* Vol. 24:1645-1652

Stevenson WG, Delacretaz E, Friedman PL & Ellison KE. (1998). Identification and ablation of macroreentrant ventricular tachycardia with CARTO electroanatomic mapping system. *Pacing Clin Electrophysiol* Vol. 21:1448-1456

Stevenson WG, Friedman PL, Kocovic D, Sager PT, Saxon LA & Pavri B. (1998). Radiofrequency catheter ablation of ventricular tachycardia after myocardial infarction. *Circulation* Vol. 98:308-314

Stevenson WG, Wilber DJ, Natale A, Jackman WM, Marchlinski FE, Talber T, GonzalesMD, Worley SJ, Daoud EG, Hwang C, Schuger C, Bump TE, Jazayeri M, Tomassoni GF, Koplelman HA, Soejima K, Nakagawa H & for the Multicenter Thermocool VT Ablation Trial Investigators. (2008). Irrigated radiofrequency catheter ablation guided by electroanatomic mapping for recurrent ventricular tachycardia after myocardial infarction. The Multicenter Thermocool Ventricular Tachycardia Ablation Trial. *Circulation* Vol. 118:2773-2782

Takatsuki S, Mitamura H & Ogawa S. (2001). Catheter ablation of monfocal premature ventricular complex trigerring idiopathic ventricular fibrillation. *Heart* Vol. 86:E3

Takahashi Y, O'Neill MD, Hocini M, Reant P, Jonsson A, Jaïs P, Sanders P, Rostock T, Rotter M, Sacher F, Laffite S, Roudaut R, Clémenty J, MD & Haïssaguerre M. (2007). Effect of stepwise ablation of chronic atrial fibrillation on atrial electrical and mechanical properties. *J Am Coll Cardiol* Vol. 49:1306-1314

Tedrow U & Stevenson WG. (2009). Strategies for epicardial mapping and ablation of ventricular tachycardia. *J Cardiovasc Electrophysiol* Vol. 20:710-713

Tian J, Jeudy J, Smith MF, Jimenez A, Yin X, Bruce PA, Lei P, Turgeman A, Abbo A, Shenkhar R, Saba M, Shorofsky S & Dickfeld T. (2001). Tree-dimensional contrast-enhanced CT for anatomic, dynamic, and perfusion characterization of abnormal myocardium to guide ventricular tachycardia ablation. *Circ Arrhythm Electrophysiol* Vol. 3:496-504

Tung R, Josephson ME, Reddy V, Reynolds MR & on behalf of the SMASH-VT investigators. (2010). Influence of clinical and procedural predictors on ventricular tachycardia ablation outcomes: An analysis from the substrate mapping and ablation in sinus rhythm to halt tachycardia trial (SMASH-VT). *J Cardiovasc Electrophysiol* Vol. 21:799-803

Wolff L, Parkinson J & White PD. (1930) Bundle-brunch block with short P-R interval in healthy young people prone to paroxysmal tachycardia. *Am Heart J* Vol. 5:685-704

Novel Technologies for Mapping and Ablation of Complex Arrhythmias

Shahnaz Jamil-Copley, Louisa Malcolme-Lawes and Prapa Kanagaratnam
Imperial College Healthcare NHS Trust, St Mary's Hospital, London,
National Heart and Lung Institute, Imperial College London,
UK

1. Introduction

1.1 The burden of complex arrhythmias

Atrial fibrillation (AF) is the most common cardiac arrhythmia, affecting about 9% of the population over 70 years of age (Feinberg, Blackshear et al. 1995). It is characterised by an irregular pulse, leading to symptoms of shortness of breath, dizziness, palpitations, chest pain, lethargy and an increased risk of stroke (Kannel, Abbott et al. 1982). Current widely accepted indications for catheter ablation of AF are significant symptoms uncontrolled by anti-arrhythmic medications, however more recent European Guidelines have suggested catheter ablation may be used as a first line treatment for symptomatic paroxysmal AF in patients with no or minimal heart disease. Randomised trials from 2003 - 2010 have shown a range of success rates for catheter ablation of AF from 56 - 89% (freedom from AF off anti-arrhythmic drugs) compared to the use of AADs alone ranging from 4 - 43% (Camm, Kirchhof et al. ; Kannel, Abbott et al. 1982).

Atrial tachycardia (AT) is relatively rare, accounting for 5-15% of all supraventricular tachycardias (SVTs). It can be encountered in patients with a structurally normal heart or those with underlying structural or scar-related heart disease. In patients with structurally normal hearts, atrial tachycardia is associated with a low mortality rate. However spontaneous resolution of symptomatic episodes is uncommon. Prolonged episodes (typically months or years) of continuous atrial tachycardia can be problematic leading to irreversible changes of the atria, including negative remodeling with atrial enlargement and myopathy causing symptomatic congestive cardiac failure. In addition, prolonged episodes can make reversion and maintenance of normal sinus rhythm more difficult. In recent years, the significance of AT in the initiation and perpetuation of atrial fibrillation has become apparent. Paradoxically AT occurs in up to 50% of patients undergoing extensive ablation for persistent AF.

Sustained ventricular tachycardia (VT) is a significant cause of morbidity and sudden death especially in patients with underlying structural heart disease. Coronary heart disease is the most common cause of clinically documented VT occurring in 76–82% of the patients (CASCADE Study 1993; Kuch et al 2000; AVID Study 1997; CIDS Study 2000). Although implantable cardioverter defibrillators (ICD) prevent sudden cardiac death and antiarrhythmic drugs reduce the frequency of VT episodes, drug side-effects and repeated device therapies can have a major impact on quality of life (Moss et al 2004, Poole et al 2008, Schron et al 2002). Recurrent VT develops in 40-60% of patients receiving an ICD for ischaemic cardiomyopathy after an episode of spontaneous sustained VT however the first ICD therapy appears to be the most important predictor of subsequent therapy in this population and is likely to occur within the first two years of implant (Koa-Wing M et al 2007). VT ablation has been shown to reduce therapies from ICDs, but in its current state, is technically challenging and time consuming with procedural times up to 8 hours (Cao et al 1996).

1.2 The challenges of complex arrhythmias

1.2.1 Atrial Fibrillation

Several models have been proposed to explain the continuous irregular atrial activation of clinical AF. It is widely accepted that the initiation of AF is from an atrial ectopic 'trigger' originating from the pulmonary veins (Haissaguerre, Jais et al. 1998). The 'trigger' can continue to act as 'a focal driver' maintaining AF or can establish a self-sustaining spiral wave (or rotor) in a localised region of the myocardium leading to fibrillatory activation in the remaining atria (Haissaguerre, Jais et al. 1998; Jalife, Berenfeld et al. 2002; Sahadevan, Ryu et al. 2004).

Pulmonary vein isolation to remove the 'trigger' has been shown to be effective in paroxysmal AF (Haissaguerre, Jais et al. 1998) (Pappone, Santinelli et al. 2004). However, triggers outside the pulmonary veins have also been identified in the superior vena cava and coronary sinus and these have been more challenging to identify and treat. Linear ablation has been performed in both paroxysmal and persistent AF along the principles of the Cox Maze surgical procedures, but these have not achieved the same success as the surgical approach (Cox, Boineau et al. 1995; Cox, Schuessler et al. 1996; Hsu, Jais et al. 2004). Linear ablation at the roof of the left atrium (Hocini, Jais et al. 2005) and the mitral isthmus between the left lower pulmonary vein and annulus has been shown to improve outcomes when there is proven conduction block of these lines (Jais, Hocini et al. 2004; Willems, Klemm et al. 2006). However, conduction block is difficult to achieve due to lack of catheter stability and failure to achieve transmurality.

More recently, catheter-based substrate modification has targeted regions of highly fractionated electrograms that others suggest as drivers for persistent AF (Lellouche, Buch et al. 2007). Nadamanee et al achieved an 81% success rate for ablation after up to 4 procedures targeting only areas of complex fractionated atrial electrograms (CFAE) (Nademanee, Schwab et al. 2008). However several other groups have failed to reproduce these success rates with CFAE ablation alone (Estner, Hessling et al. 2008). Speculation as to the mechanistic basis for CFAE has implicated regions of autonomic innervations termed the ganglionated plexi, as these were noted to be co-located with regions of CFAE in animal studies. Alternatively, they may originate from regions of atrial scarring or fibrosis, and are thought to represent a combination of wavefronts approaching the recording electrode from multiple directions. Integration of delayed-enhancment MRI imaging, particularly containing information relating to scar, may provide greater insight on the origin of CFAE. This is discussed in more detail later in this chapter.

Wide area circumferential ablation with pulmonary vein isolation, designed to encircle the PVs at a distance from the ostia, is a widely accepted technique for AF ablation and appears to achieve greater success rates than segmental PVI. (Marrouche, Martin et al. 2003; Pappone, Rosanio et al. 2003; Ouyang, Bansch et al. 2004) The most widely practiced approach is to use a 3D-navigation system to recreate a virtual left atrium and move around the chamber delivering lesions around the pulmonary veins and marking lesion points on the virtual anatomy.(Pappone, Oreto et al. 1999) The 3D geometry aids the operator in manipulating catheters around the complex anatomy of the left atrium which can vary significantly from patient to patient. This can prove particularly challenging with only 2D fluoroscopy for navigation.

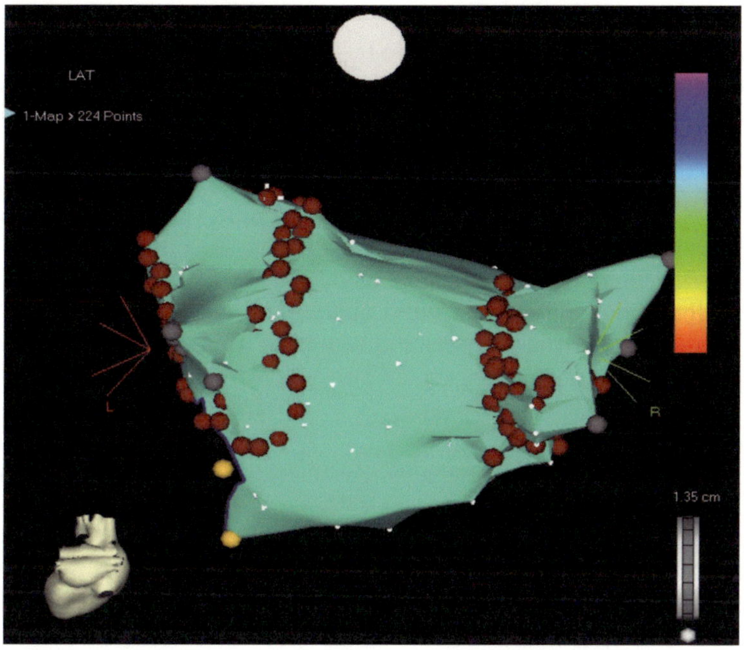

Example of virtual left atrium and points marked (red balls) during wide area circumferential ablation

Despite these novel approaches, published success rates for single procedure AF ablation range remain around 50% to 88% (Lim, Matsuo et al. 2007; Matsuo, Lim et al. 2007; Natale, Raviele et al. 2007; O'Neill, Jais et al. 2007; Marchlinski 2008) which are still not comparable to the >95% success rates expected from ablations for other arrhythmias.

1.2.2 Atrial Tachycardia

Endocardial activation allows categorisation of ATs into focal and macro-rentrant. However in the era of persistant AF ablation the presence of "micro-reentry" circuits particularly within regions of previous complex fractionated atrial electrograms (CFAE) ablation scar must be acknowledged. It is therefore imperative to clarify the mechanism of the underlying AT during electrophysiological procedures to guide ablation therapy. Currently established techniques for guiding ablation in complex atrial tachycardias include activation and/or entrainment mapping. Routinely the tachycardia is displayed as an activation map on a recreated atrial geometry from endocardial location points collected using 3-D mapping technology. However, activation mapping is limited by a point-by-point acquisition process which is not always systematic, is often time-consuming and can miss small areas crucial to the circuit. Detailed mapping often requires >150-200 points with each circuit potentially involving multiple loops and figure-of-8 circuits. In order to identify the critical isthmus maintaining the tachycardia a trained operator is required to set an accurate "window of interest" and collect activation data, which requires significant processing to ensure all collected points have been correctly annotated to the chosen reference. In addition conventionally established entrainment manoeuvres are often used to confirm the diagnosis represented by activation mapping however these can have limitations if there is a variation in the tachycardia cycle length particularly in scarred atria with multiple regions of block and slow conduction.

The most commonly recognised mechanisms seen post-AF ablation are macro re-entrant roof-dependant and mitral isthmus dependant tachycardias however with increasing linear and CFAE ablation lesions, micro-reentrant circuits must also be appreciated. In these situations diagnostic yield from mapping and entrainment can test the most skilled electrophysiologist and although acute success rates have been reported ranging from 88-100%, recurrences are disappointing with rates ranging from 0-47% over a mean follow-up of 2 to 16 months (Gerstenfeld 2004; Chugh 2005; Deisenhofer 2006; Mesas 2004; Haïssaguerre 2005).

Several other circuits capable of sustaining re-entrant tachycardias are seen following cardiac surgery, particularly congenital heart disease.

These are typically a challenge to map and ablate due to the unpredictable location and extent of the underlying iatrogenic scar exposing the limitations of the aforementioned diagnostic techniques.

1.2.3 Ventricular Tachycardia

The biggest challenge in VT ablation remains scar-related VT including ischaemic and dilated cardiomyopathy. The substrate for post-infarct VT is produced by channels of slow conduction within the scar border (the diastolic pathway), created by anatomical and functional lines of block. Identification and ablation of these diastolic pathways is required for successful VT ablation (Koa-Wing, Ho SY et al 2007; Stevenson, Khan et al 1993). Conventional techniques to identify the diastolic pathway consist of performing activation mapping followed by entrainment manoeuvres to locate areas within the scar that participate in the re-entrant circuit (Stevenson, Khan et al 1993; Huang & Wood 2006; Bogun, Good et al 2006), but non-inducibility, difficulty capturing scarred myocardium during entrainment, multiple different morphologies of VT, haemodynamic instability and circuit components deep to the sub-endocardium make this approach unreliable and prolonged with disappointingly high recurrence rates.

These limitations have led to a change in practice from targeting specific circuits to substrate modification of the scar by linear ablation in an attempt to transect potential diastolic pathways and render the VT non-inducible (Marchlinski, Callans et al 2000). Although acute ablation success rates at elimination of the "clinical" tachycardia have improved from 71-74% (Morady et al 1993, Gonska et al 1994, Kim et al 1994) in the mid-1990s to 90% in the 2000s (Sacher et al 2008) long-term outcomes remain unsatisfactory. This is despite the introduction of cardiac mapping systems, irrigated tip catheters and substrate based ablation strategies. Up to 31% of patients with an acutely successful ablation outcome of the "clinical" VT have arrhythmia recurrence. Ablation to non-inducibility of any VT has been reported with success rates approaching 65% but with recurrence rates of 29% during a median follow-up of 1 month (Sacher et al. 2008). The potential causes of recurrence or failure at the index procedure include inadequate mapping techniques of, often small, isthmi in a complex anatomic substrate and failure to achieve transmurality of lesions in those with circuits traversing the subendocardium and epicardium. Although epicardial circuits can be targeted percutaneously, this is not possible in up to 85% of patients with previous cardiac surgery (Sacher F, Roberts-Thomson K, et al. 2010).

2. Mapping

The development of intra-cardiac mapping was based on the use of individual contact catheters. Despite being able to record information from different sites using multipolar catheters, complex arrhythmias and complex substrates pose significant challenges using these techniques. 3-D electrophysiological mapping systems were developed to aid the localisation of the source of focal tachycardias and the critical isthmi of re-entrant circuits (Stevenson, Delacretaz et al 1998; Marchlinski, Callans et al 1998; Earley, Showkathali et al 2006; Schilling, Peters et al 1999; Shah, Jais et al 1997) Conventionally, these systems display electrical data from mapping catheters as either local activation time (isochronal) or local voltage (isopotential) maps. These methods indicate the parameter being displayed using a colour-scale on a 3D representation of the cardiac chamber of interest.

The current versions of these mapping systems are not only significantly more accurate but they offer many more features to facilitate mapping of complex arrhythmias; voltage mapping, propagation maps, rapid mapping using multipolar catheters and mapping of fractionated electrograms and the input of anatomical data from pre-operative CT or MRI scans of the heart or rotational angiograms. The latest feature allowing 4-dimensional mapping, 'ripple-mapping', will also be discussed in this chapter.

The use of mapping systems has not been shown to reduce the duration of the procedure or the efficacy of the procedure(Sporton, Earley et al. 2004), however, it has been shown to significantly reduce the fluoroscopy time, thereby reducing the exposure of patients and lab staff to harmful radiation.(Scaglione, Biasco et al.)

2.1 Current mapping systems

Current electroanatomic mapping systems build a 3-dimensional geometry of a cardiac chamber by recording sequential positional co-ordinates from the catheter tip in contact with the myocardium and combining this information with concomitantly acquired electrogram data. Low voltage areas and scar can be easily identified to develop a picture of the underlying substrate for arrhythmogensis. Electrogram timings with respect to a stable reference catheter, enables an activation map to be created, which is colour coded to differentiate between 'early' and 'late' signals.

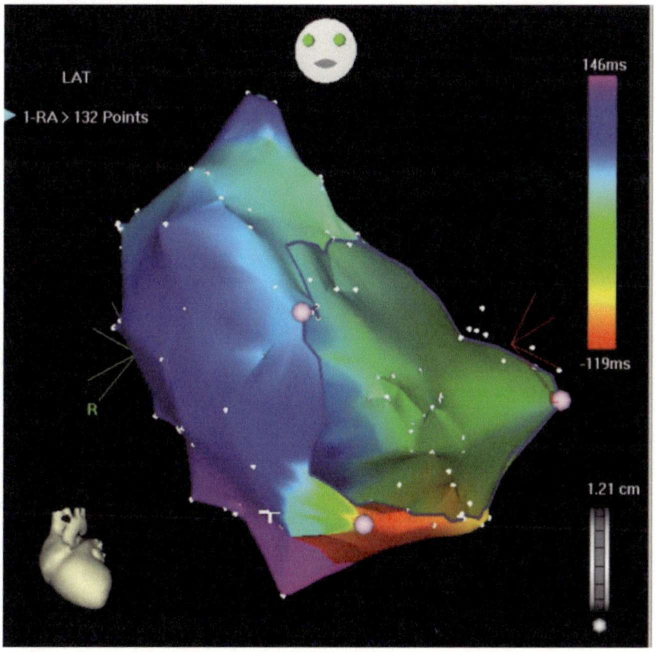

Colour coded activation map of a clockwise isthmus dependent right atrial flutter.

Alternatively, this can be displayed as a propagation map, which demonstrates activation of the excitatory wavefront as it advances across the chamber geometry. Maps can be rotated and viewed in multiple orientations at the same time so that the wavefront can be followed throughout the cardiac cycle. Electroanatomic mapping systems are primarily used for mapping stable tachycardias, however they can also facilitate substrate mapping during sinus rhythm, which is particularly useful when mapping VTs which cause significant haemodynamic compromise. Additionally, these systems facilitate encirclement of cardiac structures, the best example of which is the encirclement of pulmonary veins as part of the treatment for ablation of atrial fibrillation (AF). Areas targeted may lie between important scar boundaries (e.g. linear ablation lesions to transect the diastolic pathway in VT circuits) or between inert structures (e.g. linear ablation between the mitral valve annulus and the left inferior pulmonary vein in mitral isthmus-dependent atrial tachycardia).

2.2 Integration with robotic navigation

New Cohesion™ 3D visualisation module available with the Hansen Robotic Navigation system allows integration of the electroanatomic mapping system NavX or Velocity (St Jude Medical™) This facilitates navigation of the robotic catheter by producing an intuitive driving plane according to the orientation of the virtual geometry within the mapping system. This removes the requirement for the operator to re-orientate him or herself when using the virtual geometry of the left atrium to guide navigation. This has been tested in clinical studies and shown to reduce fluoroscopy times for robotic navigation and ablation of AF.(Steven, Servatius et al. 2009)

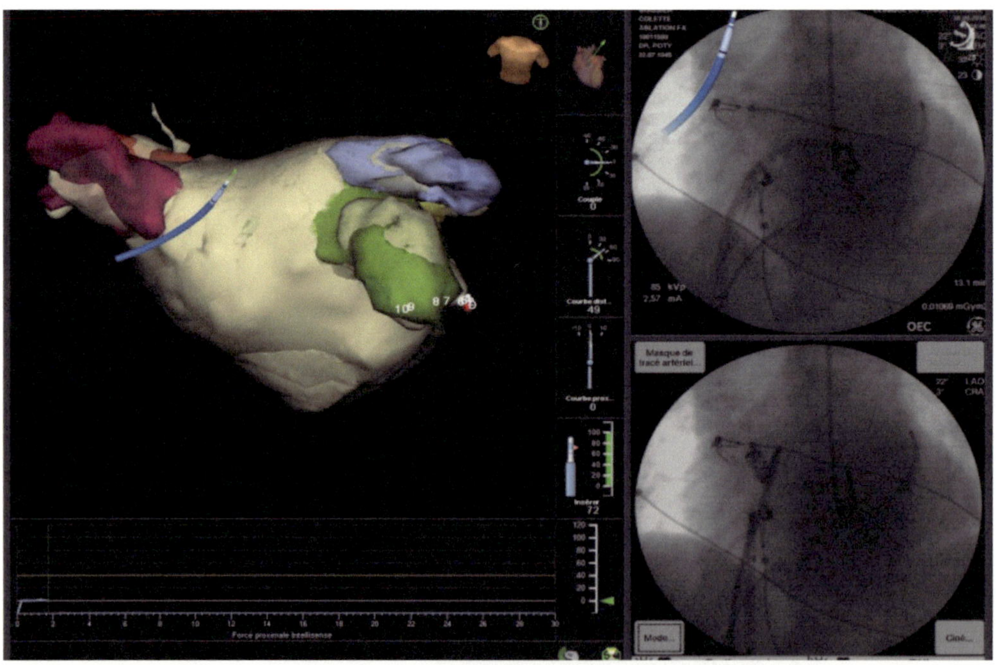

Example of Cohesion, Hansen Robotic navigation system fully integrated with NavX mapping system to provide intuitive driving in the orientation of the virtual LA geometry

2.3 Integration with MRI / CT imaging

The CARTO™ and NavX™ systems can both integrate digital computed tomography (CT) or magnetic resonance imaging (MRI) images of the heart into a mapping study, allowing navigation of "virtual" catheters within a high resolution model of the patient's anatomy.

CT / MRI studies can either be imported and segmented via the image processing platforms available in both mapping systems, or can be segmented offline by an experienced operator for direct import to the mapping system at the time of the procedure. Registration of the segmented chamber to the patient orientation is performed using fluoroscopy. Fixed anatomical landmarks close to the chamber of interest are acquired and subsequently registered with their corresponding sites on the CT/MRI image. The identified landmarks are then "merged" together to complete the registration process so that the catheter tip can be navigated within the detailed anatomical shell created on CT / MRI.

Electroanatomical mapping with CT/MRI image integration is particularly useful in patients with unusual or complex anatomy such as those with congenital heart disease and previous cardiac surgery. Detailed chamber anatomy is also helpful in pulmonary vein isolation procedures, by delineating the location, size and orientation of the pulmonary vein ostia. However, CT / MRI integration does not improve acute procedural efficacy or long term success rates.(Kistler, Rajappan et al. 2008)

2.4 Imaging of myocardial scar and integration with mapping systems

Delayed-enhanced Magnetic Resonance Imaging (DE-MRI) has been used for almost a decade to identify regions of ventricular scar. An increase in extracellular space within myocardial scar allows for an accumulation and prolonged wash-out time of the contrast agent, gadolinium.(Saraste, Nekolla et al. 2008). Information regarding ventricular or atrial scar can be obtained from voltage readings using intra-cardiac catheters. However, the integration of DE-MRI data may eliminate the need for acquisition of a detailed voltage map, and prevent inaccurate readings due to poor catheter contact.

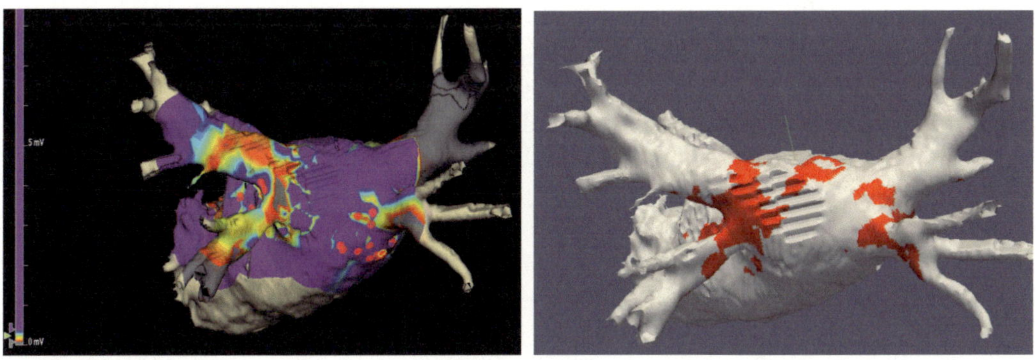

Example of similarity between endocardially collected voltage map and regions of LA scar identified by DE-MRI

2.4.1 Ventricular scar in ischaemic VT

DE-MRI enables detection, characterization and accurate quantification of acute and chronic myocardial infarction (Simonetti et al; McNamara et al 2001). Quantification of infarct size on DE-MRI has been validated against true infarct size as verified by histochemical staining in animal models (Kim RJ et al 1999). Heterogeneous tissue surrounding areas with dense LGE are hypothesized to be the imaging equivalent of slow conduction zones in patients with ischemic cardiomyopathy (Yan AT, Shayne AJ et al. 2006; Roes SD, Borleffs CJ et al 2009) although this is not a consistent finding. Until higher resolution images are possible we must accept the reality that the currently visualized "infarct core" and "heterogeneous tissue" is a mixture of true infarct core, true heterogeneous tissue, and artifacts, particularly those produced by volume averaging of infarct core with healthy tissue.

Utilising the technique described by Yan et al, Perez-David et al. demonstrated the connection between heterogeneous tissue on CMR and slow conduction zones identified by endocardial mapping. Furthermore, they confirmed that sites identified as critical VT isthmi by electrophysiological manoeuvres often reside in heterogeneous tissue identified by CMR.

2.4.2 Atrial scar in AF and AT

More recently, as scanners and scanning quality have improved, attention has turned to visualising atrial myocardium, in particular looking for regions of pre-existing fibrosis and iatrogenic scar following catheter ablation procedures.(Kim, Hillenbrand et al. 2000; Kim, Wu et al. 2000) Several recent studies have shown that high-spatial-resolution delayed enhancement MR (DE-MRI) imaging allows identification of scar induced by RF ablation in the left atrium(Peters, Wylie et al. 2007; McGann, Kholmovski et al. 2008; Badger, Adjei-Poku et al. 2009). Badger et al showed, however, that chronic atrial scar may not be formed and visible on MRI until up to 3 months following the ablation procedure. (Badger, Oakes et al. 2009) Integration of data from DE-MRI regarding location of scarred regions may benefit procedures such as repeat AF ablations and post-ablation atrial tachycardias. In particular, it may help identify the location of gaps within lines which are providing the substrate for ongoing AF / AT.

Methods for improved patient selection and non-invasive evaluation of the LA wall to assess the extent permanent tissue injury created by ablation, may be an important tool in improving ablation technique and increasing procedural success. Oakes et al demonstrated that the presence of left atrial fibrosis prior to ablation can also be detected using DE-MRI and that patients with higher levels of fibrosis had lower procedural success rates.(Oakes, Badger et al. 2009) On this basis they hypothesised that a further possible use of DE-MRI may be that of patient selection for atrial fibrillation ablation.

2.5 Novel mapping systems: CARTO Ripple

Despite the aforementioned advantages of current mapping systems there remain shortfalls and limitations to their use. The conversion of the raw electrical data to 'clean' activation maps requires operator expertise with the potential introduction of errors by incorrect assignment of local activation times or voltage thresholds. Furthermore interpolation of data within unmapped regions can lead to the display of false information. The introduction of integrated multielectrode mapping catheters should reduce this error by allowing creation of dense maps. This integration should also improve the rapidity with which maps are created with a likely increase in diagnostic yield (Patel et al 2008). Additionally, colour-spectrum isochronal maps are often converted to propagation maps that display moving activation wave fronts that are interpreted more intuitively but are mathematically extrapolated from the points collected and can give the operator a false sense of the resolution of the map. Isopotential maps created by grouping far-field reconstructed electrograms (Ensite Array) that are above a pre-specified activation threshold voltage to create activation wave fronts are prone to errors due to the subjective variation introduced by voltage threshold adjustments. In addition the hardware is limited by far-field reconstruction of low voltage electrograms.

Intracardiac electrograms provide unique site-specific data about local electrical activation and in-vitro studies have demonstrated that underlying anatomical substrate can be deduced from the electrogram morphology (Spach MS, Miller WT et al 1979). Electrograms are categorised by largely binary descriptors; simple or complex, early or late, high or low amplitude. Potentially crucial information contained within electrograms is lost to interpretation with current 3D mapping systems. CARTO does not assign any characteristics to potentials (diastolic or late systolic) within ventricular scar and is unable to appropriately display valuable data contained within complex fractionated electrograms often representing regions of slow conduction which may play a pivotal role in scar related artial arrhythmias. As the system can only assign a single value for the local activation time, isochronal and activation maps can be flawed if complex fractionated electrogams are annotated incorrectly.

ENSITE can collect simultaneous global activation data but is prone to far-field noise making low-amplitude fractionated signals difficult to differentiate from noise or repolarisation.

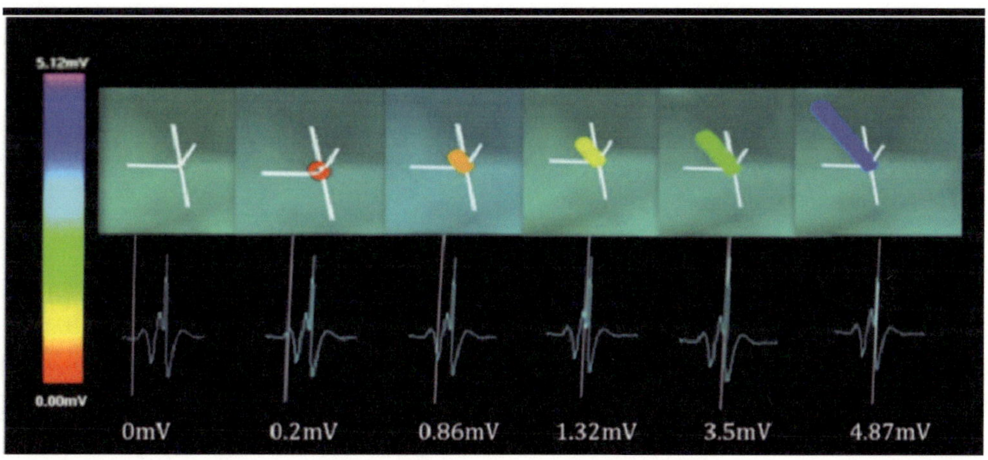

The top panel shows increasing Ripple bar height in correlation to the increasing magnitude of the electrogram voltage in the annotation window (shown in the lower window).
The bar height and colour are clearly visible. These can be correlated to the conventional reference colour bar from CARTO seen to the left of the panel with low voltage represented by red and high voltage represented by purple

The conventional 2D method for displaying electrograms is deflection from a baseline according to a voltage scale. The overall sequence of directions and rates of change and amplitudes of deflections define the electrogram "morphology". A new visualisation algorithm, Ripple Mapping, has allowed the reproduction of this 2D process on a 3D hull using a bar moving out from the cardiac surface conveying location, timing and electrogram morphology simultaneously (Linton, Koa-Wing. 2009). Multiple points collected in a small area will display bars, which change according to the local voltage change and in a temporally accurate sequence producing a 'ripple' effect which conveys the direction of wave propagation without any operator annotation. The program avoids interpolation and as it does not use a single local activation time, all the components of the electrogram are preserved and displayed. Therefore a sequence of small potentials and complex electrograms can be temporally related to adjacent electrograms. This method has the benefit of using high quality contact electrograms capable of demonstrating low amplitude signals with accurate 3D localisation, enabling the assessment of electrogram morphology within scar.

During the proof-of-concept study this novel method of cardiac mapping showed low-amplitude continuous activity in four of five tachycardias at the site of successful ablation, consistent with a re-entrant mechanism. Cardiac Ripple Mapping has been integrated onto an off-line CARTO ™ platform, which is currently undergoing validation and clinical evaluation.

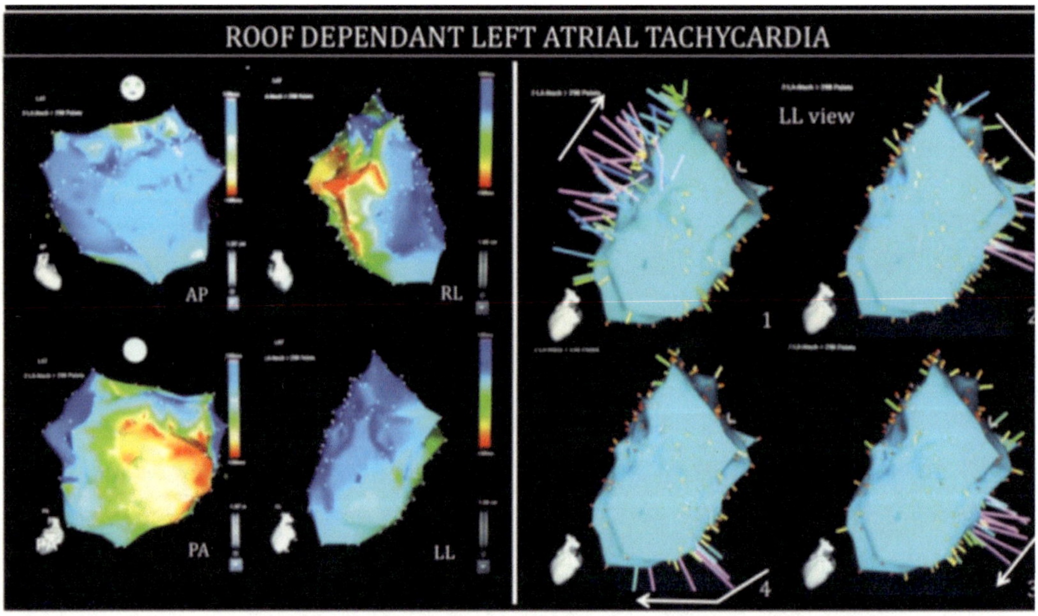

Left panel: Displays a left atrial CARTO-XP local activation time (LAT) map of a patient with left atrial tachycardia following circumferential pulmonary vein isolation for paroxysmal atrial fibrillation. Analysis of the LAT map suggests the possibility of a focal tachycardia origination from the posterior wall near the right pulmonary veins.

Right panel: The same atrial tachycardia as seen on the corresponding unaltered Ripple map (left lateral view) shows a roof dependant atrial tachycardia which was confimed by conventional entrainment manoeuvres.

3. Ablation of complex arrhythmias

The achievement of transmurality of ablation lesions for permanent VT abolition and pulmonary vein isolation is one of the ongoing challenges of ventricular tachycardia and atrial fibrillation ablation (Haissaguerre, Shah et al. 2000; Pappone, Santinelli et al.

2004);(Kosmidou, Inada et al. 2011 ; Willems, Steven et al. 2010). The Hansen™ robotic system was designed to improve catheter tip stability, lesion quality and clinical outcomes.

3.1 The Hansen robotic navigation system

The Hansen Sensei electromechanical robotic navigation system is capable of remotely steering a guide catheter to enable precise positioning and manipulation of any type of electrophysiological catheter within the heart for mapping and ablation. The Sensei system has been described in detail previously.(Saliba, Cummings et al. 2006; Kanagaratnam, Koa-Wing et al. 2008) In brief, the system comprises three linked components: the physician's workstation (Sensei™ robotic control system), remote catheter manipulator (RCM) and steerable guide catheter (Artisan™ Sheath). The steerable guide catheter comprises an outer (14F) and inner (10.5F) steerable sheath through which any 8.5F or less ablation catheter can be placed. The outer guide can be inserted, deinserted and can bend up to 90 degrees, whereas the inner guide is controlled by the 3D joystick and can be directed anywhere within the toroidal workspace. The Artisan sheath maintains the catheter position by the tensile strength of four pullwires so that the shape adopted by the sheath is uniquely suited to the point of interest to which the catheter is being positioned.(Kanagaratnam, Koa-Wing et al. 2008) This is in contrast to the manual approach, where the operator has to dynamically apply torque and flexion to prevent the catheter displacing from the point of interest. The Sensei™ robotic control system also incorporates a pressure sensor (Intellisense™), which calculates the contact force at the tip of the catheter using the differential resistance when continuously dithering the catheter in and out of the Artisan sheath. This tissue contact pressure enhances the validation of tissue contact and also provides for the ability to identify a pressure curve for optimal lesion production. (Kanagaratnam, Koa-Wing et al. 2008)

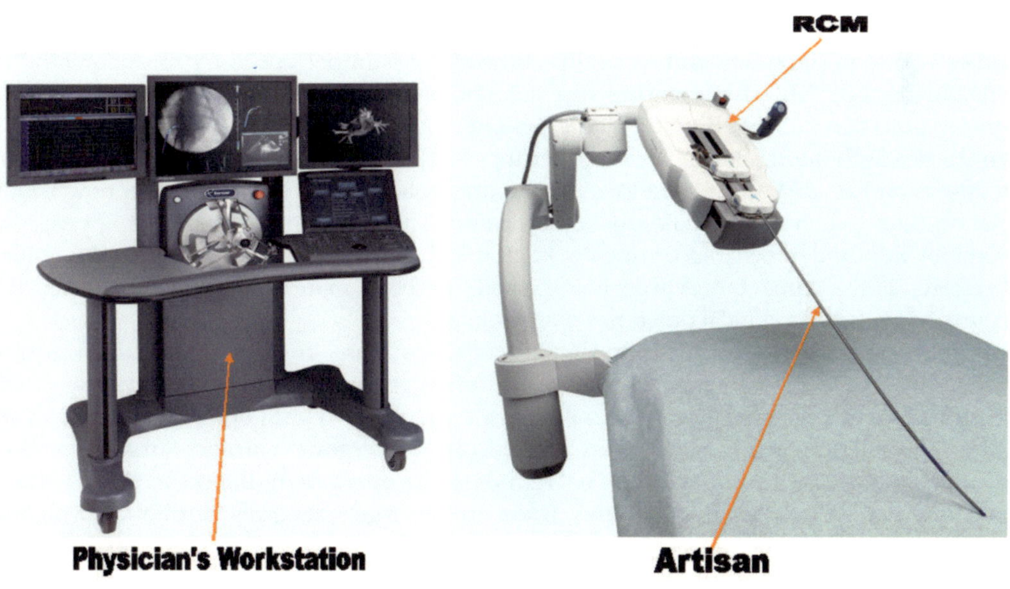

Hansen Robotic Artisan steerable sheath.

The Sensei system is currently compatible with all 8.5F or less mapping and irrigated ablation catheters. The physicians work station comprises 3 screens which can display any selected data including fluoroscopy, intracardiac echocardiography, electroanatomic mapping systems (Carto Biosense Webster, NavX St Jude Medical, Rotational Angiography imaging Philips ElectroNav etc.), and electrogram display systems (Bard Lab System Pro etc.) The free standing physician's work station and remote catheter manipulation system mounted on the patient table can be moved between laboratories and do not require any floor reinforcement such as that required for magnetic remote navigation systems.

The intended benefit of robotic catheter manipulation is that the catheter position is maintained once the physician has released the 3D joystick providing increased stability throughout the duration of RF delivery. In addition, the Intellisense system can confirm catheter contact during ablation.

3.1.1 Atrial and ventricular ablation

Several studies have been performed in animals to investigate whether the theoretical benefits of robotic ablation are translated into improved measurable parameters of lesion quality. In a study comparing robotic (Sensei) and manual ablation in 7 pig atria, robotic ablation reduced local electrogram amplitude to a greater degree than manual ablation (49+/- 2.6% vs 29 +/- 4.5% signal reduction after one minute p=0.0002) The incidence of >50% signal reduction was also greater for robotic (37%) than manual (21%) (p=0.0001).(Koa-Wing, Kojodjojo et al. 2009) Koa-Wing et al also noted that macroscopically the robotic lesions were more consistently transmural compared to the manual lesions, with no evidence of charring or perforation with either modality. In other in-vitro studies, 45W at 20-30g for 40secs, 83% of lesions were transmural, however 33% of lesions were associated with char formation. Using 30W and 20-30g pressure 0% were associated with char formation, however only 16% were associated with transmural lesion formation. (Di Biase, Natale et al. 2009),

Previous human studies comparing robotic and manual ablation have been non-randomised and have shown no significant difference in clinical outcomes. The primary aim of these studies was to prove safety and feasibility, however it is important to try to understand the potential reasons why these studies did not deliver the anticipated benefits of increased catheter precision and stability. (Willems, Steven et al 2010; Di Biase, Wang et al. 2009) The two studies both quoted using the same settings for both robotic and manual ablation (45W for 20secs and 20-25W for 60s) lesions. Interestingly, both reports comment on how robotic ablation required shorter radiofrequency duration. Therefore, in both series it appears that operators adjusted power according to anatomical location and local signal attenuation. Therefore, if the same target was being used for both manual and robotic arms, it is unsurprising that the clinical outcomes were similar.

The ability to titrate force and improve tissue contact are important attributes required during ablation in the ventricle which can be over a centimetre thick. Furthermore greater transmurality of delivered lesions should negate the need to gain epicardial access in this patient population who have often previously undergone cardiac surgery, making percutaneous access less practical. The reduction in operator radiation exposure during these long procedures is of added value. There are no large scale trials of robotic VT ablation however acute feasibility is suggested by occasional single case reports (Duncan, Johns et al 2010; Koa-Wing, Linton et al. 2009) Larger scale studies should help clarify the role of this technology in ablation of complex arrhythmias.

4. Conclusion

With the rapidly progressing field of catheter ablation, advances in mapping and ablation technologies will lead to improved therapeutic outcomes in complex cardiac arrhythmias. Innovative methods of assessing, displaying and integrating the underlying substrate of complex scar with electrophysiological data will further streamline our current practice in these challenging cases.

5. References

Anonymous (1997): A comparison of antiarrhythmic-drug therapy with implantable defibrillators in patients resuscitated from near fatal ventricular arrhythmias. The antiarrhythmics versus implantable defibrillators (AVID) Investigators. *N Engl J Med,* 337:1576- 1583.

Badger, T. J., R. S. Oakes, et al. (2009). "Temporal left atrial lesion formation after ablation of atrial fibrillation." *Heart Rhythm* 6(2): 161-8.

Badger, T. J., Y. A. Adjei-Poku, et al. (2009). "MRI in cardiac electrophysiology: the emerging role of delayed-enhancement MRI in atrial fibrillation ablation." *Future Cardiol* 5(1): 63-70.

Bogun F., Good E., Reich S., Elmouchi D., Igic P., Lemola K., Tschopp D., Jongnarangsin K., Oral H., Chugh A., Pelosi F. & Morady F. (2006) Isolated potentials during sinus rhythm and pace-mapping within scars as guides for ablation of post-infarction ventricular tachycardia. *J Am Coll.Cardiol,* 47: 2013-2019.

Calkins, H., J. Brugada, et al. (2007). "HRS/EHRA/ECAS expert Consensus Statement on catheter and surgical ablation of atrial fibrillation: recommendations for personnel, policy, procedures and follow-up. A report of the Heart Rhythm Society (HRS) Task Force on catheter and surgical ablation of atrial fibrillation." *Heart Rhythm* 4(6): 816-61.

Camm, A. J., P. Kirchhof, et al. "Guidelines for the management of atrial fibrillation: the Task Force for the Management of Atrial Fibrillation of the European Society of Cardiology (ESC)." *Europace* 12(10): 1360-420.

Cao, K. & Gonska, B. D. (1996). Catheter ablation of incessant ventricular tachycardia: acute and long-term results. *Eur Heart J.* 17:756-763.

Cappato, R., H. Calkins, et al. (2005). "Worldwide survey on the methods, efficacy, and safety of catheter ablation for human atrial fibrillation." *Circulation* 111(9): 1100-5.

Chugh A, Oral H, Lemola K, Hall B, Cheung P, Good E, Tamirisa K, Han J, Bogun F, Pelosi F, Morady F. Prevalence, mechanisms, and clinical significance of macroreentrant atrial tachycardia during and following left atrial ablation for atrial fibrillation. *Heart Rhythm*. 2005;2:464–471.

Connolly SJ, Gent M, Roberts RS, Dorian P, Roy D, Sheldon RS, Mitchell LB, Green MS, Klein GJ, O'Brien B (2000): Canadian implantable defibrillator study (CIDS): A randomized trial of the implantable cardioverter defibrillator against amiodarone. *Circulation,* 101:1297-1302.

Coumel, P. (1994). "Paroxysmal atrial fibrillation: a disorder of autonomic tone?" *Eur Heart J* 15 Suppl A: 9-16.

Coumel, P. (1996). "Autonomic influences in atrial tachyarrhythmias." *J Cardiovasc Electrophysiol* 7(10): 999-1007.

Cox, J. L., J. P. Boineau, et al. (1995). "Modification of the maze procedure for atrial flutter and atrial fibrillation. I. Rationale and surgical results." *J Thorac Cardiovasc Surg* 110(2): 473-84.

Cox, J. L., R. B. Schuessler, et al. (1996). "An 8 1/2-year clinical experience with surgery for atrial fibrillation." *Ann Surg* 224(3): 267-73; discussion 273-5.

Deisenhofer I, Estner H, Zrenner B, Schreieck J, Weyerbrock S, Hessling G, Scharf K, Karch MR, Schmitt C. Left atrial tachycardia after circumferential pulmonary vein ablation for atrial fibrillation: incidence, electrophysiological characteristics, and results of radiofrequency ablation. *Europace*. 2006;8:573–582.

Deisenhofer, I., H. Estner, et al. (2009). "Does electrogram guided substrate ablation add to the success of pulmonary vein isolation in patients with paroxysmal atrial fibrillation? A prospective, randomized study." *J Cardiovasc Electrophysiol* 20(5): 514-21.

Di Biase, L., A. Natale, et al. (2009). "Relationship between catheter forces, lesion characteristics, "popping," and char formation: experience with robotic navigation system." *J Cardiovasc Electrophysiol* 20(4): 436-40.

Di Biase, L., Y. Wang, et al. (2009). "Ablation of atrial fibrillation utilizing robotic catheter navigation in comparison to manual navigation and ablation: single-center experience." *J Cardiovasc Electrophysiol* 20(12): 1328-35.

Duncan, E., N. Johns, et al. (2010) "Robotic Catheter Navigation within the Left Ventricle." *Pacing Clin Electrophysiol*.

Earley MJ, Showkathali R, Alzetani M, et al. (2006) Radiofrequency ablation os arrhythmias guided by non-fluoroscopic catheter location: a prospective randomized trial. *Eur heart J* 27:1223-1229.

Estner, H. L., G. Hessling, et al. (2008). "Electrogram-guided substrate ablation with or without pulmonary vein isolation in patients with persistent atrial fibrillation." *Europace* 10(11): 1281-7.

Feinberg, W. M., J. L. Blackshear, et al. (1995). "Prevalence, age distribution, and gender of patients with atrial fibrillation. Analysis and implications." *Arch Intern Med* 155(5): 469-73.

Gerstenfeld EP, Callans DJ, Dixit S, Russo AM, Nayak H, Lin D, Pulliam W, Siddique S, Marchlinski FE. Mechanisms of organized left atrial tachycardias occurring after pulmonary vein isolation. *Circulation*. 2004; 110:1351–1357.

Gerstenfeld, E. P., S. Dixit, et al. (2002). "Utility of exit block for identifying electrical isolation of the pulmonary veins." *J Cardiovasc Electrophysiol* 13(10): 971-9.

Gonska D-B, Cao K, Schaumann A, Dorszewski A, von zur Muhlen F, Kreuzer H. (1994) Catheter ablation of ventricular tachycardia in 136 patients with coronary artery disease: results and long-term follow-up. *J Am Coll Cardiol.*;24:1506–1514.

Haines, D. E., D. D. Watson, et al. (1990). "Electrode radius predicts lesion radius during radiofrequency energy heating. Validation of a proposed thermodynamic model." *Circ Res* 67(1): 124-9.

Haïssaguerre M, Hocini M, Sanders P, Sacher F, Rotter M, Takahashi Y, Rostock T, Hsu LF, Bordachar P, Reuter S, Roudaut R, Clémenty J, Jaïs P. Catheter ablation of long-lasting persistent atrial fibrillation: clinical outcome and mechanisms of subsequent arrhythmias. *J Cardiovasc Electrophysiol*. 2005;16:1138 –1147.

Haissaguerre, M., D. C. Shah, et al. (2000). "Electrophysiological breakthroughs from the left atrium to the pulmonary veins." *Circulation* 102(20): 2463-5.

Haissaguerre, M., P. Jais, et al. (1998). "Spontaneous initiation of atrial fibrillation by ectopic beats originating in the pulmonary veins." *N Engl J Med* 339(10): 659-66.

Hocini, M., P. Jais, et al. (2005). "Techniques, evaluation, and consequences of linear block at the left atrial roof in paroxysmal atrial fibrillation: a prospective randomized study." *Circulation* 112(24): 3688-96.

Hsu, L. F., P. Jais, et al. (2004). "Catheter ablation for atrial fibrillation in congestive heart failure." *N Engl J Med* 351(23): 2373-83.

Huang SS, Wood MA. *Catheter Ablation of Cardiac Arrhythmias*. 1st Ed. 2006.

Jais, P., M. Hocini, et al. (2004). "Technique and results of linear ablation at the mitral isthmus." *Circulation* 110(19): 2996-3002.

Jalife, J., O. Berenfeld, et al. (2002). "Mother rotors and fibrillatory conduction: a mechanism of atrial fibrillation." *Cardiovasc Res* 54(2): 204-16.

Kanagaratnam, P., M. Koa-Wing, et al. (2008). "Experience of robotic catheter ablation in humans using a novel remotely steerable catheter sheath." *J Interv Card Electrophysiol* 21(1): 19-26.

Kannel, W. B., R. D. Abbott, et al. (1982). "Epidemiologic features of chronic atrial fibrillation: the Framingham study." *N Engl J Med* 306(17): 1018-22.

Kim, R. J., E. Wu, et al. (2000). "The use of contrast-enhanced magnetic resonance imaging to identify reversible myocardial dysfunction." *N Engl J Med* 343(20): 1445-53.

Kim, R. J., H. B. Hillenbrand, et al. (2000). "Evaluation of myocardial viability by MRI." *Herz* 25(4): 417-30.

Kistler, P. M., K. Rajappan, et al. (2008). "The impact of image integration on catheter ablation of atrial fibrillation using electroanatomic mapping: a prospective randomized study." *Eur Heart J* 29(24): 3029-36.

Koa-Wing, M., N. W. Linton, et al. (2009). "Robotic catheter ablation of ventricular tachycardia in a patient with congenital heart disease and Rastelli repair." *J Cardiovasc Electrophysiol* 20(10): 1163-6.

Koa-Wing, M., P. Kojodjojo, et al. (2009). "Robotically assisted ablation produces more rapid and greater signal attenuation than manual ablation." *J Cardiovasc Electrophysiol* 20(12): 1398-404.

Kosmidou, I., K. Inada, et al. (2011) "Role of repeat procedures for catheter ablation of postinfarction ventricular tachycardia." *Heart Rhythm* 8(10): 1516-22.

Kuck KH, Cappato R, et al. (2000). Randomized comparison of antiarrhythmic drug therapy with implantable defibrillators in patients resuscitated from cardiac arrest: The cardiac arrest study Hamburg (CASH). Circulation 102:748-754.

Lellouche, N., E. Buch, et al. (2007). "Functional characterization of atrial electrograms in sinus rhythm delineates sites of parasympathetic innervation in patients with paroxysmal atrial fibrillation." *J Am Coll Cardiol* 50(14): 1324-31.

Lim, K. T., S. Matsuo, et al. (2007). "Catheter ablation of persistent and permanent atrial fibrillation: Bordeaux experience." *Expert Rev Cardiovasc Ther* 5(4): 655-62.

Marchlinski FE, Callans DJ, Gottlieb CD, Zado E. (2000) Linear ablation lesions for control of unmappable ventricular tachycardia in patients with ischemic and nonischemic cardiomyopathy. *Circulation*. 101: 1288–1296

Marchlinski, F. E. (2008). "Atrial fibrillation catheter ablation: learning by burning continues." *J Am Coll Cardiol* 51(10): 1011-3.

Marrouche, N. F., D. O. Martin, et al. (2003). "Phased-array intracardiac echocardiography monitoring during pulmonary vein isolation in patients with atrial fibrillation: impact on outcome and complications." *Circulation* 107(21): 2710-6.

Matsuo, S., K. T. Lim, et al. (2007). "Ablation of chronic atrial fibrillation." *Heart Rhythm* 4(11): 1461-3.

McGann, C. J., E. G. Kholmovski, et al. (2008). "New magnetic resonance imaging-based method for defining the extent of left atrial wall injury after the ablation of atrial fibrillation." *J Am Coll Cardiol* 52(15): 1263-71.

Mesas CE, Pappone C, Lang CC, Gugliotta F, Tomita T, Vicedomini G, Sala S, Paglino G, Gulletta S, Ferro A, Santinelli V. Left atrial tachycardia after circumferential pulmonary vein ablation for atrial fibrillation: electroanatomic characterization and treatment. *J Am Coll Cardiol*. 2004;44:1071–1079.

Moss, A. J. *et al.* (2004). Long-term clinical course of patients after termination of ventricular tachyarrhythmia by an implanted defibrillator. *Circulation* 110: 3760–3765.

Nademanee, K., M. C. Schwab, et al. (2008). "Clinical outcomes of catheter substrate ablation for high-risk patients with atrial fibrillation." *J Am Coll Cardiol* 51(8): 843-9.

Natale, A., A. Raviele, et al. (2007). "Venice Chart international consensus document on atrial fibrillation ablation." *J Cardiovasc Electrophysiol* 18(5): 560-80.

Oakes, R. S., T. J. Badger, et al. (2009). "Detection and quantification of left atrial structural remodeling with delayed-enhancement magnetic resonance imaging in patients with atrial fibrillation." *Circulation* 119(13): 1758-67.

O'Neill, M. D., P. Jais, et al. (2007). "Catheter ablation for atrial fibrillation." *Circulation* 116(13): 1515-23.

Ouyang, F., D. Bansch, et al. (2004). "Complete isolation of left atrium surrounding the pulmonary veins: new insights from the double-Lasso technique in paroxysmal atrial fibrillation." *Circulation* 110(15): 2090-6.

Pappone, C., G. Oreto, et al. (1999). "Catheter ablation of paroxysmal atrial fibrillation using a 3D mapping system." *Circulation* 100(11): 1203-8.

Pappone, C., S. Rosanio, et al. (2003). "Mortality, morbidity, and quality of life after circumferential pulmonary vein ablation for atrial fibrillation: outcomes from a controlled nonrandomized long-term study." *J Am Coll Cardiol* 42(2): 185-97.

Pappone, C., V. Santinelli, et al. (2004). "Pulmonary vein denervation enhances long-term benefit after circumferential ablation for paroxysmal atrial fibrillation." *Circulation* 109(3): 327-34.

Patel A, d'Avila A, Neuzil P, Kim S, Mela T, Singh J, Ruskin J, ReddyV. Atrial Tachycardia After Ablation of Persistent Atrial Fibrillation : Identification of the Critical Isthmus

With a Combination of Multielectrode Activation Mapping and Targeted Entrainment Mapping. *Circ Arrhythm Electrophysiol* 2008;1;14-22.

Perez-David E, Arenal Á, Rubio-Guivernau JL, et al. (2011) Noninvasive identification of ventricular tachycardia-related conducting channels using contrast-enhanced magnetic resonance imaging in patients with chronic myocardial infarction: comparison of signal intensity scar mapping and endocardial voltage mapping. *J Am Coll Cardiol*, 57:184 -94.

Peters, D. C., J. V. Wylie, et al. (2007). "Detection of pulmonary vein and left atrial scar after catheter ablation with three-dimensional navigator-gated delayed enhancement MR imaging: initial experience." *Radiology* 243(3): 690-5.

Poole, J. E. *et al.* (2008). Prognostic importance of defibrillator shocks in patients with heart failure. *N. Engl. J. Med* 359: 1009–1017

Roes SD, Borleffs CJ, van der Geest RJ, et al. (2009) Infarct tissue hetero- geneity assessed with contrast-enhanced MRI predicts spontaneous ventricular arrhythmia in patients with ischemic cardiomyopathy and implantable cardioverter-defibrillator. *Circ Cardiovasc Imaging*, 2:183–90.

Sacher F, Roberts-Thomson K, Maury P et al. (2010) Epicardial ventricular tachycardia ablation. *J Am Coll Cardiol*, 55:2366-2372.

Sacher F, Tedrow UB, et al. (2008). Ventricular tachycardia ablation: evolution of patients and procedures over 8 years. *Circ Arrhythmia Electrophysiol.* 1: 153–16

Sahadevan, J., K. Ryu, et al. (2004). "Epicardial mapping of chronic atrial fibrillation in patients: preliminary observations." *Circulation* 110(21): 3293-9.

Saliba, W., J. E. Cummings, et al. (2006). "Novel robotic catheter remote control system: feasibility and safety of transseptal puncture and endocardial catheter navigation." *J Cardiovasc Electrophysiol* 17(10): 1102-5.

Sanders, P., P. Jais, et al. (2004). "Electrophysiologic and clinical consequences of linear catheter ablation to transect the anterior left atrium in patients with atrial fibrillation." *Heart Rhythm* 1(2): 176-84.

Saraste, A., S. Nekolla, et al. (2008). "Contrast-enhanced magnetic resonance imaging in the assessment of myocardial infarction and viability." *J Nucl Cardiol* 15(1): 105-17.

Scaglione, M., L. Biasco, et al. "Visualization of multiple catheters with electroanatomical mapping reduces X-ray exposure during atrial fibrillation ablation." *Europace* 13(7): 955-62.

Schilling RJ, Peters N, Davies W. (1999) Mapping and ablation of ventricular tachycardia with the aid of a non-contact mapping system. *Heart*, 81:570-575.

Schron, E. B. *et al.* (2002) Quality of life in the antiarrhythmics versus implantable defibrillators trial: impact of therapy and influence of adverse symptoms and defibrillator shocks. *Circulation* 105: 589–594.

Shah DC, Jais P, Haissaguerre M, et al. (1997) Three-dimensional mapping of the common atrial flutter in the right atrium. *Circulation*, 96:3904-3912.

Simonetti OP, Kim RJ, Fieno DS, et al. (2001) An improved MR imaging technique for the visualization of myocardial infarction. *Radiology*, 218:215–23.

Spach MS, Miller WT, Miller-Jones E, Warren RB, Barr RC (1979): Extracellular potentials related to intracellular action potentials during impulse conduction in anisotropic canine cardiac muscle. *Circ Res*. 45:188-204

Sporton, S. C., M. J. Earley, et al. (2004). "Electroanatomic versus fluoroscopic mapping for catheter ablation procedures: a prospective randomized study." *J Cardiovasc Electrophysiol* 15(3): 310-5.

Steven, D., H. Servatius, et al. (2009). "Reduced Fluoroscopy During Atrial Fibrillation Ablation: Benefits of Robotic Guided Navigation." *J Cardiovasc Electrophysiol.*

Stevenson W.G., Khan H., Sager P., Saxon L.A., Middlekauff H.R., Natterson P.D. & Wiener I. (1993) Identification of re-entry circuit sites during catheter mapping and radiofrequency ablation of ventricular tachycardia late after myocardial infarction. *Circulation,* 88: 1647-1670.

Stevenson WG, Delacretaz E, Friedman PL, Ellison KE. (1998) Identification and ablation of macroreentrant ventricular tachycardia with the CARTO electroanatomic mapping system. *Pacing Clin Electrophysiol,* 21:1448-1456.

Valles, E., R. Fan, et al. (2008). "Localization of atrial fibrillation triggers in patients undergoing pulmonary vein isolation: importance of the carina region." *J Am Coll Cardiol* 52(17): 1413-20.

Willems, S., D. Steven, et al. (2010) "Persistence of Pulmonary Vein Isolation After Robotic Remote-Navigated Ablation for Atrial Fibrillation and its Relation to Clinical Outcome." *JCardiovasc Electrophysiol*

Willems, S., H. Klemm, et al. (2006). "Substrate modification combined with pulmonary vein isolation improves outcome of catheter ablation in patients with persistent atrial fibrillation: a prospective randomized comparison." *Eur Heart J* 27(23): 2871-8.

Yokoyama, K., H. Nakagawa, et al. (2006). "Comparison of electrode cooling between internal and open irrigation in radiofrequency ablation lesion depth and incidence of thrombus and steam pop." *Circulation* 113(1): 11-9.

22

The Future of Cardiac Mapping

Pascal Fallavollita
Chair for Computer Aided Medical Procedures & Augmented Reality,
Technische Universität München,
Germany

1. Introduction

Severe disorders of the heart rhythm that can lead to sudden cardiac death (SCD) are often treated by radio-frequency (RF) catheter ablation. Using fluoroscopy as an imaging guide, the procedure consists of inserting a catheter inside the heart, near the area from which originates the abnormal cardiac electrical activity, then delivering RF currents through the catheter tip to ablate the arrhythmogenic area. Fluoroscopy is a conventional mapping technique that has been extremely useful in understanding and managing simpler arrhythmias. While the fluoroscopic procedure is still used in over 90% of ablations, its limitation in providing a reliable 3D geometry is evident when working upon complex cases like ventricular tachycardia (VT) or atrial fibrillation (AF) ablation. In turn, this results in impaired efficacy and length of the procedure lasting for several hours. Even though operator experience has decreased procedure times, radiation hazards still remain a major issue for the patient.

Recent 3D systems which integrate electrophysiological signals with anatomy to provide (3D+ t) geometry are extremely useful in situations where radiation needs to be limited as much as possible, and to increase the efficiency and shorten the duration of RF catheter ablation. During intracardiac mapping, it is not unusual to find sites at which the operator feels ablation is likely to succeed. Three-dimensional systems not only allow the surgeon to mark precise ablation points but also facilitate fixing reference points if the ablation process has to be repeated (Rajnish, 2009).

This chapter will summarize the most recent developments in catheter navigation and three-dimensional electroanatomic mapping. Conventional fluoroscopy techniques will be described followed by the CARTO and Ensite non-fluoroscopic mapping systems. Advances in ultrasound imaging for cardiac ablation guidance, and futuristic remote navigation technologies such as the Stereotaxis Magnetic Navigation system and the Hansen Sensei Robotic Catheter system will conclude the read.

2. Conventional catheter mapping

Every clinical electrophysiology (EP) laboratory is equipped with an X-ray system designed to provide fluoroscopic imaging of the heart. For many years this was the only form of procedural imaging available. A common characteristic of all X-ray images is that the soft tissue of the myocardium cannot be visualized (Figure 1), nevertheless, the walls of the left atrium can be indirectly assessed by bolus injection of contrast, which can be augmented by manoeuvres that minimize atrial emptying such as adenosine or rapid ventricular pacing. However, the major disadvantage of using X-ray fluoroscopy as the sole imaging modality is that all images obtained are two-dimensional representations of three-dimensional structures (D'Silva & Wright, 2011).

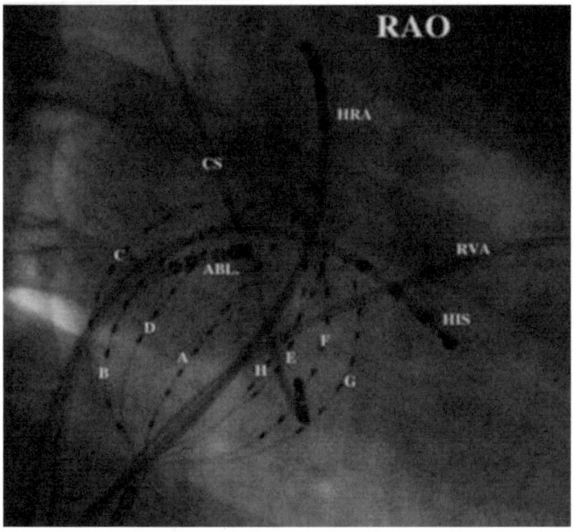

Fig. 1. A conventional fluoroscopy image showing a multielectrode basket array and other standard catheters inside the right atrium. Letters A to H identify basket splines and ABL indicates ablation catheter.
Image taken from Schmitt et al., 1999. (doi: 10.1161/01.CIR.99.18.2414).

2.1 Rotational angiography

Recently, three-dimensional rotational angiography (3DRA) has been introduced as an intraoperative modality for 3D imaging during cardiac ablation. In 3DRA, the C-arm typically performs a 200° rotation around the patient (Figure 2). Its cone-shaped radiation beam projects on a large flat-panel detector placed on the other end of the C-arm. A large number of two-dimensional projections are acquired over the course of the rotation. Reconstruction algorithms construct these into 3D images by volume or surface rendering. With adequate contrast agent administration and cardiac motion reduction (Figure 3), the image quality delivered by 3DRA has been shown to be comparable to or even exceeding classical cardiac computerized tomography (Wielandts et al., 2010). Three-dimensional rotational angiography images are more likely to represent the true anatomy than a remotely acquired image, such as CT or MRI, because of factors such as the patient's breathing and heart motion. This technique also reduces the financial and administrative burden of scheduling adjunctive and expensive imaging studies. In the case of patient movement, the geometry needs to be fully re-acquired; this can be promptly managed, but the consistent iodinated contrast agent load and radiation dose typically preclude the use of rotational angiography more than twice in a study (Casella et al., 2010).

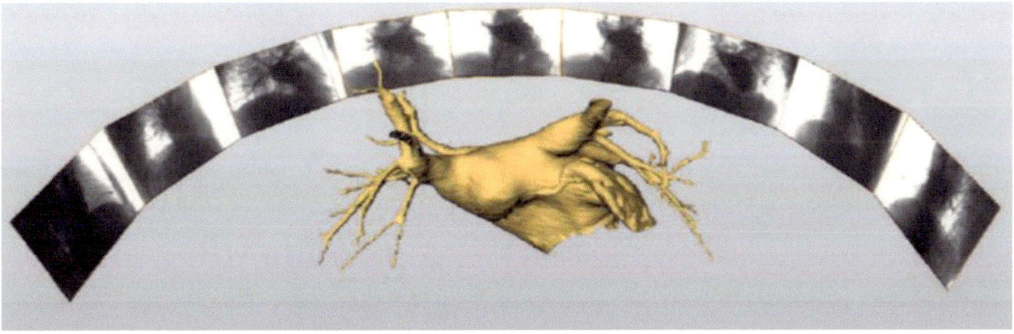

Fig. 2. A three-dimensional imaging sequence consists of 248 frames, imaged over a 200° rotation of the C-arm fluoroscope. Using advanced algorithms, a subsequent 3D volume reconstruction of the atrium is generated.
Image taken from Wielandts et al., 2010.

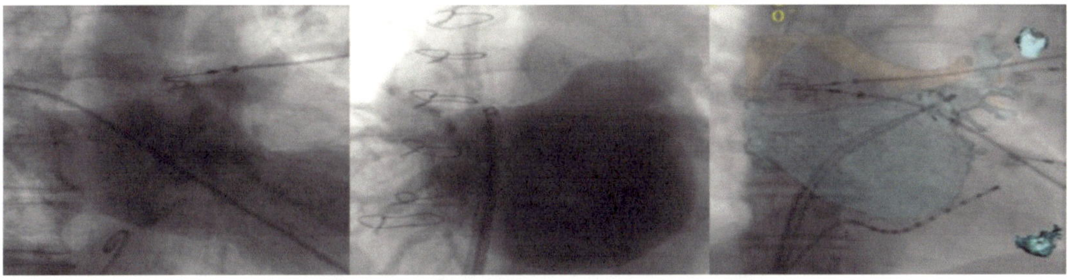

Fig. 3. Direct injection into the left atrium following segmentation of the resulting dataset. The subsequent 3D anatomical shell can then be superimposed on the live fluoroscopy.
Image taken from D'Silva & Wright, 2011.

3. Electroanatomic mapping: CARTO

CARTO (*Biosense-Webster Inc, Diamond Bar, CA*) consists of a mapping catheter with miniaturized coils at the tip, a magnetic field generator located underneath the patient, a unit which analyses the current generated by the coils in the catheter-tip and a post-processing graphical display unit. The location pad fixed beneath the patient table has three coils that generate low magnetic fields (Figure 4). The emitted fields possess well-known temporal and spatial distinguishing characteristics that encode the mapping space around the patient's chest. The location is mapped in three-dimensions with reference to a fixed point. Each of the sensor locations is determined by its distance from the location pad. Three dimensional reconstruction is performed by calculating the distance between the two sensors. In case the patient moves, the distance of each sensor from the location pad is changed; however, the distance between the sensors is retained. The three distances determine the location, orientation and rotation of the catheter (Rajnish, 2009). Accuracy of the catheter tip location has been estimated to be within 0.54 ± 0.05mm (LaPage & Saul, 2011).

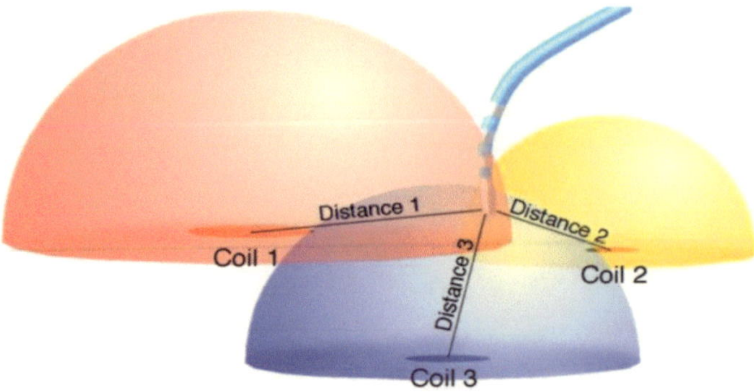

Fig. 4. Three electromagnetic fields originating from location pad coils. Spatial location of the catheter tip is accurately found by the electromagnetic fields, by determining the distance of the sensor on the catheter tip from each coil. This information is instantly computed to generate a real-time position of the catheter tip. Image courtesy of Biosense Webster.

The CARTO system is termed a point-by-point technology; multiple positions of the magnetic tip catheter are required inside the heart chamber to create a complete three-dimensional depiction of the chamber of interest (Figure 5). The activation time is referenced against an ECG lead or an intracardiac catheter (Rajnish, 2009).

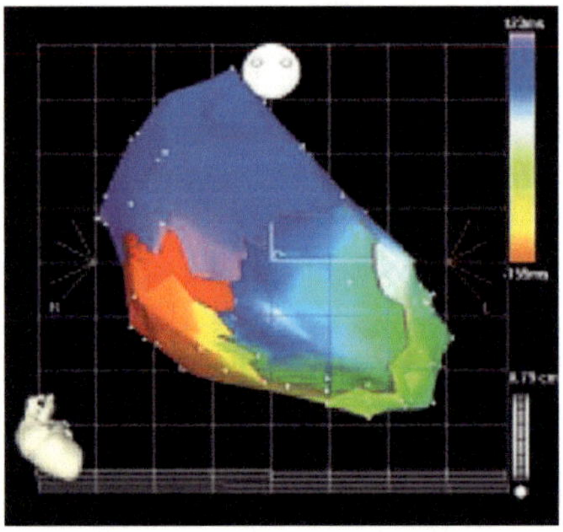

Fig. 5. Three dimensional anatomical reconstruction with superposition of activation times using the point-by-point CARTO technology. Earliest activation times are depicted in red. Image courtesy of Biosense Webster.

3.1 CARTO 3™

(Kabra & Singh, 2010) have recently reviewed the CARTO 3™ technology and some of the highlights of the system follow. First, the CARTO 3™ System is the third generation technology from Biosense Webster. Multiple catheter tips and curves can now be visualized on the electroanatomic map when compared to the traditional CARTO mapping system (Figure 6). In addition, CARTO 3™ uses a magnetic technology that calibrates the current-based technology, thereby minimizing distortions at the periphery of the electrical field. Mapping is performed in two steps. Initially, the magnetic mapping permits precise localization of the catheter with the sensor. As the catheter with the sensor moves around a chamber, multiple locations are created and stored by the system. The system then integrates the current based points with their respective magnetic locations, resulting in a calibrated current based field that permits accurate visualization of catheters and their locations (Kabra & Singh, 2010). Each electrode emits a unique frequency allowing each to be clearly distinguished, especially when in close proximity to one another. Both the catheters with and without the magnetic sensors can be visualized without spatial distortions. Lastly, CARTO 3™ has 'Fast Anatomical Mapping' (FAM) feature that permits rapid creation of anatomical maps. Unlike point-by-point electroanatomical mapping, volume data can be collected with FAM. Catheters such as the multi-polar Lasso can further enhance the collection of points and increase the mapping speed (Kabra & Singh, 2010).

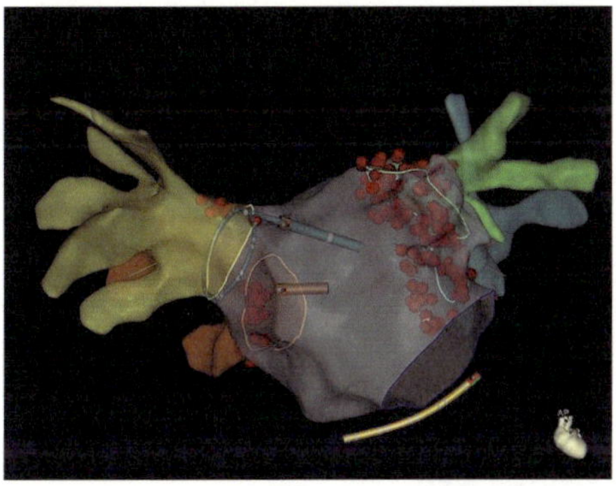

Fig. 6. The CARTO 3™ system with individually reconstructed catheters without spatial distortions. Image courtesy of Biosense Webster.

3.2 CARTOMerge

The major development for electroanatomic mapping in recent years has been the fusion of imaging technologies - MRI/CT - and electroanatomic mapping systems (Figure 7). The process of incorporating CT or MRI images into the electroanatomic mapping system involves 3D/3D registration of the catheter obtained geometry with the CT image. Typically, specific landmarks in the chamber are localized with the catheter and these points are then used to orient the CT/MRI image properly. (Rossillo et al, 2009) compared this method with a focused registration process during which they obtained multiple mapping points at each pulmonary vein using intracardiac echo guidance. They concluded that the focused registration process was a superior technique.

3.3 Advantages/disadvantages

The strengths of the CARTO technology are: (i) accurate heart chamber reconstruction, (ii) creation of linear ablations, (iii) color-coded activation maps, (iv) scar and ablation tagging capabilities. The weaknesses include: (i) incompatibility with other mapping catheters, (ii) limited utility in non-sustained arrhythmias, and (iii) orthogonal appearing volumes.

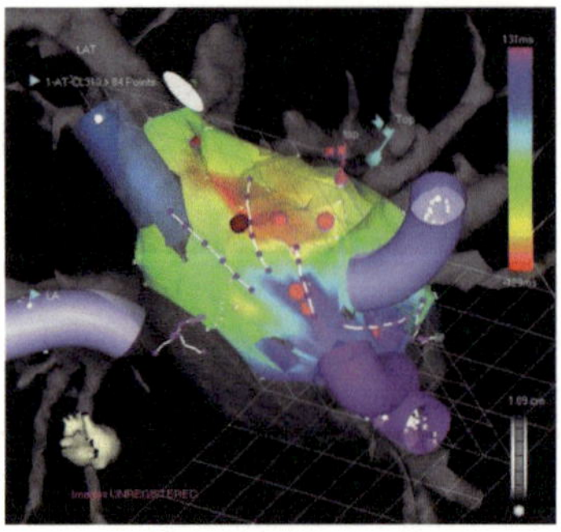

Fig. 7. The CARTOMerge technology allows the electroanatomic map of the left atrium using CARTO to be integrated with the CT/MRI images using CARTOMerge module. The circles depict the corresponding points on the two maps. Image taken from Thornton et al., 2008. (doi: doi:10.1093/europace/eun080)

3.4 Clinical study

In a recently published randomized study of 3DRA versus CARTO during atrial fibrillation ablation, the radiation exposure, procedural times and clinical outcomes at 10 months were similar in the groups investigated (Knecht et al, 2010). However the use of contrast makes it a less appealing option for patients with heart failure or renal failure. In addition, 3DRA was sensitive to patient movements during the study period. However further refinements are needed before it can be widely adopted. These include incorporation of respiratory and cardiac motion compensation and the ability to display electrogram data on the 3D (Kabra & Singh, 2010).

4. Electroanatomic mapping: ENSITE

The ENSITE system (*Endocardial Solutions, St. Jude Medical, Inc., St. Paul, MN, USA*) has two different techniques for mapping: the contact mapping system, wherein points assimilate anatomic and physiologic information in reference to five location patches applied to the skin at different places, and the non-contact mapping by a balloon array.

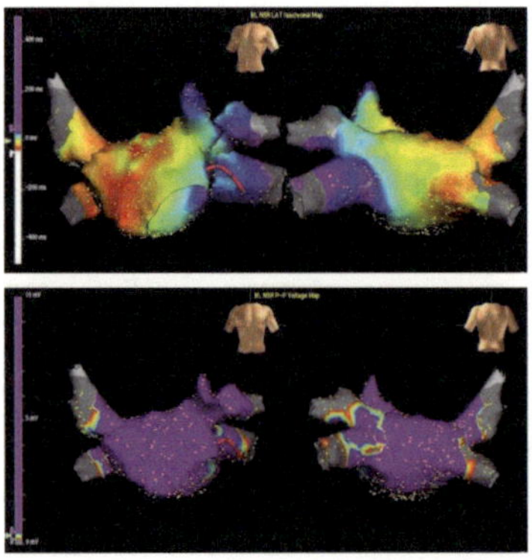

Fig. 8. Electroanatomical map acquired by the NavX system. (*Top*) Activation map of the left atrium during sinus rhythm, AP and PA views. (*Bottom*) Simultaneously-acquired voltage map of the left atrium. Image taken from Bhakta & Miller, 2008.

The contact mapping system, NavX™, is capable of displaying 3D positions of many catheters. This is achieved by applying a 5.6 kHz current through orthogonally-located skin patches on the patient. The recorded voltage and impedance at each catheter's electrodes generated from this current allows their distance from each skin patch to be triangulated with the help of a reference electrode. This determines their positions in space and the three-dimensional images of each catheter can then be displayed (Figure 8). Chamber geometry can be determined thereafter by moving a mapping catheter along the endocardial surface (Bhakta & Miller, 2008).

The non-contact mapping proceeds by using a multi electrode array (MEA). The array is comprised of 64 braided surgical-steel wires with a polyimide coating. The unipolar electrodes are created by removing a small area of insulation for each wire. The MEA is introduced into the body, like any other catheter through the femoral veins, and is inflated to 7.5 ml after positioning it at the centre of the chamber of interest (Figure 9).

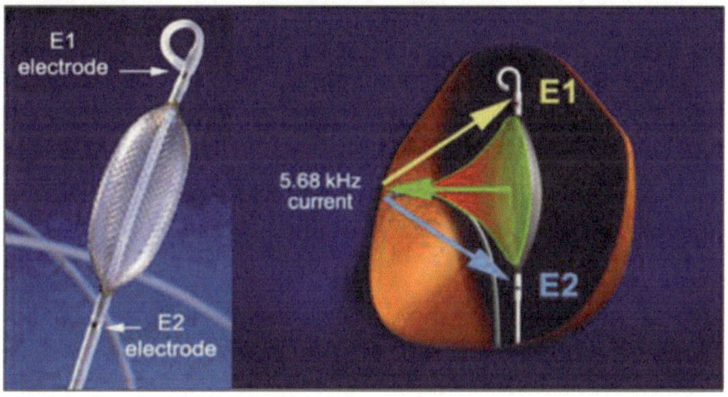

Fig. 9. Multielectrode array balloon catheter and in its deployed state. Image courtesy of Endocardial Solutions.

The balloon electrodes make galvanic contact with the blood and sense the electrical potentials induced upon them by the electrical fields generated by myocardial activity. Two ring electrodes (E1 and E2) used to build the geometry of the chamber are located on the catheter shaft about 1 cm proximal and distal to the MEA (Rajnish, 2009). A third ring electrode meant to serve as a reference for unipolar signals is located on the catheter shaft about 16 cm proximal to the MEA. The ENSITE array and a conventional catheter are placed in the heart in the same chamber. The Patient Interface Unit (PIU) sends a 5.6 kHz signal through the conventional catheter electrode, E1 and E2 alternately receive and return the signal to the PIU (Rajnish, 2009). Each of the 64 electrodes on the ENSITE array electrode senses the strength of the 5.6 kHz signal until the respective array electrode locations in three-dimensional are measured (Figure 10).

The latest version of the system, the ENSITE Velocity, has been reviewed by (Eitel et al., 2010). (Casella et al., 2009) evaluated the accuracy of the GeoMap - a new feature of Ensite Velocity that allows multipoint simultaneous geometry acquisition and activation mapping. They performed a typical point-by-point map and then a GeoMap of the right ventricle in 13 patients and compared them with MRI data from those patients. The GeoMap acquired more points in less time. The two mapping techniques disagreed in only 3% of regions and the GeoMap was more accurate at identifying low voltage correlated with areas of motion abnormality on MRI. (Schneider et al., 2010) provided one of the few recent pediatric-focused studies on noncontact mapping. They used the array in 20 patients with idiopathic ventricular tachycardia from the right ventricular outflow tract, left ventricle, or aortic root and achieved acute success in 17 of 18 patients for whom ablation was attempted with only three recurrences (LaPage & Saul, 2011). Previous versions of Ensite have been accurate within 0.7 ± 1.5mm.

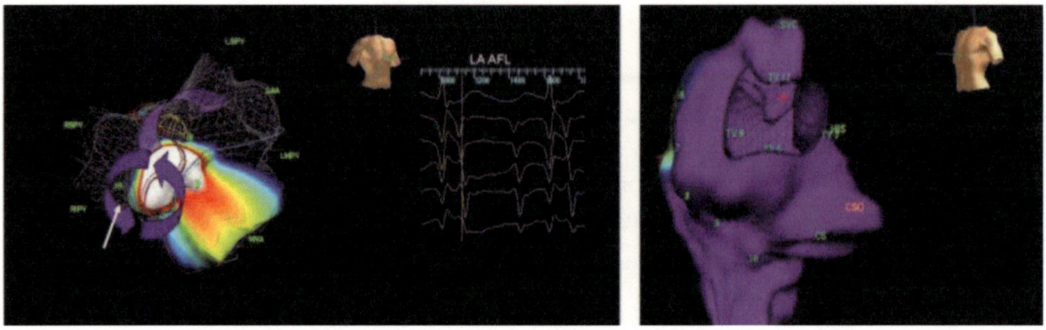

Fig. 10. Electroanatomic maps acquired by using a MEA. (*Left*) Activation map of macro-re-entrant LA flutter. The arrows depict wave front propagation within the flutter circuit. (*Right*) Anatomical reconstruction of the RA. Image taken from Bhakta & Miller, 2008.

4.1 Advantages/disadvantages

The strengths of the ENSITE technology are: (i) accurate heart chamber reconstruction, (ii) ability to use with any other catheter, (iii) respiratory and cardiac motion compensation, (iv) multiple catheter location display, and (v) useful in treating poorly sustained arrhythmias.
The weaknesses include: (i) inaccurate anatomical reconstructions, (ii) limited utility in non-sustained arrhythmias, and (iii) difficult balloon deployment.

4.2 Clinical study

Recently, two clinical studies were performed to assess the impact of the NavX mapping system when compared to conventional fluoroscopy ablation.
The first study (Kwong et al, 2011) sought to assess the impact on paediatric catheter ablation fluoroscopy times. The authors retrospectively analysed the procedural data during a 7-year period (2002 - 2008), which spanned the transition between the standard fluoroscopic mapping and adoption of routine NavX™ mapping for catheter ablation of atrioventricular nodal re-entrant tachycardia (AVNRT) and right-/left-sided accessory pathways (RAP/LAP). Overall, success rates were similar between the two mapping systems (95.7% for conventional vs. 95.9% for NavX™). Secondly, NavX™ mapping significantly reduced the ablation fluoro time (15.9 + 14.3 min vs. 11.0 + 8.9 for NavX™) with a trend towards a decrease in total fluoro time (26.4 + 15.6 min vs. 23.8 +11.1 for NavX™). Lastly, the total procedure time was not significantly different between the two methods (210.1 + 66 vs. 222.8 + 61 min for NavX™, P ¼ 0.7). (Kwong et al, 2011) concluded that the NavX™ mapping reduced ablation fluoro times during paediatric catheter ablation, particularly in accessory pathways.
The second study (Liu et al., 2011) was to probe the feasibility and safety of non-fluoroscopic radiofrequency catheter ablation of atrioventricular nodal re-entrant tachycardia guided by Ensite NavX system. Non-fluoroscopic radiofrequency catheter ablation navigated by NavX system was performed in 18 cases (mean age 52.8 + 16.1 years, range 24 - 77 years) of

atrioventricular nodal re-entrant tachycardia with normal cardiac anatomy. Using NavX, right atrial and coronary sinus geometries were reconstructed. Diagnostic electrophysiological study and radiofrequency catheter ablation were performed in all patients without use of fluoroscopy. Each site with His bundle potential were mapped and marked in the 3D geometry before ablation. The real-time position of ablation catheter was confirmed by the relative position between CS catheter and ablation catheter, which were monitored simultaneously in the Ensite NavX system. The authors show the success rate of procedure was 100%. The fluoroscopic duration of each case was zero. The average procedure duration was 97.5 + 19.8 min (55 - 125 min, the coronary sinus access was obtained in 13.4 + 7.3 min (8 - 30 min). (Liu et al., 2011) conclude that the preliminary study suggests that non-fluoroscopic catheter navigation for radiofrequency catheter ablation of atrioventricular nodal re-entrant tachycardia is safe and feasible.

5. Remote navigation systems

Is robotic guidance for cardiac ablation procedures the future? We attempt to answer this question in this section. Remote navigation systems or robotic cardiac catheter ablation was essentially developed to eliminate potential errors in catheter manipulation. Also, the use of robots could systematically decrease clinician fatigue and fluoroscopy exposure. Some electrophysiologists agree that areas between mitral valves and pulmonary veins are typically difficult to reach and position correctly the mapping catheter. Robotics can thus provide more accuracy in these cases. Currently there are two robotic systems -the Niobe Stereotaxis Magnetic Navigation System (*Stereotaxis, Inc., St Louis, Missouri, USA*) and the Hansen Sensei Robotic Catheter System (*Hansen Medical, Mountain View, California, USA*) depicted in Figure 11 and Figure 12. Both systems allow the physician to perform the mapping and ablation procedure while sitting in a control room remote from the patient [LaPage & Saul, 2011].

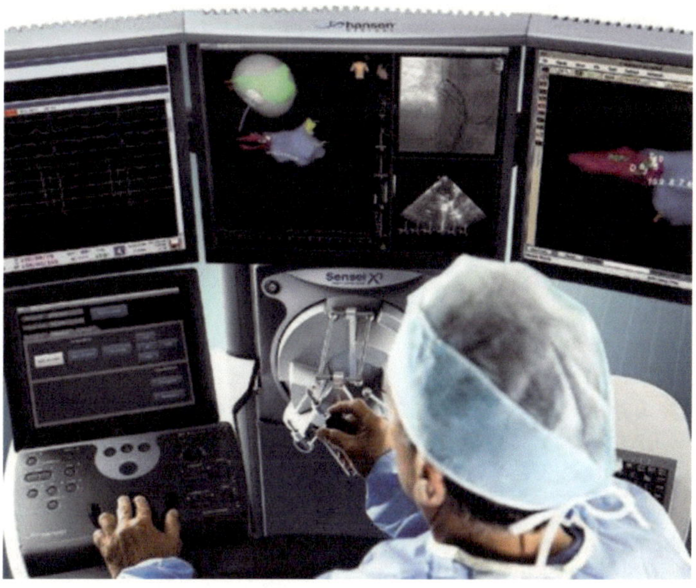

Fig. 11. The Hansen Sensei Robotic catheter system. Image taken from Hansen Medical.

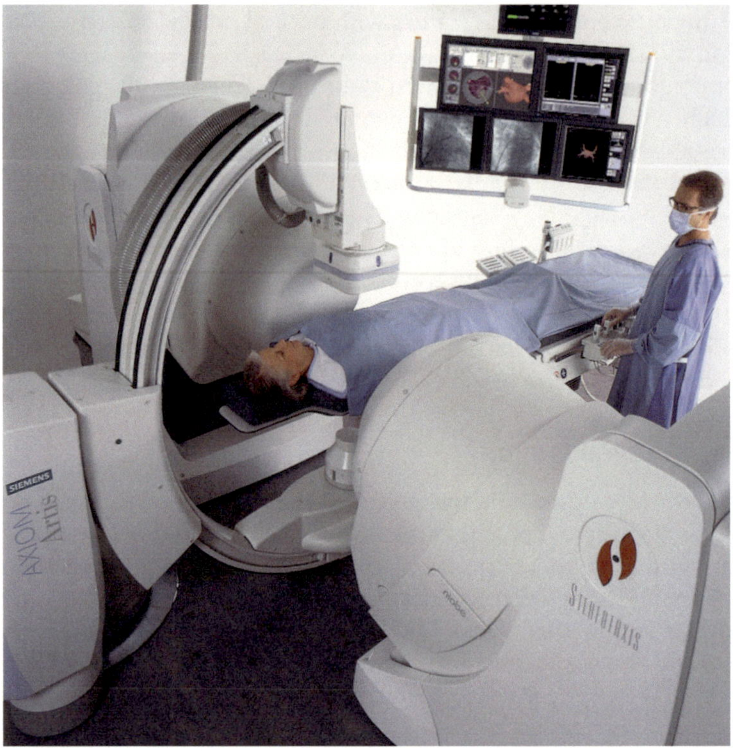

Fig. 12. Stereotaxis' Remote Magnetic Navigation System. Image taken from Stereotaxis.com.

The Stereotaxis system has been around for nearly a decade. Multiple studies have been published regarding its utility and several excellent review papers on the technology have been published (Xu et al., 2009; Wu et al., 2010 ; Thornton et al., 2010). The catheter has a magnet near the distal tip that can be oriented in any position using the fields produced by two magnets positioned bilaterally to the patient (LaPage & Saul, 2011). As an example application of Stereotaxis, (Azizian & Patel, 2011) used a magnetic tracking device to track the distal part of the ablation catheter in real time and a master-slave robot-assisted system is developed for actuation of a steerable catheter. The Sensei system facilitates catheter navigation through two coaxial sheaths steered with a pull wire mechanism controlled through a joystick remote control. The system is relatively novel and no pediatric applicable studies have been published. (Schmidt et al., 2009) achieved a high success rate using it for atrial fibrillation ablation and found the system equally compatible with both the CARTO and ENSITE systems. (LaPage & Saul, 2011) Both of these technologies have been integrated with electroanatomic mapping systems to store catheter location information for semi-automated re-navigation to regions of interest. These systems translate the operator's manipulation of a handle into precise movements of the catheter, thus allowing barely accessible regions of the heart to be reached, to create detailed electroanatomic mappings and precise ablation lesions (Casella et al., 2010).

5.1 Advantages/disadvantages

The strengths of the Sensei Hansen technology are: (i) can be used with any electroanatomic mapping system described previously, (ii) no fidelity devices or distortion effects, and (iii) catheter stability. The limitations include: (i) sheath diameter and lengths and (ii) no catheter restriction.

The strengths of the Niobe Stereotaxis technology include: (i) low risk of perforation in anatomy, (ii) numerous experiments and trials published, (iii) semiautomatic mapping, and (iv)no fidelity devices or distortion effects. The limitations include: (i) restricted to expensive magnetic catheters, (ii) non real-time movement, and (iii) patients that have implanted devices.

5.2 Clinical study

(Chong et al., 2011a) performed two clinical studies using the Niobe Stereotaxis system. The first study aimed at determining the effectiveness and safety of single magnetic-guided catheter in the ablation of outflow tract tachycardias. At the outset of the clinical study, patients with symptomatic outflow tract tachycardia on surface ECG and without structural heart disease were recruited. Electrophysiology study and ablation were performed with the use of a single Navistar RMT Thermocool 8F ablation catheter. Both activation and pace mapping of ventricular tachycardia were performed. Three dimensional localization, using CARTO, was performed during activation mapping. As comparison, the patients were compared with a cohort of similar patients undergoing conventional catheter ablation via fluoroscopy. The results demonstrated that ablation was successful in all patients. Secondly, there was no difference in median procedure time between Niobe Stereotaxis (153 min) and conventional fluoroscopy (136 min) ablation groups. Nevertheless, the median fluoroscopy time was significantly reduced in the Niobe Stereotaxis group (8 vs. 29 min). (Chong et al., 2011a) concluded that the ablation of outflow tract ventricular tachycardia with a single magnetic-guided catheter is feasible, safe, and reduces fluoroscopy time.

In their second study, (Chong et al., 2011b) aimed at outlining their experiences in the ablation of incessant ventricular tachycardia with the use of the remote Niobe Stereotaxis magnetic-guided catheter system. In the course of the 1-year study, three patients with incessant ventricular tachycardia were recruited. All underwent ablation with Navistar RMT Thermocool 8F catheter guided via the Niobe Stereotaxis system and three dimensional localization using CARTO. Upon completion of procedure two of the patients' ventricular tachycardia could no longer be induced after successful ablation, and after a 12 month period, there was no recurrence. The third patient had ventricular ectopics and non-sustained ventricular tachycardia (NSVT) noted from two further sites these were ablated as well and there were no significant complications. Total fluoroscopy time was 17.4, 18.2, and 15.2 min, respectively, whereas the total procedure time was 3, 2, and 5 h, respectively. (Chong et al., 2011b) concluded that magnetic-guided catheter ablation is effective in the ablation of patients with incessant haemodynamically stable ventricular tachycardia.

(Zvereva et al., 2011) performed a prospective study to compare the incidence of oesophageal lesions using either the remote navigation system from Hansen Sensei to a manual approach for pulmonary vein isolation using a radiofrequency catheter. A total of 33 patients were recruited, 14 of which underwent manual approach. The oesophageal probe was placed and integrated with NavX™. When temperature rose to .39 FXC, ablation was immediately stopped until temperature decreased. Lastly, endoscopy was performed within 24 h after pulmonary vein isolation. Results demonstrated that in 2 of 19 patients with Hansen Sensei treatment had an oesophageal lesion found compared to only lesion found for 1 of 14 patients using the manual approach. Altogether, patients were comparable with respect to arterial hypertension, incidence of paroxysmal and persistent atrial fibrillation, or left atrial diameter. The oesophageal lesions showed brisk healing after re-endoscopy within 2 weeks in all patients. (Zvereva et al., 2011) concluded that the incidence of oesophageal lesions in patients using Hansen Sensei compared with manually performed ablation is similar when low power settings at the posterior wall are used.

6. Ultrasound

The flexibility and ease of use of ultrasound has made it the imaging modality of choice in many intraoperative surgery rooms and laboratories worldwide. In this section we discuss specific applications of the common ultrasound instrumentation used in the electrophysiology laboratory.

6.1 CARTOSound

An extension to the CARTO mapping technology enabling ultrasound integration was created recently and termed, CARTOSound (*Biosense Webster Inc., Diamond Bar, California, USA*). It creates a three-dimensional image of a specific heart chamber undergoing cardiac ablation by utilizing an intracardiac ultrasound catheter. A first study (Schwartzman, & Zhong, 2010) evaluated the use of CARTOSound for left atrial navigation during atrial fibrillation ablation. The authors first integrated the images obtained from CARTOSound into a preoperative CT (Figure 13) and then assessed the accuracy of the CARTOSound volume representation of the left atrium from each of four different ultrasound positions (RA, left atrium, coronary sinus, and esophagus). It turns out that the most accurate representation of the chamber was obtained with the ultrasound catheter placed in the left atrium. Hence, at first sight, the CARTOSound chamber representation was found to be as accurate as the CT image (LaPage & Saul, 2011).

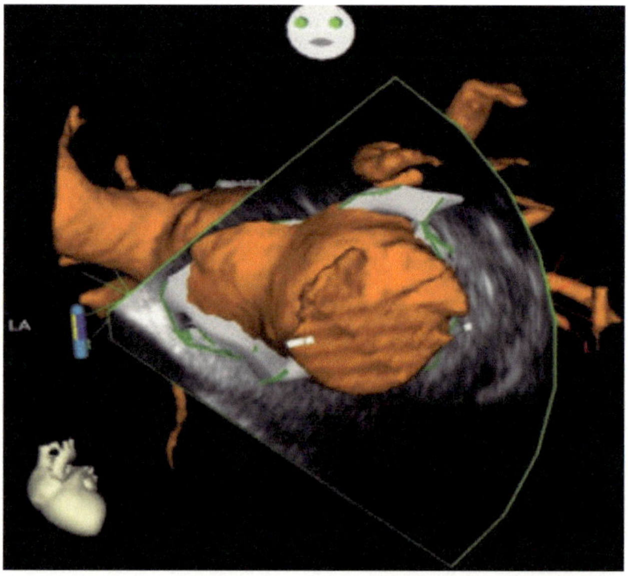

Fig. 13. The CARTOSound mapping technology that fused ultrasound images into the reconstructed volume. Image taken from Knecht et al., 2008. (doi: 10.1093/europace/eun227)

6.2 TEE imaging

Recently, real-time 3D transoesophageal echocardiography (TEE) has become available for clinical practice, offering clear and detailed rendering of the cardiac anatomy. The 3D TEE probe (*Matrix 3DTEE, Philips, Inc., Andover, MA*) allows for both 2D and 3D real-time imaging of both the left atrium and pulmonary veins. 3D TEE also provides excellent visualisation of the interatrial septum (Chierda et al., 2008a). A small study implied that 3D TEE guidance might provide safer trans-septal puncture in patients with unusual anatomy (Chierda et al., 2008b), as it offers the benefit of recognising some shapes of the atrial septum that are not well characterised by conventional two dimensional TEE. Despite these promising features, post-acquisition image processing is necessary and time-consuming. Moreover, general anaesthesia along with endotracheal intubation would be mandatory (Casella et al., 2010).

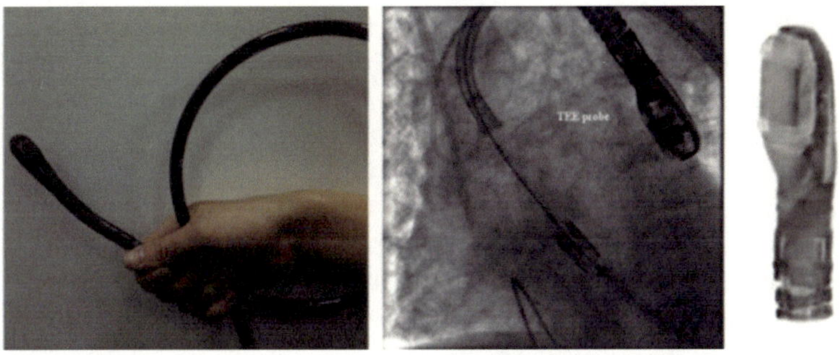

Fig. 14. The TEE probe and its tip sensor used to image left atrium or pulmonary veins during ablation procedures. Also shown is the TEE probe visible in X-ray. Image taken from King et al., 2010.

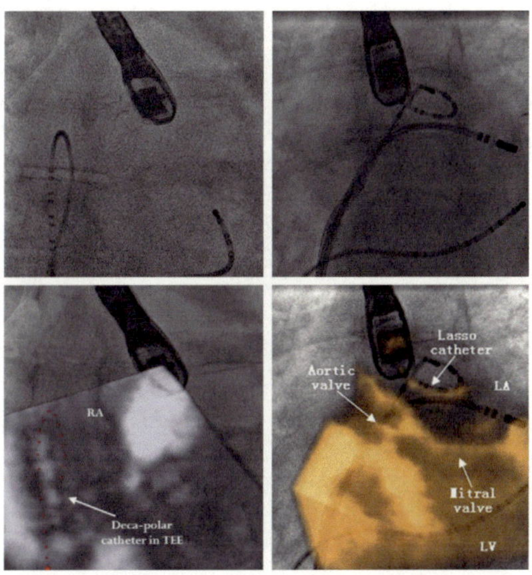

Fig. 15. (*First column*) the TEE volume shows a deca-polar catheter positioned in right atrium and dots highlight the position of the deca-polar catheter in the background of the X-ray image. (*Second column*), a lasso catheter was inserted into the left atrium with TEE volumes registered to X-ray images. Image taken from King et al., 2010.

6.3 ICE imaging

The first catheter-based 2D echocardiography systems were developed in the late 20th century for intracoronary imaging. They had high frequencies (20–40 MHz) and limited depth of penetration, making them suitable only for intravascular applications (Robinson & Hutchinson, 2010). Over the years, there has been a significant improvement in the technology with the advent of low frequency (12.5 - 9 MHz) and more recently the phased array (5.5 - 10 MHz) transducers which have been miniaturized and mounted on the catheters capable of percutaneous insertion (Pandian et al, 1990; Packer et al. 2002). Phased array ICE imaging uses a 64-element transducer on the distal end of an 8-10 French catheter. These catheters are capable of M-mode, pulsed, continuous wave and color Doppler (Daoud, 2005; Ren et al., 2002; Verma et al., 2002; Ferguson et al., 2009; Kabra & Singh, 2010.) During intervention, once transseptal access is achieved, ICE facilitates visualization of the left atrial and pulmonary venous anatomy. It also helps to assess the electrode-tissue contact. The images of ICE can be integrated with the electroanatomic mapping systems (CARTOSound) to generate the geometry of left atrium. A recent study demonstrated the feasibility of catheter ablation of atrial fibrillation without fluoroscopy using intracardiac echocardiography and electroanatomic mapping (Ferguson, 2009). Advances in intracardiac echocardiography include creation of accurate, real time three-dimensional ultrasound geometries that may obviate the need for pre-procedure CT/MRI imaging for catheter ablation of atrial fibrillation (Okumura, 2008). Other advantages over CT and MRI include ICE offering the advantage of showing the real-time detailed anatomy of the cardiac chambers that can be updated multiple times during the procedure. Furthermore, creating a 3D reconstruction without entering the LA may reduce procedural time, enhance the safety of catheter ablation procedures and eliminate geometrical distortion resulting from distension of the tissue. However, this technology bears an important financial burden because of the employment of expensive non-reusable ICE catheters (Casella et al., 2010).

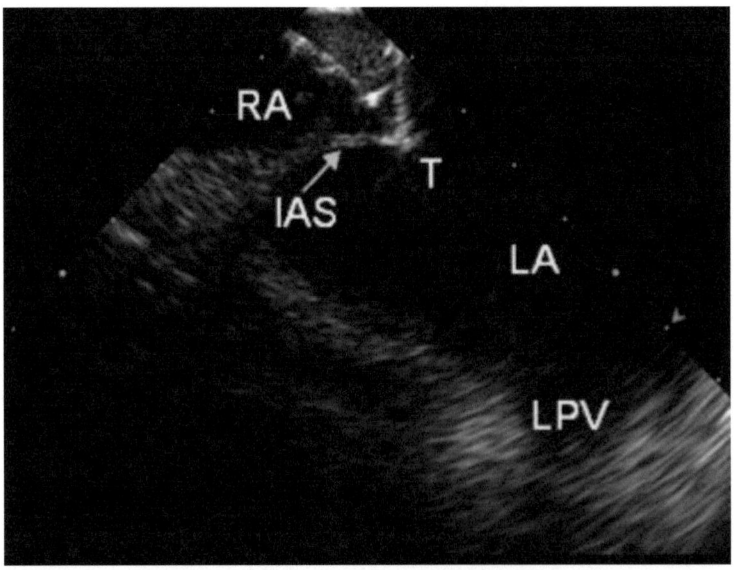

Fig. 16. ICE image showing left and right atriums, interatrial septum, needle tenting and left pulmonary veins. Image taken from Robinson & Hutchinson, 2010.

7. Conclusion

In summary, this chapter presented the latest findings involving several electroanatomical mapping systems that are available to assist electrophysiologists in treating arrhythmias. Techniques are still evolving to address the challenge of a catheter-based cure. The chapter indicates that the registration of MRI/CT images to the existing fluoroscopy image or 3D anatomical map can facilitate navigation of the ablation catheter. In addition, robotic catheter navigation is now available as well. Each method, whether it is the conventional fluoroscopic treatment or the more sophisticated remote navigation systems has its own merits and weaknesses. While all these systems provide a wealth of data and reduce fluoroscopy times slightly, they cannot replace careful interpretation of data and strict adherence to electrophysiologic principles. Although these benefits are achieved at a greater cost, there may be long-term benefits to the community and catheter laboratory staff.

8. Acknowledgment

Dr. Pascal Fallavollita would like to acknowledge the support of the Chair for Computer Aided Medical Procedures & Augmented Reality, Technische Universität München.

9. References

Azizian, M. & Patel, R. (2011). Intraoperative 3D stereo visualization for image-guided cardiac ablation.*SPIE Medical Imaging: Visualization, Image-Guided Procedures, and Modeling*, Vol. 7964, pp. 79640F

Bhakta, D. & Miller, JM. (2008). Principles of Electroanatomic Mapping. *Indian Pacing and Electrophysiology Journal,* (ISSN 0972-6292), Vol.8, Issue 1, pp. 32-50

Casella, M.; Perna, F.; Dello Russo, A.; Pelargonio, G.; Bartoletti, S.; Ricco, A.; Sanna, T.; Pieroni, M.; Forleo, G.; Pappalardo, A.; Di Biase, L.; Natale, L.; Bellocci, F; Zecchi, P.; Natale, A. & Tondo, C. (2009). Right ventricular substrate mapping using the Ensite NavX system: accuracy of high-density voltage map obtained by automatic point acquisition during geometry reconstruction. *Heart Rhythm,* Vol.6, pp. 1598–1605

Casella, M.; Perna, F.; Dello Russo, A.; Moltrasio, M.; Fassini, G.; Riva,S.; Zucchetti, M.; Majocchi,B.; Tundo,F.; Colombo, C.; De Juliis, P.; Giraldi, F.; Carbucicchio, C.; Fiorentini C. & Tondo, C. (2010). Atrial Fibrillation Ablation - New Approaches, New Technologies. *European Cardiology,* Vol.6, Issue 3, pp. 71–6

Chierchia, G.B.; Capulzini, L.; de Asmundis, C.; Sarkozy, A.; Roos, M.; Paparella, G.; Boussy, T.; Van Camp, G.; Kerkhove D. & Brugada, P. (2008a) First experience with real-time three-dimensional transoesophageal echocardiography-guided transseptal in patients undergoing atrial fibrillation ablation. *Europace,* Vol. 10, pp. 1325–8

Chierchia, G.B.; Van Camp, G., Sarkozy, A.; de Asmundis, C. & Brugada, P. (2008b). Double transseptal puncture guided by real-time three-dimensional transoesophageal echocardiography during atrial fibrillation ablation. *Europace,* Vol. 10, pp. 705–6

Chong, D.; Ching, C.K.; Liew, R.; Galalardin; Khin, M.W. & Teo, W.S. (2011a). Outflow tract ventricular tachycardia ablation with a magnetic-guided catheter is effective, safe and reduces radiation exposure. *Europace*, Vol.13, suppl 1, pp. i47-i82, poster 008

Chong, D.; Tan, B.Y.; Liew, R.; Ching, C.K. & Teo, W.S. (2011b). Ablation of incessant ventricular tachycardia using a remote magnetic-guided catheter: a tertiary centre case series. *Europace*, Vol.13, suppl 1, pp. i47-i82, poster 009

Daoud E.G. (2005). Transseptal catheterization. *Heart Rhythm*, Vol.2, pp. 212–214

D'Silva, A. & Wright, M. (2011). Advances in Imaging for Atrial Fibrillation Ablation. *Radiology Research and Practice*. Vol. 2011, Article ID 714864, 10 pages, doi:10.1155/2011/714864

Eitel, C.; Hindricks, G.; Dagres, N.; Sommer, P. & Piorkowski, C. (2010). EnSite Velocity cardiac mapping system: a new platform for 3D mapping of cardiac arrhythmias. *Expert Rev Med Devices*, Vol.7, pp.185–188

Ferguson, J.D.; Helms, A.; Mangrum, J.M.; Mahapatra, S.; Mason, P.; Bilchick, K.; McDaniel, G.; Wiggins, D. & DiMarco, J.P. (2009). Catheter ablation of atrial fibrillation without fluoroscopy using intracardiac echocardiography and electroanatomic mapping. *Circ Arrhythm Electrophysiol*, Vol. 2, pp. 611-619

Kabra, R. & Singh, J. (2010). Recent Trends in Imaging for Atrial Fibrillation Ablation. *Indian Pacing and Electrophysiology Journal*, Vol. 10, Issue5, pp. 215-227, 2010

King, A.P.; Rhode, K.S.; Ma, Y.; Yao, C.; Jansen, C.; Razavi, R. & Penney, G. (2010). Registering preprocedure volumetric images with intraprocedure 3-D ultrasound using an ultrasound imaging model. *IEEE Transactions on Medical Imaging, Vol.* 29, pp. 924 - 937

Knecht, S.; Nault, I.; Wright, M.; Matsuo, S.; Lellouche, N.; Somasundaram, P.E.; O'Neill, M.D.; Lim, K.T.; Sacher, F.; Deplagne, A.; Bordachar, P.; Mélèze, H.; Clémenty, J.; Haıssaguerre, M.; & Jaıs, P. (2008). Imaging in catheter ablation for atrial fibrillation: enhancing the clinician's view. *Europace*, Vol.10, pp. iii2–iii7

Knecht, S.; Wright, M.; Akrivakis, S.; Nault, I.; Matsuo, S.; Chaudhry, GM.; Haffajee, C.; Sacher, F.; Lellouche, N.; Miyazaki, S.; Forclaz, A.; Jadidi, AS.; Hocini, M.; Ritter, P.; Clementy, J.; Haïssaguerre, M.; Orlov, M. & Jaïs, P. (2010). Prospective randomized comparison between the conventional electroanatomical system and three-dimensional rotational angiography during catheter ablation for atrial fibrillation. *Heart Rhythm*, Vol.7, Issue 4, pp. 459-65

Kwong, W.; Neilson, AL.; Hamilton, RM.; Chiu, CC.; Stephenson, EA.: Gross, GJ.; Soucie, L. & Kirsh, JA. (2011). NavX mapping reduces ablation fluoroscopy times in paediatric catheter ablation. *Europace*, Vol.13, suppl 1, pp. i47-i82, poster 001.

LaPage, MJ. & Saul, JP. (2011).Update on rhythm mapping and catheter navigation. *Current Opinion in Cardiology*, Vol.26, pp.79–85

Liu, XQ.; Zhou, X.; Yang,G.; Zhong, GZ.; Shi, L.; Tian, Y.; Li, YB.; Wang, Au. & Yang XC. (2011). Radiofrequency catheter ablation for atrioventricular nodal re-entrant tachycardia without fluoroscopic guidance. *Europace*, Vol. 13, suppl 1, pp. i47-i82, poster 013

Okumura, Y.; Henz, B.D.; Johnson, S.B.; Bunch, T.J.; O'Brien, C.J.; Hodge, D.O.; Altman, A.; Govari, A. & Packer, D.L. (2008). Three-dimensional ultrasound for image-guided mapping and intervention: Methods, Quantitative validation, and clinical feasibility of a novel multimodality image mapping system. *Circ Arrhythm Electrophysiol*, Vol. 1, pp. 110-119

Packer, D.L.; Stevens, C.L.; Curley, M.G.; Bruce, C.J.; Miller, F.A.; Khandheria, B.K.; Oh, J.K.; Sinak, L.J. & Seward, J.B. (2002). Intracardiac phased-array imaging: methods and initial clinical experience with high resolution, under blood visualization-initial experience with intracardiac phased-array ultrasound. *J Am Coll Cardiol.* Vol.39, pp. 509-516

Pandian, N.G.; Kreis, A.; Weintraub, A.; Motarjeme, A.; Desnoyers, M.; Isner, J.M.; Konstam, M.; Salem, D.N. & Millen, V. (1990). Real-time intravascular ultrasound imaging in humans. *Am J Cardiol.* Vol. 65, pp. 1392-1396

Rajnish, J. (2009). Radiofrequency ablation for cardiac tachyarrhythmias: principles and utility of 3D mapping systems. *Current Science*, Vol.97, No.3, (August 2009), pp. 416-424

Ren, J.F.; Marchlinski, F.E.; Callans, D.J.; Zado, E.S. (2002). Intracardiac Doppler echocardiographic quantification of pulmonary vein flow velocity: an effective technique for monitoring pulmonary vein ostia narrowing during focal atrial fibrillation ablation. *J Cardiovasc Electrophysiol*, Vol.13, pp. 1076–1081

Rossillo, A.; Indiani, S.; Bonso, A.; Themistoclakis, S.; Corrado, A. & Raviele, A. (2009). Novel ICE-guided registration strategy for integration of electroanatomical mapping with three-dimensional CT/MR images to guide catheter ablation of atrial fibrillation. *J Cardiovasc Electrophysiol*, Vol 20,pp. 374–378

Schmitt, C.; Zrenner, B.; Schneider, M.; Karch, M.; Ndrepepa, G.; Deisenhofer, I.; Weyerbrock, S.; Schreieck, J. & Schömig, A. (1999). Clinical Experience with a Novel Multielectrode Basket Catheter in Right Atrial Tachycardias. *Circulation.* Vol. 99, pp. 2414-2422

Schmidt, S.; Tilz, R.R.; Neven, K.; Chun, J.K.R.; Fuernkranz, A. & Ouyang, F. (2009). Remote robotic navigation and electroanatomical mapping for ablation of atrial fibrillation: considerations for navigation and impact on procedural outcome. *Circ Arrhythmia Electrophysiol*, Vol. 2, pp. 120–128

Schneider, H.E.; Kriebel, T.; Jung, K.; Gravenhorst, V.D. & Paul, T. (2010) Catheter ablation of idiopathic left and right ventricular tachycardias in the pediatric population using noncontact mapping. *Heart Rhythm*, Vol. 7, pp.731–739.

Schwartzman, D. & Zhong, H. (2010). On the use of CartoSound for left atrial navigation. *J Cardiovasc Electrophysiol*; Vol. 21, pp. 656–664

Thornton, A.S.; Rivero-Ayerza, M. & Jordaens, L. (2008) Ablation of a focal left atrial tachycardia via a retrograde approach using remote magnetic navigation. *Europace*, Vol. 10, Issue 6, pp. 687-689

Thornton, A.S.; De Castro, C.A.; van Deel, E.; van Beusekom, H.M. & Jordaens, L.(2010). An in vivo comparison of radiofrequency cardiac lesions formed by standard and magnetically steered 4mm tip catheters. *Neth Heart J,Vol.* 18, pp. 66–71

Verma, A.; Marrouche, N.F.; Natale, A. (2002). Pulmonary vein antrum isolation: intracardiac echocardiography-guided technique. *J Cardiovasc Electrophysiol*, Vol. 15, pp. 1335–1340

Wielandts, JY.; De Buck, S.; Ector, J.; LaGerche, A.; Willems,R.; Bosmans, H. & Heidbuchel, H. (2010). Three-dimensional cardiac rotational angiography: effective radiation dose and imagequality implications. *Europace, Vol.*12, pp.194–201

Wu, J.; Pflaumer, A.; Deisenhofer, I.; Hoppmann, P.; Hess, J. & Hessling, G. (2010) Mapping of atrial tachycardia by remote magnetic navigation in postoperative patients with congenital heart disease. *J Cardiovasc Electrophysiol*, Vol. 21, pp. 751–759

Xu, D.; Yang, B.; Shan, Q.; Zou, J.; Chen, M.; Chen, C.; Hou, X.; Zhang, F.; Li, W.Q.; Cao, K. & Tse, H.F. (2009). Initial clinical experience of remote magnetic navigation system for catheter mapping and ablation of supraventricular tachycardias. *J Interv Card Electrophysiol*, Vol.25, pp. 171–174

Zvereva, V.; Rillig, A.; Meyerfeldt, U. & Jung, W. (2011). Incidence of oesophageal lesions using either a remote robotic navigation system or a manual approach for *Europace*, Vol.13, suppl 1, pp. i47-i82, poster 009

Part 6

Miscellaneous

23

Mild Induced Therapeutic Hypothermia for Survivors of Cardiac Arrest

Kevin Baker, John Prior, Karthik Sheka and Raymond A. Smego, Jr.
The Commonwealth Medical College
USA

1. Introduction

Despite advances in emergency response and critical care, good neurologic outcome after cardiac arrest is difficult to achieve, and interventions during the resuscitation phase and treatment within the first hours after the event are crucial. Although recommended by organizations such as the American Heart Association (AHA) and the International Liaison Committee on Resuscitation (ILCOR), implementation of induced mild therapeutic hypothermia for survivors of cardiac arrest in the United States has been slow, at least in part, because of the perception that this therapy is technically difficult, especially at the community level. In this chapter, we review the pathophysiology, cooling techniques, clinical evidence and uses (including costs), and effectiveness of induced mild therapeutic hypothermia in adult patients after cardiopulmonary resuscitation, using any cooling method applied within six hours of arrest. Neurologic outcome, survival and adverse events are the main outcome parameters outlined here. In addition, we also include a discussion of the applicability of mild therapeutic hypthermia for both academic health centers and community hospitals, as well as areas of uncertainty, guidelines, and recommendations.

2. Epidemiology of cardiac arrest

The incidence of out-of-hospital sudden cardiac arrest in industrialized countries is about 62 cases per 100,000 a year making sudden cardiac arrest a major cause of death in the United States amounting to more than 300,000 occurrences of cardiac arrests outside of hospital each year (Adler et al, 2011). Resuscitation is attempted on roughly 100,000 of these arrest patients but results in only 40,000 patients who survive upon arrival to the hospital (Holzer, 2010).
Despite advances in emergency medical services the mortality and morbidity associated with out-of hospital cardiac arrest is high. In 2006, the National Registry of Cardiopulmonary Resuscitation (CPR) published statistics on 19,819 adults and 524 children with return of spontaneous circulation after cardiac arrest. The mortality rates were 67% among adults and 55% among children (Jacobshagen et al, 2010). Currently, less than half of cardiac arrest patients survive to discharge and less than a third of those discharged have a good neurologic outcome as defined by the Cerebral Performance Category (CPS) Scale (Adler et al, 2011). The cost of caring for patients with poor neurologic function within the first six months alone can range anywhere from $10,000 to $300,000, with an increasing morbidity generally associated with increasing cost (Merchant et al, 2009).

3. Pathophysiology of induced mild therapeutic hypothermia

The brain receives approximately 15% of the human resting cardiac output despite comprising 1-2% of our total body weight, illustrating the high metabolic demands associated with the brain. During cardiac arrest the blood supply is interrupted leading to global cerebral ischemia.

Ischemic events are especially detrimental to the brain and are a major cause of morbidity in cardiac arrest survivors. Areas such as the hippocampus, neocortex, cerebellum, corpus striatium, and thalamus are the most vulnerable to global ischemia. Necrosis and apoptosis have both been reported in cardiac arrest victims and it still is unclear the extent to which each of these processes contribute to neuronal cell death. The brain is damaged through an ischemic cascade of events occurring on a time scale of minutes-to-days after cardiac arrest and is summarized below.

A lack of oxygen hinders the neurons ability to produce ATP. Consequently, cells switch to anaerobic metabolism which consumes glucose and produces lactic acid. As glucose concentrations are exhausted, ion transporters using ATP fail to function. Cells become depolarized allowing ions, including calcium, to flow into the cell. Due to the lack of ATPase activities, cells cannot pump calcium out of the intracellular space, and as intracellular calcium levels rise they trigger the release of excitatory neurotransmitters. Glutamate, one of the excitatory neurotransmitters, acts on AMPA and NMDA receptors to allow more calcium into cells and thereby increases the intracellular calcium leading to production of neurotoxic chemicals such as free radicals, reactive oxygen species and calcium-dependent enzyme (Sinclair & Andrews, 2010). This process is referred to as excitotoxicity. Calcium-dependent enzymes such as calpain, endonucleases, and phospholipases break down cells making them more permeable to harmful chemicals and leads to damage of the mitochondrial membrane, ultimately causing release of pro-apoptotic factors that stimulate the caspase cascade and inducing cell suicide. Cells that die due to necrosis cause a release of glutamate and other neurotoxic compounds that act on surrounding cells and perpetuate excitotoxicty.

Hypothermia exerts its effect on the ischemic cascade mentioned above to improve neurologic outcome after cardiac arrest. The following discussion will elaborate on mild therapeutic hypothermia and how it mitigates the pathologic processes involving: 1) blood-brain barrier permeability and edema, 2) inflammation, 3) metabolism, 4) excitotoxicity, 5) intracellular calcium-dependent signaling 6) cerebral vascular effects, and 7) neuronal cell death.

3.1 Blood-brain barrier permeability and edema

The blood-brain barrier displays increased permeability after ischemia and allows the entrance of water, electrolytes, and potentially toxic substances into the brain parenchyma. Hypothermia has been shown to decrease the extravasation of certain protein markers such as horseradish peroxidase from the serum into the brain. Studies have also demonstrated that treatment with hypothermia in focal ischemia results in a decrease in brain water content as measured by MRI, and leads to a reduction in the diffusion of water into the brain and a consequent reduction in vasogenic edema by alleviating blood-brain barrier injury (Sinclair & Andrews, 2010). Vasogenic edema is a result of damage to the blood-brain barrier and the passage of large osmotically-active proteins like albumin into the brain.

The attenuation of matrix metalloproteases is another effect of hypothermia that reduces the permeability of the blood-brain barrier. Matrix metalloproteases are important for the extravasation of several substances into the brain including immunologic and other inflammatory cells. Reducing movement of these cells into the brain decreases deleterious edema associated with inflammatory immune responses to ischemia and neuronal cell injury.

3.2 Inflammation and immune response

Hypothermia mitigates the inflammation response by reducing the leukocyte extravasation as well as the endogenous inflammatory response of the brain to ischemia. Astrocytes and microglia respond to tissue damage in the brain by proliferating and secreting large quantities of pro-inflammatory cytokines such as tumor necrosis factor-α and interleukin-1 which recruit cells of the immune system. Hypothermia reduces the activation of astrocytes and microglia thereby reducing the pro-inflammatory signaling and the ensuing immune response (Sinclair & Andrews, 2010).

The inflammatory response in the brain also results in the release of reactive oxygen species by astrocytes and microglia. Hypothermia, therefore, also reduces the levels of potentially damaging free radicals such as superoxide, nitric oxide, and hydroxyl radicals within the brain by decreasing their secretion from microglia and astrocytes. Hypothermia also increases the levels of superoxide dismutase, the enzyme that clears superoxide from the body, and decreases nitric oxide synthase, the enzyme responsible for production of nitric oxide. This reduction in reactive oxygen species production and increase in reactive oxygen species scavenger enzymes results in decreased neuronal damage.

3.3 Metabolism

Hypothermia has been proven to decrease glucose utilization. Studies implementing 2-deoxyglucose, a glucose analog that can be taken up by glucose transporters but not digested, has shown that hypothermia decreases utilization of glucose when compared to normothermia. Global ischemia affects the brain more than the liver due to the small stores of glycogen found in the brain compared to large stores found in the liver. Therefore, any reduction in glucose utilization will attenuate the damaging effects of poor cerebral perfusion. Hypothermia reduces the metabolic demands of the cell, preserving cellular ATP concentration more effectively when compared to normothermia. Reducing core temperature 1°C decreases metabolic rate by approximately 6%-8% (Adler et al, 2011).

The cell's ability to maintain electrochemical gradients depends heavily upon ATP concentrations. Loss of transmembrane electrochemical gradients directly precedes failure of synaptic transmission and axonal conduction. Hypothermia's ability to reduce metabolic demands, preserve ATP, and potentiate electrochemical gradients translates to better neurologic outcomes after recovery from cardiac arrest.

3.4 Excitotoxicity

The metabolic depletion of ATP associated with ischemia in cardiac arrest results in an inappropriate release of excitatory neurotransmitters such as glutamate. A reduction in the blood flow to the brain allows levels of glutamate to build up in the extracellular space around neurons. This rise in glutamate leads to activation of glutamatergic receptors AMPA (alpha-amino-3-hydroxyl-5-methyl-4-isoxazole-propionate) and NMDA (*N*-methyl d-aspartate). Glutamate acts through AMPA and NMDA to produce an influx of calcium from the extracellular fluid to the intracellular fluid. This inflow of calcium can injure the cell by initiating several cascades within the cell including, free radical generation, mitochondrial injury, and ultimately apoptosis (Nolan et al, 2008). Hypothermia inhibits the release of glutamine and dopamine while also inducing neurotrophic factors that further reduce glutamine release.

3.5 Intracellular calcium-dependent signaling

Global ischemia leads to an increase in intracellular calcium, thereby affecting normal signaling protein kinases in the cell. Proteins such as calmodulin-dependent kinase II (CaMKII) and protein kinase C (PKC) are rescued by hypothermia (Sinclair & Andrews, 2010). These proteins, as well as other signaling factors, are temperature-sensitive. Controlling signaling factors and proteins such as CaMKII and PKC through hypothermia influences neuronal injury and normal cell signaling.

3.6 Cerebral vascular and cellular effects

Hypothermia affects secretion of vasoactive substances such as endothelin, thromboxane A2, and prostaglandin I2 in the brain. Endothelin and thromboxane A2 have vasoconstrictive effects while prostaglandin I2 is a vasodilator. Thromboxane A2, endothelin, and prostaglandin I2 mediate vascular homeostasis in the brain; during ischemic and traumatic events homeostatic balance is shifted towards vasoconstriction, hypoperfusion, and thrombus formation. Hypothermia has been shown in animal models and small clinical studies to alter the response to injury by attenuating the vasconstrictive response. However, regulation of cerebral perfusion is complex and dependent on several factors including the presence or absence of cerebral autoregulation, ventilator settings, serum blood gas levels, systemic blood pressure, osmotic therapy, etc (Sinclair & Andrews, 2010).

Necrosis and apoptosis are the result of prolonged tissue ischemia and can be influenced by hypothermia. Several gene families associated with apoptosis are temperature-sensitive. Brain cells can sense irreversible injury and begin the process of self-destruction. Hypothermia leads to a delayed response of the cell to injury and this slowed response is mediated by a delay in genetic regulation (Sinclair & Andrews, 2010). Ultimately, hypothermia slows secondary injury and apoptosis through delaying the cells initial reaction to damage. Apoptosis occurs over the time frame of hours-to-days making hypothermia a major factor in mitigating apoptosis during the post-resuscitation phase.

4. Cooling methods

Several different cooling techniques are available for use in therapeutic hypothermia; however, all of the various techniques fall into two general categories: surface cooling and core cooling. Surface cooling can be carried out in two ways; the first utilizes pre-cooled pads while the second makes use of heat-exchanging mattresses or pads. Surface cooling was used in the two hallmark clinical trials carried out in 2003 in Europe and Australia that first demonstrated the beneficial effects of hypothermia on witnessed cardiac arrest survivors (Bernard et al, 2003; Holzer & Sterz, 2003).

Core cooling can be achieved with the use of intravascular cooling catheters filled with cold saline or by intravenous injection of cold fluids. Devices for core cooling and surface cooling have been specifically designed for use in therapeutic hypothermia but the ultimate goal,

whether using either surface or core cooling methods, is to rapidly cool the patient and maintain a stable temperature between 32-34°C for at least 24 hours.
Various measurements and devices may be used to monitor relevant core body temperature including esophageal probes, endotracheal tube cuff monitors, and non-invasive continuous cerebral temperature monitoring (Zeiner et al, 2010; Haugk et al, 2010). During the initial phase of head and neck cooling, jugular bulb temperature (Tjb), (which may reflect brain temperature) appears to be lower than esophageal temperature (Wandaller et al, 2009).

4.1 Surface cooling

4.1.1 Ice packs

Ice packs are an inexpensive and easy technique to initiate cooling. However, they can be messy and less effective at cooling and maintaining target temperature. Ice packs can be placed all over the body, but are more effectively placed in anatomic areas that have large heat-exchange capability due to their blood flow. These areas include the head, neck, axillae, and groin. The average temperature drop attained by using ice packs is between 0.03-0.98°C per hour (Adler et al., 2011).

4.1.2 Blankets or surface heat-exchange devices

Conventional surface cooling blankets are not ideal because of poor surface contact with the patient's skin. Generally, water-circulating cooling devices and ice packs used in combination can be effective at rapidly cooling patients. Many clinical studies have used this combination as their cooling technique. The patient is sandwiched between two blankets or cooling devices and ice packs are then applied. Once target temperature is achieved, the ice packs are removed and the blanket or cooling devices are used alone to maintain the target temperature. Newer cooling devices, specific for use in therapeutic hypothermia, use an adhesive gel to facilitate heat exchange that make them more effective at obtaining and maintaining target temperature.
Weihs and coworkers (2011) used adult, human-sized pigs to study the importance of surface area for the cooling efficacy of mild therapeutic hypothermia. Each of five adult, human-sized pigs (88-105 kg) was randomly cooled in three phases with pads that covered different areas of the body surface corresponding to humans (100% or 30% [thorax and abdomen] or 7% [neck]). The cooling pads were effective and safe for rapid induction of mild hypothermia in these porcine simulators. depending on the percentage of body surface area covered. Extrapolating to humans, covering only the neck, chest, and abdomen may achieve satisfactory cooling rates.
Convective-immersion surface cooling using a continuous shower of 2 degrees C water (ThermoSuit System) has also been found to be a rapid, effective method of inducing therapeutic hypothermia (Howes et al, 2010) and demonstrated improvement in survival and neurologic outcome in swine compared to normothermia (Weihls et al, 2008).

4.1.3 Cooling helmet

Helmet cooling devices are also available and have been used in some clinical trials. These helmets contain a solution of glycerol that facilitates heat exchange. Although this method is effective in cooling the brain it is much slower at reducing overall body temperature when compared to other methods.

4.2 Core cooling

4.2.1 Catheter-based technologies

Catheter-based technologies are usually placed in the femoral vein and provide heat exchange between the cooled saline that passes through a large coil in the catheter and the blood. The coiling provides a mechanism to increase surface area, thereby increasing the heat exchange between blood passing over the catheter. Internal cooling and rewarming is much faster and superior to other techniques in tightly regulating target temperature; it is possible to cool patients by 1.46°C - 1.59°C per hour (Jacobshagen et al, 2010). A potential advantage of using catheter-based cooling combined with anxiolytics is that it may avoid the need to use paralytics to decrease the shiver seen in surface cooling techniques.

4.2.2 Cold fluid infusion

Several studies have made use of intravenous cold fluid infusion for the induction of hypothermia. The rates of infusion differ between studies but the overall outcome is rapid cooling of the patient. Cold fluid infusion is a means of inducing hypothermia and cannot be used in the long-term maintenance of hypothermia. Usually, cold fluid infusions are used in conjunction with surface cooling methods to regulate and maintain patient body temperature. Most studies have used either normal saline or lactated Ringer solution as their cooling fluids. Evidence from reports using cold fluid infusion have not been associated with increased venous pressure, left atrial filling pressures, pulmonary pressures, pulmonary edema, cardiac arrhythmia, or other major complications.

Categories of Cooling	Techniques of Cooling	Advantages	Disadvantages
Surface Cooling	Ice packs	Inexpensive can be implemented very quickly.	Slow rate of cooling and provides poor regulation of target temperature.
	Cooling blankets and surface heat-exchange devices	Fair regulation of target temperature once it is obtained.	Slow rate of cooling unless used in conjunction with other techniques.
	Cooling helmet	Fair regulation of target temperature once it is obtained.	Slowest rate of cooling among techniques unless used in conjunction with other cooling methods.
Core Cooling	Catheter-based technologies	Rapid rate of cooling, tight target temperature regulation, minimize shiver and possible avoidance of paralytic usage.	Increased chance of thrombus formation
	Infusion of cold fluids	Rapid rate of cooling	Poor regulation of target temperature

Table 1. Cooling Technique Summary

5. Clinical evidence and uses

5.1 Clinical studies

The abovementioned landmark clinical trials from Europe and Australia, respectively, in 2003 established the benefits of hypothermia and have served as the basis for subsequent therapeutic hypothermia guidelines and clinical trials. Most clinical trials evaluate the benefits of hypothermia by scoring patients on the CPC Scale, a tool that rates a patient's neurologic status, or by measuring survival rates.

The European trial enrolled 275 patients whose cardiac arrest was caused by ventricular fibrillation or pulseless ventricular tachycardia. Patients were randomly assigned to either hypothermic (n = 137) or normothermic (n = 138) groups. Hypothermic subjects were cooled to between 32-34°C for 24 hours with a cold air mattress. The primary endpoint of this study was to establish a favorable neurologic outcome in patients six months after cardiac arrest. The authors found that 55% of surviving hypothermic patients had a favorable neurologic outcome, as defined by a score of 1 or 2 on the CPC Scale, compared to 39% of surviving normothermic patients. A secondary endpoint was to evaluate complications within the first seven days after cardiac arrest, and mortality rate at six months. The European study demonstrated that neurologic outcome, as well as patient survival at six months (55% vs. 41%), both significantly improved in the hypothermic group as compared to the normothermic group (Holzer, 2002).

In the Australian trial, 77 comatose cardiac arrest survivors with ventricular fibrillation or pulseless ventricular tachycardia as the initial rhythm were similarly assigned to normothermic (n = 34) or hypothermic (n = 43) groups based on randomization. The hypothermic group was cooled to 33°C with ice packs for 12 hours and showed a 49% survival with favorable neurologic outcome (i.e., discharged home or to a rehabilitation facility, with no or moderate disability), while the normothermic group had a 26% survival with favorable neurologic outcome at hospital discharge (Bernard et al, 2002).

In 2009, Arrich and colleagues performed a Cochrane systematic review and meta-analysis to assess the effectiveness of therapeutic hypothermia in patients after cardiac arrest. Neurologic outcome, survival and adverse events were the main outcome parameters. The authors included all randomized controlled trials assessing the effectiveness of the therapeutic hypothermia in patients after cardiac arrest without language restrictions. Studies were restricted to adult populations cooled with any cooling method applied within six hours of cardiac arrest. Four trials and one abstract reporting on 481 patients were included in the systematic review. Quality of the included studies was good in three out of five included studies. For the three comparable studies on conventional cooling methods all authors provided individual patient data. With conventional cooling methods patients in the hypothermia group were more likely to reach a best cerebral performance category score of 1 or 2 (CPC, 5-point scale; 1 -- good cerebral performance, to 5 -- brain death) during hospital stay (individual patient data; RR, 1.55; 95% CI 1.22 to 1.96) and were more likely to survive to hospital discharge (individual patient data; RR, 1.35; 95% CI 1.10 to 1.65) compared to standard post-resuscitation care. Across all studies, there was no significant difference in reported adverse events between hypothermia and control. The authors concluded that conventional cooling methods to induce mild therapeutic hypothermia seem to improve survival and neurologic outcome after cardiac arrest, and their review supports the current best medical practice as recommended by the International Resuscitation Guidelines.

Testori and colleagues (2011) retrospectively studied 347 cardiac arrest survivors aged $\geq$ 18 years suffering a witnessed out-of-hospital cardiac arrest with asystole or pulseless electric activity as the first documented rhythm, for whom hypothermia was induced in 135 patients. They found that subjects who were treated with mild therapeutic hypothermia at a temperature of 32-34°C for 24 hours were more likely to have good neurologic outcomes in comparison to patients who were not treated with hypothermia, with an odds ratio of 1.84 (95% confidence interval: 1.08-3.13). In addition, the rate of mortality was significantly lower in the hypothermia group (odds ratio: 0.56; 95% confidence interval: 0.34-0.93).

While shortening the delay from spontaneous circulation to hypothermic target temperature has been theorized as a way of improving survival and neurologic outcome, randomized controlled trials and clinical registries have not shown evidence of whether the time to target temperature correlates with neurologic outcome. A recent study has reported that in comatose cardiac arrest patients treated with therapeutic hypothermia after return of spontaneous circulation, a faster decline in body temperature to the 34°C target appears to predict an unfavorable neurologic outcome (Haugk, 2011). Among 588 survivors of cardiac arrest managed with therapeutic hypothermia, the median time from restoration of spontaneous circulation to reaching a temperature of less than 34°C was 209 minutes (interquartile range [IQR]: 130-302) in patients with favorable neurologic outcomes compared to 158 minutes (IQR: 101-230) ($p < 0.01$) in patients with unfavorable neurologic outcomes. The adjusted odds ratio for a favorable neurologic outcome with a longer time to target temperature was 1.86 (95% CI 1.03 to 3.38, $p = 0.04$). Whether faster cooling is detrimental or patients with more severe neurologic damage show a faster cooling rate has to be further evaluated.

Animal and human studies have suggested that hypothermia impairs renal function. Zeiner et al (2004) reported that 24 hours of mild therapeutic hypothermia was associated with a delayed improvement in renal function that was not reflected in serum creatinine values, and this transient impaired renal function appeared to be completely reversible within 4 weeks. In trying to determine the relationship between acute kidney injury on survivors of cardiac arrest treated with therapeutic hypothermia we found that the incidence of acute kidney injury in patients with a CPS 1 or 2 score was 13.6% compared to 86.4% in patients with a CPS score > 2 ($p < 0.001$) (J. Prior, personal communication). Stage 3 acute kidney injury correlated with poor neurologic outcome ($p = 0.04$) but there was no correlation between Stages 1 and 2 and neurologic recovery. A longer duration of cardiac arrest was predictive of the subsequent development of acute kidney injury ($p = 0.01$). In summary, the presence of acute kidney injury in survivors of cardiac arrest treated with therapeutic hypothermia appears to be associated with poorer neurologic function determined at the time of hospital discharge. Acute kidney injury in this population may serve as a marker for the severity of anoxic injury incurred during arrest.

5.2 Indications and contraindications

5.2.1 Indications

The AHA has recommended that therapeutic hypothermia is indicated in adult patients with out-of-hospital cardiac arrests and who have an initial rhthym of ventricular fibrillation or nonperfusing ventricular tachycardia, that are comatose or have a Glasgow coma score < 8, that are hemodynamically stable, and lack a verbal response. Although these are the criteria for which hypothermia is recommended, there are other patients that may benefit from therapeutic hypothermia such as post-resuscitation patients having initial rhthyms other than ventricular fibrillation or nonperfusing ventricular tachycardia, as well as in-hospital cardiac arrest patients.

Survivors of witnessed out-of-hospital cardiac arrest of suspected cardiac origin
Persons with a Glasgow Coma Scale ≤ 8
Persons with ventricular fibrillation or non-perfusing ventricular tachycardia (those with other rhythyms such as asystole or electomechanical dissociatrion *may* also benefit although firm data is lacking)
Persons who are hemodynamically stable (those in cardiac shock *may* also benefit although firm data is lacking)
Consider for survivors of in-hospital cardiac arrest (although firm data is lacking)

* Adapted from Holzer 2010.

Table 2. Summary of indications for induced therapeutic hypothermia in comatose survivors of cardiac arrest.

5.2.2 Contraindications

Exclusion criteria for the use of therapeutic hypothermia are based upon increased risks to the patient. Studies have reported increased but non-significant increases in risk for the following patients: having major surgery within the previous 14 days; having systemic infections or sepsis, in a coma which is non-cardiac in origin, having active known bleeding or inherited bleeding disorder, being pregnant or terminally ill, those with a do-no-resuscitate (DNR) order, or having a tympanic temperature < 30°C upon admission (Oommen & Menon, 2011).

6. Outcomes

Various methods have been used to try and determine the likelihood of neurologic recovery after cardiac arrest, but no single test is effective in accurately predicting neurologic outcome post-resuscitation. Clinical trials have established that combining examinations, laboratory tests and accounting for co-morbidities is often more accurate in determining neurologic outcome. Precise predictors of neurologic recovery are lacking and seriously limit the way clinicians assess patient prognosis, develop appropriate plans of care, and counsel family members. Therefore, more clinical studies are required to determine a uniform protocol for predicting neurologic outcome.

6.1 Modalities predicting neurological outcome

6.1.1 Neurologic examination

A neurologic examination is a fairly reliable predictor of neurological outcome after cardiac arrest. The presence of neurologic function during or immediately after return of spontaneous circulation (ROSC) roughly predicts a good neurologic outcome. Conversely, patients with a Glasgow Coma motor score of ≤ 2 or absent pupillary or corneal reflex at 72 hours can be predicted to have a poor neurologic outcome. The CPC Scale has also been classically used to predict patient outcome. Patients with a CPC scale score of 1 and 2 are likely to have good outcomes, while patients scoring 3, 4 or 5 have a significantly higher chance of having a poor neurologic outcome or death (Nolan et al, 2008). It is worth noting that the neurologic exam and CPC score can be influenced by the physiologic circumstances of the patient such as hypotension, shock, and severe metabolic dysfunction. Interventions such as paralytics, sedatives, and hypothermia also influence the findings of a neurologic examination and must be taken into account. Cranial nerve findings and motor response to pain are the best physical features estimating neurologic status and recovery.

1	Good cerebral performance: conscious, alert, able to work, might have mild neurologic or psychologic deficit.
2	Moderate cerebral disability: conscious, sufficient cerebral function for independent activities of daily life. Able to work in sheltered environment.
3	Severe cerebral disability: conscious, dependent on others for daily support because of impaired brain function. Ranges from ambulatory state to severe dementia or paralysis.
4	Coma or vegetative state: any degree of coma without the presence of all brain death criteria. Unawareness, even if appears awake (vegetative state) without interaction with environment; may have spontaneous eye opening and sleep/awake cycles. Cerebral unresponsiveness.
5	Brain death: apnea, areflexia, EEG silence, etc.

Note: If patient is anesthetized, paralyzed, or intubated, use "as is" clinical condition to calculate scores.

Table 3. Cerebral Performance Categories Scale (CPC Scale)

6.1.2 Neurophysiologic tests

Electroencephalography (EEG) has been used to characterize the degree of brain damage after cardiac arrest. Various EEG patterns have been associated with poor neurologic outcome such as generalized suppression, burst-suppression patterns with generalized epileptiform activity, and generalized periodic complexes on a flat background. Nevertheless, EEG alone is likely to be insufficient to prognosticate neurologic recovery. The EEG requires a physician with experience in its interpretation and knowledge of the influence of drugs and metabolic disorders on its results.

Madl & Holzer (2004) reviewed the literature on the pathophysiology of brain injury caused by cardiac arrest and the beneficial effect of therapeutic hypothermia on neurologic outcome. They summarized that electrophysiologic techniques and molecular markers of brain injury allow the accurate assessment and prognostication of long-term outcome in cardiac arrest survivors. In particular, somatosensory evoked potentials (SSEPs) appear to have the highest prognostic reliability; a systematic review of 18 studies analyzed the predictive ability of SSEPs performed early after onset of coma and found that absence of cortical SSEPs identify patients not returning from anoxic coma, with a specificity of 100%. Somatosensory-evoked potentials test the patency of the neuronal pathways, and are less affected by common drugs and metabolic disorders, making them a more reliable predictor of neurologic outcome than other modalities (Nolan et al, 2008). However, use of SSEPs in post-resuscitation patients requires advanced neurologic training which is usually restricted to specialized centers.

6.1.3 Neuroimaging

Neuroimaging is often performed to define structural brain injury related to cardiac arrest (either as a cause or consequence), including hemorrhage and cerebral vascular occlusion.

Most clinical studies evaluating neurologic outcome after use of therapeutic hypothermia do not make use of neuroimaging. The most common type of neuroimaging employed has been cranial computed tomography (CT), predominately because of the technical difficulties in performing magnetic resonance imaging (MRI) and positron emission tomography (PET) scans in the setting of arrest. Limited studies have shown that diffusion-weighted imaging (DWI), fluid attenuated inversion recovery (FLAIR), abnormalities in PET, and magnetic resonance spectroscopy can help predict poor neurologic outcome (Nolan et al, 2008).

6.1.4 Biochemical markers

Biochemical markers derived from the cerebrospinal fluid (CSF) and peripheral circulation, such as creatine phosphokinase (CPK) and neuron-specific enolase (NSE) respectively, have been used to predict neurologic outcome after cardiac arrest. The ease of obtaining blood compared to CSF has favored blood-based biochemical markers. Neuron-specific enolase is easily measured in the blood after injury to the brain and is, therefore, a good marker for neurologic outcome. Studies have shown that values of NSE > 33μg/L are predictor of poor neurologic outcome.

A calcium-binding protein from astroglia and Schwann cells, S100β, may also be a marker of neurologic outcome. An S100 β concentration > 1.2 μg/L, drawn between 24 and 48 hours after ROSC, is indicative of poor neurologic recovery (Nolan et al, 2008). Biomarker threshold values established in clinical trials vary based on the time blood and CSF are drawn after ROSC and the method for measuring the biomarker. Therefore, standardization must be applied in future clinical trials so that true threshold values can be elucidated and used to predict patient outcome.

6.1.5 Co-morbidities

We previously reported that the risk of poor neurologic outcome among patients treated with mild therapeutic hypothermia was related to the number of risk factors present (Table 4) (Vanston et al, 2010). A first rhythm of non-ventricular tachycardia/ventricular fibrillation after cardiac arrest, acute kidney injury within the first 72 hours of intensive care, and any treated cardiac arrhythmia were factors significantly associated with poor neurologic outcome and death (Table 4).

	No. patients			
	Good CPS (n = 17)	Poor CPS (n = 24)	Risk of poor CPS (%)	No. risk factors[d] (95% CI)
None	6	1	17	(0.3-52.6)
One	9	2	18	(2.3-51.8)
Any two	2	15	88[b]	(63.6-98.5)
All three	0	6	100[c]	(54.1-100)

[a] CPS. Pittsburgh Cerebral Performance Scale; C.I. = confidence intervals
[b] Significantly greater than the risk of poor neurologic outcome amongs patients with no predictive factors (p = 0.004).
[c] Significantly greater than the risk of poor neurologic outcome amongs patients with no predictive factors (p = 0.002).
[d] Include first rhythym other than ventricular fibrillation/ ventricular tachycardia, any arrhythmia, and acute kidney injury.

Table 4. Risk of poor neurologic outcome among patient treated with mild therapeutic hypothermia, according to number of risk factors present.[a]

6.2 Adverse effects

Adverse effects of mild induced therapeutic hypothermia are either directly related to the cooling device or due to hypothermia itself. In 41 clinical trials using therapeutic hypothermia the overall rate of adverse events related to a cooling device was 1% (Holzer, 2010). These adverse effects included three cases of bleeding, eight cases of infection, ten cases of deep venous thrombosis, and eight cases of pulmonary edema. The cases of deep venous thrombosis were seen in patients that were cooled with a catheter-based device, while the cases of pulmonary edema occurred in patients that were cooled with cold intravenous fluid.

Hypothermia causes a decrease in insulin secretion, as well as insulin resistance in many patients. This state of hyperglycemia requires administration of insulin to maintain glucose levels within an acceptable range. More importantly, during the re-warming phase patients can regain appropriate sensitivity to insulin rapidly, making them susceptible to hypoglycemia if insulin administration is not reduced accordingly. Glycemic lability is one of several reasons why re-warming rates after hypothermia are typically slow and controlled.

Some of the adverse effects most commonly associated with therapeutic hypothermia include pneumonia, shivering hyperglycemia, cardiac arrhythmias, seizures, and electrolyte disorders. Less frequently seen complications are sepsis, coagulopathy, and metabolic disturbances. Many of these effects can be easily managed by proper patient monitoring. In a study compiling data from major clinical trials on adverse effects unrelated to the cooling devices, such events occurred in 74% of patients who were treated with hypothermia (223 events in 300 patients) and in 71% of 285 patients given standard, normothermic treatment (Holzer, 2010). The incidences of cardiac arrhythmia, hemodynamic instability, bleeding, pneumonia, sepsis, renal failure, seizures, and pancreatitis were not significantly different between the two groups.

7. Slow implementation

Although its use is becoming more widespread, therapeutic hypothermia is still not appropriately initiated for a majority of eligible patients. Concerns with the ease of use, efficacy, and cost have limited use in the community setting. The current level of implementation of therapeutic hypothermia is difficult to measure, although hypothermia registries are attempting to bridge the gap. The AHA, along with some local communities, is advocating for the care of all patients with cardiac arrest at centers specializing in post-arrest care in order to provide the best possible outcomes. Such centers would have the capability to perform therapeutic hypothermia, perform percutaneous coronary intervention, and utilize standardized protocols for the treatment of cardiac arrest survivors, as well as pay close attention to related aspects of overall management including hemodynamic stability, ventilator support (with timely normalization of FiO_2 and pCO_2), thromboembolic prophylaxis, and glycemic control.

8. Ongoing and potential future research

8.1 Neurologic prognosis

In patients managed with therapeutic hypothermia clinical research is ongoing regarding clinical modeling and the use of aspects of the neurologic exam and acute and chronic medical co-morbidities in predicting neurologic recovery. We have previously found that several simple and reproducible clinical markers (i.e., first rhythm at cardiac arrest; the presence of acute kidney injury in the ICU; any treated cardiac arrhythmia after admission; and Glasgow Coma Score < 8 determined 12 hours after re-warming) can help predict neurologic prognosis during and after treatment, in patients managed with therapeutic hypothermia for cardiac arrest (Vanston, 2010). Additional investigation is neded to examine the potential role of other exam techniques, and electrophysiologic and neurobiochemical tests in reliably predicting neurologic outcomes, and to determine the correlation between laboratory values or exam scores and time after return of spontaneous circulation.

8.2 Non-shockable rhythms/ other cardiac

Small randomized trials and registries have begun to collect data on the use of therapeutic hypothermia in cardiac arrests with non-shockable rhythms and in-hospital cardiac arrests. Recently, in a retrospective cohort study treatment with mild therapeutic hypothermia at a temperature of 32-34°C for 24 hours was associated with improved neurologic outcome and a reduced risk of death following out-of-hospital cardiac arrest in 135 with non-shockable rhythms (Testori et al, 2011). To date, the level of evidence is inadequate to firmly recommend therapeutic hypothermia for these patients; nevertheless, many of these patients are treated with therapeutic hypothermia in the community if their arrest is thought to be of cardiac origin or if the initial rhythm after arrest is unknown. Further research is needed to determine the potential role of therapeutic hypothermia for these subsets of patients. The ILCOR currectly advocates the use of therapeutic hypothermia following perinatal asphyxia-related cardiac arrest in term newborns.

At least one study (a retrospective analysis of the Hypothermia after Cardiac Arrest (HACA) trial) suggested that cooling after successful resuscitation for ventricular fibrillation cardiac arrest did not influence infarct size (Koreny et, 2009). The authors contended that cautious interpretation of the subgroup analysis may indicate a favorable trend for early cooling, and thus additional research is indicated.

8.3 Non-cardiac applications

Clinical trials are still revealing further application of therapeutic hypothermia. It is likely that recommendations and the use of therapeutic hypothermia will expand to encompass several other pathologies such as traumatic brain and spinal cord injury and acute ischemic stroke. Currently, therapeutic hypothermia is not approved by an advisory panel for any other use besides comatose patients after return of spontaneous circulation due to ventricular fibrillation or pulseless ventricular tachycardia (Adler et al, 2011).

8.4 Aspects of treatment

Current and potential future areas of clinical research on treatment aspects of therapeutic hypothermia include, among others:

- Optimal target temperature, duration, onset, cooling rates, and re-warming rates
- Use of external, internal, or mixed modality cooling techniques
- Pharmacologic uses and standardized drug protocols i.e. (analgesics, sedatives, paralytics, etc.)

9. Areas of uncertainty

Some persistent unexposed topics that relate to the pathophysiology of therapeutic hypothermia include the precise mechanism(s) of greatest importance for good neurologic recovery, the mechanism(s) through which hypothermia exerts the most influence, the effects of co-morbidities in reducing the efficacy of therapeutic hypothermia, and the time course of cellular cascades and the ability to attenuate these processes (Holzer, 2010).

10. Guidelines

Sedation, analgesia, and paralysis should be initiated prior to hypothermia to prevent shivering which can increase oxygen consumption, promote labored breathing, increase heart rate, delay hypothermic induction, and increase patient discomfort.
The ILCOR and the AHA recommend that core body temperature of unconscious adult patients with spontaneous circulation after an out-of- hospital ventricular fibrillation cardiac arrest should be lowered to 32-34°C. The cooling process should be started in the pre-hospital setting or as soon as possible and continued for 12-24 hours. Core temperature should be continuously monitored via the esophagus, rectum, trachea or bladder. General management of hypothermia patients includes concurrent measurement of mean arterial pressure, central venous pressure, urine output, arterial blood gases, central venous oxygen saturation, serum lactate, blood glucose, electrolytes, and complete blood count, and continuous ECG monitoring and stabilization.
After hypothermia, patients should be re-warmed at a rate of 0.5°C per hour with avoidance of hyperthermia. Potassium administraction should be stopped to avoid hyperkalemia during the re-warming phase. After re-warming to 36°C, sedation and paralytic agents should be discontinued and the patient should be weened off ventilator support (Jacobshagen et al, 2010). Neurologic recovery can take several hours after discontinuation of hypothermia. Therefore, it is important to wait until the patient is completely re-warmed and stabile before evaluating patients with prognositic neurologic exams like the Glasgow Coma Scale.

11. Conclusions

Mild therapeutic hypothermia is indicated for use in witnessed out-of-hospital cardiac arrest patients with a return of spontaneous circulation, for persons with an initial rhythm of ventricular fibrillation or non-perfusing ventricular tachycardia, for persons who are comatose or have a Glasgow coma score < 8, those who are hemodynamically stable, and those who lack a verbal response. Clinical evidence has shown that mild hypothermia decreases mortality and increases the proportion of patients with a favorable neurologic outcome (score of 1 or 2 on the CPC Scale) with mininimal risk of adverse effects. Therapeutic hypothermia is a relatively inexpensive treatment modality with an incremental cost-effectiveness ratio of $47,168 (Merchant et al, 2009) and can be implemented in a variety of settings from rural community-based hospitals to specialized cardiac and neurologic centers. The indications for mild therapeutic hypothermia will broaden in the future as more clinical trials are conducted. It is important to understand the pathophysiologic processes involved in the post-cardiac arrest syndrome, as well as the concominant changes in human physiology during induced mild therapeutic hypothermia.

12. References

Adler, J., Bessman, E., Talavera, F., Setnik, G., & Halamka, J.D.. Therapeutic hypothermia. (2011). (http://emedicine.medscape.com/article/812407-overview).

Arrich, J., Holzer, M., Herkner, H., Mullner, M. (2009). Hypothermia for neuroprotection in adults after cardiopulmonary resuscitation. *Cochrane Database of Systematic Reviews* Issue 4. Art. No.: CD004128. DOI: 10.1002/14651858.CD004128.pub2

Bernard, S.A. (2002). Treatment of comatose survivors of out-of-hospital cardiac aresst with induced hypothermia. *New England Journal of Medicine* 346(8):557-563

Bernard, S., Buist, M,, Monteiro, O., Smith, K. (2003). Induced hypothermia using large volume, ice-cold intravenous fluid in comatose survivors of out-of-hospital cardiac arrest: a preliminary report. *Resuscitation* 56(1):9-13.

Haugk M, Stratil P, Sterz F, et al (2010). Temperature monitored on the cuff surface of an endotracheal tube reflects body temperature. *Crit Care Med* 38(7):1569-1573

Haugk M, Testori C, Sterz F, et al (2011). Relationship between time to target temperature and outcome in patients treated with therapeutic hypothermia after cardiac arrest. *Crit Care* 15(2):R101

Holzer, M. (2010). Targeted temperature management for comatose survivors of cardiac arrest. *New England Journal of Medicine* 363(13):1256-1264

Holzer, M., Sterz, F., Hypothermia After Cardiac Arrest Study Group. (2002). Therapeutic hypothermia after cardiopulmonary resuscitation. *Expert Rev Cardiovasc Ther* 1(2):317-25.

Howes D, Ohley W, Dorian P, et al (2010). Rapid induction of therapeutic hypothermia using convective-immersion surface cooling: safety, efficacy and outcomes. *Resuscitation* 81(4):388-392.

Hypothermia after Cardiac Arrest Study Group.(2002). Mild therapeutic hypothermia to improve the neurologic outcome after cardiac arrest. *New England Journal of Medicine* 346(8):549-556

Jacobshagen, C., Pelster, T., Pax, A., et al. (2010). Effects of mild hypothermia on hemodynamics in cardiac arrest survivors and isolated failing human myocardium. *Clinical Research in Cardiology* 99(5):267-276

Koreny M, Sterz F, Uray T, et al (2009). Effect of cooling after human cardiac arrest on myocardial infarct size. *Resuscitation* 80(1):56-60

Merchant, R.M., Becker, L.B., Abella, B.S., Asch, D.A., Groeneveld, P.W. Cost-effectiveness of therapeutic hypothermia after cardiac arrest. *Circulation: Cardiovascular Quality Outcomes*. 2009 Sep;2(5):421-428

Nolan, J.P., Morley, P.T., Vanden Hoek, T.L., & Hickey, R.W. (2003). Therapeutic hypothermia after cardiac arrest.

An advisory statement by the Advanced Life Support Task Force of the International Liaison Committee on Resuscitation. *Resuscitation* 57(3):231-235

Nolan, J.P. (2008). Post-cardiac arrest syndrome: epidemiology, pathophysiology, treatment, and prognostication. *Resuscitation* 79(3):350-379

Oommen, S.S., & Menon V. (2011). Hypothermia after cardiac arrest: beneficial, but slow to be adopted. *Cleveland Clinic Journal of Medicine* 78 (7):441-448

Prior, J., Lawhon-Triano, M., Fedor, M., et al. (2010). Community-based application of mild therapeutic hypothermia for survivors of cardiac arrest. *Southern Medical Journal* 103(4):295-300

Polderman, K.H. Mechanisms of action, physiological effects, and complications of hypothermia. (2009). *Crit Care Med* ;37(7 Suppl):S186-202

Safar, P.J., & Kochanek, P.M. (2002). Therapeutic hypothermia after cardiac arrest. *New England Journal of Medicine* 346(8):612-613

Sinclair, H.L., & Andrews, P.J.D. (2010). Bench-to-bedside review: hypothermia in traumatic brain injury. *Critical Care* 14(1):204

Testori, C., Sterz, F., Behringer, W., et al. (2011). Mild therapeutic hypothermia is associated with favourable outcome in patients after cardiac arrest with non-shockable rhythms. *Resuscitation* 82(9):1162-1167

Vanston, V.J., Lawhon-Triano, M., Getts, R., et al. (2010). Predictors of poor neurologic outcome in patients undergoing therapeutic hypothermia after cardiac arrest. *Southern Medical Journal* 103(4):301-306

Wandaller, C., Holzer, M., Sterz, F., et al. (2009). Head and neck cooling after cardiac arrest results in lower jugular bulb than esophageal temperature. *American Journal of Emergency Medicine* 27(4):460-465

Weihs, W., Schratter, A., Sterz, F., et al. (2011). The importance of surface area for the cooling efficacy of mild therapeutic hypothermia. *Resuscitation* 82(1):74-78

Zeiner, A., Klewer, J., Sterz, F., et al. (2010). Non-invasive continuous cerebral temperature monitoring in patients treated with mild therapeutic hypothermia: an observational pilot study. *Resuscitation* 81(7):861-866

24

Arrhythmias in Pregnancy

Marius Craina[1], Gheorghe Furău[2], Răzvan Nițu[1], Lavinia Stelea[1], Dan Ancuşa[1], Corina Şerban[1], Rodica Mihăescu[1] and Ioana Mozoş[1]
[1]"Victor Babeş" University of Medicine and Pharmacy, Timişoara,
[2]"Vasile Goldiş" Western University of Arad,
Romania

1. Introduction

Pregnancies, as well as the post-partum period, are characterized by important metabolic changes. A lot of physiological changes affect the circulating blood volume, peripheral vascular compliance and resistance, myocardial function, heart rate and the neuro-hormonal system. These changes are well known in normal pregnancies, due to thorough examination and intense study; however there are still some questions related to the differences between women with and without structural diseases. Tocolitic medication used in pregnancy can cause cardiac complications in a healthy woman.

The presence of cardiovascular diseases in pregnancy must not be ignored because:

- Cardiovascular diseases are top causes of non-obstetrical maternal death (Sullivan, 1990).
- The modern possibilities of investigation improved diagnosis of cardiac diseases.
- The modern therapy can help women with cardiovascular diseases to have a good pregnancy outcome. Until recently, pregnancy was forbidden in those women.
- Women with repaired congenital heart defects. These women will have an increased risk of arrhythmias during pregnancy (Tateno, 2003). These types of patients usually have fragile hemodynamics and need additional therapy in most of the cases.

2. Physiological changes during pregnancy

The antepartum period is characterized by three main changes: an increased blood volume and heart rate and a reduction in the systemic vascular resistance. The increased blood volume can be estimated by examining ventricular diastolic volume and pressure. The increase starts gradually in the 6th week of gestation and by the end of the pregnancy it will reach 50% more than in the pre-pregnant state (Lind, 1985). However, this value is not constant. Studies have shown that there are increases from 20% to 100% above pre-pregnant blood volume (Pirani, 1973). It has been demonstrated that the blood volume increases at least until mid-pregnancy. The period, when the blood pressure plateaus, is arguable: some studies consider that it plateaus in the third trimester (Rovinsky, 1965), others have found a continuous increase until term (Lund, 1967). Blood volume increases considerably in a twin pregnancy (Thomsen, 1994). The increase in the end-diastolic volume can be noticed after 10 weeks of gestation and it will peak during the third trimester (Campos O, 1996). Pregnancy is associated with "physiological anemia", as a consequence of hemodilution (there is a proportional greater increase in the plasma volume than in the red blood cell mass, the latter being around 40% above pre-pregnancy levels) (Pirani 1973). Hypervolemia is caused by hormonal factors like: prolactin, placental lactogen, growth hormone, and estrogen or peptides like the prostaglandins. Considering women without heart disease, the cardiac filling pressures are not higher in women at term compared to women 11-13 weeks' postpartum (Clark, 1989). The vascular resistance differs from one pregnancy state to another. A fall in systemic vascular resistance has been described in the 5th week of gestation; a nadir between the 20th and 32nd week was followed by a slowly increase. The overall fall in the systemic vascular resistance occurs because of the changes in the resistance and flow in multiple vascular beds, such as the uteroplacental, renal, muscular, cutaneous and mammary bed. There are no changes in the hepatic or the cerebral blood flow. Variations in the renal and unteroplacental blood flow are primarily caused by positional changes (Jurkovic, 1991). For example, in the supine position in case of a pregnant woman, there is a compression of the inferior vena cava. An obstruction of the abdominal aorta and iliac arteries may also occur because of the uterus (Bieniarz, 1969). The resistance of these vascular beds is decreased due to the great amount of secreted vasodilators for example prostacyclin.

The systemic arterial pressure has a similar behavior: it decreases in the first semester and reaches its nadir at mid-pregnancy. Thereafter it increases and, in some cases, its level is higher than the pre-pregnancy level. The cardiac output is the most common measure of cardiac performance. Cardiac output, which is dependent on the heart rate and stroke volume, is gradually increasing by about 30-50% (Clark, 1989; and Rubler S, 1977) in the 5th week of gestation, reaching its peak at approximately the end of the second trimester (Robson, 1989) or in the third trimester (Bader, 1955). Afterwards, it is either constant until term or it decreases slightly near term. Although the amount of the oxygen in the blood is proportional with the cardiac output; there is no relation between the cardiac output and oxygen consumption, the last, increasing progressively by 20-30% at term (Elkus, 1992). Studies show different results when the ejection fraction is debated: some indicate that there are no alterations in the left ventricular ejection fraction (Katz, 1978 and Geva T, 1997), meanwhile other demonstrate increases in ejection fraction (Robson, 1989). This may be a result of the different loading conditions. The ratio of early to late diastolic flow velocity has been shown to be lower during the third semester compared with postpartum (Sadaniantz, 1992).

There is a wide individual variation of heart rate; however it usually increases by 10-20 beats; peaking in the late second trimester or early third trimester. Most pregnant women remain in sinus rhythm; but premature atrial and ventricular complexes may frequently occur.

Hemodynamic changes are also a cause of neurohormonal responses. The most important are the vasodilators: nitric oxide and prostaglandins, which cause, on one hand decreases in the peripheral resistance and, on the other hand, changes in the uterine and renal blood flow. Decreased cerebral blood flow activates the sympathetic nervous system. Conversely, plasma volume expansion suppresses catecholamine levels.

Neurohormones also activate the renin-angiotensin-aldosterone system that is responsible for the regulation of the salt and water homeostasis in the body (August, 1990). Pregnancy is characterized by increased levels of renin and angiotensin. The increased level of renin is not dependent on the extracellular volume.

Natriuretic peptides (also activated by neurohormones) are associated with cardiovascular and renal functions. The level of the two main natriuretic peptides (the atrial natriuretic-ANP and the brain natriuretic-BNP) is increased during pregnancy (Yoshimura, 1994). Their release is caused by atrial and ventricular distension.

During the peripartum period the hemodynamics will radically change, due to pain, anxiety and uterine contractions. For example, uterine contractions will increase the blood volume up to 500 mL (Ueland, 1969). The blood loss will be associated to the type of delivery. If in vaginal delivery there is a 10% blood loss; in caesarian delivery there may be a loss of up to 29% of the total blood volume (Ueland, 1976). Research has demonstrated that the circulation is not influenced by the placental separation. With every contraction the cardiac output increases up to 7-15%, consequently increasing the basal blood pressure. Early after delivery, cardiac output may continue to increase to as much as 80% above pre-labour values. Cardiac output will return to pre-labour levels about 1 hour post-partum. In labour the amount of the catecholamine increase. As a result, the heart rate will have high values. These values are not constant, and depend on many factors such as: position or anesthesia. Hemodynamic parameters need around 6 months to return to their normal values. Immediately after delivery, the cardiac output increases by as much as 80%, followed by a decrease in 24 weeks. Within the first 3 days after delivery the blood volume will decrease by 20%, however the hematocrit needs 2 weeks to be stabilized. Also, within 2 weeks after delivery the systemic vascular resistance increases by 30 % (Robson, 1987), and the heart rate will return to baseline levels. Stroke volume decreases for the first 24 weeks after delivery. Systolic and diastolic blood pressures remain unaltered from late pregnancy until 12 weeks post-partum (Campos, 1996).

2.1 Prevalence of arrhythmias in pregnancy

The elevated levels of estrogen and b-choral gonadotropine appear, from experimental models, to affect the expression of cardiac ion channels. By functioning in a proarrhythmic way, pregnancy gives rise to significant problems concerning the diagnosis and treatment of certain arrhythmias, especially when drugs and/or non pharmaceutical therapeutic methods are required (Mark, 2002).

Palpitations, fatigue and syncope are common in pregnancy. The sinus rate increases by about 10 beats/minute during pregnancy, and sinus tachycardia greater than 100 beats/min is common (Conti, 2005). Extrasystoles, intermittent sinus tachycardia and non-sustained arrhythmia are encountered in more than 50% of pregnant women are investigated for symptoms of arrhythmia (Gowda, 2003). Some arrhythmias occuring during pregnancy represent a recurrence of a pre-existing problem, but a substantial number of cases appear for the first time in pregnancy. Bradyarrhythmias presenting during pregnancy are rare with a prevalence of about 1–20 000, and are usually caused by sinoatrial disease or congenital complete heart block (Lee, 1995). Atrial fibrillation and flutter are rarely encountered during pregnancy unless organic heart disease or endocrine disorders are present. Episodes of such arrhythmias appearing for the first time during pregnancy require further evaluation for possible congenital heart disease, rheumatic valvular disease or hyperthyroidism (Leung, 1998).

3. Mechanisms of arrhythmia in pregnancy

The management of the arrhythmia is not different in pregnant women. However, hemodynamic conditions should be considered.

The cardiovascular system undergoes significant changes in adaptation to pregnancy, including an increased heart rate and cardiac output, reduced systemic resistance, increased plasma catecholamine concentrations and adrenergic receptor sensitivity, atrial stretch and increased end-diastolic volumes due to intravascular volume expansion, as well as hormonal and emotional changes (Adamson, 2007). Pregnancies with abnormal uterine perfusion and subsequent pathological outcomes are paralleled by changes in ventricular repolarization, that precede clinical symptoms (Baumert, 2010). Repolarization of the ventricular myocardium might be affected in pregnancy due to changes in circulating hormones, electrolyte imbalances and increased sympathetic tone.

It is important to determine if the arrhythmia has clinical conequences such as deterioration of the underlying cardiac condition. Arrhythmogenic effects are linked to the type of arrhythmia. There is a high risk of maternal and fetal morbidity in women with repaired CHD (chronic heart diseases). Studies have demonstrated that simple tachyarrhythmia does not lead to death. However, death may occur if this type of arrhythmia is associated with structural diseases. New research suggests that women with cyanosis and CHD may experience still birth or miscarriage. In this situation, the best case scenario is a low birth weight infant.

4. Signs, investigations and diagnosis

4.1 Symptoms

Palpitations, the most common presenting symptom, are usually intermittent and only rarely indicate a serious problem. Patients with arrhythmia may also present with fatigue, breathlessness, peripheral edema and chest discomfort resulting from cardiac failure. Symptoms of thromboembolism may be the presenting feature of atrial fibrillation or atrial flutter. Patients complaining of palpitations, but without documented arrhythmia, have a low likelihood for having a life-threatening arrhythmia, and no further evaluation is warranted (Andreson, 1997). A history of previous heart disease increases the likelihood of life threatening arrythmias. Inquiry should be made about the family history, particularly with reference to cases of premature sudden death.

The severity of the symptoms allows the physician to judge whether the risks of therapy outweigh the benefits. The only difference in pregnancy is that the physician must consider the risk/benefit ratio for both the mother and the fetus. An arrhythmia that is hemodynamically compromising to the mother constitutes a major concern because of inadequate maternal, as well as placental, blood flow (Anderson, 1997).

4.2 Examination

The pulse may be abnormal during symptoms; the clinician should focus on looking for signs of heart disease that may be associated with arrhythmia, including scars from previous surgery, murmurs of structural heart disease and signs of cardiac failure. It is also important to look for systemic problems such as thyrotoxicosis that may cause arrhythmia. The diagnosis of heart disease in pregnancy is often difficult due to the anatomical and physiological changes in the cardiovascular system. Many symptoms and signs of normal pregnancy can mimic heart disease. Dyspnea is especially common, with 75% of women complaining of breathlessness by 31 weeks (Elkos, 1992). Orthopnea may also occur in the advanced stages of pregnancy and is due to pressure exerted on the diaphragm by the gravid uterus. Light-headedness and syncope can result from venocaval compression by the enlarged uterus causing supine hypotensive syndrome. Palpitations are common and are related to the increased heart rate and to women being more aware of their heart beat.

Abnormal findings which may warrant further evaluation include the following: (1) a laterally displaced apex beat (more than 2 cm beyond the mid-clavicular line) and (2) non-physiological murmurs such as diastolic murmurs, pan-systolic murmurs, late systolic murmurs, ejection systolic murmurs with intensities of grade 3 or more or those associated with ejection clicks. The radiation dose associated with a chest X-ray is very small (<0.005 rads) and the risk to the fetus is minimal with proper shielding. There should be no hesitancy in performing a chest X-ray when it is clinically indicated.

4.3 ECG

Several electrocardiographic changes have been described in pregnant patients (Gowda, 2003). Caution should be exercised when interpreting the electrocardiographic abnormalities in pregnant women, and must account for the normal physiological changes occuring in pregnancy. This may results in decreased PR, QRS, and QT intervals, but usually there is no change in the amplitude of the P wave, QRS complex, and T wave. There is an increase of the heart rate (about 10 beats/minute). The electrical axis shift can occur, more commonly leftward, due to rotation of the heart secondary to the enlargement of the gravid uterus. Premature atrial and ventricular contractions are common during pregnancy (Stein, 1999). Supraventricular tachycardia may occur as new onset paroxysmal supraventricular tachycardia or exacerbation during pregnancy, cause probably by the hyperdynamic state (Gowda, 2003). Wolf-Parkinson White (WPW) syndrome may first occur during pregnancy or the frequency of episodes may increase in women with previously diagnosed WPW syndrome. Atrial fibrillation and flutter are rare in pregnant patients and are secondary to congenital or valvular heart disease, electrolyte imbalances or metabolic disorders. Ventricular tachycardia raises usually the suspicion of underlying cardiovascular disease, but physical or physiological stresses may precipitate ventricular arrhythmias in pregnant women without structural heart disease. Bradyarrhythmias are uncommon in pregnancy.

A patient without previous heart disease will usually have a normal ECG between episodes of arrhythmia. Infrequently, a patient may have 12-lead ECG abnormalities indicative of primary 'electrical' disease, such as frequent ectopic beats or Wolff–Parkinson–White syndrome. A patient with previous heart disease may have an abnormal resting ECG, reflecting their condition and any surgical intervention they may have received in the past.

Arrhythmia symptoms are typically intermittent and a 12-lead ECG recording during symptoms may not be available. Prolonged ECG monitoring with either inpatient bedside monitoring or a portable Holter monitor may pick up an episode in a patient with frequent symptoms. Where symptoms are less frequent, it is appropriate for the patient to wear a cardiac rhythm event monitor for 7 days or longer, with a patient-activation function for use during episodes of symptoms. It is helpful for the patient to keep a diary of symptoms, which can then be related to the recorded rhythm. Most types of devices will also record asymptomatic episodes when the heart rate falls outside certain preprogrammed limits. The patient should be encouraged to pursue all her normal activities during the recording, in particular those activities that previously triggered her symptoms.

4.4 Echocardiography and Doppler

Echocardiography is of undisputed value in the diagnosis and follow-up of structural and functional heart disease, and should be considered an integral part of the investigation of any pregnant patient with arrhythmia. It is noninvasive and poses no risk to the fetus. It is the best way to exclude puerperal cardiomyopathy. Changes include slight increases in systolic and diastolic left ventricular dimensions, moderate increases in the size of the right atrium, right ventricle and left atrium, progressive dilatation of the pulmonary, tricuspid and mitral valve annuli with functional regurgitation (Campos, 2009).

4.5 Genetic testing

Several cardiac conditions increase the vulnerability to arrhythmias and have a defined genetic basis. Although routine genetic testing for these conditions is not currently available for the evaluation of arrhythmia risk in pregnancy, a detailed family history should always be taken, and include specific questioning about premature sudden death. Counseling about the risk of transmission of these conditions to offspring is essential, and it is likely that there will be an increasing role for pre-implantation diagnosis of these conditions in affected families (Ueda, 2004).

4.6 Laboratory tests

Laboratory tests are not effective in diagnosis of syncope, but it can reveal some of its causes. Blood tests like complete blood count, electrolyte panel, and chemistry panel can lead to causes of arrhythmia. The blood test count is used to detect anemia or acute blood loss. Electrolyte panel may reveal the level of hydration. As far as the chemistry panel is concerned, thyroid stimulating hormone and serum drug levels should be assessed. Studies have shown that routine blood tests are not always necessary or fruitful (Olshansky, 2008). Besides blood tests, there are more precise diagnostic tests, like HUTT used by clinicians to assess patients who present syncope (Bendit et al. 1996). Used first by the NASA, HUTT emerged in cardiology in 1980 (NASA 1999, Baron-Esquivas et al 2003). The design of the HUTT was based on the following physiological mechanism: due to gravity, in a up-ward position, the blood will be displaced downwards. Consequently, the venous system will expand. The sympathetic system will increase the PVR and the skeletal muscle tone, the latter being an important component in maintaining the upright posture and also helping the venous blood to return to the heart and brain (Brignole, 2005). The role of the HUTT is to inhibit the skeletal muscle pump in the extremities that are responsible for the upright posture or orthostatic stress. In normal conditions; skeletal muscles contraction does not occur when venous pooling starts. However, individuals presenting excessive venous pooling, difficulty with PVR or sensitivity to diminish venous return, may experience difficulty in maintaining the upright posture on HUTT. The number of HUTT protocols varies, but the main idea is to induce venous pooling either through passive upright position or using vasodilators (protenerol, nitroglycerin, and adenosine) which inhibit the innate skeletal muscle pump. Guidelines (American College of Cardiology 1996) state that HUTT is efficient in cases such as: recurrent syncope or single episode in a high-risk patient; no evidence of the structural heart disease; structural heart diseases, as long as other causes have been excluded by the diagnostic testing. There are also conditions in which HUTT has proved to be inefficient. The most common are syncope episodes without injury and not in high risk setting and syncope with identified cause and identification of NCS would not alter therapy. There are some cases in which the use of HUTT is forbidden (syncope with ventricular outflow obstruction, critical mitral stenosis, and critical cerebral vascular stenosis).

5. Treatment

Due to the fact that physiological changes of pregnancy affect drug absorption as well as the metabolism in several ways, it may be difficult to obtain adequate therapeutic drug levels and to avoid toxicity. This may explain why some women experience recurrence of symptoms of arrhythmia during pregnancy despite continuing therapy that had previously been effective (Tan, 2001).

Arrhythmias in pregnancy are treated conservatively. After determining the type of arrhythmia, the physician will evaluate for underlying causes. If symptoms are minimal, rest and vagal maneuvers may be used to help slow the heart rate. Vagal maneuvers include carotid massage, applying ice to the face, and the Valvsalva maneuver, which is the most successful in stopping tachycardias (Zu-Chi, 1998). When the arrhythmia causes symptoms or a drop in blood pressure, antiarrhythmic medications may be used. No anti-arrhythmic medication is completely safe during pregnancy; therefore medications are avoided during the first trimester, if possible, to limit risk to the fetus. Drugs with the longest safety record should be tried first. Propranolol, metoprolol, digoxin, and adenosine have been tested and shown to be well tolerated and safe during the second and third trimester (Ferrero, 2004).

When a cardiac disease is identified in a pregnant woman, we must keep in mind the following (ACOG, 1992):

- The blood volume and the cardiac output increase with approximately 50% at the beginning of the first trimester of pregnancy.
- There are big changes of the circulated volume and of the cardiac output during the birth and in the period after.
- The peripheral vascular resistance decreases in pregnancy and returns to minimum in the second trimester. After that it increases, up to 20% referred to normal, during late pregnancy.
- Hypercoagulability is present in pregnancy. This is very important, particularly in patients requiring anticoagulant therapy outside the pregnancy.

Pregnancies with any cardiac problem must be managed by a complex team, consisting of an obstetrician, a cardiologist and, if necessarily, an intensive therapy specialist and/or a fetal medicine specialist. The aforementioned are compulsory in order to obtain an excellent outcome both for mother and for the child.

5.1 Arrhythmia prevention

In pregnancy, risk of cardiac disease or arrhythmias should be eliminated by:

- *Making healthy lifestyle choices*

Living a "heart healthy" life is the best way to decrease the chances of developing heart disorders. Exercising regularly (brisk walking, running, bicycling, swimming) and eating healthy are the most important. According to the American Heart Association, a heart-healthy diet includes high amounts of fruits and vegetables (at least five servings a day) and of whole grain foods. It includes lean protein sources like fish, beans, and low-fat dairy products, derives most of its fat from unsaturated fats like olive oil, and avoids saturated fats, trans-fats, and cholesterol.

- *Maintaining a healthy weight*

It's important to balance the eaten calories with burned calories through daily activity and exercise. Obesity is linked to heart disease.

- *Smoking cessation and limiting the intake of caffeine or alcohol*

Tobacco contributes to as much as one-third of all cardiovascular disease. It is necessary to avoid or limit the intake of caffeine, alcohol, and other substances that may contribute to arrhythmias or heart disease. The American Heart Association recommends restriction of the use of alcohol to one drink a day for women and two a day for men (a drink equals 12 ounces of beer, 4 ounces of wine or 1 ounce of 100-proof spirits). A single episode of heavy consumption can trigger arrhythmias like atrial fibrillation. Stimulants, both legal and illegal, can contribute to the development of heart arrhythmias. Caffeine and nicotine may, in some cases, cause premature ventricular contractions, which, over time, may develop into more serious arrhythmias. Cocaine and amphetamines also accelerate the heart rate, in some cases leading to ventricular fibrillation and sudden death. Supplements or some herbal remedies may increase the risk of arrhythmias. For instance, Ephedra, the herbal supplement once promoted as a diet aid and energy booster, increases the risk of arrhythmia. In 2004 the FDA pulled it from the shelves for that very reason.

- *Avoiding unnecessary stress*, such as anger, anxiety or fear, and finding ways to manage or control stressful situations that cannot be avoided.
- *Avoiding stimulant medications*

Many drugs may cause arrhythmias. Over-the-counter cough and cold medicines may speed up the heart. And approximately 50 FDA-approved medications have the potential to prolong the QT interval—the measure of time it takes for the electrical system in the ventricles to recharge after each heartbeat—and thus cause the acquired form of long QT syndrome (LQTS), in which the heart's mechanical or pumping function is normal but its recharging system is slow or ineffective. Those medications include certain antibiotics, antidepressants, antifungal, antihistamines, psychotropic medications, oral hypoglycemic (medications for diabetes), anesthetic agents, and even drugs used to treat heart disease like lipid-lowing drugs and diuretics. Patients with inherited LQTS should always ask physicians and pharmacists if a prescribed drug has the potential to aggravate the condition. Women have a longer QT interval on the electrocardiogram compared to men, despite higher heart rates.

Tocolitics may induce arrhythmias. Corrected QT and Tpeak-Tend intervals were unchanged from pre-operative values after induction of spinal anaesthesia in women undergoing caesarian section, but increased significantly after oxytocin injection. The risk-benefit balance of oxytocin bolus during caesarean delivery should be discussed with women with a history of long QT syndrome. (Guillon, 2010). Women with a long QT syndrome are more susceptible to ventricular arrythmias during pregnancy, labour, delivery and postpartum (Drake, 2007; Seth, 2007).

- *Having regular physical exams* and promptly reporting any unusual symptoms to a physician. The Centers for Disease Control and Prevention suggests that families with a history of arrhythmias or sudden cardiac arrest consider screening younger family members.
- *Seeking treatment for underlying health problems* that may contribute to arrhythmias and heart disease.

Any of the following conditions can increase the likelihood of developing arrhythmias: coronary artery disease, congenital heart disease, heart failure, stroke, atherosclerosis, heart valve damage, high blood pressure, high cholesterol, diabetes, obesity, thyroid disease, advancing age

5.2 Monitoring and treating existing heart disorders

Effectively treating any existing heart disorder is the best way to prevent it from becoming more severe. This can be done by:

- Having regular check ups
- Understanding how various conditions increase the risk of arrhythmias.

- Learning about heart disorders, tests, and treatment options, and discussing them with caregivers.
- Finding out if the heart's electrical system and its ability to pump blood efficiently have been affected by heart muscle damage from a heart attack or another cause.
- Learning the importance of an ejection fraction (EF). EF is a measure of the proportion, or fraction, of blood the heart pumps out with each beat. An abnormally low EF is the single most important factor in predicting the risk of Sudden Cardiac Arrest (SCA).
- Following treatment plans.
- Reporting any new symptoms or changes in existing symptoms to physicians as soon as possible.

5.3 Treatment

When the treatment plan is conceived, the physician has to consider factors like: the severity of the arrhythmia, the severity of patient's symptoms, if the patient has other health problems/medications that the patient takes, patient's age, overall health, and personal and family medical history of the patient.

Arrhythmia treatments may include one or more of the following:

1. Medicine to prevent and control arrhythmias and to treat related conditions such as high blood pressure, coronary artery disease and heart failure
2. Anticoagulant medication to reduce the risk of blood clots and stroke
3. A pacemaker that uses batteries to help the heart to beat more regularly
4. Cardiac defibrillation and implanted cardioverter defibrillators (ICDs)
5. Cardiac ablation; cryoablation (the defective cells are detected with the help of computerized mapping techniques and destroyed with a cold probe).
6. Surgery
7. Cardioversion
8. Other therapies.

In association with the effect on the human body, heart medication is categorized into two groups: "rate control" medicines, are used to slow the heart rate to less than 100 beats per minute or "rhythm control" medications (antiarrhythmic/cardioversion drugs) used in order to restore your heart's normal sinus rhythm. The aforementioned drugs are being used less, with more care and often in conjunction with implantable cardioverter defibrillators (ICDs) or cardiac ablation.

Many of the prescription medications reviewed here are also used to treat other kinds of heart-related conditions, including heart failure, high blood pressure, and angina (chest pain).

5.3.1 Rate control heart medication

Rate control heart medicine may include beta or calcium channel blockers. The first group of medication reduces the heart rate and cardiac output by lowering the blood pressure by blocking adrenalin. The most used beta blockers are: Acebutolol, Atenolol, Betaxolol, Bisoprolol/hydrochlorothiazide, Carteolol, Esmolol, Metoprolol, Nadolol, Penbutolol, Pindolol, Propranolol and Timolol. Calcium channel blockers, also called "calcium antagonists", work by interrupting the movement of calcium into heart and blood vessel tissue, slowing the heart rate. They are used in other disorders like: angina and arrhythmias. Examples of calcium channel blockers: Amlodipine, Diltiazem, Felodipine, Isradipine, Nicardipine, Nifedipine, Nimodipine, Nisoldipine and Verapamil.

5.3.2 Rhythm control heart medications

Rhythm control medication includes sodium channel blockers, beta blockers, class III antiarrhythmics that slow the electrical conductivity of the heart to improve rhythm problems. This type of medication can be administrated intravenously in emergency situations and orally in long term situations: Amiodarone, Bepridil Hydrochloride, Disopyramide, Dofetilide, Flecainide, Ibutilide, Lidocaine, Procainamide, Propafenone, Propranolol, Quinidine, Sotalol and Tocainide.

5.3.3 Drug administration

All medications have potential side effects and risks. Antiarrhythmic drugs must be taken daily and indefinitely. There are also side effects that are hard to manage. These side effects may include proarrhythmia, which means drug-related arrhythmia. When medication proves unsuccessful, the American College of Cardiology and the American Heart Association suggest catheter (cardiac) ablation or surgical ablation as a safe and effective treatment option.

The greatest risk is however drug-induced congenital malformation, that is most prone to occur during fetal organogenesis, a process which is completed by the end of the first trimester. Thereafter, the risk is mainly of impaired growth and functional development, or direct toxicity to fetal tissues. Drugs given shortly before term or during labour may have adverse effects on labour or the neonate after delivery. Most antiarrhythmic drugs are categorized by the US Food and Drug Administration (FDA) as category C during pregnancy which signifies that: risk (to the fetus) cannot be ruled out. Adequate well-controlled human studies are lacking, and animal studies have shown a risk to the fetus or are lacking as well. There is a chance of fetal harm if the drug is administered during pregnancy; but the potential benefits may outweigh the risks (Blomstrom-Lundqvist, 2003).

Drug treatment is not required for a benign tachycardia that is well tolerated. A low dose should be used initially with titration according to response, and this must be accompanied by regular monitoring. The selection of an appropriate drug depends on knowledge of the arrhythmia mechanisms, and only drugs with a safe track record in pregnancy should be used. The most common drugs are: Adenosine, Digoxine, and Beta Blockers.

Research showed that Adenosine is useful for the emergency management of SVT and broad QRS complex tachycardias, and has been used safely in pregnant women (Blomstrom-Lundqvist, 2003). It is administered as a bolus dose and it has a very short duration of action of no more than 5–10 s. The role of this medication is to depress sinus and AV nodal function causing transient bradycardia and AV block in the mother, but it has no detectable effect on the fetal cardiac rhythm. Adenosine is contraindicated in patients with brittle asthma, in whom it may cause bronchospasm, and in those taking dipyridamole because of the risk of prolonged asystole.

There is a long history of digoxin use during pregnancy and it is considered to be safe (Blomstrom-Lundqvist, 2003). It crosses the placenta, but is not teratogenic. It is cleared by the kidney, although renal excretion is inhibited by concomitant use of amiodarone. It is mainly used for the control of ventricular rate in patients with persistent atrial fibrillation, but may also be effective in some cases of focal atrial tachycardia.

Propranolol is the beta blocker with the longest track record and is considered safe in pregnancy (Blomstrom-Lundqvist, 2003). Beta blockers are not teratogenic, but beta1-selective blockers, such as atenolol or metoprolol, may be preferred because they may interfere less with beta2-receptor-mediated uterine relaxation. However, beta1-selective agents achieve less complete cardiac beta blockade because there are functional beta2-

receptors on cardiac myocytes, and these may, therefore, be less effective anti-arrhythmic agents. There have been reports linking beta blockers to fetal bradycardia, hypotonia, hypoglycemia and intrauterine growth retardation.

Sotalol is a combined beta blocker and class III anti-arrhythmic drug. It does cross the placenta and is excreted renally. It has achieved class B classification with the FDA and its use in pregnant patients has been reported with no adverse outcome (Blomstrom-Lundqvist, 2003).

Flecainide has been used frequently during pregnancy and is a reasonable choice for patients with a structurally normal heart (Blomstrom-Lundqvist, 2003). It should probably be avoided in those with myocardial disease, and in particular patients with ventricular tachycardia or vulnerability to myocardial ischemia.

The conflict between the interests of the mother and the well-being of the fetus is thrown into sharp relief with Amiodarone. Amiodarone is a very effective anti-arrhythmic drug to treat and prevent life-threatening ventricular arrhythmias in patients with ventricular disease. Amiodarone crosses the placenta and achieves fetal concentrations of around 10% of maternal serum values (Ovadia, 1994). Maternal amiodarone use may cause a goiter, which in turn compromises the upper airway in the neonate. Amiodarone is prone to cause, neonatal hypothyroidism, and fetal growth retardation. For these reasons, amiodarone should be used only when the mother's life is significantly threatened and no other agent will do (Chow, 1998).

There are no reports of teratogenicity, but verapamil does cross the placenta and may have fetal cardiovascular effects (Klein, 1984). Intravenous verapamil is a useful alternative to adenosine for emergency termination of SVT, and oral verapamil may be used in patients to prevent SVT recurrence when beta blockers are contraindicated or not tolerated (Klein, 1984).

Anticoagulant medications help to prevent new clots appearance in the blood or existing clots from getting larger. They are often prescribed for patients with atrial fibrillation to help reduce stroke risk. Aspirin also is often recommended for these patients in addition to or instead of prescription anticoagulants.

The pacemaker is a small device that's surgically placed under the skin at the collarbone; wires lead from it to the atrium and ventricle(s). The pacemaker sends small electric signals through the wires to control the speed of the heartbeat. Most pacemakers contain a sensor that activates the device only when the heartbeat is abnormal.

An ICD (Implantable Cardioverter Defibrillator) provides automatic electrical therapy on a chronic basis for patients suffering from recurrent tachycardias. (When an episode of fast, irregular heartbeat begins, the device delivers a shock to end the tachycardia, preventing the heart from going into ventricular fibrillation, which is frequently fatal). The device is connected to leads positioned inside or on the surface of the heart. These leads sense cardiac rhythm, provide necessary electrical shocks when necessary, and at times - pace the heart as needed. Various leads are connected to a pulse generator implanted in a pouch beneath the skin of the chest or abdomen. Newer devices are smaller, with simpler lead systems and can be installed through blood vessels.

Women with an implanted cardioverter defibrillator (ICD) may undergo pregnancy successfully with a good reported outcome. Potentially threatening arrhythmias are promptly detected and automatically terminated by an ICD by, either a series of rapid pacing impulses delivered via an endocardial right ventricular pacing lead, or delivery of a synchronized shock between a coil electrode in the right ventricular cavity and a second electrode formed by the ICD box, which is located in the pre-pectoral position on the left. Prompt detection and termination of an arrhythmia by an ICD minimize the hemodynamic disturbance and thereby limit the risk of harm to the fetus. ICDs are configured to concentrate the maximal electrical field strength to the mother's ventricular myocardium, and the electrical energy to which the fetus is exposed is minimal. Delivered energies (2–40 J) are about a tenth of those used for external DC cardioversion. Research found Cardioversion safe for the entire pregnancy state therefore, it can be used, if necessary (Blomstrom, 2003). Also, there is not additional risk (excepting patients with underlying heart condition) to develop ICD complications, during pregnancy (Natale, 1997).

Ablation is a nonsurgical technique that neutralizes parts of the abnormal electrical pathway (tissue) that is causing the arrhythmia. The technique utilizes a variety of imaging and monitoring systems that navigate flexible wires (catheters) to the heart through an artery or vein, locate the abnormal electrical activity (where ablation is needed), and evaluate their progress.

Once in the heart, one or more catheters are used to pinpoint the source of the abnormal electrical signals. When the source of the arrhythmia is located, the catheter delivers bursts of high-energy waves that eliminate the abnormal areas.

There are two techniques of ablation: radiofrequency ablation and transcatheter technique. In this first technique, a catheter with an electrode at its tip is guided to the damaged portion of heart muscle and mild, painless radiofrequency energy is transmitted to the site of the pathway, killing a few cells (about 1/5 of an inch). Consequently, these cells stop conducting the extra impulses that caused the rapid heartbeats. This non-surgical procedure is used to treat patients suffering from atrial fibrillation, atrial flutter, atrial tachycardia and supraventricular tachycardia. The second technique, however, electrocauterization is performed at a targeted spot in the heart. This technique is generally used to treat supraventricular tachycardia.

Most patients who receive this treatment experience a long-term reduction in the number of episodes of arrhythmia and the severity of symptoms, or a permanent return to normal heart rhythm.

Sometimes, surgery is used to treat arrhythmia. Often this is done when surgery is already being performed for another reason, such as repair of a heart valve. One type of surgery for atrial fibrillation is called "maze" surgery. In this operation, the surgeon makes small cuts or burns in the atria, which prevent the spread of disorganized electrical signals. Ventricular resection implies the removal of a part of the heart's muscle, where the arrhythmia originates.

Coronary artery bypass surgery may be needed for arrhythmias caused by coronary artery disease. The operation improves blood supply to the heart muscle.

Cardioversion treatment can be chemical (implemented through fast-acting drugs) or electric (implemented through a direct current using paddles over the chest) and is used to restore the heart's normal rhythm. DC cardioversion may be used to terminate sustained tachycardias. It should be carried out with general anesthesia, or deep sedation with midazolam or diazepam. Traditionally, the cardioversion electrodes are placed at the right sternal edge and cardiac apex, but for atrial fibrillation, it may be more effective to use an anterior-posterior configuration. Firm downward pressure on the sternal paddle reduces the electrode separation and increases the intensity of the electrical field, thus maximizing the chance of success. A waveform that reverses polarity during delivery (biphasic waveform) achieves cardioversion at energy thresholds that are half those required when a monophasic waveform is used. For all tachyarrhythmias, except ventricular fibrillation, the shock should be synchronized to the R wave, to minimize the risk of inducing ventricular fibrillation. Patients with atrial flutter or fibrillation are particularly vulnerable to systemic thromboembolism after restoration of sinus rhythm. DC cardioversion should not be carried out on patients who have been in atrial fibrillation for longer than 24 hours unless the arrhythmia results in serious cardiovascular compromise, or the patient has been fully anticoagulated since the onset of arrhythmia, or the absence of thrombus in the left atrium has been verified by transesophageal echocardiography. Anticoagulation should be continued for a minimum of 4 weeks after DC cardioversion. DC cardioversion seems to be quite safe in all stages of pregnancy because the intensity of the electrical field to which the fetus is exposed is low. Nevertheless, the fetus should be carefully monitored throughout the procedure. In the later stages of pregnancy, full general anesthesia and intubation are used, considering the increased risk of gastric aspiration.

Vagal maneuvers are another arrhythmia treatment. These are simple exercises that sometimes can stop or slow down certain types of supraventricular arrhythmias. They stop the arrhythmia by affecting the vagus nerve, which controls the heart rate. Some vagal maneuvers include:

- Gagging
- Holding breath and bearing down (Valsalva maneuver)
- Immersing the face in ice-cold water
- Coughing
- Putting the fingers on the own eyelids and pressing down gently.

6. Management of specific arrhythmias during pregnancy, labour and delivery

Dynamic changes in maternal physiology, as well as concern for the fetal well-being, are factors that complicate the treatment of arrhythmia. Premature atrial and ventricular contractions associated with a structurally normal heart are considered to be benign. However, in order to prevent them, exacerbating factors (dehydration, caffeine, sleep deprivation) should be avoided. Also, nonpharmacologic vagal maneuvers are recommended in atrial tachycardias. In the aforementioned case, drug therapy is indicated as long as the patient present refractory symptoms. In order to prevent recurrence, digoxin and beta-blockers are recommended. If the patient does not respond to these, flecainide and propafenone should be taken into consideration. Cardioversion or intravenous adenosine is indicated in acute management. Arrhythmias in association with the Wolf-Parkinson-White syndrome should be treated with Prosainamide, during pregnancy.

Records demonstrating the safety usage of digoxin and beta-blockers have determined the specialists to use these drugs in diseases like atrial flutter and fibrillation. In these cases, there are some who appeal to a rate or rhythm control strategy, similar to the nonpregnant state.

The management of ventricular arrhythmias is closely associated to the underlying heart condition; for instance patients suffering from idiopathic ventricular tachycardia (VT), but whith a structurally normal heart will receive, as first line therapy, beta-blockers, with IC agents or sotalol as second-line agents.

In pregnancy, congenital heart diseases have a complex prognosis. In most cases, long QT or hypertrophic cardiomyopathy are associated with ventricular arrhythmias. Sustained VT can develop into peripartum cardiomyopathy or vasospastic coronary artery disease. In each case daily evaluation is compulsory. If VT is unstable hemodynamically, emergent cardioversion is recommended. Well tolerated VT is treated with lidocaine, however if VT is sustained or recurrent, procainamide, flacainide, propafenone, sotalol or amiodarone are required.

Conservatory management is the best option for asymptomatic bradycardia. In pregnancy, pacemakers' insertions are tolerated.

During labour as well as delivery, hemodynamic changes occur, due to pain, anxiety. These hemodynamic changes increase the risk of arrhythmia.

Holter monitorization of the pregnancies with arrhythmias showed a high incidence of ventricular and/or atrial extrasystoles, with no consequences on the future mother or on the child. They will gradually disappear in post-partum.

7. Conclusion

Pregnancy increases cardiac output, heart rate and prevalence of dysrrhythmias in normal healthy women. The factors that can promote arrhythmias during pregnancy are: the direct electrophysiological effects of the hormones, the increased sympathetic tone and sensitivity, hemodynamic changes, electrolyte imbalances, atrial stretch, increased end-diastolic volumes and underlying heart diseases.

The most important problem in patients diagnosed with cardiac arrhythmia in pregnancy is the early detection, a multidisciplinary monitorization and an adequate therapy. The purpose is to decrease the cardiovascular complications in pregnancy and to have a good pregnancy outcome.

8. References

Abbott, G.W.; Federico, S.; Splawski, S.I.; Marianne E Buck, Michael H Lehmann, et. al. MiRP1 forms I_{Kr} potassium channels with HERG and is associated with cardiac arrhythmia, *Cell,* Vol.97, No.2, (Aprilie, 1999), pp.175-187.

Anderson, M.H. Heart disease in pregnancy. (1997). In: Oakley C, ed. Heart disease in pregnancy. London: BMJ Publishing Group, pp. 248–81.

Adamson, D.L.; Nelson-Piercy, C. (2007). Managing palpitations and arrhythmias during pregnancy. *Heart,* Vol. 93, No.12, (December, 2007), pp. 1630–1636.

August, P.; Lenz, T.; Ales, K.L, et al. (1990). Longitudinal study of the renin–angiotensin–aldosterone system in hypertensive pregnant women: deviations related to the development of superimposed preeclampsia. *American Journal of Obstetrics and Gynecology,* vol. 163, (November, 1990), pp. 1612–1621.

Bader, R.A.; Bader, M.E.; Rose DF, Braunwald E. (1955). Hemodynamics at rest and during exercise in normal pregnancy as studies by cardiac catheterization. *Journal of Clinic Investigation,* Vol. 34, (October, 1955), pp. 1524–1536.

Baumert, M.; Seeck, A.; Faber, R., et al. (2010). Longitudinal changes in QT interval variability and rate adaptation in pregnancies with normal and abnormal uterine perfusion, *Hypertension Research,* Vol. 33, No. 6, (June, 2010), pp.555-560.

Bieniarz, J.; Yoshida, T.; Romero-Salinas, G.; Curuchet, E.; Caldeyro-Barcia, R.; Crottogini, J.J. (1969). Aortocaval compression by the uterus in late human pregnancy. IV.

Circulatory homeostasis by preferential perfusion of the placenta. *American Journal of Obstetrics and Gynecology,* Vol. 103, (January, 1969), pp. 19–31.

Blomstrom-Lundqvist, C.; Scheinman, M.M.; Aliot, E.M. et al. (2003) ACC/AHA/ESC guidelines for the management of patients with supraventricular arrhythmias. *Circulation,* Vol. 108, (October, 2003), pp. 1871–909.

Brodsky, M.; Doria, R.; Allen, B.; Sato, D.; Thomas, G.; Sada, M. (1992). Newonset ventricular tachycardia during pregnancy. *American Heart Journal,* Vol. 123, No.4, (April, 1992), pp. 933–941.

Campos, O. (1996). Doppler echocardiography during pregnancy: physiological and abnormal findings. *Echocardiography,* Vol. 13, (Mars, 1996), pp. 135–146.

Chow, T.; Galvin, J.; McGovern, B. (1998). Antiarrhythmic drug therapy in pregnancy and lactation. *American Journal of Cardiology,* Vol. 82, (August, 1998), pp. 58I–62I.

Clark, S.L.; Cotton, D.B.; Lee, W. et al. (1989). Central hemodynamic assessment of normal term pregnancy. *American Journal of Obstetrics and Gynecology,* Vol. 161, (December, 1989), pp.1439–1442.

Conti, J.B.; Curtis, A.B. (2005). Arrhythmias during pregnancy. In: Saksena S, Camm AJ (eds), Electrophysiological Disorders of the Heart. Philadelphia: Elsevier, pp. 517–532.

Drake, E.; Preston, R.; Douglas, J. (2007). Brief review: Anesthetic implications of long QT syndrome in pregnancy. *Canadian Journal of Anesthesia,* Vol. 54, No.7, (July, 2007), pp. 561-72.

Eliahou, H.E.; Silverberg, D.S.; Reisin, E.; Romem, I.; Mashiach, S.; Serr, D.M. (1978). Propranolol for the treatment of hypertension in pregnancy. *British Journal of Obstetrics and Gynaeco*logy, Vol. 85, No.6, (June, 1978), pp. 431–436.

Elkus, R.; Popovich, J. (1992). Jr. Respiratory physiology in pregnancy. *Clinics in Chest Medicine,* Vol. 13, No.4. (December, 1992), pp. 555–565.

Ferrero, S.; Colombo, B.M.; Ragni, N. (2004). Maternal arrhythmias during pregnancy. *Archives of Gynecology and Obstetrics, Vol.* 269, No. 4 (May, 2004), pp. 244-253.

Geva, T.; Mauer, M.B.; Striker, L.; Kirshon, B.; Pivarnik, J.M. (1997). Effects of physiologic load of pregnancy on left ventricular contractility and remodeling. *American Heart Journal,* Vol. 133, (January, 1997), pp. 53–59.

Gowda, R.M.; Khan IA, Mehta NJ, Vasavada BC, Sacchi TJ. (2003). Cardiac arrhythmias in pregnancy: clinical and therapeutic considerations. *International Journal of Cardiology,* Vol. 88, (April, 2003), pp.129–133.

Guillon, A.; Leyre, S.; Remerand, F.; et al. (2010). Modification of Tp-e and QTc intervals during caesarean section under spinal anaesthesia. *Anaesthesia,* Vol. 65, no. 4, (February, 2010), pp. 337-342.

Jurkovic, D.; Jauniaux, E.; Kurjak, A.; Hustin, J.; Campbell, S.; Nicolaides, K.H. (1991). Transvaginal color Doppler assessment of the uteroplacental circulation in early pregnancy. *Obstetrics and Gynecology,* Vol. 77, No.3. (March, 1977), pp. 365–369.

Katz, R.; Karliner, J.S.; Resnik, R. (1978). Effects of a natural volume overload state (pregnancy) on left ventricular performance in normal human subjects. *Circulation,* Vol. 58, (September, 1978), pp. 434–441.

Ueda, K.; Nakamura, K.; Hayashi, T. et al. (2004). Functional characterization of a trafficking- defective HCN4 mutation, D553N, associated with cardiac arrhythmia. *Journal of Biological Chemistry*, Vol. 279, No.26, (April, 2004), pp. 27194-27198.

Klein, V.; Repke, J.T. (1984). Supraventricular tachycardia in pregnancy: cardioversion with verapamil. *Obstetrics and Gynecology*, Vol. 63, Suppl. 3, (March, 1984), pp. 16S–18S.

Lee, S.H.; Chen, S.A.; Wu, T.J. et al. (1995). Effects of pregnancy on first onset and symptoms of paroxysmal supraventricular tachycardia. *American Journal of Cardiology*, Vol. 76, No.10, (October, 1995), pp.675–678.

Leung, C.; Brodsky, M. (1998). Cardiac arrhythmias and pregnancy, in Elkayam U (ed.): Cardiac Problems in Pregancy. Wiley-Liss, New York 1998; pp. 155-174.

Lind, T. (1985). Hematologic system. Maternal physiology. *Washington: CREOG*, Vol. 25, pp. 7–40.

Lydakis, C.; Lip, G.Y.; Beevers, M.; Beevers, D.G. (1999). Atenolol and fetal growth in pregnancies complicated by hypertension. *American Journal of Hypertension*, Vol.12, No.6. (June, 1999), pp. 541–547.

Mark, S.; Harris, L. (2002). Arrhythmias in pregnancy, in Wilansky S (ed.): Heart Disease in Women. Churchill Livingstone, Philadelphia, 2002; pp. 497-514.

Mashini, I.S.; Albazzaz, S.J.; Fadel, H.E. et al. (1987). Serial noninvasive evaluation of cardiovascular hemodynamics during pregnancy. *American Journal of Obstetrics and Gynecology*, Vol. 156, (May, 1987), pp. 1208–1213.

Natale, A.; Davidson, T.; Geiger, M.J.; Newby, K. (1997). Implantable cardioverter-defibrillators and pregnancy: a safe combination? *Circulation*, Vol. 96, No.9, (November, 1997), pp.2808-2012.

Onuigbo, M.; Alikhan, M. (1998). Over-the-counter sympathomimetics: a risk factor for cardiac arrhythmias in pregnancy. *South Medical Journal*, Vol.91, (December, 1998), pp.1153–1155.

Campos, O. (1996). Doppler echocardiography during pregnancy: physiological and abnormal findings. *Echocardiography*, Vol. 13, (March, 1996), pp. 135–146.

Ovadia, M.; Brito, M.; Hoyer, G.L.; Marcus, F.I. (1994). Human experience with amiodarone in the embryonic period. *American Journal of Cardiology*, Vol. 73, No.4, (February, 1994), pp. 316–317.

Pirani, B.B.; Campbell, D.M.; MacGillivray, I. (1973) Plasma volume in normal first pregnancy. *The Journal of obstetrics and gynaecology of the British Commonwealth*, Vol. 80, No.10, pp. 884–7.

Pritchard, J.A.; Rowland, R.C. (1964). Blood volume changes in pregnancy and the puerperium. III. Whole body and large vessel hematocrits in pregnant and nonpregnant women. *American Journal of Obstetrics and Gynecology*, Vol. 88, (April, 1964), pp.391–395.

Robson, S.C.; Hunter, S.; Boys, R.J.; Dunlop, W. (1989). Serial study of factors influencing changes in cardiac output during human pregnancy. *American Journal of Physiology*, Vol. 256, (April, 1989), pp. H1060–1065.

Robson, S.C.; Hunter, S.; Moore, M.; Dunlop, W. (1987). Haemodynamic changes during the puerperium: a Doppler and M-mode echocardiographic study. *British Journal of Obstetics and Gynaecology, Vol.* 94, pp. 1028–1039.

Rovinsky, J.J.; Jaffin, H. Cardiovascular hemodynamics in pregnancy. I. (1965). Blood and plasma volumes in multiple pregnancy. *American Journal of Obstetrics and Gynecology,* Vol. 93, (September, 1965), pp. 1–15.

Rubler, S.; Damani, P.M.; Pinto, E.R. (1977). Cardiac size and performance during pregnancy estimated with echocardiography. *American Journal of Cardiology,* Vol. 40, (October, 1977), pp. 534–540.

Sadaniantz, A.; Kocheril, A.G.; Emaus, S.P.; Garber, C.E.; Parisi, A.F. (1992). Cardiovascular changes in pregnancy evaluated by two-dimensional and Doppler echocardiography. *Journal of the American Society of Echocardiography,* Vol.5, (May-Jun, 1992), pp. 253–258.

Seth, R.; Moss, A.J.; Mc Nitt, S. et al. (2007). Long QT syndrome and pregnancy. *Journal of the American College of Cardiology,* Vol. 49, No. 10, (Mars, 2007), pp. 1092-1098.

Stein, P.K.; Hagley, M.T.; Cole, P.L.; Domitrovich, P.P.; Kleiger, R.E.; Rottman, J.N. (1999). Changes in 24-hour heart rate variability during normal pregnancy. *American Journal of Obstetrics and Gynecology,* Vol. 180, No.4, (April, 1999), pp. 978–985.

Tan, H.L.; Lie, K.I. (2001). Treatment of tachyarrhythmias during pregnancy and lactation. *European Heart Journal,* Vol. 22, No.6, (March, 2001), pp. 458–464.

Tateno, S.; Niwa, K.; Nakazawa, M.; Akagi, T.; Shinohara, T.; Usda, T. (2003). A Study Group for Arrhythmia Late after Surgery for Congenital Heart Disease (ALTAS- CHD). Circulation Journal. Vol. 67, no. 12, (December, 2003), pp. 992-997.

Tawam, M.; Levine. J.; Mendelson. M.; Goldberger, J.; Dyer, A.; Kadish, A. (1993). Effect of pregnancy on paroxysmal supraventricular tachycardia. *American Journal of Cardiology,* Vol. 72, No.11 (October, 1993), pp. 838–840.

Taylor, D.J.; Lind, T. (1979). Red cell mass during and after normal pregnancy. *British Journal of Obstetrics and Gynaecology,* Vol. 86, No.5, (May, 1979), pp. 364–70.

Thomsen, J.K.; Fogh-Andersen, N.; Jaszczak. P. (1994). Atrial natriuretic peptide, blood volume, aldosterone, and sodium excretion during twin pregnancy. *Acta Obstetica et Gynecologica Scandinavica,* Vol. 73, No.1, (January, 1994), pp. 14–20.

Ueland, K.; Hansen, JM. (1969). Maternal cardiovascular dynamics. 3. Labour and delivery under local and caudal analgesia. *American Journal of Obstetrics and Gynecology,* Vol.103, No.1, (January, 1969), pp.8–18.

Ueland, K. (1976). Maternal cardiovascular dynamics. VII. Intrapartum blood volume changes. *American Journal of Obstetrics and Gynecology,* Vol. 126, No.6, (November, 1976), pp. 671–677.

Yoshimura, T.; Yoshimura, M.; Yasue, H. et al. (1994). Plasma concentration of atrial natriuretic peptide and brain natriuretic peptide during normal human pregnancy and the postpartum period. *Journal of Endocrinology,* Vol. 140, No.3. (March, 1994), pp. 393–397.

Wen, Z.C.; Chen, S.A.; Tai, C.T.; Chiang, C.E.; Chiou, C.W.; Chang, M.S. (1998). Electrophysiological mechanisms and determinants of vagal maneuvers for termination of paroxysmal supraventricular tachycardia. *Circulation*, Vol. 98, No.24, (December, 1998), pp. 2716 –2723.

25

Development of Computer Aided Prediction Technology for Paroxysmal Atrial Fibrillation in Mobile Healthcare

Desok Kim[1], Jae-Hyeong Park[2] and Jun Hyung Kim[2]
[1]*Departments of Electrical Engineering and Information Communication Engineering, KAIST, Daejeon,*
[2]*Chungnam National University, School of Medicine and Hospital, Department of Cardiology, Daejeon, Korea*

1. Introduction

Atrial fibrillation (AF) is one of the major health risks for strokes, and has been found to increase the risk of ischemic stroke fivefold (Wolf et al., 1987). Strokes with AF are more severe, cause greater disability and have worse outcomes than those without (Jørgensen et al., 1996; Lin et al., 1996). Approximately 15–20% of all strokes are due to AF but the percentage increases up to 40% for patients over the age of 90 (Marini et al., 2005). As the risk of initial strokes in these patients can be reduced up to 64% by long-term treatment with anti-coagulants (Hart et al., 2007), accurate and timely detection of AF is essential in high-risk elderly populations. Paroxysmal AF (PAF) is defined as an AF episode that lasts longer than 2 min but less than 7 days. Most PAF episodes terminate spontaneously within 24 h. Although PAF is short-lived, it shares similar stroke risks with long-lasting persistent AF (Friberg et al., 2010). Furthermore, the rare and asymptomatic manifestation of AF episodes makes a definitive diagnosis of PAF even harder to provide. Holter or event recorder devices are used conventionally to capture actual episodes of AF. Using 24-h Holter monitoring, only 23% of cases were detected among PAF patients whose diagnosis was confirmed by continuous bedside electrocardiograph (ECG) monitoring (Rizos et al., 2010), which indicates an underestimated detection of PAF leading to inadequate treatment. Using 7-day event-loop recording, 5.7% of cases that were missed by 24-h Holter monitoring were revealed to be PAF (Jabaudon et al., 2004). Thus, prolonged ECG monitoring by event recorders improves the detection rates of PAF cases. However, event recorders may not be appropriate for all patients, and depend on patient compliance. The extended use of Holter monitors is not commonly practiced in clinics, and few technical guidelines are currently available for the improvement of PAF detection by a short-term use of Holter monitors.

Prediction methods have been studied in order to suppress PAF episodes through atrial pacing techniques and to provide the clinical benefit of maintaining normal sinus rhythm (NSR) in, for example, drug-refractory AF patients (Delfaut et al., 1998). Most of the methods developed were inspired by earlier physiological findings that were associated with the triggering mechanisms of PAF, namely, activated ectopic nodes in abnormal atrial tissue and the imbalance of the autonomic nervous system (ANS) via increased sympathetic or parasympathetic tone. A hypothetical transition period has been proposed during which the triggering mechanisms are activated, forcing NSR to change to PAF. During the transition, the number of premature atrial complexes (PAC), runs of atrial bigeminy and trigeminy, and length of paroxysmal atrial tachycardia were increased before PAF onset (Thong et al., 2004). Spectral analysis revealed a significant increase in ANS activity in both the sympathetic and parasympathetic branches, which were represented by increased low-frequency (LF) and high-frequency (HF) components in the power spectrum density of the heartbeat intervals (RR intervals) (Chesnokov et al., 2008; Kim et al., 2008a). Heart rate variability (HRV) features in time domain analysis were also significantly changed during the transition (Kim et al., 2008a), again indicating a change in ANS activity. The complexity of RR interval dynamics decreased before the onset of PAF episodes (Chesnokov, 2008; Vikman et al., 1999). Poincaré plots depicting the correlation between two successive RR intervals in a two-dimensional diagram were also found to be closely related to ANS activity and to exhibit highly heterogeneous patterns during the transition (Duong et al., 2009). Recently, recurrence plots representing the frequency of two RR intervals in close proximity were investigated to discover dynamic behaviors during the transition that were not uncovered by earlier methods (Mohebbi & Ghassemian, 2011). In these studies, prediction models were derived by running pattern classification algorithms on learning sets that consisted of two types of ECG data: one distant and the other immediately before the onsets, representing NSR and the transition period, respectively (available from the PhysioBank's MIT-BIH AF Prediction Database as 30-min ECG data sets). These prediction models were able to detect the transition to PAF events at rates of 70–97%. Some of PAF prediction reports are summarized in Table 1. Recent reviews of these techniques and their performance are also available (Sahoo et al., 2011; Mohebbi & Ghassemian, 2011). To apply these methods to atrial pacing techniques, ECG data need to be sampled continuously.

Authors	Feature sets	Accuracy (%)	Sensitivity (%)	Specificity (%)	Duration of ECG learning sets	Databases and their usage
Thong et al. (2004)	Number of PACs, bigeminy, and trigeminy	90	89	91	30 min	MIT-BIH AF Prediction Database as learning and test sets
Mohebbi & Ghassemi (2011)	Recurrent plots (recurrence rate, L_{max}, L_{mean}, entropy, and trapping time)		97	100	30 min	
Hickey et al. (2004)	LF, HF, and power spectral density, PAC	80.5	43.0	99.3	30 min	MIT-BIH AF Prediction Database as learning sets
	Empirical rule	100	100	100	All 30-min segments	MIT-BIH AF and NSR Database as test sets
Kikillus et al. (2008)	Poincaré plot image, SDSD	94.4	91.5	96.9	60 min	MIT-BIH AF and NSR Database as learning and test sets
Kim et al. (2008a)	HRV features		90	95	3 min	MIT-BIH AF and NSR Database as learning and test sets

Table 1. Summary of previous studies for the prediction of AF onsets and PAF subjects

Due to the low detection rates of PAF events provided by Holter devices, alternative approaches have been motivated by the physiological findings of different dynamics of heart rate controls in PAF subjects, even when AF is not actually occurring. Thus, instead of relying on the capture of PAF episodes, prediction methods have been developed to provide a diagnostic assessment of PAF cases that display either no episodes of AF or a small number of episodes (Hickey et al., 2004; Kikillus et al., 2008; Kim et al., 2008a). Although these prediction models were motivated by the similar findings and methods explained above, they were evaluated against public databases that provide long-term ECG data from PAF and NSR subjects (available from the PhysioBank's MIT-BIH AF and NSR Databases). The AF Database provides 25 ECG data sets of 10-h recordings obtained from patients with PAF. The NSR Database provides 18 ECG data sets of 24-h recordings obtained from healthy persons with no arrhythmias. Numerous approaches have been reported because multiple representations of heart rate dynamics were feasible at different time-points of the day or night. Each short segment was classified by a first-stage classifier who relied on the detection of abnormal HRV features and PAC. To incorporate prediction results made at different time-points into one assessment, a second-stage classifier inquired whether an empirical rule was satisfied. For example, a subject was classified as PAF if at least 10% of the segments were classified as PAF segments and the average probability of PAF was at least 0.35 (Hickey et al., 2004). For this approach, finding the empirical rule was critical to evaluate the performance of the classifier. The performance of this prediction model may be directly related to not only how often a PAF patient experiences a physiological condition resembling the transition period, but also how often actual PAF episodes occur immediately after the presumed transition period. However, no information is available on the frequency of a transition period being followed by an actual PAF event. Furthermore, the performance of these prediction models over a long-term monitoring period has not yet been investigated.

In contrast, if the sampling of ECG data as learning sets is not confined to the transition period, then a prediction model may be less sensitive to whether a subject experiences the transition period or not and still performs as anticipated. Instead of confining learning set samples to the transition period, 1-h ECG segments were sampled from all available time-points and evaluated by a classifier based on a risk assessment of HRV analysis and Poincaré plot analysis performed on all samples (Kikillus et al., 2008). Because the test sets included the AF episodes, the classification performance was sensitive to the length of AF episodes included in the data. Alternatively, multiple ultra-short 3-min segments were sampled from different time periods of the day and classified using two different formulas designed for day or evening time (Kim et al., 2008a, 2008b). This method did not contain AF episodes in the test data, and thus the prediction accuracy relates exclusively to detecting the transition period. In addition, transition periods were treated differently depending on the time of their occurrence (Kim et al., 2008b), which resulted in two time-dependent classifiers performing better than one classifier disregarding the occurrence time of transitions. These methods require ECG data to be continuously analyzed, that may demand some extraordinary functional capabilities from wireless devices and data networks in mobile healthcare systems. For instance, a limited battery time is common in potable wireless gateway devices such as personal data assistant (PDA) or cellular phones. Network congestion and loss should be avoided or reliably handled in a medical sensor network (MSN) (Hu & Xiao, 2009) that may monitors large number of mobile subjects. As a strategy that alleviates these requirements of future mobile healthcare devices and networks, an intermittent data sampling and its relevance to clinical decision makings could be considered. Thus, we propose that intermittently sampled ECG data (but devoid of any arrhythmic

episodes) may be used as learning sets for calculating a PAF prediction model. Our driving hypothesis remains the same as that stated in previous reports: the non-episodic state of PAF subjects is different to that of NSR subjects (Kikillus et al., 2008; Kim et al., 2008a).
The recurrence rate of silent AF is high even when the patient has undergone apparently successful ablation or drug therapy. Patients who had been treated with atrial ablation and circumferential pulmonary vein ablation were reported to have a 26.7% recurrence rate after 13 months and a rate of 31% after 19 months, respectively (Berruezo et al., 2007; Grubitzsch et al., 2008). Patients who underwent chemical or electrical cardioversion also showed high recurrence rates of 30–43% after 0.5–42 months (Aytemir et al., 1999; Lombardi et al., 2001). The recurrence of silent AF in stroke victims can also be as high as the percentage reported in these earlier studies. If clinicians and patients can be alarmed by the early diagnosis of AF to take appropriate measures and avoid the recurrence of ischemic strokes, tens of thousands of recurrent stroke victims can be saved each year. In this study, we first sought to develop a detection method for PAF subjects using HRV patterns obtained from intermittently sampled ECG. Based on this model, we then sought to predict recurrent PAF subjects among patients who had been successfully treated for AF previously and were currently under anti-arrhythmic medication. In addition, we have implemented our algorithms to a remote real-time heartbeat analysis system that consists of a portable ECG sensor with a three-axis accelerometer, a smart phone, and a data analysis server. This internet-based system should provide a developmental platform to investigate the detection of PAF further through the use of long-term monitoring.

2. Methods and subjects

2.1 Subjects and data acquisition

The 24-h ECG data of 50 cases were obtained from the archive storage in Chungnam National University Hospital, Department of Cardiology. Subjects visited the clinic due for a variety of complaints with symptoms that might have been related to underlying cardiac diseases. Data were included if the subject was older than 35 years, had visited the clinic during the past 2 years, and were free of any cardiovascular disease. All ECG data were obtained by using the same type of Holter monitors for 24 h. The use of patient ECG data was approved by the internal review board of the hospital.
Thirty-nine patients with previously diagnosed AF were recruited for 48-h Holter monitoring in the same department. Patients completed the consent form for the use of experimental data and a stress questionnaire (Koh et al., 2001). Six patients were excluded due to the failure of 48-h Holter monitoring (n = 3) and the loss of ECG data during data handling (n = 3). A total of 33 patients had been under AF management for the past 1.5 years on average (15 women: age range, 39–82 years, median age, 66 years; and 18 men: age range, 43–78 years, median age, 66 years). This experiment was approved by the internal review board of the hospital.

2.2 Data processing

2.2.1 Preparation of ECG data

ECG signals were sampled at 125 samples per second by Holter recorders (Marquette MARS PC Holter monitor, GE Healthcare) and screened for arrhythmic events first by the computer software and then by two cardiologists. A 24-h binary record (in .bin format) was transformed into four 6-h text-based records using a software tool called "rdsamp.exe" available at the Physionet. Each record represented four different time periods of the day (namely morning from 6 am to 12 noon, afternoon from noon to 6 pm, evening from 6 pm to 12 midnight, and night from midnight to 6 am). ECG segments that contained arrhythmic episodes were also removed based on medical records. Noisy parts of ECG data were automatically removed by a cut-off value that represented the maximum value of local heterogeneity of ECG signals (data not shown). The percentage of ECG signals detected as noise was also recorded.

2.2.2 RR interval detection

Time intervals between two successive QRS complexes (RR intervals) were obtained using the previous ECG analysis software for a mobile application (Salahuddin & Kim, 2006). Java-based analysis software was developed to detect RR intervals and calculate the HRV features. The analysis algorithm was mainly adapted from a derivative method (Pan & Tompkins, 1985) but several modifications had to be added to ensure the detection of true RR intervals in noisy ECG signals. Briefly, a tophat operation was performed on the band-pass waveforms to suppress noisy peaks and remove the baseline shift. A set of rules was applied to avoid detecting R peaks from unusually high or low amplitude parts and noisy parts of ECG signals. After detecting R peaks, another set of rules was applied to avoid extracting RR intervals that were too short or too long compared with average RR intervals calculated from accumulated RR intervals. The analysis algorithm was divided into three phases: a pre-processing, an R peak decision and a post-processing. During the pre-processing phase, the ECG signal (Figure 1a) was passed through a band-pass filter — a 60th order finite impulse response digital filter using a Hamming window — with a cut-off frequency ranging from 8 to 12 Hz (Figure 1b). The band-passed signal was then filtered through a tophat operation that consisted of a series of minimum and maximum operations and a subtraction operation (Figure 1c). Since the size of the tophat filter was set to equal the average width at half maximum of the R peaks (seven time-points), tophat filtering preferentially enhanced RR intervals and suppressed noisy small peaks and large T peaks. The subtraction of the minimum-maximum filtered waveforms from the original waveforms eliminated baseline drifts completely. The tophat-processed ECG signal was differentiated so that RR interval signals resulted in two wave peaks with relatively larger amplitudes (Figure 1d). The resultant signal was squared to amplify the part of the signal with larger amplitude to a greater extent (Figure 1e). An integral waveform was generated by a moving window of 30 time-points in width (Figure 1f). The integral waveform was compared with the adaptive thresholds that were continuously updated estimates of the peak signal level (Figure 1g) and the peak noise level (data not shown) (Pan & Tompkins, 1985). In our algorithm, the search back (or dual thresholds) technique (Pan & Tompkins, 1985) was not used since it did not seem to contribute significantly to the detection of the RR intervals of our ECG signals. The adaptive threshold produced a series of time-point ranges (rectangular wave tops), representing possible locations of R peak candidates (Figure 1h). The local maximum of band-passed waveform within each range was found to be an R peak candidate (shown as arrowheads in Figure 1i). During the R peak decision phase, a true R peak was found if the following two conditions were satisfied at the time-point of the R peak candidate: 1) if the amplitude of the raw signal was less than 1000; and 2) if the amplitude of tophat-filtered signal was greater than 30. During the post-processing phase, some RR intervals were often found to be unreasonably short or long due to errors such as detecting spurious peaks or missing true peaks. An RR interval was considered as valid if it satisfied the following two conditions: 1) if the RR interval was longer than 0.75 times; and 2) if the RR interval was shorter than 1.5 times the accumulated RR interval average to avoid unusually short or long RR intervals caused by noisy signals or missing R peaks, respectively.

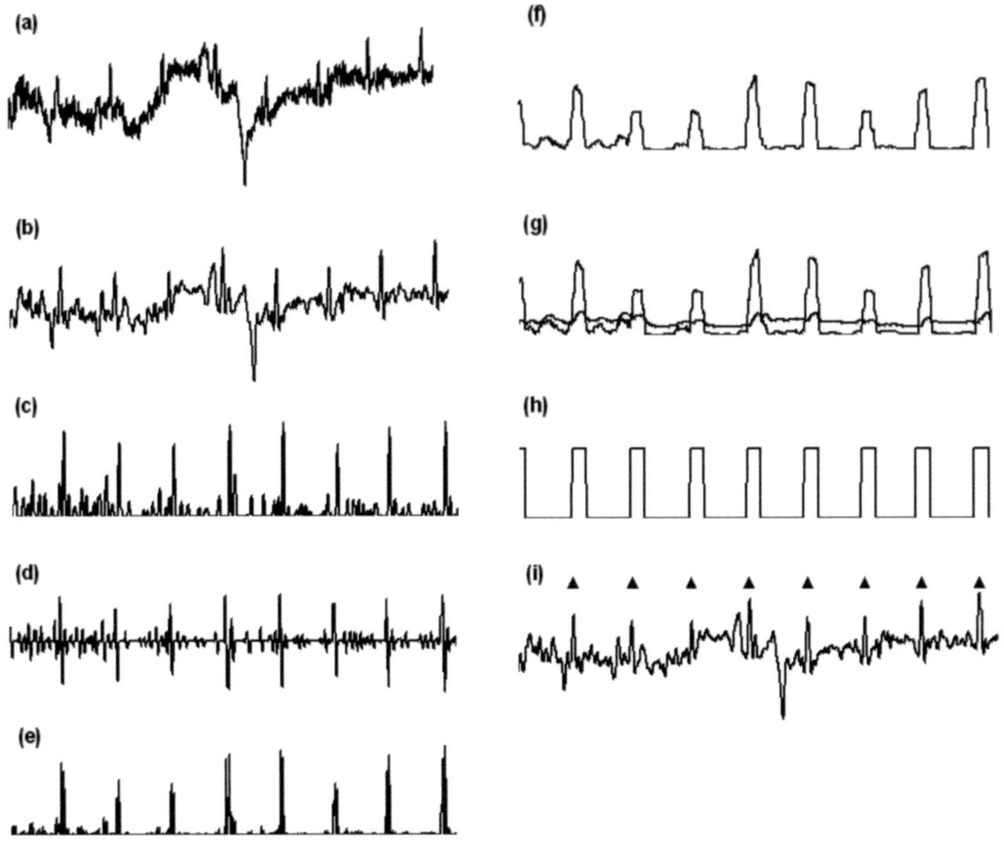

Fig. 1. Processing steps of R peak detection algorithm. (a) the input signal, (b) the output of bandpass filtering, (c) tophat, (d) differentiator, (e) squaring; (f) moving-window integration, (g) locally adaptive thresholding, (h) possible QRS complex ranges, (i) QRS complex candidates detected from band-passed waveform. (Permission from Salahuddin & Kim, 2006).

2.2.3 HRV calculation

From each 6-h RR interval record, four 30-min RR records were randomly selected. The baseline trend in heart rates introduced by postural change or movement was removed using a linear curve-fitting method. Detrended time series were cubically interpolated and re-sampled at 4 Hz, and the fast Fourier transform was windowed with 256-sample-width Hamming windows with 50% overlap. All HRV features were calculated from the detrended RR interval series.

In each RR interval set, the following HRV features were calculated using the ECG analysis software (also available at http://mhealth.kaist.ac.kr/afdectection): mean heart rate (mean HR), mean heartbeat intervals (mean RR), standard deviation of NN interval (SDNN), coefficient of variation (CV), root mean square of successive differences (RMSSD), and percentage heartbeat intervals with difference in successive heartbeat intervals greater than 50 ms (PNN50) as time domain features; HRV index (bin width of 8.0 ms), triangular interpolation of heartbeat interval histogram (TINN), and stress index (SI) (Lednev et al., 2008) as geometrical analysis features; and LF (LF 0.04-0.09 Hz), HF (HF >0.1 Hz), the ratio of LF to HF (LF/HF), normalized LF (LFnu) and normalized HF (HFnu) components as frequency domain features (Task Force, 1996). Among the HRV features, the RMSSD is worthy of further mention because it has been used to indicate the levels of mental or physical stress of a subject (Task Force, 1996). In preparing the learning sets, RMSSD was used as basis to estimate the activity level of a subject during daily activity.

2.2.4 Poincaré plot pattern analysis

The Poincaré plot is a two-dimensional scatter plot of each heartbeat interval plotted against the subsequent interval, and thus depicts the correlation between successive heartbeat intervals (Woo et al., 1992). Recently, Poincaré plots of arrhythmic ECG data were systematically investigated to discover 10 distinctive prototypical patterns that represent different kinds of arrhythmias from 24-h Holter ECG data (Esperer et al., 2008). For example, fan-shaped Poincaré plots were typical in subjects with AF; multiple side lobe patterns specified the presence of atrial premature beats or ventricular premature beats; while an island pattern was highly correlated with atrial flutter or atrial tachycardia (Esperer et al., 2008). Poincaré plots were generated to calculate Poincaré plot features and classify them into different patterns such as torped, island, multiple side lobes, and fan pattern (Duong et al., 2009). Finally, standard deviations of the minor axis (SD_1) and major axis (SD_2), the ratio of SD_1 to SD_2 (SD_1/SD_2), standard deviation of the RR intervals (SDRR), standard deviation of the successive differences of the RR intervals (SDSD), and autocorrelation function of the RR intervals (rRR) were calculated from the Poincaré plot (Brennan et al., 2001). In addition to the previously reported conventional descriptors, new cluster descriptors were calculated by analyzing the Poincaré plots as an image (Duong et al., 2009). In brief, Poincaré plot images (Figure 2A) were thresholded at the gray level of 0 (Figure 2B). Second, binary plot images were eroded once with the 3×3 structuring element, reconstructed with respect to the binary plot, and seed-filled (Figure 2C) (Serra, 1984). A cluster was defined as an isolated group of connected points containing more than 12 points that effectively represented highly correlated heartbeat interval events. Then, the cluster was described by using shape attributes, such as form factor and minor to major axis ratio; texture attributes, such as entropy and contrast; and location attributes, such as the number of clusters on the diagonal line. Torpedo, island, and multi-sided lobe patterns were classified at the accuracy of 99% using the combined set of conventional and new Poincaré plot features.

2.2.5 Circadian rhythm analysis

Circadian rhythm (CR) represents physiological phenomena repeatedly occurring during a time period of approximately 24 h. In humans, almost every physiological function displays CR to some degree and the mechanism can be endogenous, exogenous or a combination of both. The cardiovascular system also exhibits a pronounced CR which is influenced by both external stimuli and endogenous homoeostatic control mechanism with the latter playing a more important role than the former (Guo & Stein, 2002). Circadian variations are found in a number of electrophysiological parameters such as heart rate, QT interval, sinus node recovery time, and atrial refractory periods (Guo & Stein, 2002). Although detailed genetic or epigenetic mechanisms are not fully understood, numerous cardiovascular and cerebrovascular diseases show circadian variations. For example, paroxysmal and persistent atrial arrhythmia occurs more frequently during the evening time (Mitchell et al., 2002), whereas sudden cardiac death (Savopoulos et al., 2006) and myocardial ischemia (Li, 2003) occur predominantly in the morning. In previous studies, we reported circadian variations of HRV features in NSR and PAF subjects (Kim et al., 2008a) and CR parameters such as amplitudes, phase, and shift obtained from a least square fitting of sinusoidal functions to various HRV features. On the day of onset of PAF, CR of PAF subjects were affected and significantly different from those of NSR subjects. The CR parameters obtained from the non-episodic data for that day were used to detect PAF patients with an accuracy of 84.6% (Olemann & Kim, 2011).

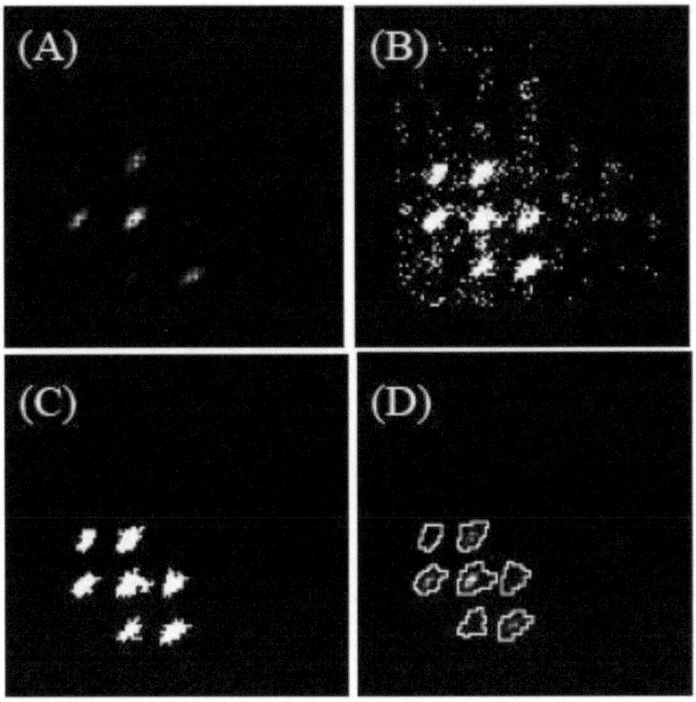

Fig. 2. The Poincaré plot of island pattern (A), its binary plot (B), opening by reconstruction and closing (C), and cluster boundary overlaid onto the binary plot (D). (Permission from Duong et al., 2009).

To obtain CR parameter patterns of HRV features, a non-linear curve-fitting method known as the Levenberg-Marquardt algorithm (Levenberg, 1944) was applied (Statgraphics Plus V4.1 Professional System®, Manugistics, Inc., Rockville, MD, USA) to each HRV feature set that consisted of at least six time-points which represents a time span of at least 6 h. The initial values for the regression were set by trial and error and were maintained constant for both the NSR and PAF group. The CR parameters obtained were the amplitude, the shift and the phase, from the following sinusoidal equation used for the curve fitting:

$$H(t) = b \times cosine\,(w\,t + p) + a \tag{1}$$

where $H(t)$ represents the HRV feature, b represents amplitude, p represents phase (in degrees), a represents shift, t represents time of the day (in hours), and w represents 15°/h. The final amplitude was obtained by taking the absolute value. The final phase was modified to restrict its phase value between 0 and 180 using the following formula:

$$Phase = 180/phi \times cosine^{-1}(b \times cosine\ (p \times phi/180\ ))/\ |b\ |) \quad (2)$$

While performing the sinusoidal curve fitting, time-points that showed unusual residuals (Studentized residual > |3.0|) were removed from the analysis.

2.3 Data analysis

2.3.1 Preparation of learning sets

Before preparing the learning sets, based on the pattern recognition algorithms of Poincaré plots, feature sets showing noisy plots that consist of most of events out of the clusters were also removed since these were caused by the poor contact of electrodes (Figure 3). Feature sets showing island, multi-sided lobe, and fan patterns were removed from learning sets of NSR group since they represent arrhythmic events (Esperer et al., 2006). However, only records showing fan shapes were removed from learning sets of PAF group. To divide learning sets according to the level of physical or mental activity, an arbitrary cut-off value of RMSSD (in sec) was selected to assign each 30-min RR interval to two types of ANS conditions: one representing the activated state of the vagal nervous system (RMSSD > 0.040 sec) and the other representing the suppressed state of the vagal nervous system due to mental or physical activity (RMSSD <0.040 sec) experienced by the subject during daily activity. HRV feature sets from different subject groups were compared by Mann-Whitney signed rank test (Statgraphics Plus V 4.1). Test results were considered significant if the p-value was less than 0.05 (95% confidence level).

From the prepared learning sets, the CR curve fittings were performed according to the procedure described in the section above. The calculated CR parameters were compared between NSR and PAF groups based on median values by the Mann-Whitney test (Statgraphics Plus V 4.1). The results were considered significantly different if p-values were less than 0.05.

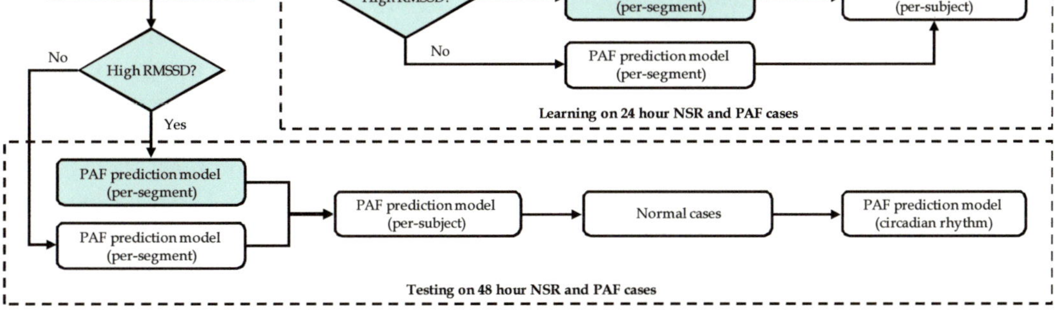

Fig. 3. Flow diagram for data processing and analysis used in the study.

2.3.2 Derivation of prediction models

Significant HRV and Poincaré plot features were selected from the learning sets by evaluating the worth of a feature based on the value of the chi-squared statistic with respect to the class (Weka 6.1, The University of Waikato, Hamilton, New Zealand). Naïve Bayesian, logistic regression, and support vector machine (SVM) analyses were performed to derive classification models that detect 30-min RR intervals of PAF subjects (Weka 6.1). Because this first classification was based on 30-min segments of RR interval data, it was called the segment-based classification. Once each 30-min segment was annotated, a second phase of classification was derived from a heuristic rule. Because annotation results for each subject were used, it was called the subject-based classification. A similar approach of two-phase classification has been reported previously (Hickey et al., 2006). According to the clinical definition of PAF, a subject would be diagnosed with PAF if at least one 30-min segment contained AF episodes. However, because our learning sets did not contain any segments with AF episodes (fan-shaped plots were removed), the empirical rule in this study was modified to classify subjects as PAF if any of four time periods had two or more segments annotated as PAF within the same time period.

Significant CR features were selected from the learning sets by the chi-squared test (Weka 6.1). Naïve Bayesian, logistic regression, and SVM analyses were performed to derive classification models that detect PAF subjects using CR features (Weka 6.1).

2.3.3 Preparation of test sets

Before preparing the test sets, the records showing noisy Poincaré plots were removed from further analysis. Testing sets were divided according to the RMSSD cut-off. The segment-based classification was performed using the classification algorithm that produced the best accuracy. These outputs were further tested using the subject-based classification rule with different segment sampling methods: two, three, or four 30-min samples per time period to determine the dependence of classification accuracy on the number of sample segments. Cases classified as NSR were tested using the CR classification (Figure 3).

3. Results

3.1 Establishment of PAF prediction models using data from the 24-h study

3.1.1 Segment-based model and subject-based model

A total of 299 and 319 items of RR interval data were obtained from 20 NSR and 24 PAF patients, respectively, and were processed for HRV calculation. HRV features that differed significantly between two types of data were initially screened by the Mann-Whitney test at a significance level of $p = 0.05$. Most HRV features were higher in the PAF groups except for SD_2, SI, and HFnu, which were lower (*data not shown*, $p<0.01$). Similar outcomes have also been reported in previous studies (Kim et al., 2008a, 2008b) using NSR and AF databases available at Physionet. These HRV features were further ranked based on their contribution to a prediction model (chi-squared feature selection method, Weka 6.1). The top nine HRV features (RMSSD, SDSD, SD_1, SDRatio, rRR, %Cluster, SDNN, CV, and PNN50) were then used to generate a prediction model that represented the segment-based classification model. The accuracy of each classification method is summarized in Table 2. The logistic regression analysis produced the highest accuracy among three classification algorithms (71.4%) and was selected for the testing.

Based on this observation, a simple heuristic rule was applied to generate the subject-based classification. Two of 24 PAF cases were misclassified as NSR (false negative) and four of 20 NSR cases (false positive) were misclassified (Table 3). False-negative cases showed only one record classified as PAF. All false-positive cases showed fan-shaped Poincaré plots.

Classification methods	Sensitivity	Specificity	Accuracy
Naïve Bayesian	39.5%	96.0%	66.8%
Logistic regression analysis	58.3%	85.3%	71.4%
Support vector machine	49.5%	89.6%	68.9%

Table 2. Performance of different classification algorithms for the segment based classification using 30-min ECG records.

Observed \ Predicted	NSR	PAF
NSR (*n=20*)	16 (80%)	4 (20%)
PAF (*n=24*)	2 (8%)	22 (92%)

Table 3. Performance of the subject based classification using the results from the segment-based classification by logistic regression analysis

3.1.2 The CR model

The phases of the HRV features of the two groups did not show significant differences (data not shown; $p > 0.05$), thereby suggesting that there was no significant difference in the time-point of HRV peak occurrence. The CR amplitudes and shifts of rRR, HF, LF, HR and RMSSD showed significant differences between the two groups (data not shown; Mann-Whitney test, $p < 0.05$). These CR features were further ranked based on their contribution to a prediction model (chi-squared feature selection method, Weka 6.1). The top three CR features (rRR shift, LF amplitude, and HR amplitude) were then used to generate a prediction model that represented the segment-based classification model. These three HRV features were curve-fitted and plotted to determine the circadian change in individual subjects (Figure 4). Logistic regression analysis was performed with the three CR features and produced an accuracy of 86% in predicting PAF cases (sensitivity of 79% classifying 19/24 PAF cases and specificity of 95% classifying 19/20 NSR cases). The false-positive subject (n=1) seemed to show greater fluctuations, whereas false-negative subjects (n=5) showed fewer fluctuations in CR amplitudes.

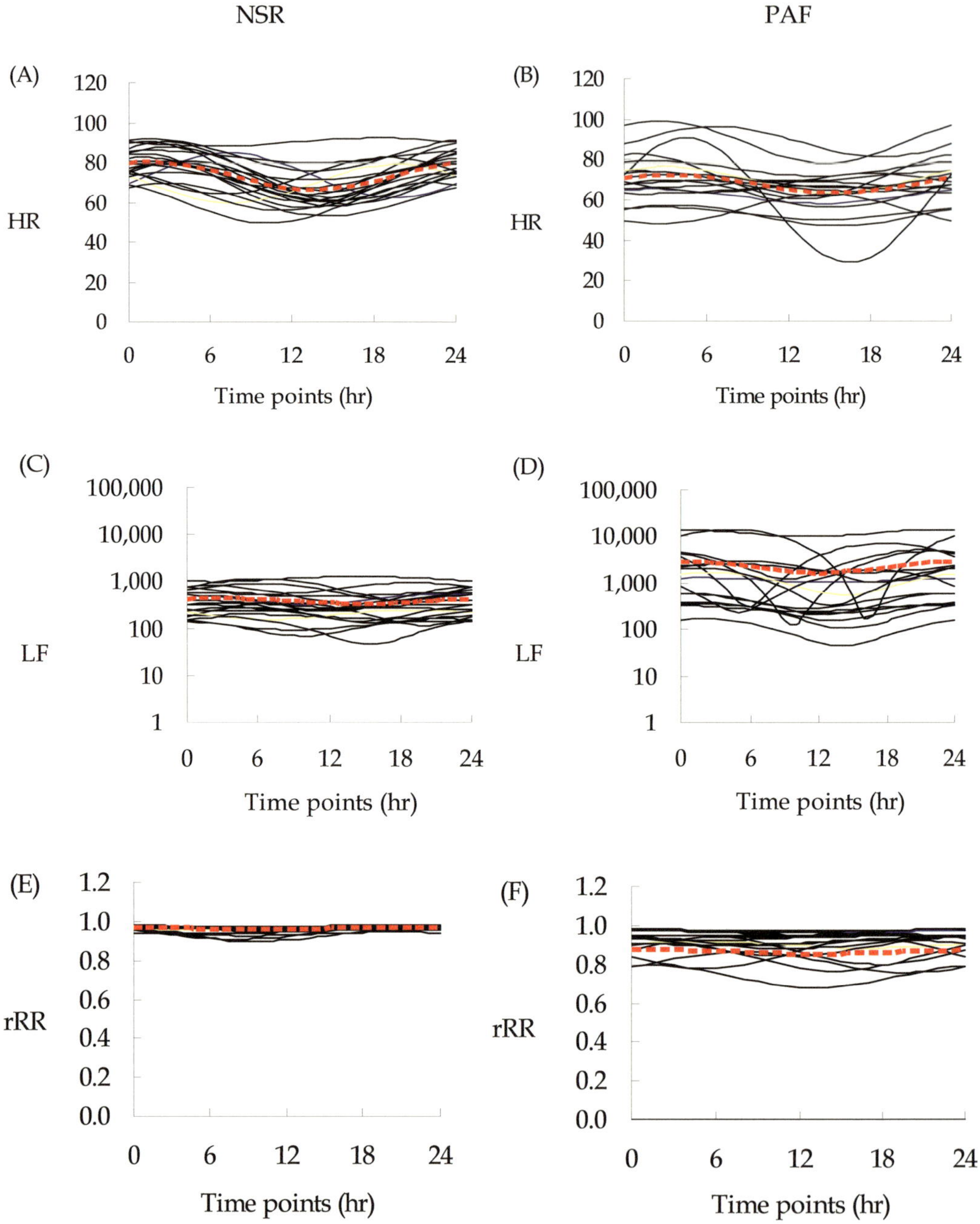

Fig. 4. Circadian rhythms of selected HRV features were significantly different between NSR and PAF cases. HR: heart rates per min, LF: low frequency area (msec^2) after logarithmic transform, and rRR: autocorrelation function of the RR intervals.

3.2 Prediction of AF recurrence using 48-h recordings

ECG data from 48-h Holter monitoring were first screened for AF episodes using the software in the Holter system and software findings for AF were confirmed by two cardiologists (JHP, JHK). Nineteen of 33 subjects were diagnosed as NSR whose heart rhythms were successfully maintained for 48 h under drug treatment (normal group). Ten subjects were diagnosed as PAF and four as persistent AF (recurrent group; recurrence rate of 42%). Normal and recurrent groups did not differ significantly different in terms of age (Mann-Whitney test, $p > 0.05$), gender, or other diseases such as diabetes, hypertension, or past strokes (chi-squared test, $p > 0.05$).
The noise detection algorithm detected four NSR cases and showed that more than 30% of the total ECG data were corrupted by noise possibly due to poor electrode contacts; these were removed from the test sets to avoid misinterpretation. When four ECG segments were sampled from each time period of ECG data, a total of 350 and 270 segments were obtained from 15 normal and 14 recurrent cases, respectively, and were processed for the calculation of HRV and Poincaré plot features. Using the segment-based classification and subject-based rule, 9/10 recurrent PAF patients were correctly identified, whereas 13/15 normal subjects were correctly identified (data not shown). In addition, four persistent AF cases were all correctly identified. An illustrative example for the subject-based rule is described in Figure 5, in which a data point represents the probability density value of the segment based model at a given time-point. Data points for an NSR case remain higher than the empirical cut-off at all time-points, whereas those for a PAF case often fall below the cut-off even during the days when no episodes were evident (Figure 5). Subjects classified as normal cases by the subject-based rule ($n = 14$) were further tested with the CR-based model. One false-negative case was correctly identified as recurrent and all normal cases were correctly confirmed as normal cases. Therefore, the final classification resulted in a sensitivity of 100% (14/14 recurrent cases) and a specificity of 86% (13/15 normal cases) (Table 4). The same classification procedure was applied to the data sets obtained by sampling two or three segments per time period and classification results are summarized in Table 4. The number of sampled segments did not change the classification outcomes drastically.

4. Conclusion and discussion

In this study, we have developed a new method for predicting PAF subjects using intermittently sampled ECG data and applied it to the identification of recurrent AF cases. The proposed method consists of an empirical rule and a CR-based classification. The empirical rule alone identified nearly 93% of recurrent cases (13/14 cases) and 86% of normal cases (13/15 cases). Because our aim was not to miss any recurrent cases, normal cases classified by the empirical rule were re-tested using the CR-based prediction model. The false-negative case was correctly identified as a recurrent case thus achieving a 100% sensitivity and no false-positive cases were generated thus maintaining the 86% specificity. Our results suggest that intermittently sampled ECG data could be used to detect the increased likelihood of PAF episodes. Since previous PAF prediction methods relied on the change during the transition from NSR to PAF, ECG needs to be analyzed continuously not to miss transition periods. Furthermore, somewhat higher degree of false positive errors may be expected in an actual implementation of long term ECG analysis since the likelihood of not having subsequent PAF episodes following a transition period is not known.

Contrary to previous prediction methods, our classification models were not designed to detect the transition period prior to PAF episodes exclusively. Instead, they were aimed to evaluate the likelihood of a 24 hour period when PAF episodes may occur. Thus, the performance of our proposed method can be less sensitive to the continuity of ECG data but allows ECG recordings to be sampled over the whole day. Two samples gave results that were as accurate as those of four samples taken during four 6-h time periods (Table 4). Furthermore, our results indicated that the proposed methods tended to show an increased likelihood of detecting PAF cases even during the days when no PAF episodes were evident (Figure 5). Therefore, we conclude that our intermittent sampling strategy is as accurate for predicting recurrent PAF as previously reported methods.

CLASS	*NSR*	*PAF*	*NSR*	*PAF*	*NSR*	*PAF*
NSR *(n = 15)*	14 (93%)	1 (7%)	13 (86%)	2 (14%)	13 (86%)	2 (14%)
PAF *(n = 10)*	0 (0%)	10 (100%)	0 (0%)	10 (100%)	0 (0%)	10 (100%)
No. of samples taken in each time period (6 hrs)	**2**		*3*		*4*	

Table 4. Performance of proposed methods for predicting PAF subjects using a subject-based rule and a CR-based classification algorithm. Performance results were obtained when two, three, or four 30-min ECG records were sampled from each of four time periods during a day.

The intermittent sampling approach might be more effective in mobile healthcare settings because the sensor may not need to be worn all day, which could effectively reduce many problems caused by poor sensor tolerance, limited battery life, and high data transmission costs of current technology. In general, mobile healthcare technology offers many attractive features such as convenient wearable ECG sensors, real-time feedback of abnormal heart rhythms, and timely intervention in the case of adverse events. However, the continuous measurement of ECG signals might not be ideal as a long-term monitoring solution in mobile healthcare settings because it requires long hours of wearing a sensor that may stigmatize a majority of patients and eventually influence the quality of the data. For example, Holter monitoring was regarded as inconvenient because of hygienic aspects, physical activity, night sleep, and skin reactions (Fensli & Boisen, 2009). Based on our understanding of current advances in low-power bioelectronics (Sarpeshkar, 2010), the proposed intermittent sampling of ECG signals is believed to provide an attractive alternative strategy to long-term monitoring in mobile healthcare settings. It could be specially adapted to work with wireless devices such as wearable sensors and gateway devices that consume battery power at high rates. In addition, the amount of data traffic would be minimized, which is also attractive in countries where wireless data transfer is costly. Thus, in developing a computer-aided prediction method for mobile healthcare settings, it seems important to consider human factors, such as patient acceptance of procedures, or device factors, such as battery time or data transfer costs.

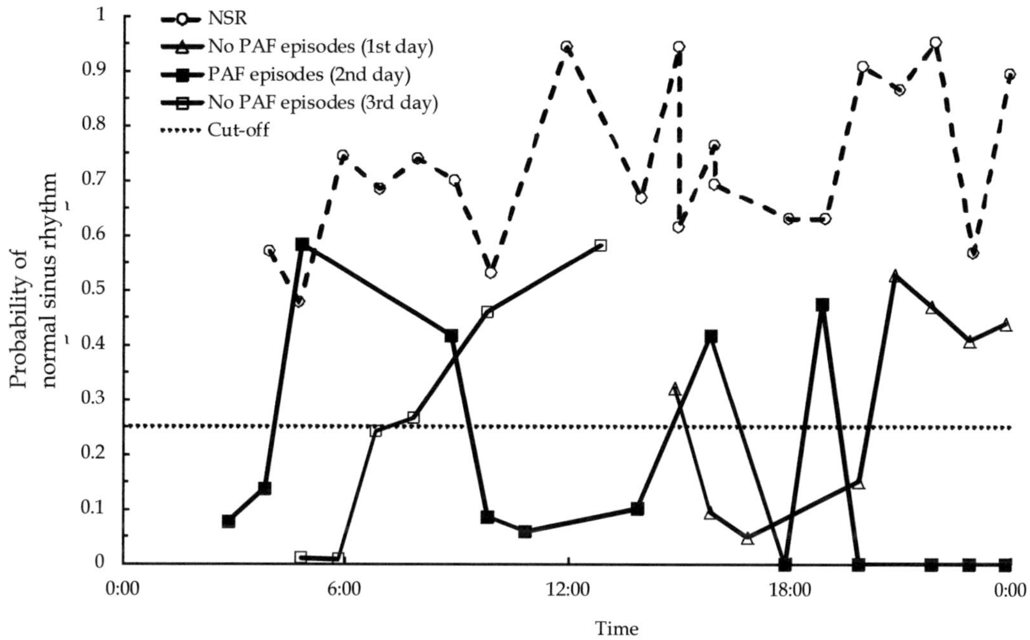

Fig. 5. Distribution of probability values from the segment-based model applied to two patient cases. Data points in the hollow circle are from a normal case (NSR). Data points in the solid square are from a PAF case on the day when PAF episodes were recorded, whereas those in the hollow square and triangle are from the same case during the previous and following days when no PAF episodes were recorded. The points in the area under the cut-off at 0.25 (broken line) were classified as PAF.

It is becoming evident that a significant proportion of cryptogenic stroke is due to intermittent AF. By using 30-day cardiac event monitors, 20% of such strokes was found to be related to AF (Elijovich et al., 2009). Warfarin treatment was given to patients after the detection of intermittent AF (despite no detection of AF on ECG or in-patient telemetry monitoring in the majority of patients). Similarly to the detection of recurrent PAF, prevention of recurrent strokes related to PAF in particular may require long-term ECG monitoring. For these applications, our proposed intermittent sampling method should also be suitable as an initial screening method that generates a real-time alarm or trend report that enables timely intervention. For example, if the incidence of abnormal segments increases, then the ECG sampling strategy may be changed to a continuous monitoring mode to capture the PAF episodes. In this way, patients can be monitored in the long term to determine recurrence after conversion treatment or the origin of strokes, so that conventional Holter monitoring can be complemented or improved. For initial screening purposes, the ECG sensor used in this study can be replaced by a heartbeat sensor because all analytic features were calculated from RR interval data rather than the morphology of ECG signals. Current advances in microelectronics have provided a variety of heartbeat sensors ranging from conventional chest belt type to Doppler radar-based non-contact types. These sensors are usually equipped with a module of wireless data communication so they can transmit the signals to the gateway device that is connected to the internet.

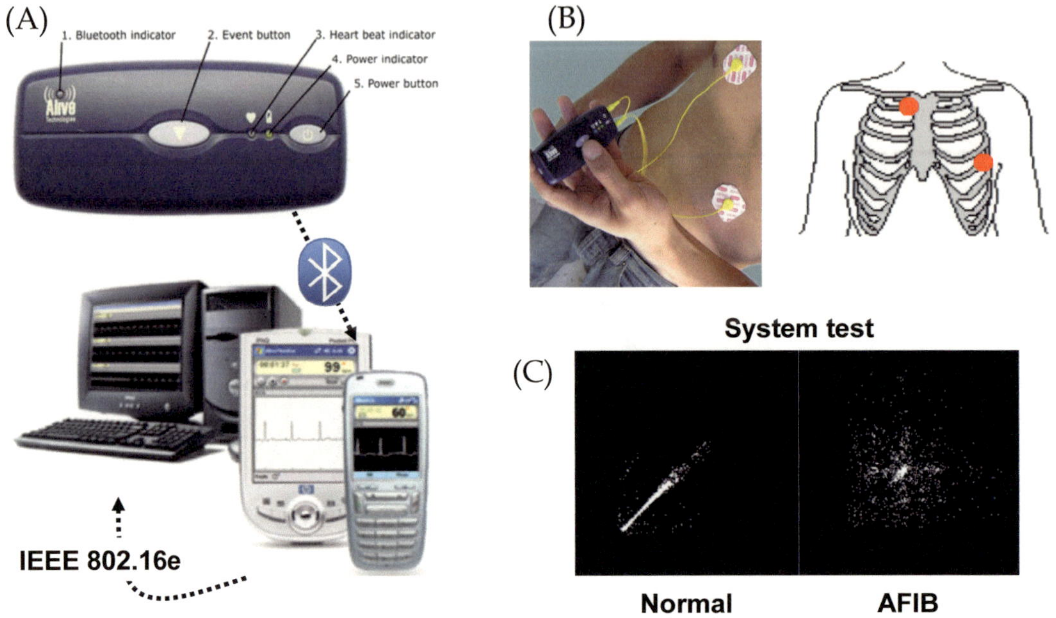

Fig. 6. (A) System components of web-based heartbeat analysis system. (B) Electrode attachment. (C) Poincaré plots were generated from wirelessly transmitted ECG data obtained from an NSR and an AF subject (Pictures in (A) and (B) were kindly provided by Alivetec Technologies Pty. Ltd.).

4.1 Development of web-based real-time heartbeat analysis

Currently, we are actively developing a remote real-time heartbeat analysis system that consists of a wearable ECG sensor (AliveECG monitor, Alive Technologies Pty. Ltd, Ashmore, Queensland, Australia) with a three-axis accelerometer, a smart phone (HD2, HTC Corporation, Taoyuan, Taiwan ROC), and a data analysis server (Microsoft Windows XP; Figure 6). The original server software (Cardiomobile, Alive Technologies) displays ECG, activity features, and global positioning system-based location in a web-based map in real time or in review mode. In addition to these functions, HRV features and outputs from a PAF prediction model are also calculated and displayed in our current version (Figure 7). A feasible scenario of using our system is that a wireless ECG sensor worn by a patient, and communicating to the smart phone through the near field Bluetooth, transmits ECG signals to the remote server through a wireless data streaming service. The remote server performs real-time analysis of transmitted ECG data and detects abnormal events (or trends). In the case of PAF prediction, a cardiology specialist at the hospital may be notified to interpret the remote monitoring and confirm the diagnosis. Compared with conventional Holter monitoring systems, a mobile healthcare solution can be designed to enable the patient to carry out normal daily activities, while still being under continuous monitoring.

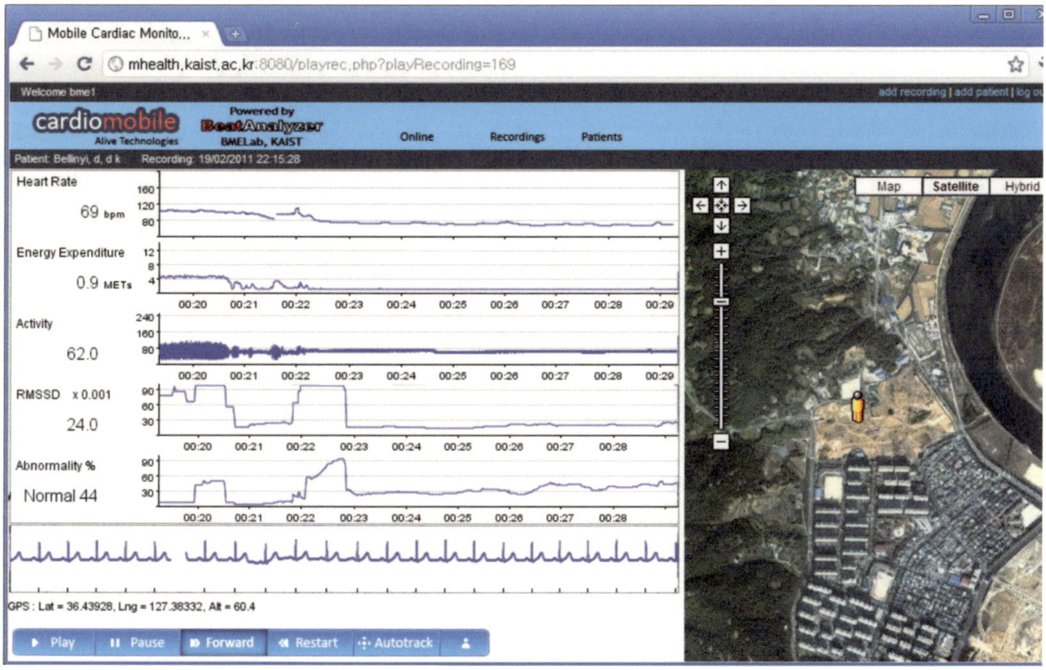

Fig. 7. Real-time heartbeat analysis system for remote monitoring of ECG and HRV of patients. Heart rates, energy expenditure, physical activity, HRV (RMSSD), and abnormal heartbeats (Abnormality %) can be monitored by remote clinical staff in real time while a patient is exercising outdoors during daily activity. In the case of advent events, user location data from the global positioning system can be provided to paramedic staff (user's current position is indicated by the avatar on the web-based map) (Cardiomobile is the trademark of Alivetec Technologies Pty. Ltd.
The server software was kindly provided to be modified by us.)

Since the patient may experience an arrhythmic episode during physical activity, mobile solutions may enhance the quality of data measured by enabling the patient to carry out normal daily routines. Currently, we are also implementing the CR analysis of HRV features and its related PAF prediction. This prototype system should help us to discover the "real problem" and the users' requirements, demonstrate the actual functionality of a device, and provide many insights on how to design and build a more advanced system that should enable long-term ECG monitoring. The future system is being designed to provide additional benefits for stroke or heart disease rehabilitation patients.

5. Acknowledgement

We would like to express sincere gratitude to Mrs. Young Mi Choi who participated in patient recruitment and data retrieval, Ms. Yoon Ju Na who developed a batch run software, and Dr. Seung Hwan Kim who initially suggested this collaboration. This work was partly supported by Science and Technology Fundamental Frontier Research fund at KAIST ICC, Korea.

6. References

Aytemir, K., Aksoyek, S., Yildirir, A., Ozer, N., & Oto, A. (1999). Prediction of Atrial Fibrillation Recurrence After Cardioversion by P Wave Signal-averaged Electrocardiography. *International Journal of Cardiology*, Vol. 70, No. 1, pp. 15.

Berruezo, A., Tamborero, D., Mont, L., Benito, B., Tolosana, J.M., Sitges, M., Vidal, B., Arriagada, G., Méndez, F., Matiello, M., Molina, I., & Brugada, J. (2007). Pre-procedural Predictors of Atrial Fibrillation Recurrence After Circumferential Pulmonary Vein Ablation. *European Heart Journal,* Vol. 28, No. 7, pp. 836.

Brennan, M., Palaniswami, M., & Kamen, P. (2001). Do existing Measures of Poincaré Plot Geometry Reflect Nonlinear Features of Heart rate Variability? *IEEE Transactions on Biomedical Engineering,* Vol. 48, No. 11, pp. 1342.

Chesnokov, Y.V. (2008). Complexity and Spectral Analysis of the Heart Rate Variability Dynamics for Distant Prediction of Paroxysmal Atrial Fibrillation with Artificial Intelligence Methods. *Artificial Intelligence in Medicine,* Vol. 43, No. 2, pp. 151.

Delfaut, P., Saksena, S., Prakash, A., & Krol, R.B. (1998). Long-term Outcome of Patients with Drug-refractory Atrial Flutter and Fibrillation after Single- and Dual-site Right Atrial Pacing for Arrhythmia Prevention. *Journal of the American College of Cardiology,* Vol. 32, No. 7, pp. 1900.

Duong, N.D., Jeong, H., Youn, C.-H. & Kim, D. (2009). Development of New Cluster Descriptors for Image Analysis of Poincare Plots In: *World Congress on Medical Physics and Biomedical Engineering, Vol. 25/IV Image Processing, Biosignal Processing, Modelling and Simulation, Biomechanics,* pp. 1661, Munich, Germany.

Elijovich, L., Josephson. S.A., Fung, G.L., & Smith, W.S. (2009). Intermittent Atrial Fibrillation May Account for a Large Proportion of Otherwise Cryptogenic Stroke: A Study of 30-day Cardiac Event Monitors. *Journal of Stroke Cerebrovascular Disease,* Vol. 18, No. 3, pp. 185.

Esperer, H.D., Esperer, C., & Cohen, R.J. (2008). Cardiac Arrhythmias Imprint Specific Signatures on Lorenz Plots. *Annals of Noninvasive Electrocardiology,* Vol. 13, No. 1, pp. 44.

Fensli, R. & Boisen, E. (2009). Human Factors Affecting the Patient's Acceptance of Wireless Biomedical Sensors, Biomedical Engineering Systems and Technologies. *Communications in Computer and Information Science,* Vol. 25, No. 4, pp. 402.

Friberg, L., Hammar, N., & Rosenqvist, M. (2010). Stroke in Paroxysmal Atrial Fibrillation: Report from the Stockholm Cohort of Atrial Fibrillation. *Eurorpean Heart Journal,* Vol. 31, No. 8, pp. 967.

Grubitzsch, H., Grabow, C., Orawa, H., & Konertz, W. (2008). Factors Predicting the Time until Atrial Fibrillation Recurrence After Concomitant Left Atrial Ablation. *European Journal of Cardiothoracic Surgery,* Vol. 34, No. 1, pp. 67.

Guo, Y.F. & Stein, P.K. (2002). Circadian Rhythm in the Cardiovascular System: Considerations in Non-invasive Electrophysiology. *Cardiac Electrophysiology Review,* Vol. 6, No. 3, pp. 267.

Hu, F. & Xiao, Y. (2009). Congestion Aware, Loss-Resilient Bio-Monitoring Sensor Networking for Mobile Health Applications. *IEEE Journal on Selected Areas in Communications,* Vol. 27, No. 4, pp. 450.

Hart, R.G., Pearce, L.A., & Aguilar, M.I. (2007). Meta-analysis: antithrombotic therapy to prevent stroke in patients who have nonvalvular atrial fibrillation. *Ann Intern Med.* Vol. 146, No. 12, pp. 857.

Hickey, B., Heneghan, C., & De Chazal, P. (2004). Non-episode-dependent Assessment of Paroxysmal Atrial Fibrillation Through Measurement of RR Interval Dynamics and Atrial Premature Contractions. *Annals of Biomedical Engineering,* Vol. 32, No. 5, pp. 677.

Jabaudon, D., Sztajzel, J., Sievert, K., Landis, T., Sztajzel, R. (2004). Usefulness of ambulatory 7-day ECG monitoring for the detection of atrial fibrillation and flutter after acute stroke and transient ischemic attack. *Stroke,* Vol. 35, No. 7, pp. 1647.

Jørgensen, H.S., Nakayama, H., Reith, J., Raaschou, H.O., & Olsen, T.S. (1996) Acute Stroke with Atrial Fibrillation. The Copenhagen Stroke Study. *Stroke,* Vol. 27, pp. 1765.

Kikillus, N. , Schweikert, M., & Bolz, A. (2008). Identifying Patients Suffering from Atrial Fibrillation During Atrial Fibrillation and Non-atrial Fibrillation Episodes. In: *4th European Conference of the International Federation for Medical and Biological Engineering 2008,* Vol. 22, pp. 1349–1352, Antwerp, Belgium.

Kim, D., Seo, Y., Jung, W., & Youn, C.-H. (2008a). Detection of Long Term Variations of Heart Rate Variability in Normal Sinus Rhythm and Atrial Fibrillation ECG Data. In: *Biomedical Engineering and Informatics 2008,* Sanya, Hainan, China.

Kim, D., Seo, Y., & Youn, C.-H. (2008b). Prediction of Atrial Fibrillation Onsets by Multiple Formulas Based on Long Term Variation of Heart Rate Variability. In: *Healthcom 2008,* Singapore.

Koh, K.B., Park, J.K., Kim, C.H., & Cho, S. (2001). Development of the Stress Response Inventory and Its Application in Clinical Practice. *Psychosomatic Medicine,* Vol. 63, pp. 668.

Lednev, V.V., Belova, N.A., Ermakov, A.M., Akimov, E.B., & Tonevitsky, A.G. (2008). Modulation of Cardiac Rhythm in the Humans Exposed to Extremely Weak Alternating Magnetic Fields. *Biophysics,* Vol. 53, No. 6, pp. 648.

Levenberg, K. (1944). A Method for the Solution of Certan Non-linear Problems in Least Squares. *The Quarterly of Applied Mathematics,* Vol. 2, pp. 164.

Li, J.J. (2003). Circadian Variation in Myocardial Ischemia: The Possible Mechanisms Involving in This Phenomenon. *Medical Hypotheses,* Vol. 61, No. 2, pp. 240.

Lin, H.J., Wolf, P.A., Kelly-Hayes, M., Beiser, A.S., Kase, C.S., Benjamin, E.J., & D'Agostino, R.B. (1996). Stroke Severity in Atrial Fibrillation: The Framingham study. *Stroke,* Vol. 6, No. 27, pp. 1760.

Lombardi, F., Colombo, A., Basilico, B., Ravaglia, R., Garbin, M., Vergani, D., Battezzati, P.M., & Fiorentini, C.J. (2001). Heart Rate Variability and Early Recurrence of Atrial Fibrillation after Electrical Cardioversion. *Journal of the American College of Cardiol*ogy, Vol. 37, No. 1, pp. 157.

Marini, C., De Santis, F., Sacco, S., Russo, T., Olivieri, L., Totaro, R., & Carolei, A. (2005). Contribution of Atrial Fibrillation to Incidence and Outcome of Ischemic Stroke: Results from a Population Based Study. *Stroke,* Vol. 36, pp. 1115.

Mitchell, A.R., Spurrell, P.A., & Sulke, N. (2002). Circadian Variation of Arrhythmia Onset Patterns in Patients with Persistent Atrial Fibrillation. *American Heart Journal,* Vol. 6, No. 3, pp. 262.

Mohebbi, M. & Ghassemian, H. (2011). Prediction of Paroxysmal Atrial Fibrillation Using Recurrence Plot-based Features of the RR-interval Signal. *Physiological Measurement,* Vol. 32, pp. 1147.

Olemann, A. & Kim, D. (2011). Detection of Paroxysmal Atrial Fibrillation Subjects based on Circadian Rhythm Parameters of Heart Rate Variability. In: IEEE International Conference on Bioinformatics and Biomedicine, Atlanta, GA (2011) (*in press*).

Pan, J. & Tompkins, W.J. (1985). A Real-time QRS Detection Algorithm. *IEEE Transactions on Biomedical Engineering*, Vol. 32, No. 3, pp. 230.

Rizos, T., Rasch, C., Jenetzky, E., Hametner, C., Kathoefer, S., Reinhardt, R., Hepp, T., Hacke, W., & Veltkamp, R. (2010). Detection of Paroxysmal Atrial Fibrillation in Acute Stroke Patients. *Cerebrovascular Dis*eases, Vol. 30, No. 4, pp. 410.

Sahoo, S.K., Lu, W., Teddy, S.D., Kim, D. & Feng, M. (2011). Detection of Atrial Fibrillation from Non-Episodic ECG Data: A Review of Methods. In: *33rd Annual International IEEE EMBS Conference,* Boston, MA, USA (in press).

Salahuddin, L. & Kim, D. (2006). Detection of Acute Stress by Heart Rate Variability Using a Prototype Mobile ECG Sensor. In: *Hybrid Information Technology, ICHIT' 06,* Vol. 2, pp. 453-459, Jeju, Korea.

Sarpeshkar, R. (2010). *Ultra Low Power Bioelectronics: Fundamentals, Biomedical Applications, and Bio-Inspired Systems.* Cambridge University Press, New York, NY, USA.

Savopoulos, C., Ziakis, A., Hatzitolios, A., Delivoria, C., Kournanis, A., Mylonas, S., Tsougas, M. & Psaroulis, D. (2006). Circadian Rhythm in Sudden Cardiac Death : A Retrospective Study of 2,665 Cases. *Angiology,* Vol. 57, No. 2, pp. 197.

Serra, J. (1984) *Image Analysis and Mathematical Morphology.* Academic Press, New York, NY, USA.

Task Force (Task Force of the European Society of Cardiology and the North American Society of Pacing and Electrophysiology) (1996) Heart Rate Variability: Standards of Measurement, Physiological Interpretation and Clinical Use. *European Heart Journal,* Vol. 17, pp. 1043.

Thong, T., McNames, J., Aboy, M. & Goldstein, B. (2004). Prediction of Paroxysmal Atrial Fibrillation by Analysis of Atrial Premature Complexes. *IEEE Transactions on Biomedical Eng*ineering, Vol. 51, pp. 561.

Vikman, S., Mäkikallio, T.H., Yli-Mäyry, S., Pikkujämsä, S., Koivisto, A.-M., Reinikainen, P., Airaksinen, K.E.J. & Huikuri, H.V. (1999). Altered Complexity and Correlation Properties of R-R Interval Dynamics Before the Spontaneous Onset of Paroxysmal Atrial Fibrillation. *Circulation,* Vol. 100, pp. 2079.

Wolf, P.A., Abbott, R.D., & Kannel, W.B. (1987). Atrial Fibrillation: A Major Contributor to Stroke in the Elderly. The Framingham Study. *Archhives of Internal Medicine,* Vol. 147, pp. 1561.

Woo, M.A., Stevenson, W.G., Moser, D.K., Trelease, R.B., & Haper, R.M. (1992). Patterns of Beat to Beat Heart Rate Variability in Advanced Heart Failure. *American Heart Journal,* Vol. 123, No. 3, pp. 704.